Cutting Edge Therapies for Cancer in the 21st Century

Edited By

Pier Paolo Claudio
Marshall University
Joan C. Edwards School of Medicine
McKown Translational Research Genomic Institute
Department of Biochemistry and Microbiology
& Department of Surgery
USA

&

Paraskevi Vogiatzi
Thomas Jefferson University
Department of Cancer Biology
Kimmel Cancer Center
USA

DEDICATION

This book is dedicated to my father Francesco, mentor of a lifetime and friend, to my lovely wife Candace and kids Carley and Franco for their love and encouragement, to my mother Paola, and my parents-in-law Minnie and Dan for their support.

Pier Paolo Claudio

This book is dedicated to my husband, Marco for the encouragement to improve my knowledge and move my career forward and my kids, Antonio, Maria Aikaterini and Olga Evangelia, who are just about the best children a mom could hope for: happy, loving, and fun to be with.

Paraskevi Vogiatzi

CONTENTS

FOREWORD

It is a pleasure to introduce "Cutting Edge Therapies for Cancer in the 21st Century". As the Vice-Dean for Clinical and Translational Research at the Joan C Edwards School of Medicine of Marshall University I have had opportunity to interact with the principal author, Dr. Pier Paolo Claudio. He is an outstanding investigator performing cutting edge translational cancer research at our cancer center. His enthusiasm for his work is infectious! The book by Dr. Claudio and his former student, Dr. Vogiatzi, has a great breadth and depth of knowledge and fully meets the needs of medical students and cancer researchers.

The book is penned by professionals highly regarded in the field and addresses complex clinical and translational research in cancer with clarity. One could feel the excitement of the authors as one reads the latest advances in Caveolin-1, Stat3/5, Interferon, Interleulin-6, Leptin, Omega-3 fatty acids, and Gastrokin-1; neuroendocrine, oral, respiratory and abdominal malignancies, and the latest therapeutic advances in radiation therapy, nuclear medicine, epigenetic modifying drugs, and the emerging concepts of theranostics (therapeutic and diagnostics combined modalities) and ultrasound-mediated gene therapy.

The study of cancer is a dynamic field both diagnostically and therapeutically and this book carefully reviews the pertinent topics. It provides a logical framework for robust learning of the on-going research and critical appraisal of recently published relevant manuscripts. I unequivocally recommend this book; it is educational, insightful, and instructive.

Uma Sundaram
Marshall University
USA

PREFACE

What's the purpose of this book? In the face of the large volume of cancer literature, when so many texts flood the bookstores, why offer another one? Mainly for our greatest passion for cancer research, the motivation to learn more, and share this kind of knowledge as well.

Cancer is a broad group of diseases involving unregulated cell growth with elevated death rates since more people live in old age with mass lifestyle changes occurring in the developing world. The causes of cancer are diverse, complex, and still only partially understood. The chances of surviving the disease vary remarkably by the type and location of the malignancy and the extent of disease at the start of treatment. Early cancer detection is proving to be a valid approach. Cancer can be detected in a number of ways, including the presence of certain signs and symptoms, screening tests, or medical imaging. Cancer therapy is dynamically changing and revision and change in patient management is constant. Cancer is routinely treated with chemotherapy, radiation therapy and surgery. Tailored cancer targeted therapy is becoming an emerging objective of today.

Here, a constructive group of cancer research experts worked together with a shared vision, to give an extensive and realistic view of individual tumors, such as breast, oral, prostate, gastric, and neuroendocrine tumors. New terms and concepts in genetics and epigenetics, diet, and anticancer delivery systems are introduced aiming to present experimental strategies and key findings that enhance our understanding of cancer. It is our hope that for undergraduates, medical students, PhDs, cancer researchers, and also cancer families this text will be concise and palatable, and even conceive a curiosity about the subjects presented that will lead to further study. Material used in this book was reviewed at various stages to improve clarity and include relevant sources. A tremendous amount of work went into this text and we thank the authors for their selfless contributions.

Pier Paolo Claudio
Marshall University
USA

Paraskevi Vogiatzi
Thomas Jefferson University
USA

List of Contributors

Ana L. Romero-Weaver

Department of Radiation Oncology, University of Pennsylvania School of Medicine, Philadelphia, PA 19104, USA

Candace M. Howard

Department of Biochemistry and Microbiology, McKown Translational Genomic Research Institute, Marshall University, Huntington, WV, 25755, USA

Caterina Cinti

Institute of Clinical Physiology, National Research Council, Consiglio Nazionale delle Ricerche, Siena, 53100, Italy

Chiara S. di Stadio

Department of Biochemistry and Medical Biotechnologies, University of Naples Federico I and CEINGE, Advanced Biotechnologies, Naples, Italy

Daniela Trani

Department of Radiation Oncology (MaastRO Lab/Maastro Clinic), GROW-School for Oncology and Developmental Biology, Maastricht University Medical Centre, 6200 MD Maastricht, The Netherlands

David T. Hoang

Department of Cancer Biology, Kimmel Cancer Center, Thomas Jefferson University, Philadelphia, PA 19107, USA

Elaine W. Hardman

Department of Biochemistry and Microbiology, McKown Translational Genomic Research Institute, Marshall University, Huntington, WV, 25755, USA

Emili Rippa

Department of Biochemistry and Medical Biotechnologies, University of Naples Federico I and CEINGE, Advanced Biotechnologies, Naples, Italy

Faizan Alawi

Department of Pathology, School of Dental Medicine, University of Pennsylvania, Philadelphia, PA 19104, USA

Filomena Altieri

Department of Biochemistry and Medical Biotechnologies, University of Naples Federico I and CEINGE, Advanced Biotechnologies, Naples, Italy

Giuseppina Miselli

Department of Biochemistry and Medical Biotechnologies, University of Naples Federico I and CEINGE, Advanced Biotechnologies, Naples, Italy

Gloria Bonuccelli

Departments of Stem Cell Biology and Regenerative Medicine and Cancer Biology; Kimmel Cancer Center; Thomas Jefferson University; Philadelphia, PA, USA

Ilaria Naldi

Institute of Clinical Physiology, Consiglio Nazionale delle Ricerche, Siena, 53100, Italy

Johannes F. Fahrmann

Department of Biochemistry and Microbiology, McKown Translational Genomic Research Institute, Marshall University, Huntington, WV, 25755, USA

John J. Sauk

J.R. Brown Cancer Center, University of Louisville, Cancer Center, Louisville, KY 40202, USA

Juan C. T. Pardo

Institute of Clinical Physiology, Consiglio Nazionale delle Ricerche, Siena, 53100, Italy

Laslo Otvos

PeptheRx, Inc., 801 Mockingbird Lane, Audubon, PA 19403, USA

Marco Durante

GSI Helmholtzzentrum für Schwerionenforschung, Biophysics Department, Planckstraße 1, 64291 Darmstadt, Germany

Maria I. Scarano

Department of Biochemistry and Microbiology, McKown Translational Genomic Research Institute, Marshall University, Huntington, WV, 25755, USA

Marja T. Nevalainen

Department of Cancer Biology, Kimmel Cancer Center, Thomas Jefferson University, Philadelphia, PA 19107, USA

Michael P. Lisanti

Breakthrough Breast Cancer Research Unit, Institute of Cancer Sciences, University of Manchester, M20 4BX, United Kingdom (UK)

Monia Taranta

Institute of Clinical Physiology, Consiglio Nazionale delle Ricerche, Siena, 53100, Italy

Paolo Arcari

Department of Biochemistry and Medical Biotechnologies, University of Naples Federico I and CEINGE, Advanced Biotechnologies, Naples, Italy

Paraskevi Vogiatzi

Department of Cancer Biology, Kimmel Cancer Center, Thomas Jefferson University, Philadelphia, PA 19107, USA

Philippe G. Frank

Departments of Stem Cell Biology and Regenerative Medicine and Cancer Biology; Kimmel Cancer Center; Thomas Jefferson University; Philadelphia, PA, USA

Pier P. Claudio

Department of Biochemistry and Microbiology, Department of Surgery, McKown Translational Genomic Research Institute, Marshall University, Huntington, WV, 25755, USA

Pipitska Valsamaki

Nuclear Medicine Department, "Alexandra" University General Hospital, Athens, Greece

Rounak Nande

Department of Biochemistry and Microbiology, McKown Translational Genomic Research Institute, Marshall University, Huntington, WV, 25755, USA

Shilpa Gupta

Department of Medical Oncology, Thomas Jefferson University, Philadelphia, PA 19107, USA

Sonia Godoy-Tundidor

Department of Urology, Innsbruck Medical University, Anichstrasse 35, A-6020, Innsbruck, Austria

Sucharitha Balasubramaniam

Department of Cancer Biology, Thomas Jefferson University, Philadelphia, PA 19107, USA

Theodore R. Witte

Department of Biochemistry and Microbiology, McKown Translational Genomic Research Institute, Marshall University, Huntington, WV, 25755, USA

Zoran Culig

Department of Urology, Innsbruck Medical University, Anichstrasse 35, A-6020, Innsbruck, Austria

1

Send Orders for Reprints to reprints@benthamscience.net
Cutting Edge Therapies for Cancer in the 21st Century, 2014, 3-27

CHAPTER 1

Role of Caveolin-1 in Cancer and Therapeutic Implications

Gloria Bonuccelli, Philippe G. Frank and Michael P. Lisanti*

Breakthrough Breast Cancer Research Unit, Institute of Cancer Sciences, University of Manchester, M20 4BX, United Kingdom (UK)

Abstract: Caveolae are flask-shaped plasma membrane invaginations that represent a subset of the well-known lipid raft. These organelles are characterized by the presence of the caveolin-1 (Cav-1) protein that plays an important role in the regulation of several signal transduction pathways. More than ten years ago, *in vitro* experiments showed that downregulation of Cav-1 drives cell transformation and hyperactivation of the Ras-p42/44 MAP kinase cascade. In addition, it was shown that Cav-1 functions as a repressor of cyclin D1, possibly explaining its tumor suppressor activity in cultured cells. Later on, *in vivo* experiments showed that Cav-1 was involved in tumor development. In particular, the absence of Cav-1 in mouse skin increased the susceptibility to carcinogen-induced epidermal hyperplasia and tumor formation. Moreover, loss of Cav-1 expression caused the development of dysplastic mammary lesions in tumor-prone transgenic mice where cyclin D1 expression levels were dramatically elevated. These studies were the first *in vivo* demonstrations showing that caveolin-1 could function as a tumor suppressor gene. However, other investigators have shown that certain cancer cells show up-regulation of caveolin-1 that results in more metastatic and aggressive tumor like in bladder, thyroid, and prostate carcinomas. Taken together, these data suggest that Cav-1 is implicated in both tumor suppression and oncogenesis.

Keywords: Caveolae, caveolin-1, breast cancer, prostate cancer, melanoma, metalloproteins, MMP-2, MMP-9, estrogen receptor, P132L, EGFR, Her2/Neu, PDGF receptor tyrosine kinases, Ras, MAP kinase, PI-3-kinase, Warburg effect, Reverse Warburg effect.

1. INTRODUCTION

Caveolae are cellular invaginations of the plasma membrane that were first identified in 1953 (Palade, 1953). These vesicular structures are a special type of lipid rafts and appear as small (50 -100 nm) caves enriched in proteins as well as

***Address correspondence to Michael P. Lisanti:** Breakthrough Breast Cancer Research Unit, Institute of Cancer Sciences, University of Manchester, M20 4BX, United Kingdom (UK); Tel: +44(0) 161 446 8478; Fax: +44(0) 161 446 8000; E-mail: michaelp.lisanti@gmail.com

Pier Paolo Claudio and Paraskevi Vogiatzi (Eds)

lipids such as cholesterol and sphingolipids (Anderson, 1998, Brown and London, 1998, Galbiati, Razani and Lisanti, 2001). Importantly, there is a set of proteins present in the caveolae but absent in lipid rafts, the caveolins. The caveolin protein family is composed of three distinct integral membrane proteins, caveolin-1, -2, and -3 (Cav-1, -2,-3) (Glenney, 1992, Rothberg, Heuser, Donzell *et al.*, 1992, Scherer, Okamoto, Chun *et al.*, 1996, Tang, Scherer, Okamoto *et al.*, 1996). Caveolins are integral proteins inserted into the cell membrane. Both the C-terminus and the N-terminus face the cytoplasmic side of the membrane. Cav-1 is commonest member of this family (Fig. **1**). There are two isoforms of caveolin-1: caveolin-1α and caveolin-1β. The first 31 residues of caveolin-1α are absent in caveolin-1β (Sargiacomo, Scherer, Tang *et al.*, 1995).

Cav-1 and -2 form hetero-oligomeric complexes and are co-expressed in many cell types particularly in endothelial cells, adipocytes, and type I pneumocytes, (Scherer, Lewis, Volonte *et al.*, 1997), while Cav-3 is exclusively expressed in skeletal, cardiac and smooth muscle cells (Scherer, Lisanti, Baldini *et al.*, 1994, Scherer, Okamoto, Chun *et al.*, 1996, Tang, Scherer, Okamoto *et al.*, 1996).

Caveolae play a role in endocytosis, and cholesterol homeostasis, and have several functions in signal transduction and oncogenesis. Previous studies have revealed that cells can use caveolae for the uptake of small molecules and full size proteins such as albumin and alkaline phosphatase (Anderson, Kamen, Rothberg and Lacey, 1992, Parton, Joggerst and Simons, 1994, Predescu, Predescu and Palade, 1997, Schnitzer, Oh, Pinney and Allard, 1994). Moreover, in certain cell-types, caveolae are also involved in the uptake of viruses (*e.g.* simian virus 40) and bacteria (*e.g.* specific strains of *E. coli*) (Anderson, Chen and Norkin, 1996, Montesano, Roth, Robert and Orci, 1982, Shin, Gao and Abraham, 2000).

Research has shown that caveolin-1 binds cholesterol both *in vitro* (Murata, Peranen, Schreiner *et al.*, 1995) and *in vivo* (Thiele, Hannah, Fahrenholz and Huttner, 2000). In addition, a role has been suggested for caveolin-1 in the regulation of the intracellular movement of cholesterol as well as in its cellular uptake and efflux (Babitt, Trigatti, Rigotti *et al.*, 1997, Frank, Marcel, Connelly *et al.*, 2002, Smart, Ying, Donzell and Anderson, 1996, Uittenbogaard, Ying and Smart, 1998).

Regarding the role of caveolae in signal transduction, various signaling molecules have been shown to concentrate within these organelles *via* an interaction between the "caveolin-scaffolding domain" (caveolin-1 amino acids 82-101) and a "caveolin-binding motif" present in these associated proteins (Lisanti, Scherer, Tang and Sargiacomo, 1994, Mercier, Jasmin, Pavlides *et al.*, 2009, Okamoto, Schlegel, Scherer and Lisanti, 1998). The signaling molecules include H-ras, src-family tyrosine kinases, heterotrimeric G-proteins, eNOS, *etc.* (Lisanti, Scherer, Vidugiriene *et al.*, 1994, Smart, Ying, Donzell and Anderson, 1996).

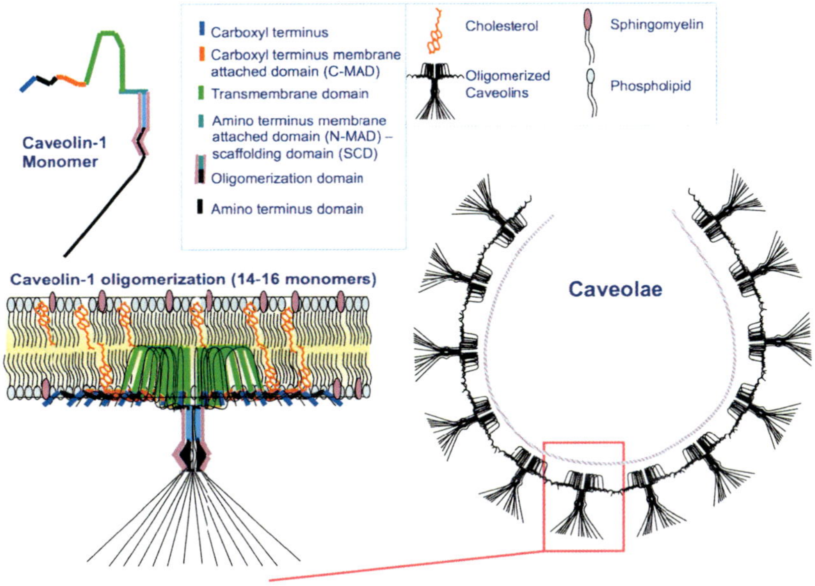

Figure 1: Caveolin-1 domain organization and caveolar assembly. Caveolin-1 is the principal component of caveolae membranes. Among its several domains is included the "caveolin-scaffolding domain" (SCD) through which various classes of signaling molecules bind Cav-1. Note that Cav-1 forms oligomers (14-16 monomers) modeling an umbrella shape and associates with cholesterol and sphingolipids leading to the formation of caveolae. Adapted and reproduced with permission from Mercier *et al.,* 2009.

Moreover, several proteins localized within caveolae play important roles in pro-proliferative/anti-apoptotic signaling, and their impairment can result in cells with hyperactive cell cycles and eventually tumor formation. These proteins are inhibited by Cav-1 and they include EGFR, Her2/Neu, and PDGF receptor tyrosine kinases, components of the Ras/p42/44 MAP kinase cascade, and members of the PI-3-kinase cascade (Couet, Sargiacomo and Lisanti, 1997,

Engelman, Chu, Lin *et al.*, 1998, Liu, Ying, Ko and Anderson, 1996, Yamamoto, Toya, Jensen and Ishikawa, 1999, Zundel, Swiersz and Giaccia, 2000).

Importantly, caveolae and Cav-1 have been suggested to be essential for cell tumor suppression since they are able to down regulate tumorigenic signals. Interestingly, it has been observed that caveolae are absent or reduced in number and Cav-1 is transcriptionally down-regulated in numerous cancers (Engelman, Lee, Karnezis *et al.*, 1998, Koleske, Baltimore and Lisanti, 1995, Lee, Reimer, Oh, Campbel and Schnitzer, 1998, Razani, Altschuler, Zhu *et al.*, 2000). In addition, both human Cav-1 and Cav-2 genes map to 7q31.1 that is a region of chromosome 7 found to be frequently deleted in several epithelial cancers - *e.g.* (breast, lung, renal, and ovary) (Kerr, Leary, Hurst *et al.*, 1996, Shridhar, Sun, Miller *et al.*, 1997, Zenklusen, Bieche, Lidereau and Conti, 1994).

Finally, generation of mice deficient in caveolin-1 [Cav-1 knockout (KO) mice] has provided an important tool for studying the role of caveolin-1 *in vivo*.

2. ROLE OF CAV-1 IN BREAST CANCER

Many studies have provided evidence for the tumor suppressor effect of Cav-1 on pro-proliferative signaling pathways. One of these pathways is the ERK-1/2 pathway that has been shown to contribute to mammary epithelial hyperplasia and tumor initiation (Sotgia, Rui, Bonuccelli *et al.*, 2006).

MAP kinases or extracellular-signal-regulated kinases (ERKs) are protein kinase intracellular signaling molecules that play key roles in the regulation of meiosis, mitosis, and postmitotic functions in different cells. ERK-1/2 has been localized to caveolae membrane (Liu, Ying and Anderson, 1997, Smart, Ying, Mineo and Anderson, 1995) and has been shown to be directly inhibited by Cav-1, both *in vitro* and *in vivo* (Engelman, Chu, Lin *et al.*, 1998, Zhang, Razani, Altschuler *et al.*, 2000). On the other hand, activation of the Ras-p42/44 MAP kinase cascade caused the downregulation of Cav-1 expression in NIH-3T3 cells (mouse embryonic fibroblasts) and in the mammary gland (Engelman, Zhang, Razani, Pestell and Lisanti, 1999). Finally, hyperactivation of ERK-1/2 occurs in Cav-1(-/-) mouse cells and tissues (Capozza, Williams, Schubert *et al.*, 2003, Cohen, Razani, Wang *et al.*,

2003, Williams, Lee, Cheung *et al.*, 2004). Thus, these findings, suggest that Cav-1 functions as an inhibitor of the p42/44 MAP kinase cascade.

In addition, *in vitro* evidences have shown that the cyclin D1 gene is transcriptionally repressed by overexpression of the caveolin-1 protein. The cyclin D1 protein is able to phosphorylate and inactivate the tumor suppressor retinoblastoma (Rb) protein (Kato, Matsushime, Hiebert, Ewen and Sherr, 1993, Lundberg and Weinberg, 1998, Sicinski, Donaher, Parker *et al.*, 1995) promoting cell cycle progression. Thus, inhibition of the cyclin D1 gene by caveolin-1 expression may contribute to the inhibition of cellular transformation.

Estrogen receptors (ER; ERα and ERβ) are members of a nuclear receptor family and ligand activated transcription factors. Estrogens are important mitogens of normal mammary epithelial cells, and ERα is expressed at low levels in the normal breast but is up-regulated in premalignant hyperplasia and during carcinoma development.

One-third of ERα-positive breast cancers harbor Cav-1 mutations, which have never been found associated with ERα-negative breast tumors. The most common mutation of Cav-1, (P132L), is a proline to leucine change at position 132 within the putative transmembrane domain of Cav-1 (Li, Sotgia, Vuolo *et al.*, 2006). Importantly, patients with breast cancer carrying Cav-1 mutations are more susceptible to undergo recurrence and metastasis, despite the good prognosis that usually is associated with ER positivity.

The P132L mutation behaves in a dominant negative manner with respect to wild-type cav-1 expression, since both proteins are retained in a perinuclear ER/Golgi like compartment preventing the correct targeting of wild-type Cav-1 to the plasma membrane. However, the Cav-1 (P132L) mutation acts as a gain-of-function mutation in the context of cell migration, invasion, and experimental metastasis (Bonuccelli, Casimiro, Sotgia *et al.*, 2009). Interestingly, based on gene expression profiling (DNA microarray analysis), the Cav-1 (P132L) mutation was shown to activate several signaling pathways implicated in cell migration, invasion, and metastasis. These findings mechanistically explain why breast cancer patients with Cav-1 mutations are more susceptible to disease recurrence (Bonuccelli, Casimiro, Sotgia *et al.*, 2009).

Previous studies have shown that Cav-1 suppresses breast cancer metastasis. In fact, it has been found that an absence of caveolin-1 results in evident increases in the frequency of distant lung metastases from the primary site of origin. Metastatic mammary tumor cells that recombinantly express Cav-1 showed significant reductions in matrigel invasion and dramatically reduced MMP-9/MMP-2 activities (Sloan, Stanley and Anderson, 2004, Williams, Medina, Badano *et al.*, 2004). It has been described that MMPs activity enhances tumor invasiveness and metastasis (Coussens and Werb, 1996). Moreover, MMP-2 and MMP-9 are clearly linked to breast cancer metastatic potential since MMP-2- and MMP-9-deficient mice are both much less susceptible to metastasis formation (Itoh, Tanioka, Matsuda *et al.*, 1999, Itoh, Tanioka, Yoshida *et al.*, 1998).

All together, these findings indicate that Cav-1 gene therapy may have an important application in the treatment of metastatic human breast cancer.

Finally, in normal breast tissue, Cav-1 is a regulator of proliferation and apoptosis, the highly programmed cell death. It has been described that in mouse embriogenic fibroblasts and epithelial cells, overexpression of caveolin-1 induced apoptotic cell death through inhibition of PI3-kinase and/or activation of caspase-3 (Liu, Lee, Galbiati, Kitsis and Lisanti, 2001, Zundel, Swiersz and Giaccia, 2000). However, upregulation of Cav-1 in the rat fibroblast cell line Rat1A, and in the human prostate cancer cell line LNCaP, causes resistance to apoptosis. Moreover, antisense downregulation of Cav-1 increases apoptosis in prostate cancer cells (Li, Ren, Tahir, Ren and Thompson, 2003, Li, Yang, Ebara *et al.*, 2001, Nasu, Timme, Yang *et al.*, 1998).

In conclusion, caveolin-1 has a complicated and controversial dual role of caveolin-1 in the apoptotic process, depending on the cell type or cellular context.

2.1. Perspectives

The theory that was proposed, and accepted, by Otto Warburg during the 1930s regarding the Warburg effect is now considered to be only partially accurate.

Warburg indicated that aerobic glycolysis does occur inside cancer cells, however it has recently been proved to be also found in the stromal cells, called cancer associated fibroblasts, and not just in cancer epithelial cells. This is because cancer researchers used isolated tumor cells in their studies on cancer. Now, mounting evidences have shown that when cancer cells were put back into their stromal environment, they were critically dependent on fibroblasts for their survival (Martinez-Outschoorn, Pavlides, Whitaker-Menezes *et al.*, 2010). These new studies showed that cancer cells promote oxidative stress that can cause fibroblasts to begin eating themselves. This process, termed autophagy, provides recycled nutrients that fuel cancer growth and explains the dramatic weight loss frequently observed in cancer patients. Without the nutrients provided by fibroblasts, tumor cells become fragile and die.

Based on this data, a new tumor growth theory has recently been proposed, and named "The Reverse Warburg Effect" (Fig. **2**). Essentially, epithelial cancer cells induce the Warburg effect (aerobic gylcolysis) in proximity to stromal fibroblasts. In particular, MCF7 cells when co-cultured with fibroblasts induced oxidative stress in the neighboring cells, mimicking hypoxia, where ROS (Reactive oxygen Species) triggered transcription factors like HIF1α and NFκB to signal fibroblasts mitochondria to break down (a process called "catabolism"). MCF7 cells then take nutrients from the broken-down mitochondria from the fibroblasts. Oxidative stress causes autophagy and mitophagy, producing recycled cell nutrients through glycolysis. Epithelial cancer cells are able to take up the above mentioned energy metabolites and use them in the mitochondrial TCA cycle, promoting energy production generating ATP *via* oxidative phosphorylation. The final result is a higher proliferative capacity causing tumor growth (as well as protecting cancer cells from apoptosis) and metastasis formation (Bonuccelli, Tsirigos, Whitaker-Menezes *et al.*, 2010, Pavlides, Whitaker-Menezes, Castello-Cros *et al.*, 2009). Cancer associated fibroblasts undergo myo-fibroblastic differentiation, and produce lactate, pyruvate and ketones. We have previously reported that cancer cells, *via* oxidative stress, induce downregulation of Cav-1 in adjacent fibroblasts in breast cancer and in ductal carcinoma *in situ* (DCIS) patients (Martinez-Outschoorn, Pavlides, Whitaker-Menezes *et al.*, 2010). It has been shown that Cav-1 (-/-) deficient stromal cells have characteristics of myo-fibroblasts overexpressing different myo-fibroblasts protein markers and also several glycolytic enzymes including the M2-isoform of pyruvate kinase and lactate dehydrogenase (Bonuccelli, Whitaker-Menezes, Castello-Cros *et al.*, 2010, Pavlides, Whitaker-Menezes, Castello-Cros *et al.*, 2009).

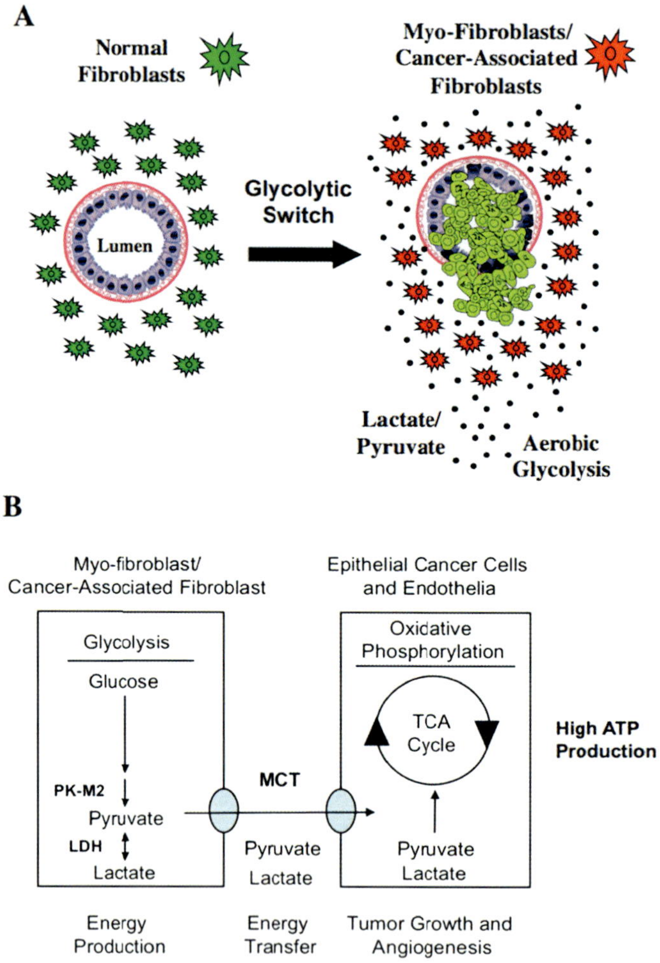

Figure 2: The Reverse Warburg Effect. These diagrams (A and B) summarize the new model developed for a better understanding of the Warburg effect (aerobic glycolysis) in tumor metabolism. Our hypothesis is that cancer epithelial cells induce aerobic glycolysis in cancer-associated fibroblasts (CAFs). CAFs then undergo myo-fibroblastic differentiation and produce lactate and pyruvate. Epithelial cancer cells use these energy-rich metabolites in the mitochondrial TCA cycle, promoting high ATP production leading to an increased proliferative capacity and metastasis formation. Transfer of pyruvate and lactate from CAFs to epithelial cancer cells and endothelia occurs *via* a mono-carboxylate transporter (MCT). Adapted and reproduced with permission from Pavlides *et al.*, 2009.

Cav-1 (-/-) deficient stromal cells also share characteristics with human breast cancer associated fibroblast as shown by studies of genome expression (Sotgia, Del Galdo, Casimiro *et al.*, 2009). Furthermore, Cav-1 (-/-) mammary stromal fibroblast over expressed growth factors like PGDF, VEGF, TGF-β, and IL-6 that are associated with cancer-associated fibroblasts and can stimulate the EMT (epithelial to mesenchymal transition) in normal mammary epithelial cells (Sotgia, Del Galdo, Casimiro *et al.*, 2009).

Recently, it has been demonstrated that loss of stromal expression of Cav-1 in human breast cancers is associated with poor clinical outcome (Witkiewicz, Dasgupta, Nguyen *et al.*, 2009, Witkiewicz, Dasgupta, Sotgia *et al.*, 2009). These findings were validated using human breast cancer tissues lacking stromal expression of Cav-1. Notably, in these human samples, M2-isoform of pyruvate kinase and lactate dehydrogenase, that are both Warburg-related glycolytic enzymes, were highly expressed in cancer-associated fibroblast in the tumor stroma, but not in the adjacent cancer cells. Consequently, it has been shown that loss of stromal Cav-1 is a powerful predictive biomarker for breast cancer, and all together these findings suggest that the presence of aerobic glycolysis in the tumor stroma may be very important to predict patient survival.

Interestingly, proteomics analysis revealed that Cav-1 (-/-) deficient stromal cells showed upregulation of two antioxidant proteins (peroxiredoxin 1 and catalase) normally associated with reactive oxygen species (ROS) production and oxidative stress. In addition, loss of stromal Cav-1 induces oxidative stress (Pavlides, Whitaker-Menezes, Castello-Cros *et al.*, 2009). Moreover, proteomics studies performed on Cav-1 (-/-) stromal cells have shown HIF-mediated transcriptional activation, showing the upregulation of 45 known HIF-target genes. Several NFkB target genes were also transcriptionally upregulated (Pavlides, Tsirigos, Vera *et al.*, 2010).

Taken together, these findings offer a clear and exhaustive scenario of the new theory, about cancer cell metabolism, that can be renamed "The autophagic tumor stroma model of cancer" (Chiavarina, Whitaker-Menezes, Migneco *et al.*, 2010, Martinez-Outschoorn, Trimmer, Lin *et al.*, 2010, Martinez-Outschoorn, Whitaker-Menezes, Pavlides *et al.*, 2010, Pavlides, Tsirigos, Migneco *et al.*, 2010).

Importantly, it could potentially lead to better diagnostics and therapies for high-risk cancer patients. The simple habit of taking daily anti-oxidants can combat the oxidative stress. The most effective antioxidant available in the local health-food store is NAC (N-acetyl cysteine). NAC prevents ROS from being generated in the mitochondria, preventing autophagy and starving cancer cells. New hopes for the development of new therapies are also generated by the use of drugs that can potentially break the "parasitic" connection between tumor cells and fibroblasts, effectively starving cancer cells. This new theory can now explain why the idea, already well accepted by the cancer research community, that a cancer cell's local environment is important for tumor growth.

3. CAV-1 AND MELANOMA

Malignant melanoma is the most dangerous type of skin cancer and it is the leading cause of death from skin disease. Its incidence has been dramatically increasing in the last few decades. It involves cells called melanocytes, which produce a skin pigment called melanin.

Cav-1 is known to exert a complex and ambiguous role as oncogene or tumor suppressor depending on the cellular microenvironment. The role of Cav-1 in malignant melanoma is still poorly understood. Different groups reported conflicting results for the role of Cav-1 in melanoma transformation and invasion. For example, a group characterized mouse melanoma B16-F10 cells, a metastatic cell model with low endogenous caveolin-1 and E-cadherin levels. In these cells, caveolin-1-mediated down-regulation of survivin in the presence of E-cadherin, and this effect caused increased apoptosis. Thus, the results described in this manuscript underline the ability of caveolin-1 to activate pathways potentially relevant to its role as a tumor suppressor (Torres, Tapia, Rodriguez *et al.*, 2007).

On the contrary, another independent study investigated Cav-1 expression and function in a panel of melanomas at different stages. They found that Cav-1 was expressed in all the cell lines. However, melanomas in neoplasias group displayed higher Cav-1 expression in primary tumors and/or distant metastases compared to the corresponding normal tissues (Felicetti, Parolini, Bottero *et al.*, 2009). Moreover, the down-regulation of Cav-1 in metastatic Cav-1-expressing melanomas was associated with reduced proliferative rates as well as tumorigenicity.

In addition, as first reported and accurately demonstrated for prostate cancer (Ayala, Dai, Tahir *et al.*, 2006, Tahir, Yang, Ebara *et al.*, 2001), where serum levels of Cav-1 were proposed as diagnostic and prognostic markers (Tahir, Frolov, Hayes *et al.*, 2006), the same study detected a fraction of Cav-1 that was secreted by melanomas. Thus, these *in vitro* experimental studies showed the Cav-1 ability to stimulate *in vitro* anchorage independence, migration and invasion in a paracrine/autocrine fashion (Felicetti, Parolini, Bottero *et al.*, 2009).

Overall, Cav-1 appears to exert a prominent role in melanoma progression, thus suggesting the future opportunity of utilizing it as a new diagnostic and/or prognostic molecular marker, as already hypothesized in metastatic prostate cancer (Tahir, Yang, Goltsov *et al.*, 2008). Moreover, Cav-1 might eventually represent a new target for innovative clinical setting, particularly relevant in those types of cancer, such as melanoma, still lacking effective traditional therapies.

Finally, recent studies have reported that Cav-1 expression inhibited the motility of B16-F10 melanoma cells employed as an *in vitro* system. In addition, it has been shown that Cav-1 suppression reduced the ability of B16F10 cells to form lung metastases *in vivo* (Trimmer, Whitaker-Menezes, Bonuccelli *et al.*, 2010). Interestingly, Cav-1 expression promoted proliferation whereas it suppressed the formation of lung metastasis. Primary melanoma tissue samples and cell lines showed significant Cav-1 expression compared with normal human melocytes, whereas metastatic cell lines and tissue samples showed complete loss or a striking reduction in Cav-1 levels. Cav-1 expression contributed to primary tumor growth, whereas its loss was an important factor in metastatic progression. These findings provide the first evidence that Cav-1 may function as an anti-metastatic gene in malignant melanoma. Finally, a mechanistic explanation of this behavior was proposed. Indeed, Cav-1 expression suppressed the expression and activity of Src and FAK proteins following integrins engagement (Trimmer, Whitaker-Menezes, Bonuccelli *et al.*, 2010). Notably, this study showed that Cav-1 expression is also reduced in human metastatic melanoma cell lines and human tissue samples derived from metastatic lesions. All together, these findings suggest that Cav-1 expression in melanoma is stage dependant, and loss of cav-1 is a late event in melanoma progressions. Thus, Cav-1 may be involved in regulating mechanisms that affect the metastatic process.

In conclusion, it seems evident that Cav-1 has a biphasic expression pattern in melanoma, where it is up-regulated in primary tumors and lost in melanoma metastasis. This is the first study that links the role of Cav-1 to promote cell proliferation and suppress metastatic potential in melanoma, altering integrins/Src/FAK signaling.

Currently, patients with metastatic disease have very few treatment options available. Taken together, these results suggest that Cav-1 may function as an anti-metastatic gene in melanoma, and it could be critical for the development of new therapeutics in this type of cancer.

4. CAV-1 AND PROSTATE CANCER

As previously mentioned, several studies have shown that Cav-1 functions as a tumor suppressor and is down-regulated in different type of human tumors, including lung cancer (Racine, Belanger, Hirabayashi *et al.*, 1999), breast cancer (Lee, Reimer, Oh, Campbell and Schnitzer, 1998), and ovary cancer (Wiechen, Diatchenko, Agoulnik *et al.*, 2001), colon adenocarcinoma (Bender, Reymond, Bron and Quest, 2000, Wiechen, Diatchenko, Agoulnik *et al.*, 2001) and sarcomas (Wiechen, Sers, Agoulnik *et al.*, 2001). However, other evidence suggests a role for Cav-1 in promoting tumorigenesis and metastasis in other human neoplasias, including bladder, esophageal, and prostate carcinomas (Fong, Garcia, Gwynn *et al.*, 2003, Hu, Lam, Law, Wong and Srivastava, 2001, Kato, Hida, Miyamoto *et al.*, 2002, Rajjayabun, Garg, Durkan *et al.*, 2001, Satoh, Yang, Egawa *et al.*, 2003, Yang, Truong, Timme *et al.*, 1998).

Prostate cancer (PCa) is the second leading cause of male deaths in Western countries (Jemal, Siegel, Ward *et al.*, 2008, Linton and Hamdy, 2003). PCa is, in most cases, slow-growing and symptom-free. It is a life threatening cancer and the high mortality is caused by the presence of occulted metastasis that eliminates the benefit of prostate cancer therapy. Prostate cancer most commonly metastasizes to the bones, lymph nodes, rectum, and bladder.

The first *in vivo* molecular genetic evidence showing that Cav-1 had a role as a promoter of mouse tumor development was reported by a group that utilized an animal model obtained by interbreeding Cav-1 (-/-) null mouse with a TRAMP (transgenic adenocarcinoma of mouse prostate) mouse (Williams, Hassan, Li *et al.*, 2005). In fact, prostate tumors from the well-characterized TRAMP mouse model (Gingrich, Barrios, Morton *et al.*, 1996, Greenberg, DeMayo, Finegold *et al.*, 1995, Kaplan-Lefko, Chen, Ittmann *et al.*, 2003) demonstrated an up-regulation of Cav-1 expression, like in human prostate cancers. Importantly, ablation of one or both Cav-1 alleles resulted in decrease of primary tumor burden and metastatic disease.

Cav-1 expression has been demonstrated at very low levels in normal human prostate epithelium, and there is a well-established correlation between its expression and prostate cancer progression. Indeed, it appears that elevated caveolin-1 protein levels are present in higher prostate carcinoma grade leading to a negative outcome in clinical studies. In human prostate cancers, Cav-1 levels correlate positively with the Gleason score (GS), which is one of the most important predictors of poor clinical outcome, extra-prostatic extension, and lymph node involvement (Satoh, Yang, Egawa *et al.*, 2003, Yang, Truong, Wheeler and Thompson, 1999). In addition, Cav-1 is expressed at higher levels in primary and metastatic human prostate cancer after androgen ablation therapy (Li, Yang, Ebara *et al.*, 2001). In mouse prostatic metastasis-derived cell lines, Cav-1 expression was up-regulated compared with primary tumor-derived cells (Yang, Truong, Timme *et al.*, 1998). *In vitro* studies have also confirmed that Cav-1 up-regulation increases androgen independence (Li, Yang, Ebara *et al.*, 2001, Nasu, Timme, Yang *et al.*, 1998). Interestingly, it has been demonstrated that androgen-insensitive human prostate cancer cells express and secrete Cav-1 that possess autocrine or paracrine tumor-promoting functions (Tahir, Yang, Ebara *et al.*, 2001). Experiments performed on PC-3 cells, suggested that Cav-1 is secreted by prostate cancer cell through a particular mechanism based on "prostasomes" which are vesicular organelles containing raft components (Llorente, de Marco and Alonso, 2004). A previous study, has shown that prostate cancer cell-derived Cav-1 mediated angiogenesis (Yang, Addai, Wheeler *et al.*, 2007). Recently, another study showed evidences that recombinant Cav-1 is taken up by prostate cancer and endothelial cells *in vitro*, and that recombinant Cav-1 increases angiogenesis *in vitro* and *in vivo* (Tahir, Yang, Goltsov *et al.*, 2008, Thompson, Tahir, Li *et al.*). This angiogenic alteration of the tumor microenvironment by secreted Cav-1 occurs through the PI3K-Akt-eNOS signaling pathway (Tahir, Yang, Goltsov *et al.*, 2008). It is important to note that Akt activation has been demonstrated to have an important role in prostate cancer progression (Li, Ittmann, Ayala *et al.*, 2005). Furthermore, a direct association has been reported between Cav-1 expression and Akt in prostate cancer through the scaffolding domain binding site interactions (Li, Ren, Tahir, Ren and Thompson, 2003).

Recent studies have shown that Akt activity regulates the expression of fatty acid synthase (FASN). FASN is a cytoplasmic enzyme producing long chain fatty acids in the form of palmitate, myristate, oleate and stearate. This enzyme has been implicated in prostate cancer progression, and Cav-1 has been demonstrated to be upstream of the control of FASN expression (Di Vizio, Sotgia, Williams *et al.*, 2007). After this work, the same group provided the first evidence showing that FASN and Cav-1 are both overexpressed in human prostate cancer tissues and that the two proteins directly interact. Importantly, their overexpression correlates with tumor grade and is predictive of metastatic potential, independently of the hormone responsive state (Di Vizio, Adam, Kim *et al.*, 2008). All these evidences, suggest that overexpression of Cav-1 may promote prostate tumor progression by elevating FASN levels (Di Vizio, Sotgia, Williams *et al.*, 2007).

Finally, as reported in this chapter, an absence of Cav-1 may be a marker of the cancer-associated fibroblast phenotype, as it relates to DCIS progression and breast cancer metastasis (Mercier, Casimiro, Wang *et al.*, 2008, Sloan, Ciocca, Pouliot *et al.*, 2009, Sotgia, Del Galdo, Casimiro *et al.*, 2009, Witkiewicz, Casimiro, Dasgupta *et al.*, 2009, Witkiewicz, Dasgupta, Nguyen *et al.*, 2009, Witkiewicz, Dasgupta, Sotgia *et al.*, 2009). Deletion of the Cav-1 gene is sufficient to confer the cancer-associated fibroblast phenotype in cultured mammary stromal fibroblasts (Sotgia, Del Galdo, Casimiro *et al.*, 2009). Recently, it was shown that loss of stromal Cav-1 is a marker of advanced prostate cancer and metastatic disease (Di Vizio, Morello, Sotgia *et al.*, 2009). An absence of stromal Cav-1 directly correlates with increased Gleason score. Moreover, stromal

Cav-1 expression was inversely correlated with the epithelial expression levels of Cav-1 and epithelial levels of phospho-Akt (Di Vizio, Morello, Sotgia *et al.*, 2009). Thus, an absence of stromal cav-1 is predictive of increased epithelial Cav-1 expression and activated epithelial Akt signaling, both in human primary prostate cancers and metastatic tumor tissue. These results indicate that loss of stromal Cav-1 may be a biomarker applicable for a type of cancer different from breast cancer.

4.1. Perspectives

Concerning the management of prostate cancer, radical prostatectomy is a valid therapy for treatment of early clinical stage PCa that is confined to the gland. Local radiotherapy can be used as adjuvant therapy. Chemical castration is made with treatment using gonadotropin-releasing hormone (GRH) superagonist to inhibit testosterone secretion from the testes (Labrie, Dupont, Belanger *et al.*, 1986). Surgery like orchidectomy/orchiectomy is also effective in most cases (Bennett, Hooper, Lee and Gobe, 2009). Inoperable malignant PCa, particularly associated with metastasis, is treated with androgen deprivation where the protein target is the androgen receptor (AR). In normal prostatic epithelial cells, AR expression is regulated by androgens such as 5a-dihydrotestosterone (DHT) and testosterone. Androgen deprivation therapies are often used in combination with orchidectomy or GRH agonists to produce the highest level of androgen deprivation (Bennett, Hooper, Lee and Gobe, 2009). However, possible effect of androgen deprivation is that recurrent tumors after this treatment evolve to a castrate-resistant phenotype, always with presence of metastasis, resulting in patient death within 5 years. Currently, there is not an effective treatment for this form of the disease.

Previously, a group presented results showing that serum Cav-1 levels in men affected by localized prostate cancers were significantly higher than those observed in healthy control men and in men with clinical benign prostatic hyperplasia (Tahir, Ren, Timme *et al.*, 2003). Interestingly, the expression and secretion of Cav-1 by prostate cancer represent an opportunity for the development of Cav-1 based biomarkers for prostate cancer (Thompson, Tahir, Li *et al.*, 2010). Particularly, high serum Cav-1 concentrations may identify men with PCa who will likely evolve toward tumor recurrence, following radical prostatectomy. Finally, the same authors consider the possibility of developing a therapy for prostate cancer targeting secreted Cav-1 (Thompson, Tahir, Li *et al.*, 2010).

Additional avenues relative to the prognostic value of Cav-1 as biomarker are offered from the research involving the role of stromal Cav-1. In fact, Cav-1 as a stromal biomarker can be proposed not only for ductal carcinoma *in situ* (DCIS) and breast cancer but also for prostate cancer. As discussed before, a loss of stromal Cav-1 predicts poor clinical outcome in DCIS, breast cancer and prostate cancer patient. Importantly, in all these three cases, a loss of Cav-1 could be used to identify high-risk cancer patients at diagnosis, facilitating stratification and clinical management. Thus, prostate cancer can also fit in the new paradigm recently proposed "The autophagic tumor stroma model of cancer" where a loss of stromal Cav-1 we believe represents a new biomarker for hypoxia, oxidative stress, autophagy and the "Reverse Warburg effect" (Fig. **3**).

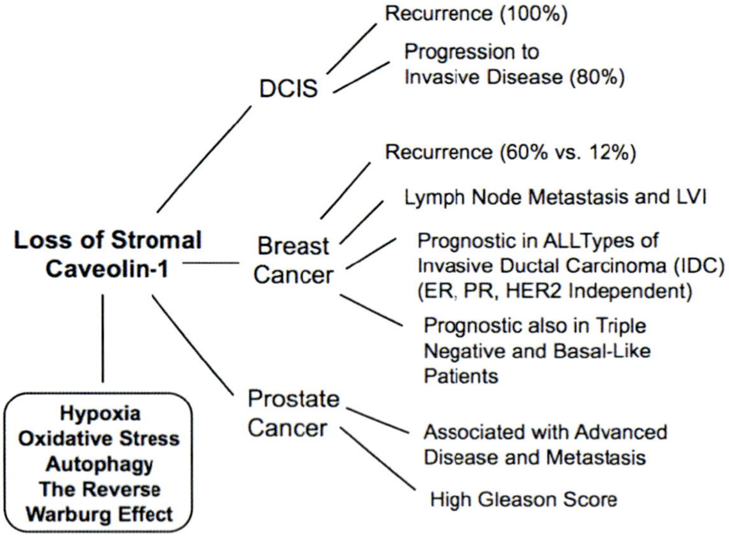

Figure 3: Cav-1 is a stromal biomarker for DCIS, breast cancer and prostate cancer. Loss of stromal Cav-1 effectively predicts poor clinical outcome in DCIS, breast cancer and prostate cancer patients. This diagram summarizes that loss of Cav-1 is a new biomarker for hypoxia, oxidative stress, autophagy and the "Reverse Warburg effect". Thus, stromal Cav-1 could be used to identify high-risk cancer patients and facilitate treatment stratification and clinical therapy. Adapted and reproduced with permission from Martinez-Outschoorn *et al.,* 2010c.

5. CONCLUSIONS

Studies have clearly established the notion that Cav-1 is a protein with two opposing roles depending on the stage of tumor progression (Williams and Lisanti, 2005). Interestingly, Cav-1 has a role as a "tumor and metastasis-modifying gene" and has tissue or cell type specific roles regarding tumorigenesis. Because of the heterogeneity of Cav-1 expression, therapies targeting Cav-1 must consider its specific role or function within a particular type of cancer (Williams and Lisanti, 2005).

Finally, we believe that cancer starts with oxidative stress. Cancer cells use stromal autophagy as a metabolic fuel source to become more aggressive. Effective cancer chemotherapy should eliminate this fuel supply, with powerful anti-oxidants and mitochondrial inhibitors (*i.e.*, N-acetyl cysteine, quercetin or metformin) as well as systemic modulators of autophagy (*i.e.*, chloroquine or rapamycin and its derivatives). Undoubtedly, these discoveries offer exciting opportunities to develop new anti-cancer therapies.

ACKNOWLEDGEMENTS

Dr. Lisanti's current affiliation is the University of Manchester (United Kingdom), where he receives funding from Breakthrough Breast Cancer (BBC), The European Research Council (ERC), and the Manchester Cancer Research Centre (MCRC), as well as the University. Previously, Dr. Lisanti was supported by the resources of Thomas Jefferson University in Philadelphia, USA.

CONFLICT OF INTEREST

The authors confirm that this chapter content has no conflict of interest.

REFERENCES

Anderson, H. A., Chen, Y. & Norkin, L. C. 1996. Bound simian virus 40 translocates to caveolin-enriched membrane domains, and its entry is inhibited by drugs that selectively disrupt caveolae. *Mol. Biol. Cell,* 7, 1825-1834.

Anderson, R. G. W. 1998. The caveolae membrane system. *Ann. Rev. Biochem.,* 67, 199-225.

Anderson, R. G. W., Kamen, B. A., Rothberg, K. G. & Lacey, S. W. 1992. Potocytosis: sequestration and transport of small molecules by caveolae. *Science,* 255, 410-411.

Ayala, G. E., Dai, H., Tahir, S. A., Li, R., Timme, T., Ittmann, M., Frolov, A., Wheeler, T. M., Rowley, D. & Thompson, T. C. 2006. Stromal antiapoptotic paracrine loop in perineural invasion of prostatic carcinoma. *Cancer Res,* 66, 5159-64.

Babitt, J., Trigatti, B., Rigotti, A., Smart, E. J., Anderson, R. G. W., Xu, S. & Krieger, M. 1997. Murine SR-BI, a high density lipoprotein receptor that mediates selective lipid uptake, is N-glycosylated and fatty acylated and colocalizes with plasma membrane caveolae. *J. Biol. Chem.,* 272, 13242-13249.

Bender, F. C., Reymond, M. A., Bron, C. & Quest, A. F. 2000. Caveolin-1 levels are down-regulated in human colon tumors, and ectopic expression of caveolin-1 in colon carcinoma cell lines reduces cell tumorigenicity. *Cancer Res,* 60, 5870-8.

Bennett, N., Hooper, J. D., Lee, C. S. & Gobe, G. C. 2009. Androgen receptor and caveolin-1 in prostate cancer. *IUBMB Life,* 61, 961-70.

Bonuccelli, G., Casimiro, M. C., Sotgia, F., Wang, C., Liu, M., Katiyar, S., Zhou, J., Dew, E., Capozza, F., Daumer, K. M., Minetti, C., Milliman, J. N., Alpy, F., Rio, M. C., Tomasetto, C., Mercier, I., Flomenberg, N., Frank, P. G., Pestell, R. G. & Lisanti, M. P. 2009. Caveolin-1 (P132L), a common breast cancer mutation, confers mammary cell invasiveness and defines a novel stem cell/metastasis-associated gene signature. *Am J Pathol,* 174, 1650-62.

Bonuccelli, G., Tsirigos, A., Whitaker-Menezes, D., Pavlides, S., Pestell, R. G., Chiavarina, B., Frank, P. G., Flomenberg, N., Howell, A., Martinez-Outschoorn, U. E., Sotgia, F. & Lisanti, M. P. 2010a. Ketones and lactate "fuel" tumor growth and metastasis: Evidence that epithelial cancer cells use oxidative mitochondrial metabolism. *Cell Cycle,* 9, 3506-14.

Bonuccelli, G., Whitaker-Menezes, D., Castello-Cros, R., Pavlides, S., Pestell, R. G., Fatatis, A., Witkiewicz, A. K., Vander Heiden, M. G., Migneco, G., Chiavarina, B., Frank, P. G., Capozza, F., Flomenberg, N., Martinez-Outschoorn, U. E., Sotgia, F. & Lisanti, M. P. 2010b. The reverse Warburg effect: Glycolysis inhibitors prevent the tumor promoting effects of caveolin-1 deficient cancer associated fibroblasts. *Cell Cycle,* 9.

Brown, D. A. & London, E. 1998. Functions of lipid rafts in biological membranes. *Ann. Rev. Cell Dev. Biol.,* 14, 111-136.

Capozza, F., Williams, T. M., Schubert, W., Mcclain, S., Bouzahzah, B., Sotgia, F. & Lisanti, M. P. 2003. Absence of caveolin-1 sensitizes mouse skin to carcinogen-induced epidermal hyperplasia and tumor formation. *Am J Pathol,* 162, 2029-39.

Chiavarina, B., Whitaker-Menezes, D., Migneco, G., Martinez-Outschoorn, U. E., Pavlides, S., Howell, A., Tanowitz, H. B., Casimiro, M. C., Wang, C., Pestell, R. G., Grieshaber, P., Caro, J., Sotgia, F. & Lisanti, M. P. 2010. HIF1-alpha functions as a tumor promoter in cancer associated fibroblasts, and as a tumor suppressor in breast cancer cells: Autophagy drives compartment-specific oncogenesis. *Cell Cycle,* 9, 3534-51.

Cohen, A. W., Razani, B., Wang, X. B., Combs, T. P., Williams, T. M., Scherer, P. E. & Lisanti, M. P. 2003. Caveolin-1-deficient mice show insulin resistance and defective insulin receptor protein expression in adipose tissue. *Am J Physiol Cell Physiol,* 285, C222-35.

Couet, J., Sargiacomo, M. & Lisanti, M. P. 1997. Interaction of a receptor tyrosine kinase, EGF-R, with caveolins. Caveolin binding negatively regulates tyrosine and serine/threonine kinase activities. *J. Biol. Chem.,* 272, 30429-30438.

Coussens, L. M. & Werb, Z. 1996. Matrix metalloproteinases and the development of cancer. *Chem Biol,* 3, 895-904.

Di Vizio, D., Adam, R. M., Kim, J., Kim, R., Sotgia, F., Williams, T., Demichelis, F., Solomon, K. R., Loda, M., Rubin, M. A., Lisanti, M. P. & Freeman, M. R. 2008. Caveolin-1 interacts with a lipid raft-associated population of fatty acid synthase. *Cell Cycle,* 7, 2257-67.

Di Vizio, D., Morello, M., Sotgia, F., Pestell, R. G., Freeman, M. R. & Lisanti, M. P. 2009. An absence of stromal caveolin-1 is associated with advanced prostate cancer, metastatic disease and epithelial Akt activation. *Cell Cycle,* 8, 2420-4.

Di Vizio, D., Sotgia, F., Williams, T. M., Hassan, G. S., Capozza, F., Frank, P. G., Pestell, R. G., Loda, M., Freeman, M. R. & Lisanti, M. P. 2007. Caveolin-1 is required for the upregulation of fatty acid synthase (FASN), a tumor promoter, during prostate cancer progression. *Cancer Biol Ther,* 6, 1263-8.

Engelman, J. A., Chu, C., Lin, A., Jo, H., Ikezu, T., Okamoto, T., Kohtz, D. S. & Lisanti, M. P. 1998a. Caveolin-mediated regulation of signaling along the p42/44 MAP kinase cascade *in vivo*. A role for the caveolin-scaffolding domain. *FEBS Lett.,* 428, 205-211.

Engelman, J. A., Lee, R. J., Karnezis, A., Bearss, D. J., Webster, M., Siegel, P., Muller, W. J., Windle, J. J., Pestell, R. G. & Lisanti, M. P. 1998b. Reciprocal regulation of Neu tyrosine kinase activity and caveolin-1 protein expression *in vitro* and *in vivo*. Implications for mammary tumorigenesis. *J. Biol. Chem.,* 273, 20448-20455.

Engelman, J. A., Zhang, X. L., Razani, B., Pestell, R. G. & Lisanti, M. P. 1999. p42/44 MAP kinase-dependent and -independent signaling pathways regulate caveolin-1 gene expression. Activation of Ras-MAP kinase and protein kinase a signaling cascades transcriptionally down-regulates caveolin-1 promoter activity. *J Biol Chem,* 274, 32333-41.

Felicetti, F., Parolini, I., Bottero, L., Fecchi, K., Errico, M. C., Raggi, C., Biffoni, M., Spadaro, F., Lisanti, M. P., Sargiacomo, M. & Care, A. 2009. Caveolin-1 tumor-promoting role in human melanoma. *Int J Cancer,* 125, 1514-22.

Fong, A., Garcia, E., Gwynn, L., Lisanti, M. P., Fazzari, M. J. & Li, M. 2003. Expression of caveolin-1 and caveolin-2 in urothelial carcinoma of the urinary bladder correlates with tumor grade and squamous differentiation. *Am J Clin Pathol,* 120, 93-100.

Frank, P. G., Marcel, Y. L., Connelly, M. A., Lublin, D. M., Franklin, V., Williams, D. L. & Lisanti, M. P. 2002. Stabilization of caveolin-1 by cellular cholesterol and scavenger receptor class B type I. *Biochemistry,* 41, 11931-40.

Galbiati, F., Razani, B. & Lisanti, M. P. 2001. Emerging themes in lipid rafts and caveolae. *Cell,* 106, 403-11.

Gingrich, J. R., Barrios, R. J., Morton, R. A., Boyce, B. F., Demayo, F. J., Finegold, M. J., Angelopoulou, R., Rosen, J. M. & Greenberg, N. M. 1996. Metastatic prostate cancer in a transgenic mouse. *Cancer Res,* 56, 4096-102.

Glenney, J. R. 1992. The sequence of human caveolin reveals identity with VIP 21, a component of transport vesicles. *FEBS Lett.,* 314, 45-48.

Greenberg, N. M., Demayo, F., Finegold, M. J., Medina, D., Tilley, W. D., Aspinall, J. O., Cunha, G. R., Donjacour, A. A., Matusik, R. J. & Rosen, J. M. 1995. Prostate cancer in a transgenic mouse. *Proc Natl Acad Sci U S A,* 92, 3439-43.

Hu, Y. C., Lam, K. Y., Law, S., Wong, J. & Srivastava, G. 2001. Profiling of differentially expressed cancer-related genes in esophageal squamous cell carcinoma (ESCC) using human cancer cDNA arrays: overexpression of oncogene MET correlates with tumor differentiation in ESCC. *Clin Cancer Res,* 7, 3519-25.

Itoh, T., Tanioka, M., Matsuda, H., Nishimoto, H., Yoshioka, T., Suzuki, R. & Uehira, M. 1999. Experimental metastasis is suppressed in MMP-9-deficient mice. *Clin Exp Metastasis,* 17, 177-81.

Itoh, T., Tanioka, M., Yoshida, H., Yoshioka, T., Nishimoto, H. & Itohara, S. 1998. Reduced angiogenesis and tumor progression in gelatinase A-deficient mice. *Cancer Res,* 58, 1048-51.

Jemal, A., Siegel, R., Ward, E., Hao, Y., Xu, J., Murray, T. & Thun, M. J. 2008. Cancer statistics, 2008. *CA Cancer J Clin,* 58, 71-96.

Kaplan-Lefko, P. J., Chen, T. M., Ittmann, M. M., Barrios, R. J., Ayala, G. E., Huss, W. J., Maddison, L. A., Foster, B. A. & Greenberg, N. M. 2003. Pathobiology of autochthonous prostate cancer in a pre-clinical transgenic mouse model. *Prostate,* 55, 219-37.

Kato, J., Matsushime, H., Hiebert, S. W., Ewen, M. E. & Sherr, C. J. 1993. Direct binding of cyclin D to the retinoblastoma gene product (pRb) and pRb phosphorylation by the cyclin D-dependent kinase CDK4. *Genes Dev,* 7, 331-42.

Kato, K., Hida, Y., Miyamoto, M., Hashida, H., Shinohara, T., Itoh, T., Okushiba, S., Kondo, S. & Katoh, H. 2002. Overexpression of caveolin-1 in esophageal squamous cell carcinoma correlates with lymph node metastasis and pathologic stage. *Cancer,* 94, 929-33.

Kerr, J., Leary, J. A., Hurst, T., Shih, Y. C., Antalis, T. M., Friedlander, M., Crawford, E., Khoo, S. K., Ward, B. & Chenevix-Trench, G. 1996. Allelic loss on chromosome 7q in ovarian adenocarcinomas: two critical regions and a rearrangement of the PLANH1 locus. *Oncogene,* 13, 1815-1818.

Koleske, A. J., Baltimore, D. & Lisanti, M. P. 1995. Reduction of caveolin and caveolae in oncogenically transformed cells. *Proc Natl Acad Sci U S A,* 92, 1381-5.

Labrie, F., Dupont, A., Belanger, A., St-Arnaud, R., Giguere, M., Lacourciere, Y., Emond, J. & Monfette, G. 1986. Treatment of prostate cancer with gonadotropin-releasing hormone agonists. *Endocr Rev,* 7, 67-74.

Lee, S. W., Reimer, C. L., Oh, P., Campbel, L. D. B. & Schnitzer, J. E. 1998a. Tumor cell growth inhibition by caveolin re-expression in human breast cancer cells. *Oncogene,* 16, 1391-1397.

Lee, S. W., Reimer, C. L., Oh, P., Campbell, D. B. & Schnitzer, J. E. 1998b. Tumor cell growth inhibition by caveolin re-expression in human breast cancer cells. *Oncogene,* 16, 1391-7.

Li, L., Ittmann, M. M., Ayala, G., Tsai, M. J., Amato, R. J., Wheeler, T. M., Miles, B. J., Kadmon, D. & Thompson, T. C. 2005. The emerging role of the PI3-K-Akt pathway in prostate cancer progression. *Prostate Cancer Prostatic Dis,* 8, 108-18.

Li, L., Ren, C. H., Tahir, S. A., Ren, C. & Thompson, T. C. 2003. Caveolin-1 maintains activated Akt in prostate cancer cells through scaffolding domain binding site interactions with and inhibition of serine/threonine protein phosphatases PP1 and PP2A. *Mol Cell Biol,* 23, 9389-404.

Li, L., Yang, G., Ebara, S., Satoh, T., Nasu, Y., Timme, T. L., Ren, C., Wang, J., Tahir, S. A. & Thompson, T. C. 2001. Caveolin-1 mediates testosterone-stimulated survival/clonal growth and promotes metastatic activities in prostate cancer cells. *Cancer Res,* 61, 4386-92.

Li, T., Sotgia, F., Vuolo, M. A., Li, M., Yang, W. C., Pestell, R. G., Sparano, J. A. & Lisanti, M. P. 2006. Caveolin-1 mutations in human breast cancer: functional association with estrogen receptor alpha-positive status. *Am J Pathol,* 168, 1998-2013.

Linton, K. D. & Hamdy, F. C. 2003. Early diagnosis and surgical management of prostate cancer. *Cancer Treat Rev,* 29, 151-60.

Lisanti, M. P., Scherer, P. E., Tang, Z. & Sargiacomo, M. 1994a. Caveolae, caveolin and caveolin-rich membrane domains: a signalling hypothesis. *Trends Cell Biol,* 4, 231-5.

Lisanti, M. P., Scherer, P. E., Vidugiriene, J., Tang, Z., Hermanowski-Vosatka, A., Tu, Y. H., Cook, R. F. & Sargiacomo, M. 1994b. Characterization of caveolin-rich membrane domains isolated from an endothelial-rich source: implications for human disease. *J Cell Biol,* 126, 111-26.

Liu, J., Lee, P., Galbiati, F., Kitsis, R. N. & Lisanti, M. P. 2001. Caveolin-1 expression sensitizes fibroblastic and epithelial cells to apoptotic stimulation. *Am J Physiol Cell Physiol,* 280, C823-35.

Liu, P., Ying, Y. & Anderson, R. G. 1997. Platelet-derived growth factor activates mitogen-activated protein kinase in isolated caveolae. *Proc Natl Acad Sci U S A,* 94, 13666-70.

Liu, P., Ying, Y., Ko, Y.-G. & Anderson, R. G. W. 1996. Localization of the PDGF-stimulated phosphorylation cascade to caveolae. *J. Biol. Chem.,* 271, 10299-10303.

Llorente, A., De Marco, M. C. & Alonso, M. A. 2004. Caveolin-1 and MAL are located on prostasomes secreted by the prostate cancer PC-3 cell line. *J Cell Sci,* 117, 5343-51.

Lundberg, A. S. & Weinberg, R. A. 1998. Functional inactivation of the retinoblastoma protein requires sequential modification by at least two distinct cyclin-cdk complexes. *Mol Cell Biol,* 18, 753-61.

Martinez-Outschoorn, U. E., Pavlides, S., Whitaker-Menezes, D., Daumer, K. M., Milliman, J. N., Chiavarina, B., Migneco, G., Witkiewicz, A. K., Martinez-Cantarin, M. P., Flomenberg, N., Howell, A., Pestell, R. G., Lisanti, M. P. & Sotgia, F. 2010a. Tumor cells induce the cancer associated fibroblast phenotype *via* caveolin-1 degradation: Implications for breast cancer and DCIS therapy with autophagy inhibitors. *Cell Cycle,* 9.

Martinez-Outschoorn, U. E., Trimmer, C., Lin, Z., Whitaker-Menezes, D., Chiavarina, B., Zhou, J., Wang, C., Pavlides, S., Martinez-Cantarin, M. P., Capozza, F., Witkiewicz, A. K., Flomenberg, N., Howell, A., Pestell, R. G., Caro, J., Lisanti, M. P. & Sotgia, F. 2010b. Autophagy in cancer associated fibroblasts promotes tumor cell survival: Role of hypoxia, HIF1 induction and NFkappaB activation in the tumor stromal microenvironment. *Cell Cycle,* 9, 3515-33.

Martinez-Outschoorn, U. E., Whitaker-Menezes, D., Pavlides, S., Chiavarina, B., Bonuccelli, G., Casey, T., Tsirigos, A., Migneco, G., Witkiewicz, A., Balliet, R., Mercier, I., Wang, C., Flomenberg, N., Howell, A., Lin, Z., Caro, J., Pestell, R. G., Sotgia, F. & Lisanti, M. P. 2010c. The autophagic tumor stroma model of cancer or "battery-operated tumor growth": A simple solution to the autophagy paradox. *Cell Cycle,* 9, 4297-306.

Mercier, I., Casimiro, M. C., Wang, C., Rosenberg, A. L., Quong, J., Minkeu, A., Allen, K. G., Danilo, C., Sotgia, F., Bonuccelli, G., Jasmin, J. F., Xu, H., Bosco, E., Aronow, B., Witkiewicz, A., Pestell, R. G., Knudsen, E. S. & Lisanti, M. P. 2008. Human breast cancer-associated fibroblasts (CAFs) show caveolin-1 downregulation and RB tumor suppressor functional inactivation: Implications for the response to hormonal therapy. *Cancer Biol Ther,* 7, 1212-25.

Mercier, I., Jasmin, J. F., Pavlides, S., Minetti, C., Flomenberg, N., Pestell, R. G., Frank, P. G., Sotgia, F. & Lisanti, M. P. 2009. Clinical and translational implications of the caveolin gene family: lessons from mouse models and human genetic disorders. *Lab Invest,* 89, 614-23.

Montesano, R., Roth, J., Robert, A. & Orci, L. 1982. Non-coated membrane invaginations are involved in binding and internalization of cholera and tetanus toxins. *Nature (Lond.),* 296, 651-653.

Murata, M., Peranen, J., Schreiner, R., Weiland, F., Kurzchalia, T. & Simons, K. 1995. VIP21/caveolin is a cholesterol-binding protein. *Proc. Natl. Acad. Sci., USA,* 92, 10339-10343.

Nasu, Y., Timme, T. L., Yang, G., Bangma, C. H., Li, L., Ren, C., Park, S. H., Deleon, M., Wang, J. & Thompson, T. C. 1998. Suppression of caveolin expression induces androgen sensitivity in metastatic androgen-insensitive mouse prostate cancer cells. *Nat Med,* 4, 1062-4.

Okamoto, T., Schlegel, A., Scherer, P. E. & Lisanti, M. P. 1998. Caveolins, A family of scaffolding proteins for organizing "pre-assembled signaling complexes" at the plasma membrane. *J. Biol. Chem., (Mini-review),* 273, 5419-5422.

Palade, G. E. 1953. An electron microscope study of the mitochondrial structure. *J Histochem Cytochem,* 1, 188-211.

Parton, R. G., Joggerst, B. & Simons, K. 1994. Regulated internalization of caveolae. *J. Cell Biol.,* 127, 1199-1215.

Pavlides, S., Tsirigos, A., Migneco, G., Whitaker-Menezes, D., Chiavarina, B., Flomenberg, N., Frank, P. G., Casimiro, M. C., Wang, C., Pestell, R. G., Martinez-Outschoorn, U. E., Howell, A., Sotgia, F. & Lisanti, M. P. 2010a. The autophagic tumor stroma model of cancer: Role of oxidative stress and ketone production in fueling tumor cell metabolism. *Cell Cycle,* 9, 3485-505.

Pavlides, S., Tsirigos, A., Vera, I., Flomenberg, N., Frank, P. G., Casimiro, M. C., Wang, C., Fortina, P., Addya, S., Pestell, R. G., Martinez-Outschoorn, U. E., Sotgia, F. & Lisanti, M. P. 2010b. Loss of stromal caveolin-1 leads to oxidative stress, mimics hypoxia and drives inflammation in the tumor microenvironment, conferring the "reverse Warburg effect": A transcriptional informatics analysis with validation. *Cell Cycle,* 9.

Pavlides, S., Whitaker-Menezes, D., Castello-Cros, R., Flomenberg, N., Witkiewicz, A. K., Frank, P. G., Casimiro, M. C., Wang, C., Fortina, P., Addya, S., Pestell, R. G., Martinez-Outschoorn, U. E., Sotgia, F. & Lisanti, M. P. 2009. The reverse Warburg effect: aerobic glycolysis in cancer associated fibroblasts and the tumor stroma. *Cell Cycle,* 8, 3984-4001.

Predescu, S. A., Predescu, D. N. & Palade, G. E. 1997. Plasmalemmal vesicles function as transcytotic carriers for small proteins in the continuous endothelium. *Am J Physiol,* 272, H937-49.

Racine, C., Belanger, M., Hirabayashi, H., Boucher, M., Chakir, J. & Couet, J. 1999. Reduction of caveolin 1 gene expression in lung carcinoma cell lines. *Biochem Biophys Res Commun,* 255, 580-6.

Rajjayabun, P. H., Garg, S., Durkan, G. C., Charlton, R., Robinson, M. C. & Mellon, J. K. 2001. Caveolin-1 expression is associated with high-grade bladder cancer. *Urology,* 58, 811-4.

Razani, B., Altschuler, Y., Zhu, L., Pestell, R. G., Mostov, K. E. & Lisanti, M. P. 2000. Caveolin-1 expression is down-regulated in cells transformed by the human papilloma virus in a p53-dependent manner. Replacement of caveolin-1 expression suppresses HPV-mediated cell transformation. *Biochemistry,* 39, 13916-24.

Rothberg, K. G., Heuser, J. E., Donzell, W. C., Ying, Y., Glenney, J. R. & Anderson, R. G. W. 1992. Caveolin, a protein component of caveolae membrane coats. *Cell,* 68, 673-682.

Sargiacomo, M., Scherer, P. E., Tang, Z.-L., Kubler, E., Song, K. S., Sanders, M. C. & Lisanti, M. P. 1995. Oligomeric structure of caveolin: Implications for caveolae membrane organization. *Proc. Natl. Acad. Sci., USA,* 92, 9407-9411.

Satoh, T., Yang, G., Egawa, S., Addai, J., Frolov, A., Kuwao, S., Timme, T. L., Baba, S. & Thompson, T. C. 2003. Caveolin-1 expression is a predictor of recurrence-free survival in pT2N0 prostate carcinoma diagnosed in Japanese patients. *Cancer,* 97, 1225-33.

Scherer, P. E., Lewis, R. Y., Volonte, D., Engelman, J. A., Galbiati, F., Couet, J., Kohtz, D. S., Van Donselaar, E., Peters, P. & Lisanti, M. P. 1997. Cell-type and tissue-specific expression of caveolin-2. Caveolins 1 and 2 co-localize and form a stable hetero-oligomeric complex *in vivo*. *J Biol Chem,* 272, 29337-46.

Scherer, P. E., Lisanti, M. P., Baldini, G., Sargiacomo, M., Corley-Mastick, C. & Lodish, H. F. 1994. Induction of caveolin during adipogenesis and association of GLUT4 with caveolin-rich vesicles. *J. Cell Biol.,* 127, 1233-1243.

Scherer, P. E., Okamoto, T., Chun, M., Nishimoto, I., Lodish, H. F. & Lisanti, M. P. 1996. Identification, sequence and expression of caveolin-2 defines a caveolin gene family. *Proc. Natl. Acad. Sci., USA,* 93, 131-135.

Schnitzer, J. E., Oh, P., Pinney, E. & Allard, J. 1994. Filipin-sensitive caveolae-mediated transport in endothelium: Reduced transcytosis, scavenger endoctytosis, and capillary permeability of select macromolecules. *J. Cell Biol.,* 127, 1217-1232.

Shin, J. S., Gao, Z. & Abraham, S. N. 2000. Involvement of cellular caveolae in bacterial entry into mast cells. *Science,* 289, 785-8.

Shridhar, V., Sun, Q. C., Miller, O. J., Kalemkerian, G. P., Petros, J. & Smith, D. I. 1997. Loss of heterozygosity on the long arm of human chromosome 7 in sporadic renal cell carcinomas. *Oncogene,* 15, 2727-33.

Sicinski, P., Donaher, J. L., Parker, S. B., Li, T., Fazeli, A., Gardner, H., Haslam, S. Z., Bronson, R. T., Elledge, S. J. & Weinberg, R. A. 1995. Cyclin D1 provides a link between development and oncogenesis in the retina and breast. *Cell,* 82, 621-30.

Sloan, E. K., Ciocca, D. R., Pouliot, N., Natoli, A., Restall, C., Henderson, M. A., Fanelli, M. A., Cuello-Carrion, F. D., Gago, F. E. & Anderson, R. L. 2009. Stromal cell expression of caveolin-1 predicts outcome in breast cancer. *Am J Pathol,* 174, 2035-43.

Sloan, E. K., Stanley, K. L. & Anderson, R. L. 2004. Caveolin-1 inhibits breast cancer growth and metastasis. *Oncogene,* 23, 7893-7.

Smart, E. J., Ying, Y.-S., Donzell, W. C. & Anderson, R. G. W. 1996a. A role for caveolin in transport of cholesterol from endoplasmic reticulum to plasma membrane. *J. Biol. Chem.,* 271, 29427-29435.

Smart, E. J., Ying, Y., Donzell, W. C. & Anderson, R. G. 1996b. A role for caveolin in transport of cholesterol from endoplasmic reticulum to plasma membrane. *J Biol Chem,* 271, 29427-35.

Smart, E. J., Ying, Y. S., Mineo, C. & Anderson, R. G. 1995. A detergent-free method for purifying caveolae membrane from tissue culture cells. *Proc Natl Acad Sci U S A,* 92, 10104-8.

Sotgia, F., Del Galdo, F., Casimiro, M. C., Bonuccelli, G., Mercier, I., Whitaker-Menezes, D., Daumer, K. M., Zhou, J., Wang, C., Katiyar, S., Xu, H., Bosco, E., Quong, A. A., Aronow, B., Witkiewicz, A. K., Minetti, C., Frank, P. G., Jimenez, S. A., Knudsen, E. S., Pestell, R. G. & Lisanti, M. P. 2009. Caveolin-1-/- null mammary stromal fibroblasts share characteristics with human breast cancer-associated fibroblasts. *Am J Pathol,* 174, 746-61.

Sotgia, F., Rui, H., Bonuccelli, G., Mercier, I., Pestell, R. G. & Lisanti, M. P. 2006. Caveolin-1, mammary stem cells, and estrogen-dependent breast cancers. *Cancer Res,* 66, 10647-51.

Tahir, S. A., Frolov, A., Hayes, T. G., Mims, M. P., Miles, B. J., Lerner, S. P., Wheeler, T. M., Ayala, G., Thompson, T. C. & Kadmon, D. 2006. Preoperative serum caveolin-1 as a prognostic marker for recurrence in a radical prostatectomy cohort. *Clin Cancer Res,* 12, 4872-5.

Tahir, S. A., Ren, C., Timme, T. L., Gdor, Y., Hoogeveen, R., Morrisett, J. D., Frolov, A., Ayala, G., Wheeler, T. M. & Thompson, T. C. 2003. Development of an immunoassay for serum caveolin-1: a novel biomarker for prostate cancer. *Clin Cancer Res,* 9, 3653-9.

Tahir, S. A., Yang, G., Ebara, S., Timme, T. L., Satoh, T., Li, L., Goltsov, A., Ittmann, M., Morrisett, J. D. & Thompson, T. C. 2001. Secreted caveolin-1 stimulates cell survival/clonal growth and contributes to metastasis in androgen-insensitive prostate cancer. *Cancer Res,* 61, 3882-5.

Tahir, S. A., Yang, G., Goltsov, A. A., Watanabe, M., Tabata, K., Addai, J., Fattah El, M. A., Kadmon, D. & Thompson, T. C. 2008. Tumor cell-secreted caveolin-1 has proangiogenic activities in prostate cancer. *Cancer Res,* 68, 731-9.

Tang, Z.-L., Scherer, P. E., Okamoto, T., Song, K., Chu, C., Kohtz, D. S., Nishimoto, I., Lodish, H. F. & Lisanti, M. P. 1996. Molecular cloning of caveolin-3, a novel member of the caveolin gene family expressed predominantly in muscle. *J. Biol. Chem.,* 271, 2255-2261.

Thiele, C., Hannah, M. J., Fahrenholz, F. & Huttner, W. B. 2000. Cholesterol binds to synaptophysin and is required for biogenesis of synaptic vesicles. *Nat Cell Biol,* 2, 42-9.

Thompson, T. C., Tahir, S. A., Li, L., Watanabe, M., Naruishi, K., Yang, G., Kadmon, D., Logothetis, C. J., Troncoso, P., Ren, C., Goltsov, A. & Park, S. 2010. The role of caveolin-1 in prostate cancer: clinical implications. *Prostate Cancer Prostatic Dis,* 13, 6-11.

Torres, V. A., Tapia, J. C., Rodriguez, D. A., Lladser, A., Arredondo, C., Leyton, L. & Quest, A. F. 2007. E-cadherin is required for caveolin-1-mediated down-regulation of the inhibitor of apoptosis protein survivin *via* reduced beta-catenin-Tcf/Lef-dependent transcription. *Mol Cell Biol,* 27, 7703-17.

Trimmer, C., Whitaker-Menezes, D., Bonuccelli, G., Milliman, J. N., Daumer, K. M., Aplin, A. E., Pestell, R. G., Sotgia, F., Lisanti, M. P. & Capozza, F. 2010. CAV1 inhibits metastatic potential in melanomas through suppression of the integrin/Src/FAK signaling pathway. *Cancer Res,* 70, 7489-99.

Uittenbogaard, A., Ying, Y. & Smart, E. J. 1998. Characterization of a cytosolic heat-shock protein-caveolin chaperone complex. Involvement in cholesterol trafficking. *J Biol Chem,* 273, 6525-32.

Wiechen, K., Diatchenko, L., Agoulnik, A., Scharff, K. M., Schober, H., Arlt, K., Zhumabayeva, B., Siebert, P. D., Dietel, M., Schafer, R. & Sers, C. 2001a. Caveolin-1 is down-regulated in human ovarian carcinoma and acts as a candidate tumor suppressor gene. *Am J Pathol,* 159, 1635-43.

Wiechen, K., Sers, C., Agoulnik, A., Arlt, K., Dietel, M., Schlag, P. M. & Schneider, U. 2001b. Down-regulation of caveolin-1, a candidate tumor suppressor gene, in sarcomas. *Am J Pathol,* 158, 833-9.

Williams, T. M., Hassan, G. S., Li, J., Cohen, A. W., Medina, F., Frank, P. G., Pestell, R. G., Di Vizio, D., Loda, M. & Lisanti, M. P. 2005. Caveolin-1 promotes tumor progression in an autochthonous mouse model of prostate cancer: genetic ablation of Cav-1 delays advanced prostate tumor development in tramp mice. *J Biol Chem,* 280, 25134-45.

Williams, T. M., Lee, H., Cheung, M. W., Cohen, A. W., Razani, B., Iyengar, P., Scherer, P. E., Pestell, R. G. & Lisanti, M. P. 2004a. Combined loss of INK4a and caveolin-1 synergistically enhances cell proliferation and oncogene-induced tumorigenesis: role of INK4a/CAV-1 in mammary epithelial cell hyperplasia. *J Biol Chem,* 279, 24745-56.

Williams, T. M. & Lisanti, M. P. 2005. Caveolin-1 in oncogenic transformation, cancer, and metastasis. *Am J Physiol Cell Physiol,* 288, C494-506.

Williams, T. M., Medina, F., Badano, I., Hazan, R. B., Hutchinson, J., Muller, W. J., Chopra, N. G., Scherer, P. E., Pestell, R. G. & Lisanti, M. P. 2004b. Caveolin-1 gene disruption promotes mammary tumorigenesis and dramatically enhances lung metastasis *in vivo*. Role of Cav-1 in cell invasiveness and matrix metalloproteinase (MMP-2/9) secretion. *J Biol Chem,* 279, 51630-46.

Witkiewicz, A. K., Casimiro, M. C., Dasgupta, A., Mercier, I., Wang, C., Bonuccelli, G., Jasmin, J. F., Frank, P. G., Pestell, R. G., Kleer, C. G., Sotgia, F. & Lisanti, M. P. 2009a. Towards a new "stromal-based" classification system for human breast cancer prognosis and therapy. *Cell Cycle,* 8, 1654-8.

Witkiewicz, A. K., Dasgupta, A., Nguyen, K. H., Liu, C., Kovatich, A. J., Schwartz, G. F., Pestell, R. G., Sotgia, F., Rui, H. & Lisanti, M. P. 2009b. Stromal caveolin-1 levels predict early DCIS progression to invasive breast cancer. *Cancer Biol Ther,* 8, 1071-9.

Witkiewicz, A. K., Dasgupta, A., Sotgia, F., Mercier, I., Pestell, R. G., Sabel, M., Kleer, C. G., Brody, J. R. & Lisanti, M. P. 2009c. An absence of stromal caveolin-1 expression predicts early tumor recurrence and poor clinical outcome in human breast cancers. *Am J Pathol,* 174, 2023-34.

Yamamoto, M., Toya, Y., Jensen, R. A. & Ishikawa, Y. 1999. Caveolin is an inhibitor of platelet-derived growth factor receptor signaling. *Exp Cell Res,* 247, 380-8.

Yang, G., Addai, J., Wheeler, T. M., Frolov, A., Miles, B. J., Kadmon, D. & Thompson, T. C. 2007. Correlative evidence that prostate cancer cell-derived caveolin-1 mediates angiogenesis. *Hum Pathol,* 38, 1688-95.

Yang, G., Truong, L. D., Timme, T. L., Ren, C., Wheeler, T. M., Park, S. H., Nasu, Y., Bangma, C. H., Kattan, M. W., Scardino, P. T. & Thompson, T. C. 1998. Elevated expression of caveolin is associated with prostate and breast cancer. *Clin Cancer Res,* 4, 1873-80.

Yang, G., Truong, L. D., Wheeler, T. M. & Thompson, T. C. 1999. Caveolin-1 expression in clinically confined human prostate cancer: a novel prognostic marker. *Cancer Res,* 59, 5719-23.

Zenklusen, J. C., Bieche, I., Lidereau, R. & Conti, C. J. 1994. (C-A)n microsatellite repeat D7S522 is the most commonly deleted region in human primary breast cancer. *Proc Natl Acad Sci U S A,* 91, 12155-12158.

Zhang, W., Razani, B., Altschuler, Y., Bouzahzah, B., Mostov, K. E., Pestell, R. G. & Lisanti, M. P. 2000. Caveolin-1 inhibits epidermal growth factor-stimulated lamellipod extension and cell migration in metastatic mammary adenocarcinoma cells (MTLn3). Transformation suppressor effects of adenovirus-mediated gene delivery of caveolin-1. *J Biol Chem,* 275, 20717-25.

Zundel, W., Swiersz, L. M. & Giaccia, A. 2000. Caveolin 1-mediated regulation of receptor tyrosine kinase-associated phosphatidylinositol 3-kinase activity by ceramide. *Mol Cell Biol,* 20, 1507-14.

Send Orders for Reprints to reprints@benthamscience.net

 Cutting Edge Therapies for Cancer in the 21st Century, 2014, 28-80

CHAPTER 2

Role of Epigenetic Alterations in the Pathogenesis of Cancer: Recent Clinical Trials in Epigenetic Therapy

Caterina Cinti*, Monia Taranta, Ilaria Naldi and Juan Carlos Trivino Pardo

Institute of Clinical Physiology, National Research Council, Consiglio Nazionale delle Ricerche, Siena, Italy

Abstract: The pattern of gene expression can vary in each cell without changes in the DNA sequence. This is accomplished by reversible chemical modifications of the chromatin, which are generally indicated with the term "epigenetics". Chromatin remodeling caused by DNA methylation and histone modifications, especially at the site of genes promoters, are the major epigenetic events enabling transcriptional regulation. It is known that alterations of epigenetic signals are important early events for cancer development. These changes profoundly influence gene expression and are at the basis of malignant transformation. Specific pathways of genes are proficiently turned on or off by cancer cells to achieve uncontrolled proliferation. Genes playing key roles in DNA damage responses, apoptosis signaling and DNA repair are in fact frequently silenced by epigenetic modifications, while those involved in cell proliferation are often overexpressed. But the appealing feature of epigenetic changes is that they can be potentially reverted. This peculiarity has opened the way to new therapeutic possibilities to fight tumors that might be collectively termed "epigenetic therapy". Here we will discuss the basic aspects of epigenetic alterations, and in particular those events involving critical genes implicated in carcinogenesis, and the current relevance of DNA methyltransferase and histone deacetylase inhibitors for cancer therapy.

Keywords: Cancer, DNA, methylation, CpG islands, chromatin, eterochromatin, euchromatin, histones, histone deacetylase, histone acetylation, histone acetyltransferases, epigenetic therapy, demethylating agents, deacetylating agents, DNA methyltransferases, multi-drug resistance associated protein, clinical trials, metalloproteinases, inhibitor of metalloproteinase, computational epigenetics.

1. INTRODUCTION

All the cells in a human body have the same DNA content, but the pattern of gene expression can be very different. This is due to finely coordinated mechanisms which establish, read and erase epigenetic marks. The term *"epigenetics"*

***Address correspondence to Caterina Cinti:** Institute of Clinical Physiology, National Research Council, c/o Siena Biotech, Strada del Petriccio e Belriguardo 35, 53100 Siena, Italy; Tel: + 39 0577 381294; Fax: +39 0577 381298; E-mail ccinti@ifc.cnr.it

Pier Paolo Claudio and Paraskevi Vogiatzi (Eds)

suggests a kind of information that is "*over*" (from Greek "*epi*") the primary DNA sequence but that, like DNA, is heritable. Epigenetic modifications in somatic cells, indeed, can be mitotically transmitted to daughter cells, and those in the germ line transmitted to the offspring.

The epigenetic control on gene expression is carried out by modulating the organization of DNA into chromatin, and thus its accessibility to the transcriptional machinery factors. In the chromatin, about 146 bp of DNA are wrapped twice around a core of eight histone proteins to form nucleosomes. Nucleosomes are then packed into even more compact structures by other histone and non-histone proteins. Epigenetic modifications involve essentially four mechanisms. First, DNA can be methylated by covalent addition of methyl groups. Second, histones in the nucleosome core can undergo different chemical modifications in their amino-terminal tails, mostly through methylation, acetylation, phosphorylation and ubiquitination. Third, in accordance with these two processes, also non-coding RNAs play an important role in regulating chromatin accessibility. Then, other complementary mechanisms control the higher order of chromatin organization *via* long-range interactions. The orchestrated work of these epigenetic marks defines the chromatin accessibility and consequently its transcriptional activity. Indeed, while highly condensed regions of chromatin (heterochromatin) are transcriptionally silenced, lightly packed chromatin (euchromatin) allows gene expression (Fig. **1**).

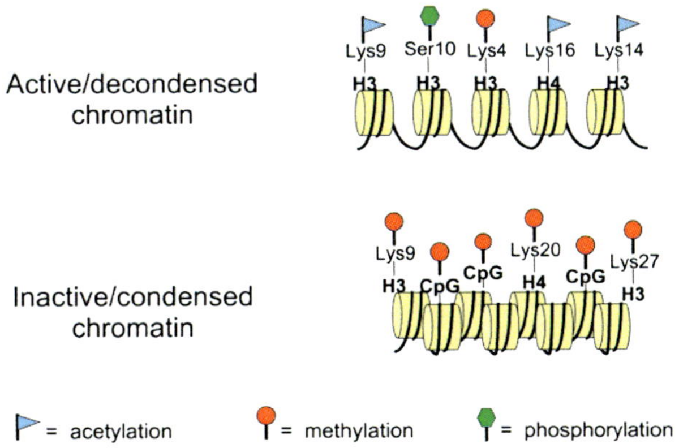

Figure 1: Chromatin remodeling by DNA and histone modifications. Examples of combinatorial DNA and histone modifications characteristic of either active or inactive chromatin.

An important epigenetic phenomenon is represented by genomic imprinting. This term refers to a process in which the expression of a given gene specifically depends on the parent of origin. Some genes, in fact, receive parent of origin epigenetic marks which allow the specific expression of only one allele. Genes can receive a maternal or a paternal imprint, but never both. In germ cells and early embryos, epigenetic markers are genome-wide erased and re-established, according on the individual sex, so that all genes will be properly imprinted in the next generation. Epigenetic reprogramming is in fact pivotal to establish nuclear totipotency and generate cells with a broad developmental potential (Morgan, *et al.*, 2005).

1.1. DNA Methylation

One of the best known epigenetic marker is DNA methylation, that is the covalent binding of a methyl group to the cytosine base within a CpG dinucleotide. CpG dinucleotides are under represented in the genome. However, there are some regions, called CpG islands, in which these dinucleotides are even five times more frequent than the rest of the genome. Methylation of CpG islands is associated with a repressive state of chromatin, whereas the lack of methylation coincides with regions of gene activity. Repeated sequences involving up to 35% of the genome are generally hypermethylated, while CpG dinucleotides within the promoter regions and first exon of house-keeping and tissue-specific genes are commonly not methylated (Bird, 1992).

DNA methylation is catalyzed by different DNA methyltransferases (DNMTs). DNMT3a and DNMT3b are required for establishing the *de novo* methylation, while DNMT1, recognizing hemimethylated sequences of DNA following replication, is primarily responsible for maintaining the pre-existing methylation patterns through mitosis (Bestor, 2000; Okano, *et al.*, 1999; Rhee, *et al.*, 2002; Kim, *et al.*, 2002).

The different epigenetic markers are not independent but cooperate to regulate chromatin accessibility. Methylated DNA, in fact, is interpreted by methyl-binding domain (MBD) proteins, which are important "translators" between DNA methylation and histone modifications to establish a transcriptionally inactive environment.

1.2. Histone Modifications

Chromatin remodeling at the promoter sites, by histone modifications, is another crucial mechanism of transcriptional regulation. This nucleosome reorganization involves numerous post-translational histone modifications such as acetylation, methylation, phosphorylation, ubiquitination, sumoylation, ADP-ribosylation, glycosylation, biotinylation and carbonylation. It has been observed that certain histone epigenetic marks tend to be associated with an active state of chromatin, and others with a repressive one. The overall of these modifications generate a "histone code" which is read and interpreted by different proteins that, governing chromatin dynamics, regulate gene expression.

Histone acetylation is modulated by the activity of two family of enzymes, called histone acetyltransferases (HATs) and deacetylases (HDACs). In general, it can be said that acetylated histones tend to be associated to transcriptionally active chromatin. Differently, histone methylation, governed by histone methyltransferases (HMTs) and demetylase (HDMTs), is found associated to both active and inactive chromatin, depending on the specific residue involved. Trimethylation of histone H3 at lysine 4, for example, is commonly found in active chromatin, whereas trimethylation of histone H3 at lysine 9 is associated to repressed genes (Fig. **1**).

As already said, there is a close interconnection between DNA and histone modifications (Das and Singal, 2004). In fact, hypermethylated DNA promoters are often coupled with histone modifications characterized by specific hypoacetylation and methylation (An, 2007). DNMTs are able to recruit both HDACs and HMTs to modify specific histone residues (Fuks, *et al.*, 2003). This active recruitment of multiple factors leads to a characteristic repressive pattern characterized by histone H3 and H4 deacetylation, lysine 9 of histone H3 trimethylation, and demethylation of histone H3 at lysine 4 (Stirzaker, *et al.*, 2004).

1.3. Non-Coding RNA

In the cells, the DNA information is transcribed into RNA molecules, of which only about 3% are translated into proteins; the remaining are considered non-coding RNAs (ncRNAs). Some of these are functional molecules, such as tRNAs and rRNAs, which play different roles in mRNAs translation, and snRNAs, which are involved in RNA splicing. Other ncRNAs are instead implicated in gene regulation, by tampering with different phases of the full process, including mRNA expression, maturation, degradation and translation (Kaikkonen, *et al.*, 2011). As regards the mRNA expression, there is even more frequent evidence that regulatory ncRNAs can control gene expression by altering chromatin conformation (Mattick, 2009). These ncRNAs are both long ncRNAs (lncRNAs) and small ncRNAs such as endogenous small-interfering RNAs (siRNAs), microRNAs (miRNAs) and Piwi-interacting RNAs (piRNAs).

A classical example of lncRNA involved in gene silencing by heterochromatin formation is *Xist*, which has a key role in the X chromosome inactivation process (Lee, 2009). But beyond *Xist*, also other lncRNAs have been demonstrated to have a role in altering chromatin structure (Ponting *et al.*, 2009).

Among small ncRNA, miRNAs are known to regulate gene expression by targeting specific mRNAs for degradation. However, it has been more recently discovered that they can also recruit chromatin-modifying factors, altering chromatin conformation (Carthew and Sontheimer, 2009). However, the participation of ncRNAs in chromatin remodeling is only just coming to light and many aspects of this process are still to be discovered.

1.4. Epigenetic Modifications in Human Cancer

Cancer development can result from inherited germ line mutations, or from genetic changes occurring in somatic cells during life. These mutations can cause the inaction of tumor suppressor genes or the abnormal enhancement of proto-oncogenes. However, changes in DNA methylation of promoters or first exons of tumor suppressor genes or of proto-oncogenes can have the same effect of genetic mutations. In numerous cancers, in fact, a growing number of tumor suppressor and other cancer-related genes have been demonstrated to be silenced by aberrant methylation (Baylin and Herman, 2000). In contrast to normal cells, the methylation pattern in cancer cells is altered: there is a global DNA hypomethylation, together with a region-specific DNA hypermethylation. The hypomethylation of commonly silenced regions can contribute to tumorigenesis by causing activation of proto-oncogenes, latent retrotrasposons and other genes involved in genomic instability, cell proliferation, invasion and metastasis (Bayani, *et al*., 2007). At the same time, the hypermethylation occurs at CpG islands near promoters of genes involved in cell cycle control (Baylin, *et al*., 2001; Toyota and Issa, 2005; Costello, *et al.,* 2000). Their inactivation removes checkpoints of normal proliferation, increasing the risk of a malignant transformation.

An example of gene activation by DNA demethylation is provided by the insulin-like growth factor 2 (*Igf2*). In normal cells, *Igf2* is expressed only from one allele due to genetic imprinting. DNA hypomethylation causes the second allele reactivation and the overexpression of this growth factor induces malignant cell proliferation (Vu, *et al*., 2003).

Long Interspersed Nuclear Elements (LINEs) are strongly methylated retrotransposons found in all human cells. Methylation of these elements is a host defense mechanisms to make them silent. In colon cancer and chronic lymphocytic leukemia it has been observed that global hypomethylation can cause LINEs activation and consequent genomic instability that contributes to malignancy development (Carnell and Goodman, 2003).

On the other hand, the *p16INK4a* gene, encoding a cyclin dependent kinase (CDK) inhibitor, which negatively regulates G1–S transition of the proliferating cells, is hypermethylated in many solid tumors, including colorectal, lung, and breast carcinomas (Herman, *et al*., 1995), but also in leukemias and lymphomas (Kusy *et al*., 2004). Inactivation of this gene by methylation allows the cells to undergo an uncontrolled proliferation.

Another example is the decreased expression of the tissue inhibitor of metalloproteinase-3 (*TIMP3*), due to CpG island methylation, that has been observed in a variety of tumors. Matrix metalloproteinases are involved in degradation of the extracellular matrix, and inactivation of *TIMP3* gene increases its turnover, which is considered a key event in the local invasion and metastasis of many tumors (Chambers and Matrisian, 1997). Aberrant methylation of *TIMP3* occurs in primary cancers of the kidney, brain, colon, breast and lung, and is particularly frequent in renal cancer (Baker, *et al*., 1999).

Also other genes involved in crucial cellular pathways have been found methylated. Examples are genes involved in the cell cycle regulation, such as *p14arf* and *p73*, in the DNA repair, such as *hMLH1, MGMT* and *BRCA1*, in apoptosis, such as *DAPK*, and in the cancer genesis process, such as *APC,* and metabolic enzymes such as *GSTP1*. Methylation of some of these genes, like, *MGMT* and *DAPK* has a wide distribution among many tumors (Sanchez-Cespedes, *et al*., 2000); alteration of other genes is instead more tumor-specific, reflecting their peculiar involvement in selected tumor types or groups of tumors (Hanahan and Weinberg, 2000). Inactivation of *p14arf* and *APC*, for example, is often found in gastrointestinal tumors (Esteller, *et al*., 2000a), whereas methylation of *GSTP1* is characteristic of breast, liver, and prostate cancers (Esteller, *et al*., 1998; Esteller, *et al*., 2000b). *BRCA1* is commonly methylated in breast and ovarian carcinomas (Esteller, *et al*., 2000b), whereas hypermethylation of the mismatch repair gene *hMLH1* is restricted to three sporadic tumor types: colorectal, endometrial, and gastric tumors with microsatellite instability (Kane, *et al*., 1997). In any given tumor it is possible to find simultaneous alteration of several pathways. For example, in colorectal tumor, cell cycle control, DNA repair, and metastasis-related processes can be damaged by hypermethylation of *p16INK4a*, *hMLH1* and *TIMP3* respectively, whereas in mammary tumor, similar objectives can be accomplished by silencing *p16INK4a*, *BRCA1* and *CDH1*, and in lung tumor by inactivating *p16INK4a*, *MGMT* and *DAPK* (Esteller, *et al*., 2002).

It is interesting to note that in various cancer types, epigenetic inactivation of many genes correlates with an increased expression of DNMT1 and DNMT3B (Ahluwalia *et al*., 2001, Mizuno *et al*., 2001). Downregulation of these enzymes has been demonstrated to reduce DNA methylation, with the consequent re-expression of inactivated genes (Rhee *et al*., 2002).

By now it is clear that cancer is a stepwise process of accumulation of genetic and epigenetic changes, and it is just the synergy of these two processes to drive tumor progression and malignancy. *De novo* methylation of CpG islands in the promoter region of tumor suppressor genes may cause transcriptional silencing through a complex process involving histone deacetylation and chromatin condensation. This tumorigenic event is functionally equivalent to genetic changes, like mutation and deletion (Jones and Laird, 1999). However, unlike genetic mutations, epigenetic alterations are potentially reversible. Moreover, for some genes, the promoter methylation may be the only type of gene inactivation, since mutations of multiple genes are rare events. These observations provide the rationale for the utilization of DNA demethylating and chromatin remodeling agents for cancer therapy.

1.5. Epigenetics and Drug Resistance of Tumors

One of the major causes of failure in the treatment of cancer is multi-drug resistance that many cancer cells develop, causing resistance to chemotherapy. Tumors often are made of a mix of malignant cells, some of which are drug sensitive while others resist to drugs. Chemotherapy kills drug sensitive cells, leaving behind the resistant ones. As a consequence, the remaining resistant cells make the tumor grow again, causing chemotherapy failure. The development of drug resistance is in fact one of the major challenges in cancer therapy and a limiting factor in patient survival. Both intrinsic and acquired drug resistance in tumors can be the result of an alteration in gene expression, which, in some cases, can be due to aberrant epigenetic regulation. Numerous studies suggest a direct role for epigenetic inactivation of genes in determining tumor chemosensitivity (Balch, *et al.*, 2004; Teodoridis, *et al.*, 2004; Baker and El-Osta, 2003). To understand the mechanisms underlying drug resistance, many efforts have been made to identify the cellular pathways that are triggered in tumor cells following drug or radiation therapy (Ferriera, *et al.*, 2002). Since cell death induced by chemotherapy and radiotherapy is mainly the result of apoptosis activation, it has been suggested that inhibition of this pathway should be crucial for drug response (Shah and Schwartz, 2001).

p53 is a tumor suppressor factor well-known to play an important role in modulating cell response to various damages and stress. Since it regulates a large number of genes required for the apoptotic response (Isoldi, *et al.*, 2005), it is not surprising that its gene is inactivated in many type of cancers. The *p53* family members are also mediators of cytotoxicity of chemotherapeutic drugs, and for this reason loss of their function often contributes to both tumor aggressiveness and drug resistant phenotype (La Sala, *et al.*, 2003). Whereas in cancer cells *p53* is commonly inactivated by genetic mutations, *p73* is generally silenced by epigenetic alterations. For example, in many cases of aggressive hematological neoplasm, it has been noted that epigenetic silencing of *p73* is related to poor response to therapy (Martinez-Delgado, *et al.*, 2002). Another example is given by osteosarcoma. Here cells bearing mutations in both *p53* and *Rb1* tumor suppressor genes, following drug treatment, can still undergo apoptosis in a p73-dependent manner (Hansen, 1991). However, in about 35% of cases, these cells show resistance after few chemotherapeutic treatments, since *p73* transcription is repressed by methylation (La Sala, *et al.*, 2003), determining the failure of therapy.

Metastatic melanoma is another example of cancer that usually does not respond to conventional chemotherapy. In this case, drug resistance seems to be due, at least in part, to *Apaf-1* inactivation through epigenetic alterations. This gene encodes for a cell-death effector that binds to cytochrome c to activate caspase-9 and induce apoptosis. Some studies have demonstrated that *Apaf-1* expression can be restored by treatment with the DNA methylation inhibitor 5-aza-2'-deoxycytidine, and that restoration of physiological levels of this cell-death effector enhances chemosensitivity (Fu, *et al.*, 2003). At the same manner, in various tumors also *caspase-8* is frequently inactivated by methylation and treatment with demethylating agents can restore its expression, increasing chemosensitization (Fulda, *et al.*, 2001).

Another protein that has been demonstrated to be important to determine chemotherapeutics sensitivity is hMLH1, which is a member of the human DNA mismatch repair system (Fink, *et al.*, 1998; Buermeyer, *et al.*, 1999 ; Toft, *et al.*, 1999; Mackay, *et al.*, 2000). In many cases, including sporadic colon (Herman, *et al.*, 1998), gastric (Leung, *et al.*, 1999), endometrial (Gurin, *et al.*, 1999) and ovarian cancers (Strathdee, *et al.*, 1999), it has been observed a high frequency of *hMLH1* promoter methylation, and treatment with the demethylating agent 5-aza-2'-deoxycytidine has demonstrated to restore sensitization to DNA damaging agents (Buermeyer, *et al.*, 1999; Strathdee, *et al.*, 1999).

FancF is an important factor for the activation of a DNA repair complex, and alterations of this pathway has demonstrated an increased susceptibility to develop cancer due to a reduced capability to repair DNA damages (Olopade and Wei, 2003). Inactivation of *FancF* gene through promoter methylation has been observed in many malignancies including ovarian cancer (Taniguchi, *et al.*, 2003), acute myeloid leukemia, lung and head and neck cancers (Marsit, *et al.*, 2004). Even for this gene, treatment with 5-aza-2'-deoxycytidine has been demonstrated to restore cisplatin sensitivity (Taniguchi, *et al.*, 2003).

In tumors, epigenetic events probably contribute to chemoresistance at several steps of drug response pathways. In ovarian cancer, for example, drug resistance is mediated by epigenetic down regulation of different genes, such as *FancF, hMLH1, Apaf-1, p16INK4* and *p73*, together with the upregulation of other genes, such as *MDR1, MRP1, MRP2* and *BCRP* (Gottesman, 2002 ; Balch, *et al.*, 2004). *MDR1* encodes for a transmembrane protein, which enhances drugs efflux in an energy dependent manner (Langmann, *et al.*, 2003). It is a member of the ATP-binding cassette transporter proteins (ABC), which collectively are able to transport a vast array of toxicants. The overexpression of *MDR1*, together with the multi-drug resistance associated protein 1 (*MRP1*) and 2 (*MRP2*), and the breast cancer resistance protein (*BCRP*) is related to an increased efflux of chemotherapeutics, such as anthracyclines, epipodophyllotoxins and vinca-alkaloids, thus resulting in multi-drug resistance (Gottesman, 2002; Baker and El-Osta, 2003).

As observed, in cancer cells, the two coexisting processes of global hypomethylation and regional hypermethylation confer a selective advantage by turning on and off different sets of genes with opposite roles. Regional hypermethylation causes the downregulation of genes whose products are required to suppress tumorigenesis, while global hypomethylation induces activation of genes with pivotal roles in the transformation process. It is obvious that single gene alteration is not sufficient neither for cancer development nor for drug resistance acquirement, but it is rather the concerted work of several genes that eventually determines the cell state and the drug fate inside the tumor cell. Even among cells clonally derived from the same one it is possible to find different patterns of gene alteration. This phenomenon may explain the existence of cross-resistance to different types of chemotherapeutics (Gottesman, 2002), and by now it is clear that epigenetic changes have key roles within this context.

2. COMPUTATIONAL EPIGENETICS

For several years, there has been an exponential growth of the amount of life science data, for example, mass spectroscopy data, 3D structures, sequenced complete genomes and DNA/Protein chips. These data must be combined together and processed by bioinformatics tools and algorithms deployed on efficient infrastructure to permit the full integration of these biological knowledge and, guiding the analysis of data, to help in the process of cancer interpretation as biological complex system. With the completion of the human genome sequence and the development of high-throughput technologies, that have permitted to study human transcriptome and proteome, and other typologies of genomic knowledge, such as single nucleotide polymorphisms or the functional annotation of genome, it is possible to develop computational approaches that can contribute to understand the epigenetic mechanism associated to cancer and open up novel approaches for early diagnosis and treatment of this disease (Jones and Baylin, 2007).

In this part of the chapter, we discuss arising bioinformatic challenges, and show how computational methods have contributed and will continue to contribute answering important epigenetic questions.

2.1. Generation and Processing of Epigenetic Data

Different computational, mathematical and statistical methods, based on data-mining, sequence analysis, molecular interactions, text mining, 3D structure predictions, have been proposed in the last years, to obtain epigenetic information associated to cancer. Traditional sequence analysis tools, such as BLAST (Altschul, *et al.*, 1990), BLAT(BLAST-Like Alignment Tool) (Kent, 2002) and MEGA(Molecular Evolutionary Genetics Analysis) (Kumar, *et al.*, 2008) allow for the inference of structural and functional information of DNA and protein sequences. Furthermore, based on this typology of information, it has been used different methods applied to ortholog searches, homology modeling of protein associated to epigenetics events (Koudan, *et al.*, 2004), 3D protein predictions (Chang, *et al.*, 2010), molecular dynamics simulations and docking (Wang, *et al.*, 2005). Various experimental techniques have been developed for genome-wide mapping of epigenetic information. These typology of experimental methods for epigenome mapping generate large amounts of data and require efficient ways of processing and interpretation.

ChIP-on-chip is a technique which combines chromatin immunoprecipitation (ChiIP) with microarray technology (chip) (Buck and Lieb, 2004). ChIP-on-chip is used to investigate the enrichment and the identified genomic DNA sequences bound by regulatory proteins, as well as to identify sites of histone and DNA modification. The main computational tools, which have been developed for Chip-on-chip analysis, are focused on the identification of Chip enrichment site, for example, Chromatin Immuno Precipitation On Tiled arrays (ChIPOTle) (Buck, *et al*., 2005), Ringo (Toedling, *et al*., 2007), rMAT (Droit, *et al*., 2010) and TileMap (Ji and Wong, 2005). ChIP-seq technology combines chromatin immunoprecipitation (ChIP) with high-throughput DNA sequencing and it is used to analyze protein interactions with DNA (Mikkelsen, *et al*., 2007). This method has two advantages over ChIP-on-chip (Bock and Lengauer, 2008): (i) data normalization is less of an issue because sequencing results in absolute read count rather than relative hybridization scores (Barski, *et al*., 2007); (ii) recent progress in sequencing-by-synthesis methods, for example, Roche, Solexa, Makes ChIP-seq apparatus highly cost-efficient. The key bioinformatic step of ChIP-seq is the fast and accurate mapping of short sequence reads to the reference genome. In the last years, different specialized algorithms have been developed for short-read assembly, for example, Qpalma (De Bona, *et al*., 2008) or AMOScmp (Pop, *et al*., 2004). The technology of bisulfite sequencing is based on bisulfite treatment of DNA and it is useful to determine the pattern of DNA methylation (Pop, *et al*., 2004; Hajkova, 2002; Lewin, *et al*., 2004), the genome-wide comparison of histone modification site identified by various epigenome mapping initiatives (Xu, *et al*., 2008) or the analysis of DNA methylation patterns of different tissue types (Tost, *et al*., 2003).

2.2. Data Sources for Epigenetic Research

The development of experimental technologies and bioinformatic methodologies has enabled the exponential growth in the amount of data relevant for epigenetic research. These amount of biological information must be stored and integrated by specialized epigenetic databases to facilitate the discovery of new fact, interpretation of results and design of experiments.

DNA methylation databases contain information on DNA methylation genes and patterns across different individuals, tissue, cell types and phenotypes. Important sources of this typology of information include MethDB (Negre and Grunau, 2006) and MethPrimerDB (Pattyn, *et al.*, 2006). Respect specific cancer methylation databases, the major sources include MethyCancer (He, *et al.*, 2008), PubMeth (Ongenaert, *et al.*, 2008) and MeInfoText (Fang, *et al.*, 2008) which contains information on gene methylation profiles of specific cancer types.

Histone databases are important for research in the compaction and accessibility of eukaryotic genomic DNA, post translational modifications (PTM), structures of histones, proteins containing the histone fold motif, enzymes responsible for the PTMs and their relevance to various diseases. Important sources of this typology of information include The National Human Genome Research Institute (NHGRI)'s Histone Database (Sullivan, *et al.*, 2002), HHMD (Zhang, *et al.*, 2010) and HistoneHits (Huang, *et al.*, 2009).

The National Center of Biotechnology Information (NCBI)'s Gene Expression Omnibus (GEO) is a central repository for high-throughput gene expression data, functional genomic, chromatin structure, methylation status and transcription factor binding (Barrett, *et al.*, 2009).

2.3. Computational Tools for Epigenetic Research

A substantial amount of bioinformatic tools has been development to the prediction of epigenetic information from genome sequences. Such predictions serve as dual propose (Bock and Lengauer, 2008). First, accurate epigenome predictions are relevant for discovered epigenetic mechanisms. Promoter prediction is an important topic in bioinformatic. Promoters are crucial control regions for transcriptional activation of every gene, and are characterized by an open and permissive chromatin structure. The promoters exhibit specific epigenetic properties such as the presence of the CpG islands, the absence of DNA methylation and the enrichment of histone acetylation. Different promoter predictions have been developed in the last years, some of them based in CpG island prediction. The over-representation of GC and CpG frequencies using different methodologies, for example, CpG island searcher (Takai and Jones, 2003), CpGProD (Ponger and Mouchiroud, 2002), CpGcluster (Hackenberg, *et al.*, 2006) or CG clusters (Glass, *et al.*, 2007) have been used in this typology of analysis.

Second, prediction algorithms build statistical models of epigenetic information from training data and can act as a first approximation toward quantitative modeling of an epigenetic mechanism. A variety of methods for the prediction of DNA methylation have been reported in the literature. Some of them include algorithms based on support vector machines (SVM), hidden Markov models (HMM), ANNs, logistic regression, K-nearest neighbours, naïve bayes and decision trees (Bhasin, *et al.*, 2005; Chen, *et al.*, 2006; Shao, *et al.*, 2009). Other typologies of algorithms are based on the integration of the results of DNA methylation with other biological knowledge (Bock, *et al.*, 2007; Chen, *et al.*, 2007). Another important process in the analysis of epigenetic events is the study of histone modification. Histone proteins are the main components of chromatin and play a key role in the compaction and accessibility of genome. There is intense interest in the analysis, modeling and prediction of histones modification in DNA sequences. These modifications, such as methylation, acetylation, phosphorylation, sumoylation or ubiquitination can affect chromosome function in different ways. For the study of these modifications, different algorithms have been designed, some of them based in machine-learning (Won, *et al.*, 2008; Miranda-Saavedra, *et al.*, 2007), HMM applied to ChIP-on-chip and ChIP-seq databases (Xu, *et al.*, 2008) or structural techniques as Quantitative Structure-Activity Relationship (QSAR) (Chen, *et al.*, 2009).

2.4. Computational Epigenetic, Toward Therapy and Early Diagnosis of Cancer

DNA methylation play an important role in the regulation of genomic stability, cellular plasticity and it is associated with numerous and functional process including cancer. The importance of epigenetic mechanisms for cancer development has been reported in the last years. It is now clear that the epigenetic deregulation can silence tumor suppressor genes and may program cells for cancer-like-behaviour (Jones and Baylin, 2007). Information on epigenetic modification opens new perspectives for diagnosis and therapy of cancer. The analysis of specific genomic areas that exhibit epigenetic differences between tumor cells and normal cells or between different subtypes of cancer is one of the main area of study. Different groups have applied several bioinformatic methods based on integration of biological knowledge with different mathematical and statistical algorithms, such as the over-representation Gene Ontology terms, sequences motifs discovery or genomic clustering (Keshet, *et al.*, 2006; Loss, *et al.*, 2010; Goh, *et al.*, 2007), to identify patterns of epigenetic regulations. The analysis of the epigenetically silenced genes in cancer opens the possibility of detect new candidates of cancer-specific hypermethylation.

The discovery and validation of biomarkers is also an important challenge for cancer diagnosis, prognosis and therapy optimization. The role of the bioinformatic in this typology of analysis is: 1) to maximize the genomic coverage in the early stages of the biomarkers search; 2) to identify and to optimize a small number of highly promising candidates; 3) to validate biomarker performance and computational prediction between candidate drugs and active site of the epigenetic related proteins (Fig. **2**). Different biomarkers have been identified by means of technologies that combine clustering algorithms, visualization tools and high-throughput gene expression data using various case-control models (Andrechek, *et al.*, 2009). Popular bioinformatics tools for biomarkers search include MAGMA for statistical analysis (Rehrauer, *et al.*, 2007), CARMAweb for microarray analysis (Rainer, *et al.*, 2006), GenePattern for expression data analysis (GenePattern, 2010) and OmniBiomarker (Osunkoya, *et al.*, 2009) for developing biomarkers in oncology.

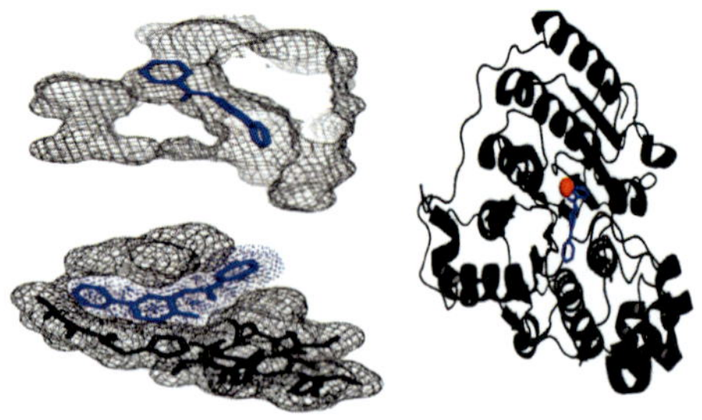

Figure 2: The bioinformatic study of docking allows predicting possible candidate drugs associated to epigenetic events. Bioinformatic validation of the binding between N-(2-amino-5-substituted phenyl)benzamide (blue structure), an inhibitor of HDAC2, and Histone deacetylase.

3. DNA HYPOMETHYLATING AGENTS AND HISTONE DEACETHYLASE INHIBITORS AS THERAPEUTIC TOOLS IN CANCER

Due to their potential reversibility, epigenetic changes involved in tumor development and progression provide the rationale for the use of DNA demethylating and chromatin remodeling compounds in cancer therapy, with the consequent reactivation of silenced genes.

3.1. Epigenetic Therapy – A New Development in Pharmacology

At the moment, epigenetic therapy represents an important branch of pharmacology. Epigenetic profile can influence the response to chemotherapeutic treatment in patients. There is a unique stage of promoter hypermethylation for silenced genes in human cancer and it is now emerging the pharmaco-epigenetics, a new branch of personalized medicine, which studies the treatment response in each cancer patient. This therapy is based on personalized epigenetic differences, to improve the individual response to the treatment (Herranz and Esteller, 2007). Potentially reversible epigenetic abnormalities have encouraged the development of DNA methyltransferase (DNMT) and histone deacetylase (HDAC) inhibitors as anti-cancer treatments. DNMT inhibitors target DNA hypermethylation, instead HDAC inhibitors target histone deacetylation (Table **1A** and **B**).

Table 1A: Classification of Epigenetic DNMT inhibitors According to Potential Therapeutic Use and Clinical Trials

DNMT Inhibitors				
Nucleoside Analogue Inhibitors				
Inhibitor	***Alternate Name***	***Use***	***State of Development***	***Reference***
5-azacytidine	5-Aza-CR Azacytidine Vidaza	MDS	Phase III/IV (FDA)	Raffoux, *et al.*, 2010; Kornblith, *et al.*, 2002; ClinicalTrials.gov, 2010
		leukemia	Phase II	Raffoux, *et al.*, 2010; Goffin and Eisenhauer, 2002
		AML	Phase II	ClinicalTrials.gov, 2010
		CML	Phase II	ClinicalTrials.gov, 2010

Table 1: contd...

		myelofibrosis	Phase II	ClinicalTrials.gov, 2010
		thalassemia	Phase II	ClinicalTrials.gov, 2010
		lymphoma	Phase II	ClinicalTrials.gov, 2010
		solid tumors (*e.g.* lung and prostate)	Phase I/II	ClinicalTrials.gov, 2010; Egger, *et al.*, 2004; Goffin and Eisenhauer, 2002
		head and neck cancer	Phase I	ClinicalTrials.gov, 2010
5-aza-2'-deoxycytidine	DAC 5-Aza-CdR Decitabine Dacogen	MDS	Phase III/IV (FDA)	ClinicalTrials.gov, 2010; Egger, *et al.*, 2004
		leukemia	Phase III	ClinicalTrials.gov, 2010; Goffin and Eisenhauer, 2002
		AML	Phase II	ClinicalTrials.gov, 2010
		CML	Phase II	ClinicalTrials.gov, 2010
		beta thalassemia	Phase II	ClinicalTrials.gov, 2010
		solid tumors (*e.g.* kidney and ovarian)	Phase I/II	ClinicalTrials.gov, 2010; Goffin and Eisenhauer, 2002
		myelofibrosis	Phase I	ClinicalTrials.gov, 2010
		lymphoma	Phase I	ClinicalTrials.gov, 2010
		melanoma	Phase I	ClinicalTrials.gov, 2010
		mesothelioma	Phase I	ClinicalTrials.gov, 2010
		neuroblastoma	Phase I	ClinicalTrials.gov, 2010
5,6-dihydro-5-azacytidine	DHAC	melanoma	Phase II	Goffin and Eisenhauer, 2002; Creagan, *et al.*, 1993
		mesothelioma	Phase II	Dhingra, *et al.*, 1991; Samuels, *et al.*, 1998
		solid tumors (eg. ovarian)	Phase I/II	Curt, *et al.*, 1985
		lymphoma	Phase I/II	Boothman, *et al.*, 1989

Table 1: contd…

		leukemia	Preclinical	Goffin and Eisenhauer, 2002
5-fluoro-2'-deoxycytidine	FdCyd	MDS	Phase II	ClinicalTrials.gov, 2010
		AML	Phase II	ClinicalTrials.gov, 2010
		solid tumors (*e.g.* breast)	Phase I	ClinicalTrials.gov, 2010
1-hydrazinylphthalazine	Hydralazine hydrochloride Apresoline	hypertension	Phase IV	ClinicalTrials.gov, 2010
		cardiovascular and heart diseases	Phase II	ClinicalTrials.gov, 2010
		solid tumors (*e.g.* cervix and breast)	Phase II	ClinicalTrials.gov, 2010
NSC 309132	Zebularine	solid tumors (*e.g.* bladder and ovarian)	Preclinical	Cheng, *et al.*, 2003; Yoo, *et al.*, 2004; Balch, *et al.*, 2005
		glioma	Preclinical	Dote, *et al.*, 2005
		leukemia	Preclinical	Lemaire, *et al.*, 2009; Herranz, *et al.* 2006
arabinosyl-5-azacytidine	Fazarabine	leukemia	Phase I/II	Goffin and Eisenhauer, 2002; Wilhelm, *et al.*, 1999
		CML	Phase I	Wilhelm, *et al.*, 1999
		solid tumors (*e.g.* lung)	Preclinical	Goffin and Eisenhauer, 2002; Heideman, *et al.*, 1998
Non-Nucleoside Analogue Inhibitors				
Inhibitor	***Alternate Name***	***Use***	***State of Development***	***Reference***
procainamide	Pronestyl Procan-SR Procanbid	cardiovascular diseases	Phase III/IV	ClinicalTrials.gov, 2010
		prostate carcinoma	Preclinical	Lin, *et al.*, 2001
procaine hydrochloride	Novocain SP01A	HIV	Phase I/II	ClinicalTrials.gov, 2010
		breast cancer	Preclinical	Villar-Garea, *et al.*, 2003

Table 1: contd...

epigallocatechin-3gallate	EGCG	-	Phase I	Fang, *et al.*, 2003; Chow, *et al.*, 2003
		solid tumors (*e.g.* prostate and cervix)	Preclinical	Lee, *et al.*, 2008
Small Molecules				
Inhibitor	***Alternate Name***	***Use***	***State of Development***	***Reference***
RG108	-	-	Preclnical	Brueckner, *et al.*, 2005
Antisense Oligonucleotides				
Inhibitor	***Alternate Name***	***Use***	***State of Development***	***Reference***
MG98	MethylGene	head and neck cancer	Phase II	Davis, *et al.*, 2003
		solid tumors (*e.g.* kidney)	Phase I/II	ClinicalTrials.gov, 2010 - Zhang, 2001
		MSD	Phase I	Klisovic, *et al.*, 2008
		AML	Phase I	Klisovic, *et al.*, 2008

Table 1B: Classification of Epigenetic HDAC inhibitors According to Potential Therapeutic Use and Clinical Trials

HDAC Inhibitors				
Hydroxamates				
Inhibitor	***Alternate Name***	***Use***	***State of Development***	***Reference***
trichostatin A	TSA	breast cancer	Preclinical	Monneret, 2007; Yoshida, *et al.*, 1990; Kim, *et al.*, 2010
		SMA	Preclinical	Avila, *et al.*, 2007
		cornal haze	Preclinical	Sharma, *et al.*, 2009
		cloned calves	Preclinical	Wang, *et al.*, 2010

Table 1: contd…

suberoylanilide hydroxamic acid	SAHA Vorinostat Zolinza	CTCL	Phase IV (FDA)	-
		NSCLC	Phase II/III	ClinicalTrials.gov, 2010
		lymphoma	Phase II/III	ClinicalTrials.gov, 2010
		STS	Phase II	ClinicalTrials.gov, 2010
		blood and bone marrow diseases	Phase II	ClinicalTrials.gov, 2010
		anaplastic glioma	Phase II	ClinicalTrials.gov, 2010
		melanoma	Phase II	ClinicalTrials.gov, 2010
		AML	Phase II	ClinicalTrials.gov, 2010
		Sezary syndrome	Phase II	ClinicalTrials.gov, 2010
		head and neck cancer	Phase II	ClinicalTrials.gov, 2010
		kidney cancer	Phase II	ClinicalTrials.gov, 2010
		MM and plasma cell neoplasm	Phase I/II	ClinicalTrials.gov, 2010
		breast cancer	Phase I/II	ClinicalTrials.gov, 2010
		MDS	Phase I/II	ClinicalTrials.gov, 2010
		leukemia	Phase I/II	ClinicalTrials.gov, 2010
		brain and CNS tumors	Phase I/II	ClinicalTrials.gov, 2010
		solid tumors (*e.g.* prostate and ovarian)	Phase I	ClinicalTrials.gov, 2010

Table 1: contd…

		hematological tumors	Phase I	Kelly, *et al.*, 2003
		colorectal carcinoma	Preclinical	Folkvord, *et al.*, 2009
suberoyl-3-aminopyridinamine hydroxamic acid	PXD101 PX105684 Belinostat Pyroxamide	lymphoma	Phase I/II	ClinicalTrials.gov, 2010
		solid tumors (e.g ovarian)	Phase I/II	ClinicalTrials.gov, 2010
		MDS	Phase I	ClinicalTrials.gov, 2010
		CML	Phase I	ClinicalTrials.gov, 2010
		leukemia	Phase I	ClinicalTrials.gov, 2010
		MM and plasma cell neoplasm	Phase I	ClinicalTrials.gov, 2010
		solid tumors (*e.g.* ovarian and colon)	Preclinical	Paoluzzi, *et al.*, 2010; Plumb, *et al.*, 2003; Qian, *et al.*, 2006; Agus, *et al.*, 1999
oxamflatin	Metacept 3	melanoma	Preclinical	Kim, *et al.*, 1999
		HIV	-	-
LAQ824	Dacinostat NVP-LAQ824	solid tumors	Phase I	Subramaniam, *et al.*, 2010
		hematological tumors	Phase I	Atadja, *et al.*, 2004a; Atadja, *et al.*, 2004b
		leukemia	Preclinical	Atadja, *et al.*, 2004b
		MM	Preclinical	Catley, *et al.*, 2003
LBH-589	LBN-589 NVP-LBH589 Panobinostat	CTCL	Phase II/III	ClinicalTrials.gov, 2010
		Hodgkin's lymphoma	Phase II/III	ClinicalTrials.gov, 2010
		CML	Phase II/III	ClinicalTrials.gov, 2010

Table 1: contd…

		primary myelofibrosis	Phase II/III	ClinicalTrials.gov, 2010
		SCLC	Phase II	ClinicalTrials.gov, 2010
		STS	Phase II	ClinicalTrials.gov, 2010
		glioblastoma	Phase II	ClinicalTrials.gov, 2010
		glioma	Phase II	ClinicalTrials.gov, 2010
		melanoma	Phase II	ClinicalTrials.gov, 2010
		leukemia	Phase II	ClinicalTrials.gov, 2010
		adult T-cell leukemia/lymphoma	Phase II	ClinicalTrials.gov, 2010
		GVHD	Phase II	ClinicalTrials.gov, 2010
		MM and plasma cell neoplasm	Phase II	ClinicalTrials.gov, 2010
		AML	Phase I/II	ClinicalTrials.gov, 2010
		lymphoma	Phase I/II	ClinicalTrials.gov, 2010
		solid tumors (*e.g.* breast and prostate)	Phase I/II	Atadja, 2009
		MDS	Phase I	ClinicalTrials.gov, 2010
		GIST	Preclinical	Floris, *et al.*, 2009
cyclic hydroxamic-acid-containing peptide 1	CHAP1	murine melanoma	Preclinical	Komatsu, *et al.*, 2001; Furumai, *et al.*, 2001
cyclic hydroxamic-acid-containing peptide 31	CHAP31	solid tumors	Preclinical	Komatsu, *et al.*, 2001

Table 1: contd…

suberic hydroxamic acid	SBHA	MTC	Preclinical	Ning, *et al.*, 2008
		murine malaria	Preclinical	Andrews, *et al.*, 2000
PCI-24781	CRA-02478 CRA-024781	lymphoma	Phase I/II	ClinicalTrials.gov, 2010
		sarcoma	Phase I	ClinicalTrials.gov, 2010; Rivera-Del Valle, *et al.*, 2010; Adimoolam, *et al.*, 2007; Banuelos, *et al.*, 2007
		hematological tumors	Phase I	ClinicalTrials.gov, 2010
		MM	Phase I	ClinicalTrials.gov, 2010
		CML	Phase I	ClinicalTrials.gov, 2010
		-	Preclinical	Rivera-Del Valle, *et al.*, 2010; Adimoolam, *et al.*, 2007; Banuelos, *et al.*, 2007
ITF2357	Givinostat Gavinostat	myeloproliferative diseases (PV ET MF)	Phase II	ClinicalTrials.gov, 2010; Rambaldi, *et al.*, 2010
		SOJIA	Phase II	ClinicalTrials.gov, 2010
		MM	Phase II	ClinicalTrials.gov, 2010; Golay, *et al.*, 2007; Galli, *et al.*, 2010
		CLL	Phase II	ClinicalTrials.gov, 2010
		Hodgkin's lymphoma	Phase I/II	ClinicalTrials.gov, 2010
		Crohn's disease	Phase I/II	ClinicalTrials.gov, 2010
		systemic inflammation	Preclinical	Leoni, *et al.*, 2005

Table 1: contd…

SB939	-	MDS	Phase I	ClinicalTrials.gov, 2010
		solid tumors (*e.g.* prostate)	Phase I	ClinicalTrials.gov, 2010
		hematological tumors	Phase I	ClinicalTrials.gov, 2010
m-carboxycinnamic acid bishydroxamide	CBHA	neuroblastoma	Preclinical	Coffey, *et al.*, 2001
scriptaid	-	solit tumors (*e.g.* breast and colon)	Preclinical	Su, *et al.*, 2000; Johnson, *et al.*, 2005; Keen, *et al.*, 2003; Lee, *et al.*, 2008
Aliphatic Acids (Short-Chain Fatty Acid)				
Inhibitor	*Alternate Name*	*Use*	*State of Development*	*Reference*
sodium butyrate	NaB SB Phenylbutyrate Buphenyl	diabetes insulin resistance	Phase IV (FDA)	ClinicalTrials.gov, 2010
		urea cycle disorder	Phase II/III	ClinicalTrials.gov, 2010
		ASA	Phase II	ClinicalTrials.gov, 2010
		Huntington's disease	Phase II	ClinicalTrials.gov, 2010
		brain and CNS tumors	Phase II	ClinicalTrials.gov, 2010
		solid tumors (*e.g.* lung and prostate)	Phase II	ClinicalTrials.gov, 2010
		leukemia	Phase II	ClinicalTrials.gov, 2010
		lymphoma	Phase II	ClinicalTrials.gov, 2010
		MDS	Phase II	ClinicalTrials.gov, 2010

Table 1: contd…

		thalassemia major	Phase II	ClinicalTrials.gov, 2010
		head and neck cancer	Phase I/II	ClinicalTrials.gov, 2010
		ALS	Phase I/II	ClinicalTrials.gov, 2010
		cystic fibrosis	Phase I	ClinicalTrials.gov, 2010
		SMA	Phase I	ClinicalTrials.gov, 2010
valproic acid	VPA dipropylacetic acid myproic acid Divalproex Depakote Depakene	epilepsy	Phase IV (FDA)	ClinicalTrials.gov, 2010
		bipolar disorders	Phase IV	ClinicalTrials.gov, 2010
		schizophrenia	Phase IV	ClinicalTrials.gov, 2010
		PTSD	Phase IV	ClinicalTrials.gov, 2010
		depression	Phase IV	ClinicalTrials.gov, 2010
		mania	Phase IV	ClinicalTrials.gov, 2010
		post cerebral hemorrahge	Phase IV	ClinicalTrials.gov, 2010
		mental retardation	Phase IV	ClinicalTrials.gov, 2010
		developmental disabilities	Phase IV	ClinicalTrials.gov, 2010
		attention deficit hyperactivity disorder	Phase IV	ClinicalTrials.gov, 2010
		alcoholism	Phase IV	ClinicalTrials.gov, 2010
		drug dependence	Phase IV	ClinicalTrials.gov, 2010

Table 1: contd…

		obesity	Phase IV	ClinicalTrials.gov, 2010
		bronchial asthma	Phase III/ IV	ClinicalTrials.gov, 2010
		Alzheimer's disease	Phase III	ClinicalTrials.gov, 2010
		migraine	Phase III	ClinicalTrials.gov, 2010
		partial seizure disorder	Phase III	ClinicalTrials.gov, 2010
		ALS	Phase III	ClinicalTrials.gov, 2010
		neuropathic peripheral pain	Phase II/III	ClinicalTrials.gov, 2010
		CML	Phase II	ClinicalTrials.gov, 2010
		leukemia	Phase II	ClinicalTrials.gov, 2010
		MDS	Phase II	ClinicalTrials.gov, 2010
		AML	Phase II	ClinicalTrials.gov, 2010
		SMA	Phase II	ClinicalTrials.gov, 2010; Kuendgen, *et al.*, 2006
		solid tumors (*e.g.* cervix and breast)	Phase II	ClinicalTrials.gov, 2010
		PSP	Phase II	ClinicalTrials.gov, 2010; Gottlicher, *et al.*, 2001; Atmaca, *et al.*, 2007
		autism	Phase II	ClinicalTrials.gov, 2010
		HIV	Phase I/II	ClinicalTrials.gov, 2010

Table 1: contd...

		melanoma	Phase I/II	ClinicalTrials.gov, 2010
		advanced cancers	Phase I	ClinicalTrials.gov, 2010
		brain and CNS tumors	Phase I	ClinicalTrials.gov, 2010
		lymphoma	Phase I	ClinicalTrials.gov, 2010
AN-9	Pivaloyloxymethyl butyrate Pivanex	NSCLC	Phase II	ClinicalTrials.gov, 2010
		CLL	Phase II	ClinicalTrials.gov, 2010
		melanoma	Phase I/II	ClinicalTrials.gov, 2010
OSU-HDAC42	AR-42	solid tumors (*e.g.* prostate and breast)	Preclinical	Sargeant, *et al.*, 2008; Weng, *et al.*, 2009
		HCC	Preclinical	Lu, *et al.*, 2007
Cyclic Tetrapeptides and Analogues				
Inhibitor	***Alternate Name***	***Use***	***State of Development***	***Reference***
depsipeptide	FK228 FR901228 Romidepsin Istodax	CTCL	Phase II	ClinicalTrials.gov, 2010
		PTCL	Phase II	ClinicalTrials.gov, 2010
		MM and plasma cell neoplasm	Phase II	ClinicalTrials.gov, 2010
		melanoma	Phase II	ClinicalTrials.gov, 2010
		head and neck cancer	Phase II	ClinicalTrials.gov, 2010
		MDS	Phase II	ClinicalTrials.gov, 2010
		leukemia	Phase II	ClinicalTrials.gov, 2010

Table 1: contd…

		lymphoma	Phase II	ClinicalTrials.gov, 2010
		pancreatic cancer	Phase II	ClinicalTrials.gov, 2010
		brain and CNS tumors	Phase II	ClinicalTrials.gov, 2010
		NSCLC	Phase I	ClinicalTrials.gov, 2010
		SCLC	Phase I	ClinicalTrials.gov, 2010
		mesothelioma	Phase I	ClinicalTrials.gov, 2010
		prostate cancer	Preclinical	Lai, *et al.*, 2008
apicidin	-	trypanopsomiasis	Preclinical	Murray, *et al.*, 2001
		HCC	Preclinical	Lai, *et al.*, 2009
		Ishikawa endometrial cancer	Preclinical	Ahn, *et al.*, 2010
		murine malaria	Preclinical	Darkin-Rattray, *et al.*, 1996
trapoxin A	TPX A	-	Preclinical	-
HC-toxin	-	-	Preclinical	Brosch, *et al.*, 1995
chlamydocin	-	-	-	-
Benzamides				
Inhibitor	***Alternate Name***	***Use***	***State of Development***	***Reference***
MS-275	SNDX-275 MS-27-275 BAY86-5274 Entinostat Benzamidine	solid tumors (*e.g.* breast)	Phase II	ClinicalTrials.gov, 2010]
		melanoma	Phase II	ClinicalTrials.gov, 2010
		MDS	Phase I/II	Hu, *et al.*, 2003; Riester, *et al.*, 2007; Bouchain, *et al.*, 2003

Table 1: contd...

		AML	Phase I/II	Hu, *et al.,* 2003; Riester, *et al.*, 2007; Bouchain, *et al.*, 2003
		CML	Phase I/II	Hu, *et al.,* 2003; Riester, *et al.*, 2007; Bouchain, *et al.*, 2003
		NSCLC	Phase I/II	ClinicalTrials.gov, 2010; Hu, *et al.,* 2003; Riester, *et al.*, 2007; Bouchain, *et al.*, 2003
		leukemia	Phase I	ClinicalTrials.gov, 2010
		lymphoma	Phase I	ClinicalTrials.gov, 2010
		MM and plasma cell neoplasm	Phase I	ClinicalTrials.gov, 2010
CI-994	PD-123654 GOE-5549 N-acetyl-dinaline Tacedinaline Acetyldinaline	solid tumors (*e.g.* lung)	Phase III	ClinicalTrials.gov, 2010; Kraker, *et al.*, 2003
		pancreatic cancer	Phase II	Shore, *et al.*, 2003; Richards, *et al.*, 2005
		MM and plasma cell neoplasm	Phase II	ClinicalTrials.gov, 2010
pimelic diphenylamide	-	FRDA	Preclinical	Rai, *et al.*, 2010
BML-210	CAY10433	leukemia	-	Borutinskaite, *et al.*, 2006; Savickiene, *et al.*, 2006; Herman, *et al.*, 2006
M344	D237	solid tumors (*e.g.* ovarian)	-	Riessland, *et al.*, 2006; Jung, *et al.*, 1999
		SMA	-	Riessland, *et al.*, 2006; Jung, *et al.*, 1999
MGCD0103	Mocetinostat	MDS	Phase II	ClinicalTrials.gov, 2010
		AML	Phase II	ClinicalTrials.gov, 2010

Table 1: contd...

		CLL	Phase II	ClinicalTrials.gov, 2010
		Hodgkin's lymphoma	Phase II	ClinicalTrials.gov, 2010
		non Hodgkin's lymphoma	Phase II	ClinicalTrials.gov, 2010
		solid tumors (*e.g.* breast and prostate)	Phase I/II	Riester, *et al.*, 2007; Tan, *et al.*, 2010
		hematological tumors	Phase I/II	ClinicalTrials.gov, 2010
		NSCLC	Phase I	ClinicalTrials.gov, 2010

Among the DNMT inhibitors (Table **1A**), there are several epigenetic drugs working like nucleoside analogue inhibitors. The precursor of this class of molecules is 5-azacytidine (5-Aza-CR, Azacitidine, Vidaza), a simple derivative of the nucleoside cytidine, while the other well-known drug 5-aza-2'-deoxycytidine (5-Aza-CdR, Decitabine, Dacogen) is the deoxyribose analogue. They both are the most extensively studied in clinical trials for the treatment of several type of cancers, such as leukemia and lymphoma (ClinicalTrials.gov, 2010), and they were approved by the U.S. Food and Drug Administration (FDA) as chemotherapeutic agents for myelodysplastic syndromes (MDS) (Raffoux, *et al.*, 2010; Kornblith, *et al.*, 2002; ClinicalTrials.gov, 2010). The 5-Aza-CdR active form is tri-phosphorylated and then it is incorporated into replicating DNA. A covalent complex is formed with active sites of DNMTs, and this results in the demethylation of DNA. Both 5-azacytidine and 5-aza-2'-deoxycytidine result very instable in neutral aqueous solution and they can cause myelotoxicity as side effects.

More stable cytidine analogues have been developed and they are undergoing Phase I and II studies for the treatment of several malignancies, such as melanoma and solid tumors (Egger, *et al.*, 2004;ClinicalTrials.gov, 2010; Creagan, *et al.*, 1993; Samules, *et al.*, 1998). It has been observed some toxic effects for 5-fluoro-2'-deoxycytidine, probably due to its metabolites (Curt, *et al.*, 1985; Boothman, *et al.*, 1989). Apresoline (hydrazine hydrochloride) is used in Phase II clinical trials for cervical and breast cancers (ClinicalTrials.gov, 2010). The most recent addition to this group is Zebularine (NSC 309132), a novel cytosine analogue, which is very stable, less toxic and can be orally administered for the treatment of solid tumors, glioma and leukemia in preclinical studies (Cheng, *et al*., 2003; Yoo, *et al*., 2004; Balch, *et al*., 2005; Dote, *et al*., 2005; Lemaire, *et al*., 2009). However, it is much less effective than Azacitidine and Decitabine and, therefore, higher doses of this drug per administration are needed (Foubister, 2003), leading important consequences for its clinical potential (Yoo, *et al*., 2004). Another important molecule in this class is Fazarabine, that is under investigation in clinical trials for the treatment of several types of leukemia since few years (Goffin and Eisenhauer, 2002; Wilhelm, *et al*., 1999).

The myelotoxicity of these epigenetic drugs, associated with their incorporation into DNA, is the reason why it has been developed and identified another class of molecules, the non-nucleoside analogue inhibitors. Procainamide (Pronestyl, Procanbid) and procaine hydrochloride (Novocain) are structurally different from cytosine and inhibit DNMTs by perturbing interactions between the protein and its target sites. Both these drugs are investigated in preclinical trials because of their anti-proliferative effects in prostate and breast cancers (Lin, *et al*., 2001; Villar-Garea, *et al*., 2003). Another non-nucleoside analogous is a natural product derived from green tea, the epigallocatechin-3-gallate (EGCG), which can block and consequently inhibit the human DNMT (Fang, *et al*., 2003). It is used *in vivo* studies for the treatment of solid tumors, like prostate and cervical carcinomas (Lee, *et al*., 2008b).

In the class of small molecules, RG108 is a novel epigenetic drug that blocks the DNMT active site, but does not affect methylation of centromeric satellite sequences. This compound may become particularly useful for new drug development (Brueckner, *et al*., 2005).

Most DNMT inhibitors are not specific for a given DNMT enzyme and they frequently cause adverse toxicity. Thus, new selective compounds for DNMT have been improved. MG98 (MethyGene), an antisense oligonucleotide, is complementary to mRNA for human DNMT1 and able to block the translation of it. MG98 is undergoing clinical trials, involving the treatment of head and neck cancer, solid tumors, MDS and acute myeloid leukemia (AML) (Zhang, 2001; Davis, *et al*., 2003; Klisovic, *et al*., 2008).

HDAC inhibitors are several molecules, either with natural origins or recently synthesized, and they have been characterized playing an anticancer activity in preclinical and clinical studies. These compounds are heterogeneous, and their classification is based on their chemical nature and mechanism of inhibition, such as their affinity for the HDACs of classes 1, 2, 4. Among HDAC inhibitors (Table **1B**), the most important class of molecules is hydroxamates; they are very effective, although their inhibition is reversible and their binding is strong to the HDAC catalytic site (Monneret, 2007).

Trichostatin A (TSA) is a well known hydroxamic acid derivative and it was first developed as an antifungal agent. This molecule is active in several *in vivo* studies, at nanomolar concentrations (Yoshida, *et al.*, 1990; Kim, *et al.*, 2010; Avila, *et al.*, 2007; Sharma, *et al.*, 2009; Wang, *et al.*, 2010). TSA is an organic compound that inhibits both class 1 and 2 HDACs, leading to an increase in histone acetylation.

Another compound in this class is suberoylanilide hydroxamic acid (SAHA, Vorinostat, Zoliza), which has been approved for cutaneous T-cell lymphoma (CTCL) treatment, and it is undergoing investigation in clinical trials for several other tumors (ClinicalTrials.gov, 2010; Kelly, *et al.*, 2003). It binds directly to the catalytic site of the enzyme, thereby blocking substrate access. It inhibits class I and class II HDACs at nanomolar concentrations.

Pyroxamide (PXD101, Belinostat) is a strong cytotoxic hydroxamate-type inhibitor of histone deacetylase activity and it was found to inhibit *in vitro* cancer multidrug-resistant cell growth, synergy working in combination with relevant chemotherapeutics. It is under investigation in clinical trials Phase I and II in many cancers, like lymphoma, solid tumors and few types of leukemia (ClinicalTrials.gov, 2010; Paoluzzi, *et al.*, 2010), and it can delay cell growth in xenograft models of ovarian and colon cancer (Plumb, *et al.*, 2003; Qian, *et al.*, 2006; Agus, *et al.*, 1999). Oxamflatin (Metacept 3) is a hydroxamates used in preclinical treatment of melanoma (Kim, *et al.*, 1999).

The molecule NVP-LAQ824 (Dacinostat) is a very strong DHAC inhibitor and it is undergoing Phase I in solid and hematologic tumors (Subramaniam, *et al.*, 2010; Atadja, *et al.*, 2004a; Atadja, *et al.*, 2004b).

The epigenetic drug LBH589 (Panobinostat) is a hydroxamic acid based HDAC inhibitor, with a similar structure to Vorinostat, but with a longer half-life. *In vitro* it induces cell cycle arrest and apoptosis in various tumor cell types, while *in vivo* it inhibits tumor angiogenesis. Panobinostat is used in several clinical trials for the treatment of CTCL, Hodgkin's lymphoma, myelofibrosis, glioma, leukemia and many other tumors (ClinicalTrials.gov, 2010; Atadja, 2009).

The cyclic hydroxamic-acid-containing peptides (CHAPs) compounds derived from TSA and cyclic tetrapeptides. They inhibit HDACs at very low concentrations (Santini, *et al.*, 2007), and they are used *in vivo* experiments for cancer treatment (Komatsu, *et al.*, 2001; Furumai, *et al.*, 2001). The hydroxamate SBHA is used indeed in preclinical studies for medullary thyroid cancer and for murine malaria (Ning, *et al.*, 2008; Andrews, *et al.*, 2000).

The molecule PCI-24781 (CRA-02748) is a specific broad spectrum phenyl hydroxamic acid-based inhibitor of multiple HDAC isoforms and it is an orally bioavailable compound, used in Phase I and II for cancer therapy in lymphoma, sarcoma and hematological diseases (ClinicalTrials.gov, 2010; Rivera-Del Valle, *et al.*, 2010; Adimoolam, *et al.*, 2007; Banuelos, *et al.*, 2007). PCI-24781 has an optimized half life, oral bioavailability, potency, and duration of exposure compared to competitor drugs (*e.g.* Zolinza or LBH-589) to achieve an ideal balance of efficacy with minimal toxicity.

ITF2357 (Givinostat) is a new synthetic inhibitor of class I and II histone deacetylases, with a high anti-proliferative and pro-apoptotic activity. It is 2-10-fold stronger than vorinostat, and it is used for myeloproliferative diseases, active systemic onset juvenile idiopathic arthritis (SOJIA) and multiple myeloma in Phase I and II, and for the cure of systemic inflammation *in vivo* (ClinicalTrials.gov, 2010; Rambaldi, *et al.*, 2010; Golay, *et al.*, 2007; Galli, *et al.*, 2010; Leoni, *et al.*, 2005).

SB939 is a molecule used in clinical trials for MDS, solid and hematological tumors (ClinicalTrials.gov, 2010).

CBHA is a member of a recently synthesized family of hybrid polar compounds, that have been shown to be inhibitors of HDAC and potent inducers of transformed cell growth arrest and terminal differentiation at micromolar (LD50 range, 1–4 μM) concentrations. CBHA is used in preclinical experiments or neuroblastoma (Coffey, *et al.*, 2001).

The new hydroxamate scriptaid is a new synthetized HDAC inhibitor with a relatively low toxicity, and it is undergoing preclinical investigation for the treatment of solid tumors (Su, *et al.*, 2000; Johnson, *et al.*, 2005; Keen, *et al.*, 2003; Lee, *et al.*, 2008).

Another widely used and clinically efficacious class of HDAC inhibitor is short chain fatty acids (SCFA), although it has a weaker mechanism of action comparing other molecules. Phenylbutyrate (Sodium butyrate, Buphenyl) and valproic acid (VPA, Divalproex, Depakote, Depakene) are relatively old drugs and they have been used as treatments in pathology other than cancer since several years (ClinicalTrials.gov, 2010; Kuendgen, *et al.*, 2006; Gottlicher, *et al.*, 2001; Atmaca, *et al.*, 2007). Sodium butyrate is the most common and physiologic member of HDAC inhibitors, because it is formed in the colon by fermentation of dietary fibers. It is able to induce cell cycle arrest, differentiation and apoptosis in various cancer cells. The compound in millimolar concentrations causes an accumulation of acetylated histone species in a variety of vertebrate cell lines. VPA has been used in the treatment of epilepsy for almost 30 years. Recently, both sodium butyrate and valproid acid were put under investigation for cancer therapy, due to their activities as HDAC inhibitors (ClinicalTrials.gov, 2010; Monneret, 2007). Their acyl group is able to bind the catalytic HDAC zinc ion, but because of their very short side chains, it cannot make significant contact with the catalytic pocket. Therefore, these HDAC inhibitors work at relatively high concentrations.

Other SCFA molecules are AN-9 (Pivanex), that is under investigation in Phase II for the treatment of non-small cell lung carcinoma (NSCLC), and other tumors, while OSU-HDAC42 is used in preclinical studies for solid tumors, like prostate and breast cancers, and hepatocellular carcinoma (HCC) (ClinicalTrials.gov, 2010; Sargeant, *et al.*, 2008; Weng, *et al.*, 2009; Lu, *et al.*, 2007).

Cyclic tetrapeptides is another class of HDAC inhibitors. This includes depsipeptide (FK-228, Romidepsin, Istodax), apicidin and trapoxin A. Depsipeptide is a pro-drug, activated by reduction upon cellular uptake and it is able to inhibit class I HDACs, though the mechanism of its action is still unclear (Furumai, *et al.*, 2002). It is undergoing investigation in Phase I and II in the treatment of several tumors, like CTCL, lymphoma and leukemia (ClinicalTrials.gov, 2010). Apicidin is a reversible HDAC inhibitor at very low doses, with an alkylketone residue that is supposed to chelate the catalytic HDAC zinc ion (Murray, *et al.*, 2001). It is used in preclinical investigation for HCC, Ishikawa endometrial cancer and murine malaria (Lai, *et al.*, 2006; Ahn, *et al.*, 2010; Darkin-Rattray, *et al.*, 1996). Trapoxin A is able to irreversibly inactivate HDAC by covalent interaction between its epoxide group and the catalytic site of the enzyme; it is used in preclinical studies, like HC-toxin (Brosch, *et al.*, 1995).

The fourth class of HDAC inhibitors are the benzamides, which bind the active zinc in the HDAC catalytic site. MS-275 (Entinostat, Benzamidine) is a synthetic molecule that preferentially inhibits HDAC1 at micromolar concentrations. The amine group of the benzanilide half part might act as a hydrogen bond donor or could be involved in other electrostatic interactions, which are necessary for inhibitory activity. It is under investigation in Phase I and II for the treatment of solid tumors, MDS, AML and other types of cancer (ClinicalTrials.gov, 2010; Hu, *et al.*, 2003; Riester, *et al.*, 2007; Bouchain, *et al.*, 2003). The epigenetic drug CI-994 (N-acetyl-dinaline, Tacedinaline) was originally used as an anticonvulsant agent, and it is actually a novel orally active compound, with a wide spectrum of antitumor activity in preclinical models, *in vitro* and *in vivo*. CI-944 is a relatively weak HDAC inhibitor and the mechanism of action remains unclear. It is undergoing Phase II and III for the treatment of solid tumors, like lung and pancreatic cancers, and MM and plasma cell neoplasm (ClinicalTrials.gov, 2010; Kraker, *et al.*, 2003; Shore, *et al.*, 2003; Richards, *et al.*, 2005).

Pimelic diphenylamide is a quite recent molecule and it is used for the treatment of Friedreich's Ataxia (FRDA) in preclincal trials (Rai, *et al.*, 2010); the novel histone deacetylase inhibitor BML-210 (CAY10433) is for leukemia (Borutinskaite, *et al.*, 2006; Savickiene, *et al.*, 2006; Herman, *et al.*, 2006) and the new synthesized molecule M344 (D237) is for solid tumors and spinal muscular atrophy (SMA)

(Riessland, *et al*., 2006; Jung, *et al*., 1999). MGCD0103 (Mocedinostat) is in clinical trials Phase II for the treatment of MDS, AML, Hodgkin's lymphoma and solid tumors (ClinicalTrials.gov, 2010; Riester, *et al*., 2007; Tan, *et al*., 2010). Promising characteristics of hydroxamic acids are their tolerability and oral absorption, while their therapeutic potential is hampered by their short half-life.

Hypomethylating and Deacetylating Agents in Clinical Trials

Clinical application of molecules able to revert epigenetic aberrations is a favorable strategy for cancer treatment. As previously described both *in vitro* and *in vivo*, many agents are able to inhibit DNA methylation and histone deacetylation. However, their therapeutic significance will be established by ongoing clinical trials.

Some old drugs have been used as therapeutics for cancers and other diseases, while other new generation compounds have been evaluated for a possible epigenetic therapy. Currently, some DNMT inhibitors are under investigation in Phase I, II and II clinical trials, whereas no HDAC inhibitors are approved for cancer therapy, with the exception of SAHA, which is considered a new drug application for CTCL.

HDACs are approved for pathologies other than cancer, including phenylbutyrate for urea cycle disorders and valproic acid for seizures and epilepsy. Although there are several clinical reports with valproic acid, it has some limitations, such as low potency and specificity. There are severe dose-related side effects that impede valproic acid administration at theoretically therapeutic anticancer doses.

In preclinical studies, peak plasma levels higher than those expected *in vitro* could be achieved with single iv or oral doses of depsipeptide and they could be sustained with iv infusion (Chan, *et al*., 1997). These studies predicted severe side effects, but depsipeptide was well tolerated in patients with non- or relative mild-hematological toxicity (Sandor, *et al*., 2002).

The use of trichostatin A is limited because of its extremely instability, so other hydroxamic acids have been identified and used, like SAHA, that is currently under investigation in both iv infusion and oral administration. In a Phase I study the safety and activity of oral SAHA were evaluated. The maximum tolerated dose (MTD) was 200 mg twice a day or 250 mg three times a day. It presents many dose-related side effects, like fatigue, nausea, vomiting, and diarrhea (Garcia-Manero, *et al.*, 2008).

In a Phase I study of MS-275, a cohort of daily treated patients presented severe toxicity, such as elevated liver enzymes, hypophosphatemia, hypoalbuminemia and pleural effusion. Analysis of pharmacokinetic showed a long half-life of MS-275. The experimental design was modified to assess the real MS-275 half-life and the drug was dispensed either weekly or bi-weekly. The observed side effects included fatigue, nausea, vomiting, hypoalbuminemia, anxiety, dyspepsia, anemia, fever and dysgeusia (Ryan, *et al.*, 2005).

Chronic administration of acetyldinaline CI-994 was investigated in Phase I clinical trial (Prakash, *et al.*, 2001). The drug was orally administered once a day for 2 months to patients with non-small lung cancer, and the highest tolerated dose was $8mg/m^2/d$. Dose limiting toxicities were neutropenia and thrombocytopenia and several side effects including leukopenia, nausea, vomiting, diarrhea, fatigue and anorexia were reported. An adaptation phenomenon of the platelet count was observed during this study, which rebounded after the first month of therapy.

The promising features of the benzamides involve their tolerability and oral absorption. While the surprisingly long half-life of these therapeutics may be a favorable aspect, the best schedule has yet to be established.

Several issues still persist unsolved concerning the ideal evaluation and use of HDAC inhibitors for cancer prevention and cure. However, it is not evident up to now whether the therapeutic effects of HDAC inhibitors are the consequences of changes of histone acetylation patterns or of increased nonhistone proteins acetylation, which regulates alterations in growth regulatory pathways. Due to the presence of several different HDACs, it is decisive to realize the specificity of the current HDAC inhibitors as well as to develop selective inhibitors that target individual enzymes. Many compounds have been discovered acting as efficient anti-cancer drugs with a well-established value, comparing the HDAC inhibitors.

The dose limiting toxicity for both Vidaza and Decitabine is characterized by myelosuppression, and nausea and vomiting are commonly reported as non-hematologic adverse effects. In lung cancer patients, toxicity resulted both dose and schedule dependent, and decitabine turned out to be less myelosuppressive if the same dose was administered over a shorter treatment period than over a longer period (Momparler, *et al.*, 1997).

The patient group treated with demethylating agents showed higher response rates in comparison to the group that received only supportive care, and also the quality of life was significantly improved (Silverman, *et al.*, 2002; Issa, 2005). These results led to FDA approval of 5-azacytidine for treatment of all myelodysplastic syndromes subtype and to the fast-track status of 5-aza-2'deoxycytidine for myelodysplastic syndromes (Kaminskas, *et al.*, 2005).

Although these demethylating agents have demonstrated clinical benefit, there are several limitations concerning their clinical application. The mechanism of DNMTs inhibition, demethylation and gene reactivation is not completely understood. These demethylating agents are normally not specific for a particular DNMT or gene, and in some cases toxicity is due essentially to the covalent trapping of DNMT rather than to DNA demethylation (Juttermann, *et al.*, 1994). Toxicity might be overtaken by optimizing treatment schedules, for example by giving lower doses over longer time periods (Issa, 2005), or by developing non-nucleoside inhibitors that should result less toxic since they will not be incorporated into DNA.

To target epigenetic gene regulation, maybe it should be more efficient to use of a combination of chromatin modifying agents instead of only one. Today, based on numerous experimental results, many investigators believe that some of these drugs might work better together than individually. The reactivation of gene expression *in vitro* has demonstrated to be more efficient if HDAC inhibitors were administered together with DNMT inhibitors, and therefore there is the possibility that these molecules will be synergistic also in clinical practice. In a clinical trial, a demethylating agent administered in combination with a HDAC inhibitor to patients with hematological and solid tumors has demonstrated complete and partial remission (Rudek, *et al.*, 2005; Gore, *et al.*, 2006).

In conclusion, targeting of cancer through DNA demethylation and histone acetylation is an exiting area of cancer therapy. The development of second generation inhibitors of DNA methyltrasferase and HDACs is in progress and their efficacy as anti-tumoral drugs will ultimately require evaluation both in monotherapy and in combination.

ACKNOWLEDGEMENT

This work was supported by CNR funding.

CONFLICT OF INTEREST

The authors confirm that this chapter content has no conflict of interest.

REFERENCES

Adimoolam, S., Sirisawad, M., Chen, J., Thiemann, P., Ford, J.M. and Buggy, J.J., 2007. HDAC inhibitor PCI-24781 decreases RAD51 expression and inhibits homologous recombination. *Proceedings of the National Academy of Sciences*, Vol. 104 (49), pp. 19482-7.

Agus, D.B., Cordon-Cardo, C., Fox, W., Drobnjak, M., Koff, A., Golde, D.W. and Scher, H.I., 1999. Prostate cancer cell cycle regulators: response to androgen withdrawal and development of androgen indipendence. *Journal of the National Cancer Institute*, 91, pp. 1869-76.

Ahluwalia A, Hurteau J.A., Bigsby R.M., Nephew K.P., 2001. DNA methylation in ovarian cancer. II. Expression of DNA methyltransferases in ovarian cancer cell lines and normal ovarian epithelial cells. *Gynecologic Oncology*, 82, pp. 299-304.

Ahn, M.Y., Chung, H.Y., Choi, W.S., Lee, B.M., Yoon, S., Kim, H.S., 2010. Anti-tumor effect of apicidin on Ishikawa human endometrial cancer cells both *in vitro* and *in vivo* by blocking histone deacetylase 3 and 4. *International Journal of Oncology*, 36, pp. 125-31.

Altschul, S.F., Gish, W., Miller, W., Myers, E.W. and Lipman, D.J., 1990. Basic local alignment search tool. *Journal of Molecular Biology*, 215 (3), pp. 403-10.

An, W., 2007. Histone acetylation and methylation: combinatorial players for transcriptional regulation. *Sub-cellular Biochemistry*, 41, pp. 351-69.

Andrechek, E.R., Cardiff, R.D., Chang, J.T., Gatza, M.L., Acharya, C.R., Potti, A. and Nevins, J.R., 2009. Genetic heterogeneity of Myc-induced mammary tumors reflecting diverse phenotypes including metastatic potential. *Proceedings of the National Academy of Sciences*, 106 (38), pp. 16387-92.

Andrews, K.T., Walduck, A., Kelso, M.J., Fairlie, D.P., Saul, A. and Parsons, P.G., 2000. Anti-malarial effect of histone deacetylation inhibitors and mammalian tumour cytodifferentiating agents. *International Journal for Parasitology*, 30, pp. 761-8.

Atadja, P., 2009. Development of the pan-DAC inhibitor panobinostat (LBH589): Successes and challenges. *Cancer Letters*, 280, pp. 233-41.

Atadja, P., Gao, L., Kwon, P., Trogani, N., Walker, H., Hsu, M., Yeleswarapu, L., Chandramouli, N., Perez, L., Versace, R., Wu, A., Sambucetti, L., Lassota, P., Cohen, D., Bair, K., Wood, A. and Remiszewski, S., 2004 b. Selective growth inhibition of tumor cells by a novel histone deacetylase inhibitor, NVP-LAQ824. *Cancer Research*, 64, pp. 689-95.

Atadja, P., Hsu, M., Kwon, P., Trogani, N., Bhalla, K. and Remiszewski, S., 2004 a. Molecular and cellular basis for the anti-proliferative effects of the HDAC inhibitor LAQ824. *Novartis Foundation Symposium*, 259, pp. 249-66.

Atmaca, A., Al-Batran, S.E., Maurer, A., Neumann, A., Heinzel, T., Hentsch, B., Schwarz, S.E., Hövelmann, S., Göttlicher, M., Knuth, A. and Jäger, E., 2007. Valproic acid (VPA) in patients with refractory advanced cancer: a dose escalating phase I clinical trial. *British Journal of Cancer*, 97(2), pp. 177-82.

Avila, A.M., Burnett, B.G., Taye, A.A., Gabanella, F., Knight, M.A., Hartenstein, P., Cizman, Z., Di Prospero, N.A., Pellizzoni, L., Fischbeck, K.H., Sumner, C.J., 2007. Trichostatin A increases SMN expression and survival in a mouse model of spinal muscular atrophy. *Journal of Clinical Investigation*, 117, pp. 659-71.

Baker, A.H., George, S.J., Zaltsman, A.B., Murphy, G. and Newby, A.C., 1999. Inhibition of invasion and induction of apoptotic cell death of cancer cell lines by overexpression of TIMP-3. *British Journal of Cancer*, 79 (9/10), pp. 1347-55.

Baker, E.K. and El-Osta, A., 2003. The rise of DNA methylation and the importance of chromatin on multidrug resistance in cancer. *Experimental Cell Research*, 290 (2), pp.177-94.

Balch, C., Huang, T.H., Brown, R. and Nephew, K.P., 2004. The epigenetics of ovarian cancer drug resistance and resensitization. *American Journal of Obstetrics and Gynecology*, 191 (5), pp. 1552-72.

Balch, C., Yan, P., Craft, T., Young, S., Skalnik, D.G., Huang, T.H. and Nephew, K.P., 2005. Antimitogenic and chemosensitizing effects of the methylation inhibitor zebularine in ovarian cancer. *Molecular Cancer Therapeutics*, 4, pp. 1505-14.

Banuelos, C.A., Banáth, J.P., MacPhail, S.H., Zhao, J., Reitsema, T. and Olive, P.L., 2007. Radiosensitization by the Histone Deacetylase Inhibitor PCI-24781. *Clinical Cancer Research*, Nov (13), pp. 6816-26.

Barrett, T., Troup, D.B., Wilhite, S.E., Ledoux, P., Rudnev, D., Evangelista, C., Kim, I.F., Soboleva, A., Tomashevsky, M., Marshall, K.A., Phillippy, K.H., Sherman, P.M., Muertter, R.N. and Edgar, R., 2009. NCBI GEO: archive for high-throughput functional genomic data. *Nucleic Acids Research*, 37. pp. D885-90.

Barski, A., Cuddapah, S., Cui, K., Roh, T.Y., Schones, D.E., Wang, Z., Wei, G., Chepelev, I. and Zhao, K., 2007. High-Resolution Profiling of Histone Methylations in the Human Genome. *Cell*, 129 (4), pp. 823-37.

Bayani, J., Selvarajah, S., Maire, G., Vukovic, B., Al-Romaih, K., Zielenska, M. and Squire, J.A., 2007. Genomic mechanisms and measurement of structural and numerical instability in cancer cells. *Seminars in Cancer Biology*, 17 (1), pp. 5-18.

Baylin, S.B. and Herman, J.G., 2000. DNA hypermethylation in tumorigenesis: epigenetics joins genetics. *Trends in Genetics*, 16 (4), pp. 168-74.

Baylin, S.B., Esteller, M., Rountree, M.R., Bachman, K.E., Schuebel, K. and Herman, J.G., 2001. Aberrant patterns of DNA methylation, chromatin formation and gene expression in cancer. *Human Molecular Genetics*,10 (7), pp. 687-92.

Bestor, T.H., 2000. The DNA methyltransferases of mammals. *Human Molecular Genetics*, 9 (16), pp. 2395-402.

Bhasin, M., Zhang, H., Reinherz, E.L. and Reche, P.A., 2005. Prediction of methylated CpGs in DNA sequences using a support vector machine. *FEBS Letters*, 579 (20), 4302-8.

Bird, A., 1992. The essentials of DNA methylation, *Cell*, 70 (1), pp. 5-8.

Bock, C. and Lengauer, T. 2008. Computational epigenetics. *Bioinformatics*, 24 (1), pp. 1-10.

Bock, C., Walter, J., Paulsen, M. and Lengauer, T., 2007. CpG island mapping by epigenome prediction. *PLoS Computational Biology*, 3(6), pp. e110.

Boothman, D.A., Briggle, T.V. and Greer, S. 1989. Exploitation of elevated pyrimidine deaminating enzymes for selective chemotherapy. *Pharmacology and Therapeutics*, 42, pp. 65-88.

Borutinskaite, V.V., Navakauskiene, R. and Magnusson, K.E., 2006. Retinoic acid and histone deacetylase inhibitor BML-210 inhibit proliferation of human cervical cancer HeLa cells. *Annals of the New York Academy of Sciences*, 1091, pp. 346-55.

Bouchain, G., Leit, S., Frechette, S., Khalil, E.A., Lavoie, R., Moradei, O., Woo, S.H., Fournel, M., Yan, P.T., Kalita, A., Trachy-Bourget, M.C., Beaulieu, C., Li, Z., Robert, M.F., MacLeod, A.R., Besterman, J.M. and Delorme, D., 2003. Development of Potential Antitumor Agents. Synthesis and Biological Evaluation of a New Set of Sulfonamide Derivatives as Histone Deacetylase Inhibitors. *Journal of Medical Chemistry*, 46, pp. 820-30.

Brosch, G., Ransom, R., Lechner, T., Walton, J.D. and Loidl, P., 1995. Inibition of Maize Histone Deacetylases by HC Toxin, the Host-Selective toxin of Cochlioboluscarbonum. *The Plant Cell*, 7, pp. 1941-50.

Brueckner, B., Garcia Boy, R., Siedlecki, P., Musch, T., Kliem, H.C., Zielenkiewicz, P., Suhai, S., Wiessler, M. and Lyko, F., 2005. Epigenetic reactivation of tumor suppressor genes by a novel small-molecule inhibitor of human DNA methyltransferases. *Cancer Research*, 65, pp. 6305-11.

Buck, M.J. and Lieb, J.D., 2004. ChIP-chip: considerations for the design, analysis, and application of genome-wide chromatin immunoprecipitation experiments. *Genomics*, 83, pp. 349-360.

Buck, M.J., Nobel, A.B. and Lieb, J.D., 2005. ChIPOTle: a user-friendly tool for the analysis of ChIP-chip data. *Genome Biology*, 6 (11), R97.

Buermeyer, A.B., Wilson-Van Patten, C., Baker, S.M. and Liskay, R.M., 1999. The human MLH1 cDNA complements DNA mismatch repair defects in Mlh1-deficient mouse embryonic fibroblasts. *Cancer Research*, 59, pp. 538-41.

Carnell A.N., Goodman J.I. 2003. The long (LINEs) and the short (SINEs) of it: altered methylation as a precursor to toxicity. *Toxicological Sciences*, 75, pp. 229-235.

Carthew RW, Sontheimer EJ. 2009. Origins and mechanisms of miRNAs and siRNAs. *Cell*, 136, pp 642–55.

Catley, L., Weisberg, E., Tai, Y.T., Atadja, P., Remiszewski, S., Hideshima, T., Mitsiades, N., Shringarpure, R., LeBlanc, R., Chauhan, D., Munshi, N.C., Schlossman, R., Richardson, P., Griffin, J. and Anderson, K.C., 2003. NVP-LAQ824 is a potent novel histone deacetylase inhibitor with significant activity against multiple myeloma. *Blood*, 102, pp. 2615-22.

Chambers, A.F. and Matrisian, L.M., 1997. Changing views of the role of matrix metalloproteinases in metastasis. *Journal of the National Cancer Institute*, 89 (17), pp. 1260-1270.

Chan, K.K., Bakhtiar, R. and Jiang, C., 1997. Depsipeptide (FR901228, NSC-630176) pharmacokinetics in the rat by LC/MS/MS. *Investigational New Drugs*, 15 (3), pp. 195-206.

Chang, Y., Ganesh, T., Horton, J.R., Spannhoff, A., Liu, J., Sun, A., Zhang, X., Bedford, M.T., Shinkai, Y., Snyder, J.P. and Cheng, X., 2010. Adding a lysine mimic in the design of potent inhibitors of histone lysine methyltransferases. *Journal of Molecular Biology*, 400 (1), pp. 1-7.

Chen, H., Xue, Y., Huang, N., Yao, X. and Sun, Z., 2006. MeMo: a web tool for prediction of protein methylation modifications. *Nucleic Acids Research*, 34, pp. W249-53.

Chen, Y., Blackwell, T.W., Chen, J., Gao, J., Lee, A.W. and States, D.J., 2007. Integration of genome and chromatin structure with gene expression profiles to predict c-MYC recognition site binding and function. *PLoS Computational Biology*, 3 (4), pp. e63.

Chen, Y., Li, H., Tang, W., Zhu, C., Jiang, Y., Zou, J., Yu, Q. and You, Q., 2009. 3D-QSAR studies of HDACs inhibitors using pharmacophore-based alignment. *European Journal of Medical Chemistry*, 44 (7), pp. 2868-76.

Cheng, J.C., Matsen, C.B., Gonzales, F.A., Ye, W., Greer, S., Marquez, V.E., Jones, P.A., Selker, E.U., 2003. Inhibition of DNA Methylation and Reactivation of Silenced Genes by Zebularine. *Journal of the National Cancer Institute*, Vol. 95, 5, pp. 399-409.

Chow, H.H., Cai, Y., Hakim, I.A., Crowell, J.A., Shahi, F., Brooks, C.A., Dorr, R.T., Hara, Y. and Alberts, D.S., 2003. Pharmacokinetics and Safety of Green Tea Polyphenols after Multiple-Dose Administration of Epigallocatechin Gallate and Polyphenon E in Healthy Individuals. *Clinical Cancer Research*, Vol. 9, pp. 3312-9.

ClinicalTrials.gov 2010 Available at: http://clinicaltrials.gov/

Coffey, D.C., Kutko, M.C., Glick R.D., Butler, L.M., Heller, G., Rifkind, R.A., Marks, P.A., Richon, V.M., La Quaglia, M.P., 2001. The histone deacetylase inhibitor, CBHA, inhibits growth of human neuroblastoma xenografts. *Cancer Research*, 61, pp. 3591-4.

Costello, J.F., Frühwald, M.C., Smiraglia, D.J., Rush, L.J., Robertson, G.P., Gao, X., Wright, F.A., Feramisco, J.D., Peltomäki, P., Lang, J.C., Schuller, D.E., Yu, L., Bloomfield, C.D., Caligiuri, M.A., Yates, A., Nishikawa, R., Su Huang, H., Petrelli, N.J., Zhang, X., O'Dorisio, M.S., Held, W.A., Cavenee, W.K. and Plass, C., 2000. Aberrant CpGisland methylation has non-random and tumour-type-specific patterns. *Nature Genetics*, 24 (2), pp. 132-8.

Creagan, E.T., Schaid, D.J., Hartmann, L.C. and Loprinzi, C.L., 1993. A phase II study of 5,6-dihydro-5-azacytidine hydrochloride in disseminated malignant melanoma. *American Journal of Clinical Oncology*, 16, pp. 243-4.

Curt, G.A., Kelley, J.A., Fine, R.L., Huguenin, P.N., Roth, J.S., Batist, G., Jenkins, J. and Collins, J.M., 1985. A phase I and pharmacokinetic study of dihydro-5-azacytidine (NSC 264880). *Cancer Research*, 45, pp. 3359-63.

Darkin-Rattray, S.J., Gurnett, A.M., Myers, R.W., Dulski, P.M., Crumley, T.M., Allocco, J.J., Cannova, C., Meinke, P.T., Colletti, S.L., Bednarek, M.A., Singh, S.B., Goetz, M.A., Dombrowski, A.W., Polishook, J.D. and Schmatz D.M., 1996. Apicidin: A novel antiprotozoal agent that inhibit parasite histone deacetylase. *Proceedings of the National Academy of Sciences of the USA*, 93, pp. 13143–7.

Das, P.M. and Singal, R, 2004. DNA methylation and cancer. *Journal of Clinical Oncology*, 22 (22), pp.4632-42.

Davis, A.J., Gelmon, K.A., Siu, L.L., Moore, M.J., Britten, C.D., Mistry, N., Klamut, H., D'Aloisio, S., MacLean, M., Wainman, N., Ayers, D., Firby, P., Besterman, J.M., Reid, G.K. and Eisenhauer, E.A., 2003. Phase I and pharmacologic study of the human DNA methyltransferase antisense oligodeoxynucleotide MG98 given as a 21-day continuous infusion every 4 weeks. *Investigational New Drugs*, 21, pp. 85-97.

De Bona, F., Ossowski, S., Schneeberger, K. and Rätsch, G., 2008. Optimal spliced alignments of short sequence reads. *Bioinformatics*, 24 (16), pp. i174-80.

Dhingra, H.M., Murphy, W.K., Winn, R.J., Raber, M.N. and Hong, W.K., 1991 Phase II trial of 5,6-dihydro-5-azacytidine in pleural malignant mesothelioma. *Investigational New Drugs*, 9, pp 69-72.

Dote, H., Cerna, D., Burgan, W.E., Carter, D.J., Cerra, M.A., Hollingshead, M.G., Camphausen, K. and Tofilon, P.J., 2005. Enhancement of *In vitro* and *In vivo* Tumor Cell Radiosensitivity by the DNA Methylation Inhibitor Zebularine. *Clinical Cancer Research*, 11, pp. 4571-9.

Droit, A., Cheung, C. and Gottardo, R., 2010. rMAT--an R/Bioconductor package for analyzing ChIP-chip experiments. *Bioinformatics*, 26 (5), pp. 678-9.

Egger, G., Liang, G., Aparicio, A. and Jones, P.A., 2004. Epigenetics in human disease and prospects for epigenetic therapy. *Nature*, 429, pp. 457-63.

Esteller, M., Corn, P.G., Urena, J.M., Gabrielson, E., Baylin, S.B. and Herman, J.G., 1998. Inactivation of glutathione S-transferase P1 gene by promoter hypermethylation in human neoplasia. *Cancer Research*, 58 (20), pp. 4515-8.

Esteller, M., Loda, M., Gaida, G.M., Lipman, J., Mishra, R., Goldman, H., Jessup, J.M. and Kolodner, R., 2002. Hypermethylation of the DNA repair gene O(6)-methylguanine DNA methyltransferase and survival of patients with diffuse large B-cell lymphoma. *Journal of the National Cancer Institute*, 94 (1), pp. 26-32.

Esteller, M., Silva, J.M., Dominguez, G., Bonilla, F., Matias-Guiu, X., Lerma, E., Bussaglia, E., Prat, J., Harkes, I.C., Repasky, E.A., Gabrielson, E., Schutte, M., Baylin, S.B. and Herman J.G., 2000b. Promoter Hypermethylation and BRCA1 Inactivation in Sporadic Breast and Ovarian Tumors. *Journal of the National Cancer Institute*, 92 (7), pp. 564-9.

Esteller M, Tortola, S., Toyota, M., Capella, G., Peinado, M.A., Baylin, S.B. and Herman, J.G., 2000a. Hypermethylationassociated inactivation of p14(ARF) is independent of p16(INK4a) methylation and p53 mutational status. *Cancer Research*, 60 (1), pp. 129- 33.

Fang, M.Z., Wang, Y., Ai, N., Hou, Z., Sun, Y., Lu, H., Welsh, W. and Yang, C.S., 2003. Tea polyphenol (-)-epigallocatechin-3-gallate inhibits DNA methyltransferase and reactivates methylation-silenced genes in cancer cell lines. *Cancer Research*, 63, pp. 7563-70.

Fang, Y.C., Huang, H.C. and Juan, H.F., 2008. MeInfoText: associated gene methylation and cancer information from text mining. *BMC Bioinformatics*, 9, 22.

Fink, D., Aebi, S. and Howell, S.B., 1998. The role of DNA mismatch repair in drug resistance. *Clinical Cancer Research*, 4, pp. 1-6.

Floris, G., Debiec-Rychter, M., Sciot, R., Stefan, C., Fieuws, S., Machiels, K., Atadja, P., Wozniak, A., Faa, G. and Schöffski, P., 2009. High efficacy of panobinostat towards human gastrointestinal stromal tumors in a xenograft mouse model. *Clinical Cancer Research*, 5(12), pp. 4066-76.

Folkvord, S., Ree, A.H., Furre, T., Halvorsen, T. and Flatmark, K., 2009. Radiosensitization by SAHA in Experimental Colorectal Carcinoma Models - *In Vivo* Effects and Relevance of Histone Acetylation Status. *International Journal of Radiation Oncology*, Vol. 74 (2), pp. 546-52.

Fu, W.N., Bertoni, F., Kelsey, S.M., McElwaine, S.M., Cotter, F.E., Newland, A.C. and Jia, L., 2003. Role of DNA methylation in the suppression of Apaf-1 protein in human leukaemia. *Oncogene*, 22 (3), pp. 451-5.

Fuks, F., Hurd, P.J., Deplus, R. and Kouzarides T., 2003. The DNA methyltransferases associate with HP1 and the SUV39H1 histone methyltransferase. *Nucleic Acids Research*, 31 (9), pp. 2305-12.

Fulda, S., Küfer, M.U., Meyer, E., van Valen, F., Dockhorn-Dworniczak, B. and Debatin, K.M., 2001. Sensitization for death receptor- or drug-induced apoptosis by re-expression of caspase-8 through demethylation or gene transfer. *Oncogene*, 20, pp. 5865-77.

Furumai, R., Komatsu, Y., Nishino, N., Khochbin, S., Yoshida, M., Horinouchi, S., 2001. Potent histone deacetylase inhibitors built from trichostatin A and cyclic tetrapeptide antibiotics including trapoxin. *Proceedings of the National Academy of Sciences*, Vol. 98 (1), pp. 87-92.

Galli, M., Salmoiraghi, S., Golay, J., Gozzini, A., Crippa, C., Pescosta, N. and Rambaldi, A., 2010. A phase II multiple dose clinical trial of histone deacetylase inhibitor ITF2357 in patients with relapsed or progressive multiple myeloma. *Annals of Hematology*, 89, pp. 185-90.

Garcia-Manero, G., Yang, H., Bueso-Ramos, C., Ferrajoli, A., Cortes, J., Wierda, W.G., Faderl, S., Koller, C., Morris, G., Rosner, G., Loboda, A., Fantin, V.R., Randolph, S.S., Hardwick, J.S., Reilly, J.F., Chen, C., Ricker, J.L., Secrist, J.P., Richon, V.M., Frankel, S.R. and Kantarjian, H.M., 2008. Phase I study of the histone deacetylase inhibitor vorinostat (suberoylanilide hydroxamic acid, SAHA) in patients with advanced leukemia and myelodysplastic syndromes. *Blood*, 111 (3), pp. 1060-6.

GenePattern 2010 Available at: https://cabig.nci.nih.gov/tools/GenePattern

Glass, J.L., Thompson, R.F., Khulan, B., Figueroa, M.E., Olivier, E.N., Oakley, E.J., Van Zant, G., Bouhassira, E.E., Melnick, A., Golden, A., Fazzari, M.J. and Greally, J.M., 2007. CG dinucleotide clustering is a species-specific property of the genome. *Nucleic Acids Research*, 35, pp. 6798–807.

Goffin, G. and Eisenhauer, E., 2002. DNA methiltransferase inhibitors-state of the art. *Annals of Oncology*, 13, pp. 1699-716.

Goh, L., Murphy, S.K., Muhkerjee, S. and Furey, T.S., 2007. Genomic sweeping for hypermethylated genes. *Bioinformatics*, 23 (3), pp. 281-8.

Golay, J., Cuppini, L., Leoni, F., Micò, C., Barbui, V., Domenghini, M., Lombardi, L., Neri, A., Barbui, A.M., Salvi, A., Pozzi, P., Porro, G., Pagani, P., Fossati, G., Mascagni, P., Introna M. and Rambaldi A., 2007. The histone deacetylase inhibitor ITF2357 has anti-leukemic activity *in vitro* and *in vivo* and inhibits IL-6 and VEGF production by stromal cellsAnti-leukemic activity of the new HDAC inhibitor ITF2357. *Leukemia*, 21, pp. 1892-1900.

Gore, S.D., 2006. Six (or more) drugs in search of a mechanism: DNA methyltransferase and histone deacetylase inhibitors in the treatment of myelodysplastic syndromes. *Journal of the National Comprehensive Cancer Network*, 4 (1), pp. 83-90.

Gottesman, M.M., 2002. Mechanisms of cancer drug resistance. *Annual Review of Medicine*, 53, pp. 615-27.

Gottlicher, M., S, Zhu, P., Krämer, O.H., Schimpf, A., Giavara, S., Sleeman, J.P., Lo Coco, F., Nervi, C., Pelicci, P.G. and Heinzel, T., 2001. Valproic acid defines a novel class of HDAC inhibitors inducing differentiation of transformed cells. *EMBO Journal*, 20, pp. 6969-78.

Gurin, C.C., Federici, M.G., Kang, L. and Boyd, J., 1999. Causes and consequences of microsatellite instability in endometrial carcinoma. *Cancer Research*, 59, pp. 462-6.

Hackenberg, M., Previti, C., Luque-Escamilla, P.L., Carpena, P., Martínez-Aroza, J. and Oliver, J.L., 2006. CpGcluster: a distance-based algorithm for CpG-island detection. *BMC Bioinformatics*, 7, pp. 446.

Hajkova, P., 2002. DNA-methylation analysis by the bisulfite-assisted genomic sequencing method. *Methods in Molecular Biology*, 200, pp. 143-54.

Hanahan, D. and Weinberg, R.A., 2000. The hallmarks of cancer. *Cell*, 100 (1), pp. 57-70.

Hansen, M.F., 1991. Molecular genetic considerations in osteosarcoma. *Clinical Orthopaedics & Related Research*, 270, pp. 237-46.

He, X., Chang, S., Zhang, J., Zhao, Q., Xiang, H., Kusonmano, K., Yang, L., Sun, Z.S., Yang, H. and Wang, J., 2008. MethyCancer: the database of human DNA methylation and cancer. *Nucleic Acids Research*, 36, pp. D836-41.

Heideman, R.L., Balis, F.M., McCully, C. and Poplack, D.G., 1998. Preclinical Pharmacology of Arabinosyl-5-azacytidine in Nonhuman Primates. *Cancer Research*, 48, pp. 4294-8.

Herman, D., Jenssen, K., Burnett, R., Soragni, E., Perlman, S.L. and Gottesfeld, J.M., 2006. Histone deacetylase inhibitors reverse gene silencing in Friedreich's ataxia. *Nature Chemical Biology*, 2, pp. 551-8.

Herman, J.G., Merlo, A., Mao, L., Lapidus, R.G., Issa, J.P., Davidson, N.E., Sidransky, D. and Baylin, S.B., 1995. Inactivation of the CDKN2/p16/MTS1 gene is frequently associated with aberrant DNA methylation in all common human cancers. *Cancer Research*, 55, pp. 4525-30.

Herman, J.G., Umar, A., Polyak, K., Graff, J.R., Ahuja, N., Issa, J.P., Markowitz, S., Willson, J.K., Hamilton, S.R., Kinzler, K.W., Kane, M.F., Kolodner, R.D., Vogelstein, B., Kunkel, T.A. and Baylin, S.B., 1998. Incidence and functional consequences of hMLH1 promoter hypermethylation in colorectal carcinoma. *Proceedings of the National Academy of Sciences of USA*, 95 (12), pp. 6870-5.

Herranz, M. and Esteller, M., 2007. DNA methylation and histone modifications in patients with cancer: potential prognostic and therapeutic targets. *Methods in Molecular Biology*, 361, pp. 25-62.

Herranz, M., Martín-Caballero, J., Fraga, M.F., Ruiz-Cabello, J., Flores, J.M., Desco, M., Marquez, V. and Esteller, M., 2006. The novel DNA methylation inhibitor zebularine is effective against the development of murine T-cell lymphoma. *Blood*, Vol. 107 (3), pp. 1171-7.

Hu, E., Dul, E., Sung, C.M., Chen, Z., Kirkpatrick, R., Zhang, G.F., Johanson, K., Liu, R., Lago, A., Hofmann, G., Macarron, R., de los Frailes, M., Perez, P., Krawiec, J., Winkler, J. and Jaye, M., 2003. Identification of novel isoform-selective inhibitors within class I histone deacetylases. *Journal of Pharmacology and Experimental Therapeutics*, 307, pp. 720-8.

Huang, H., Maertens, A.M., Hyland, E.M., Dai, J., Norris, A., Boeke, J.D. and Bader, J.S., 2009. HistoneHits: a database for histone mutations and their phenotypes. *Genome Research*, 19 (4), pp. 674-81.

Isoldi, M.C., Visconti, M.A. and Castrucci, A.M., 2005. Anti-cancer drugs: molecular mechanisms of action. *Mini-Reviews in Medical Chemistry*, 5 (7), pp. 685-95.

Issa, J.P., 2005. Optimizing therapy with methylation inhibitors in myelodysplastic syndromes: dose, duration, and patient selection. *Nature Clinical Practice Oncology*, 2, pp. S24-9.

Johnson, J., Hunter, R., McElveen, R., Qian, X.H., Baliga, B.S. and Pace, B.S., 2005. Fetal hemoglobin induction by the histone deacetylase inhibitor, scriptaid. *Cellular and Molecular Biology (Noisy-le-grand)*, 51, pp. 229-38.

Jones, P.A. and Baylin, S.B., 2007. The epigenomics of cancer. *Cell*, 128 (4), pp. 683-92.

Jones, P.A. and Laird, P.W., 1999. Cancer epigenetics comes of age. *Nature Genetics*, 21 (2), pp. 163-7.

Jung, M., Brosch, G., Kölle, D., Scherf, H., Gerhäuser, C. and Loidl, P., 1999. Amide Analogues of Trichostatin A as Inhibitors of Histone Deacetylase and Inducers of Terminal Cell Differentiation. *Journal of Medicinal Chemistry*, 42, pp. 4669-79.

Juttermann, R., Li, E. and Jaenisch, R., 1994. Toxicity of 5-aza-2'-deoxycytidine to mammalian cells is mediated primarily by covalent trapping of DNA methyltransferase rather than DNA demethylation. *Proceedings of the National Academy of Sciences of USA*, 91 (25), pp. 11797-801.

Kaikkonen MU, Lam MT, Glass CK. 2011. Non-coding RNAs as regulators of gene expression and epigenetics. *Cardiovascular Research*, 90, pp. 430–40.

Kaminskas, E., Farrell, A., Abraham, S., Baird, A., Hsieh, L.S., Lee, S.L., Leighton, J.K., Patel, H., Rahman, A., Sridhara, R., Wang, Y.C., and Pazdur, R., 2005. FDA Approval summary: azacitidine for treatment of myelodysplastic syndrome subtypes. *Clinical Cancer Research*, 11 (10), pp. 3604-8.

Kane, M.F., *et al.*, 1997. Methylation of the hMLH1 promoter correlates with lack of expression of hMLH1 in sporadic colon tumors and mismatch repair-defective human tumor cell lines. *Cancer Research*, 57 (5), pp. 808-11.

Keen, J.C., Yan, L., Mack, K.M., Pettit, C., Smith, D., Sharma, D. and Davidson, N.E., 2003. A novel histone deacetylase inhibitor, Scriptaid, enhances expression of functional estrogen receptor α (ER) in ER negative human breast cancer cells in combination with 5-aza 2'-deoxycytidine. *Breast Cancer Research and Treatment*, 81, pp. 177-86.

Kelly, W.K., Richon, V.M., O'Connor, O., Curley, T., MacGregor-Curtelli, B., Tong, W., Klang, M., Schwartz, L., Richardson, S., Rosa, E., Drobnjak, M., Cordon-Cordo, C., Chiao, J.H., Rifkind, R., Marks, P.A. and Scher, H., 2003. Phase I Clinical Trial of Histone Deacetylase Inhibitor: Suberoylanilide Hydroxamic Acid Administered Intravenously. *Clinical Cancer Research*, 9, pp. 3578-88.

Kent, W.J., 2002. BLAT--the BLAST-like alignment tool. *Genome Research*, 12 (4), pp. 656-64.

Keshet, I., Schlesinger, Y., Farkash, S., Rand, E., Hecht, M., Segal, E., Pikarski, E., Young, R.A., Niveleau, A., Cedar, H. and Simon, I., 2006. Evidence for an instructive mechanism of *de novo* methylation in cancer cells. *Nature Genetics*, 38 (2), pp. 149-53.

Kim, G.D., Ni, J., Kelesoglu, N., Roberts, R.J. and Pradhan, S., 2002. Co-operation and communication between the human maintenance and *de novo* DNA (cytosine-5) methyltransferases. *The EMBO Journal*, 21, pp. 4183-95.

Kim, S.H., Kang, H.J., Na, H. and Lee M.O., 2010. Trichostatin A enhances acetylation as well as protein stability of ERα through induction of p300 protein. *Breast Cancer Research*, 12: R22.

Kim, Y.B., Lee, K.H., Sugita, K., Yoshida, M., Horinouchi, S., 1999. Oxamflatin is a novel antitumor compound that inhibits mammalian histone deacetylase. *Oncogene*, 18, pp. 2461-70.

Klisovic, R.B., Stock, W., Cataland, S., Klisovic, M.I., Liu, S., Blum, W., Green, M., Odenike, O., Godley, L., Burgt, J.V., Van Laar, E., Cullen, M., Macleod, A.R., Besterman, J.M., Reid, G.K., Byrd, J.C. and Marcucci, G., 2008. A Phase I Biological Study of MG98, an

Oligodeoxynucleotide Antisense to DNA Methyltransferase 1, in Patients with High-Risk Myelodysplasia and Acute Myeloid Leukemia. *Clinical Cancer Research*, 14, pp. 2444-9.

Komatsu, Y., Tomizaki, K.Y., Tsukamoto, M., Kato, T., Nishino, N., Sato, S., Yamori, T., Tsuruo, T., Furumai, R., Yoshida, M., Horinouchi, S. and Hayashi, H., 2001. Cyclic Hydroxamic-acid-containing Peptide 31, a Potent Synthetic Histone Deacetylase Inhibitor with Antitumor Activity. *Cancer Research*, 61, pp. 4459-66.

Kornblith, A.B., Herndon, J.E. 2nd, Silverman, L.R., Demakos, E.P., Odchimar-Reissig, R., Holland, J.F., Powell, B.L., DeCastro, C., Ellerton, J., Larson, R.A., Schiffer, C.A. and Holland, J.C., 2002. Impact of Azacytidine on the Quality of Life of Patients With Myelodysplastic Syndrome Treated in a Randomized Phase III Trial: A Cancer and Leukemia Group B Study. *Journal of Clinical Oncology*, Vol. 20 (10), pp. 2441-52.

Koudan, E.V., Bujnicki, J.M. and Gromova, E.S., 2004. Homology modeling of the CG-specific DNA methyltransferase SssI and its complexes with DNA and AdoHcy. *Journal of Biomolecular Structure & Dynamics*, 22 (3), pp. 339-45.

Kraker, A.J., Mizzen, C.A., Hartl, B.G., Miin, J., Allis, C.D., and Merriman R.L., 2003. Modulation of Histone Acetylation by [4-(Acetylamino)-N-(2-Amino-henyl) Benzamide] in HCT-8 Colon Carcinoma. *Molecular Cancer Therapeutics*, 2, pp. 401-8.

Kuendgen, A., Schmid, M., Schlenk, R., Knipp, S., Hildebrandt, B., Steidl, C., Germing, U., Haas, R., Dohner, H. and Gattermann, N., 2006. The Histone Deacetylase (HDAC) Inhibitor Valproic Acid as Monotherapy or in Combination with All-*Trans* Retinoic Acid in Patients with Acute Myeloid Leukemia. *Cancer*, Vol. 106 (1), pp. 1-235.

Kumar, S., Nei, M., Dudley, J. and Tamura, K., 2008. MEGA: A biologist-centric software for evolutionary analysis of DNA and protein sequences. *Briefings in Bioinformatics*, 9(4), pp. 299–306.

Kusy S, Larsen C.J., Roche J., 2004. p14ARF, p15INK4b and p16INK4a methylation status in chronic myelogenous leukemia. *Leukemia & Lymphoma,*45 (10), pp 1989-94.

La Sala, D., Macaluso, M., Trimarchi, C., Giordano, A. and Cinti, C., 2003. Triggering of p73-dependent apoptosis in osteosarcoma is under the control of E2Fs-pRb2/p130 complexes. *Oncogene*, 22 (23), pp. 3518-29.

Lai, J.P., Sandhu, D.S., Moser, C.D., Cazanave, S.C., Oseini, A.M., Shire. A.M., Shridhar, V., Sanderson, S.O. and Roberts, L.R., 2009. Additive effect of apicidin and doxorubicin in sulfatase 1 (SULF1)-expressing hepatocellular carcinoma *in vitro* and *in vivo*. *Journal of Hepatology*, 50, pp. 1112-21.

Lai, M.T., Yang, C.C., Lin, T.Y., Tsai, F.J. and Chen, W.C., 2008. Depsipeptide (FK228) inhibits growth of human prostate cancer cells. *Urologic Oncology*, 26 (2), 182-9.

Langmann, T., *et al.*, 2003. Real-time reverse transcription-PCR expression profiling of the complete human ATP-binding cassette transporter superfamily in various tissues. *Clinical Chemistry*, 49, pp. 230-8.

Lee, E.J., Lee, B.B., Kim, S.J., Park, Y.D., Park, J., Kim, D.H., 2008a. Histone deacetylase inhibitor scriptaid induces cell cycle arrest and epigenetic change in colon cancer cells. *International Journal of Oncology*, 33, pp. 767-76.

Lee J.T., 2009. Lessons from X-chromosome inactivation: long ncRNA as guides and tethers to the epigenome. *Genes Development*, 23, pp 1831–42.

Lee, S.C., Chan, W.K., Lee, T.W., Lam, W.H., Wang, X., Chan, T.H. and Wong, Y.C., 2008b. Effect of a Prodrug of the Green Tea Polyphenol(-)-Epigallocatechin-3-Gallate on thecGrowth of Androgen-Independent Prostate Cancer *In Vivo*. *Nutrition and Cancer*, 60, pp. 483-91.

Lemaire, M., Momparler, L.F., Raynal, N.J., Bernstein, M.L. and Momparler, R.L., 2009. Inhibition of cytidine deaminase by zebularine enhances the antineoplastic action of 5-aza-2'-deoxycytidine. *Cancer Chemotherapy and Pharmacology*, 63, pp. 411-6.

Leoni, F., Fossati, G., Lewis, E.C., Lee, J.K., Porro, G., Pagani, P., Modena, D., Moras, M.L., Pozzi, P., Reznikov, L.L., Siegmund, B., Fantuzzi, G., Dinarello, C.A. and Mascagni, P., 2005. The Histone Deacetylase Inhibitor ITF2357 Reduces Production of Pro-Inflammatory Cytokines *In Vitro* and Systemic Inflammation *In Vivo*. *Molecular Medicine*, 11, pp. 1-15.

Leung, S.Y., Yuen, S.T., Chung, L.P., Chu, K.M., Chan, A.S. and Ho, J.C., 1999. hMLH1 promoter methylation and lack of hMLH1 expression in sporadic gastric carcinomas with high-frequency microsatellite instability. *Cancer Research*, 59, pp. 159-64.

Lewin, J., Schmitt, A.O., Adorján, P., Hildmann, T. and Piepenbrock, C., 2004. Quantitative DNA methylation analysis based on four-dye trace data from direct sequencing of PCR amplificates. *Bioinformatics*, 20 (17), pp. 3005-12.

Lin, X., Asgari, K., Putzi, M.J., Gage, W.R., Yu, X., Cornblatt, B.S., Kumar, A., Piantadosi, S., DeWeese, T.L., De Marzo, A.M. and Nelson, W.G., 2001. Reversal of GSTP1 CpG island hypermethylation and reactivation of pi-class glutathione Stransferase (GSTP1) expression in human prostate cancer cells by treatment with procainamide. *Cancer Research*, 61, pp. 8611-6.

Loss, L.A., Sadanandam, A., Durinck, S., Nautiyal, S., Flaucher, D., Carlton, V.E., Moorhead, M., Lu, Y., Gray, J.W., Faham, M., Spellman. P. and Parvin, B., 2010. Prediction of epigenetically regulated genes in breast cancer cell lines. *BMC Bioinformatics*, 11, pp. 305.

Lu, Y.S., Kulp, S.K., Wang, Y.C., Wang, D., Hung, J.H., Tang, M., Lin, Z.Z., Chen, T.J., Cheng, A.L. and Chen, C.S., 2007. Efficacy of a novel histone deacetylase inhibitor in murine models of hepatocellular carcinoma. *Hepatology*, 46, pp. 1119-30.

Mackay, H.J., Cameron, D., Rahilly, M., Mackean, M.J., Paul, J., Kaye, S.B. and Brown, R., 2000. Reduced MLH1 expression in breast tumors after primary chemotherapy predicts diseasefree survival. *Journal of Clinical Oncology*, 18, 87-93.

Marsit, C.J., Liu, M., Nelson, H.H., Posner, M., Suzuki, M. and Kelsey, K.T., *et al.*, 2004. Inactivation of the Fanconi anemia/BRCA pathway in lung and oral cancers: implications for treatment and survival. *Oncogene*, 23 (4), pp.1000-4.

Martinez-Delgado, B., Melendez, B., Cuadros, M., Jose Garcia, M., Nomdedeu, J., Rivas, C., Fernandez-Piqueras, J. and Benítez, J., 2002. Frequent inactivation of the p73 gene by abnormal methylation or LOH in non-Hodgkin's lymphomas. *International Journal of Cancer*, 102 (1), pp. 15-9.

Mattick JS. 2009. The genetic signatures of noncoding RNAs. *PLoS Genetics,* 5 (4) e1000459.

Mikkelsen, T.S., Ku, M., Jaffe, D.B., Issac, B., Lieberman, E., Giannoukos, G., Alvarez, P., Brockman, W., Kim, T.K., Koche, R.P., Lee, W., Mendenhall, E., O'Donovan, A., Presser, A., Russ, C., Xie, X., Meissner, A., Wernig, M., Jaenisch, R., Nusbaum, C., Lander, E.S. and Bernstein, B.E., 2007. Genome-wide maps of chromatin state in pluripotent and lineage-committed cells. *Nature*, 44 (7153), pp. 553-60.

Miranda-Saavedra, D. and Barton, G.J., 2007. Classification and functional annotation of eukaryotic protein kinases. *Proteins*, 68 (4), pp. 893-914.

Mizuno S., Chijiwa T., Okamura T., Akashi K., Fukumaki Y., Niho Y., Sasaki H., 2001. Expression of DNA methyltransferases DNMT1, 3A, and 3B in normal hematopoiesis and in acute and chronic myelogenous leukemia. *Blood*, 97, pp. 1172-1179.

Momparler, R.L., Bouffard, D.Y., Momparler, L.F., Dionne, J., Bélanger, K. And Ayoub, J., 1997. Pilot phase I-II study on 5-aza-2'-deoxycytidine (Decitabine) in patients with metastatic lung cancer. *Anticancer Drugs*, 8 (4), pp. 358-68.

Monneret, C., 2007. Histone deacetylase inhibitors for epigenetic therapy of cancer. *Anticancer Drugs*, 18, pp. 363-70

Morgan, H.D., Santos, F., Green, K., Dean, W. and Reik, W., 2005. Epigenetic reprogramming in mammals. *Human Molecular Genetics*, 14 (1), pp. R47-58.

Murray, P.J., Kranz, M., Ladlow, M., Taylor, S., Berst, F., Holmes, A.B., Keavey, K.N., Jaxa-Chamiec, A., Seale, P.W., Stead, P., Upton, R.J., Croft, S.L., Clegg, W. and Elsegood, M.R., 2001. The synthesis of cyclic tetrapeptoid analogues of the antiprotozoal natural product apicidin. *Bioorganic and Medicinal Chemistry Letters*, 11, pp. 773-6.

Negre, V. and Grunau, C., 2006 The MethDB DAS server: adding an epigenetic information layer to the human genome. *Epigenetics*, 1 (2), pp.101-5.

Ning, L., Jaskula-Sztul, R., Kunnimalaiyaan, M. and Chen, H., 2008. Suberoyl Bishydroxamic Acid Activates Notch1 Signaling and Suppresses Tumor Progression in an Animal Model of Medullary Thyroid Carcinoma. *Annals of Surgical Oncology*, 15, pp. 2600-5.

Okano, M., Bell, D.W., Haber, D.A. and Li, E., 1999. DNA methyltransferases Dnmt3a and Dnmt3b are essential for *de novo* methylation and mammalian development. *Cell*, 99 (3), pp. 247-57.

Olopade, O.I. and Wei, M., 2003. FANCF methylation contributes to chemoselectivity in ovarian cancer. *Cancer Cell*, 3, pp. 417-20.

Ongenaert, M., Van Neste, L., De Meyer, T., Menschaert, G., Bekaert, S. and Van Criekinge, W., 2008. PubMeth: a cancer methylation database combining text-mining and expert annotation. *Nucleic Acids Research*, 36, pp. D842-6.

Osunkoya, A.O., Yin-Goen, Q., Phan, J.H., Moffitt, R.A., Stokes, T.H., Wang, M.D. and Young, A.N., 2009. Diagnostic biomarkers for renal cell carcinoma: selection using novel bioinformatics systems for microarray data analysis. *Human Pathology*, 40, pp. 1671-8.

Paoluzzi, L., Scotto, L., Marchi, E., Zain, J., Seshan, V.E. and O'Connor, O.A., 2010. Romidepsin and belinostat synergize the antineoplastic effect of bortezomib in mantle cell lymphoma. *Clinical Cancer Research*, 16, pp. 554-65.

Pattyn, F., Hoebeeck, J., Robbrecht, P., Michels, E., De Paepe, A., Bottu, G., Coornaert, D., Herzog, R., Speleman, F. and Vandesompele, J., 2006. methBLAST and methPrimerDB: web-tools for PCR based methylation analysis. *BMC Bioinformatics*,7, 496.

Plumb, J.A., Finn, P.W., Williams, R.J., Bandara, M.J., Romero, M.R., Watkins, C.J., La Thangue, N.B. and Brown, R., 2003. Pharmacodynamic response and inhibition of growth of human tumor xenografts by the novel histone deacetylase inhibitor PXD101. *Molecular Cancer Therapeutics*, 2, pp. 721-8.

Ponger, L. and Mouchiroud, D., 2002. CpGProD: identifying CpG islands associated with transcription start sites in large genomic mammalian sequences. *Bioinformatics*, 18 (4), pp. 631-3.

Ponting CP, Oliver PL, Reik W. 2009. Evolution and functions of long noncoding RNAs. *Cell*, 136, pp 629–41.

Pop, M., Phillippy, A., Delcher, A.L. and Salzberg, S.L., 2004. Comparative Genome Assembly. *Briefings in Bioinformatics*, 5 (3), pp. 237-48.

Prakash, S., Foster, B.J., Meyer, M., Wozniak, A., Heilbrun, L.H., Flaherty, L., Zalupski, M., Radulovic, L., Valdivieso M. and LoRusso P.M., 2001. Chronic oral administration of CI-994: a phase 1 study. *Investigational New Drugs*, 19 (1), pp. 1-11.

Qian, X., LaRochelle, W.J., Ara, G., Wu, F., Petersen, K.D., Thougaard, A., Sehested, M., Lichenstein, H.S. and Jeffers, M., 2006. Activity of PXD101, a histone deacetylase inhibitor, in preclinical ovarian cancer studies. *Molecular Cancer Therapeutics*, 5, pp. 2086-95.

Raffoux, E., Cras, A., Recher, C., de Labarthe, A., Turlure, P., Reman, O., Gardin, C., Victor, M., Maury, S., Malfuson, J.V., Maarek, O., Daniel, M.T., Fenaux, P., Degos, L., Chomienne, C., Chevret, S. and Dombret, H., 2010. Phase 2 clinical trial of 5-azacitidine, valproic acid, and all-*trans* retinoic acid in patients with high-risk acute myeloid leukemia or myelodysplastic syndrome. *OncoTaget*, May, pp. 34-42.

Rai, M., Soragni, E., Chou, C.J., Barnes, G., Jones, S., Rusche, J.R., Gottesfeld, J.M. and Pandolfo, M., 2010. Two New Pimelic Diphenylamide HDAC Inhibitors Induce Sustained Frataxin Upregulation in Cells from Friedreich's Ataxia Patients and in a Mouse Model. *PloS One*, Vol. 5, e8825.

Rainer, J., Sanchez-Cabo, F., Stocker, G., Sturn, A. and Trajanoski, Z., 2006. CARMAweb: comprehensive R- and bioconductor-based web service for microarray data analysis. *Nucleic Acids Research*. 34 (Web Server issue): W498-503.

Rambaldi, A., Dellacasa, C.M., Finazzi, G., Carobbio, A., Ferrari, M.L., Guglielmelli, P., Gattoni, E., Salmoiraghi, S., Finazzi, M.C., Di Tollo, S., D'Urzo, C., Vannucchi, A.M, Barosi, G. and Barbui, T., 2010. A pilot study of the Histone-Deacetylase inhibitor Givinostat in patients with JAK2V617F positive chronic myeloproliferative neoplasms. *British Journal of Haematology*, Vol. 150 (4), pp. 446-55.

Rehrauer, H., Zoller, S. and Schlapbach, R., 2007. MAGMA: analysis of two-channel microarrays made easy. *Nucleic Acids Research*, 35 (Web Server issue): W86–W90.

Rhee, I., Bachman, K.E., Park, B.H., Jair, K.W., Yen, R.W., Schuebel, K.E., Cui, H., Feinberg, A.P., Lengauer, C., Kinzler, K.W., Baylin, S.B. and Vogelstein, B., 2002. DNMT1 and DNMT3b cooperate to silence genes in human cancer cells. N*ature*, 416, pp. 552-6.

Richards, D.A., Oettle, H., Vervenne, W. L., Saif, M. W., Thomas, J. P., Spitzer, G., Visseren-Grul, C., Enas, N., Weitzman, A., 2005. Randomized double-blind phase II trial comparing gemcitabine (GEM) plus LY293111 *vs.* GEM plus placebo in advanced adenocarcinoma of the pancreas. *Journal of Clinical Oncology*, 23, pp. 4092-9.

Riessland, M., Brichta, L., Hahnen, E. and Wirth, B., 2006. The benzamide M344, a novel histone deacetylase inhibitor, significantly increases SMN2 RNA/protein levels in spinal muscular atrophy cells. *Human Genetics*, 120, pp. 101-10.

Riester, D., Hildmann, C. and Schwienhorst, A., 2007. Histone deacetylase inhibitors-turning epigenic mechanisms of gene regulation into tools of therapeutic intervention in malignant and other diseases. *Applied Microbiology and Biotechnology*, 75, pp. 499-514.

Rivera-Del Valle, N., Gao, S., Miller, C.P., Fulbright, J., Gonzales, C., Sirisawad, M., Steggerda, S., Wheler, J., Balasubramanian, S., Chandra, J., 2010. PCI-24781, a Novel Hydroxamic Acid HDAC Inhibitor, Exerts Cytotoxicity and Histone Alterations *via* Caspase-8 and FADD in Leukemia Cells. *International Journal of Cell Biology*, Vol. 2010, Article ID 207420.

Rudek, M.A., M., He, P., Hartke, C., Gilbert, J., Gore, S.D., Carducci, M.A. and Baker S.D., 2005. Pharmacokinetics of 5-Azacitidine administered with phenylbutyrate in patients with refractory solid tumors or hematologic malignancies. *Journal of Clinical Oncology*, 23 (17), pp. 3906-11.

Ryan, Q.C., Headlee, D., Acharya, M., Sparreboom, A., Trepel, J.B., Ye, J., Figg, W.D., Hwang, K., Chung, E.J., Murgo, A., Melillo, G., Elsayed, Y., Monga, M., Kalnitskiy, M., Zwiebel, J. and Sausville, E.A., 2005. Phase I and pharmacokinetic study of MS-275, a histone deacetylase inhibitor, in patients with advanced and refractory solid tumors or lymphoma. *Journal of Clinical Oncology*, 23 (17), pp. 3912-22.

Samuels, B., Herndon, J.E. 2nd, Harmon, D.C., Carey, R., Aisner, J., Corson, J.M., Suzuki, Y., Green, M.R. and Vogelzang, N.J., 1998. Dihydro-5-Azacytidine and Cisplatin in the Treatment of Malignant Mesothelioma. A Phase II Study by the Cancer and Leukemia Group B. *Cancer*, 82, pp. 1578-84.

Sanchez-Cespedes M, Esteller, M., Wu, L., Nawroz-Danish, H., Yoo, G.H., Koch, W.M., Jen, J., Herman, J.G. and Sidransky, D., 2000. Gene promoter hypermethylation in tumors and serum of head and neck cancer patients. *Cancer Research*, 60, pp. 892-5.

Sandor, V., Bakke, S., Robey, R.W., Kang, M.H., Blagosklonny, M.V., Bender, J., Brooks, R., Piekarz, R.L., Tucker, E., Figg, W.D., Chan, K.K., Goldspiel, B., Fojo, A.T., Balcerzak, S.P. and Bates, S.E., 2002. Phase I trial of the histone deacetylase inhibitor, depsipeptide (FR901228, NSC 630176), in patients with refractory neoplasms. *Clinical Cancer Research*, 8 (3), pp. 718-28.

Sargeant, A.M., Rengel, R.C., Kulp, S.K., Klein, R.D., Clinton, S.K., Wang, Y.C. and Chen, C.S., 2008. OSU-HDAC42, a Histone Deacetylase Inhibitor, Blocks Prostate Tumor Progression in the Transgenic Adenocarcinoma of the Mouse Prostate Model. *Cancer Research*, 68, pp. 3999-4009.

Savickiene, J., Borutinskaite, V.V., Treigyte, G., Magnusson, K.E. and Navakauskiene, R., 2006. The novel histone deacetylase inhibitor BML-210 exerts growth inhibitory, proapoptotic and differentiation stimulating effects on the human leukemia cell lines. *European Journal of Pharmacology*, 549 (1-3), pp 9-18

Shah, A.M. and Schwartz, G.K., 2001. Cell cycle-mediated drug resistance: an emerging concept in cancer therapy. *Clinical Cancer Research*, 7, pp. 2168-81.

Shao, J., Xu, D., Tsai, S.N., Wang, Y. and Ngai, S.M., 2009. Computational identification of protein methylation sites through bi-profile Bayes feature extraction. *PLoS One*, 4 (3), pp. e4920.

Sharma, A., Mehan, M.M., Sinha, S., Cowden, J.W. and Mohan, R.R., 2009. Trichostatin a inhibits corneal haze *in vitro* and *in vivo*. *Investigative Ophthalmology & Visual Science*, 50, pp. 2695-701.

Shore, S., Raraty, M.G., Ghaneh, P. and Neoptolemos, J.P., 2003. Chemotherapy for Pancreatic Cancer: Chemotherapy Agents in Advanced Pancreatic Cancer. *Alimentary Pharmacology and Therapeutics*, 18, pp. 1049-69.

Silverman, L.R., Demakos, E.P., Peterson, B.L., Kornblith, A.B., Holland, J.C., Odchimar-Reissig, R., Stone, R.M., Nelson, D., Powell, B.L., DeCastro, C.M., Ellerton, J., Larson, R.A., Schiffer, C.A. and Holland J.F., 2002. Randomized controlled trial of azacitidine in patients with the myelodysplastic syndrome: a study of the cancer and leukemia group B. *Journal of Clinical Oncology*, 20 (10), pp. 2429-40.

Stirzaker, C., Song, J.Z., Davidson, B. and Clark, S.J., 2004. Transcriptional gene silencing promotes DNA hypermethylation through a sequential change in chromatin modifications in cancer cells. *Cancer Research*, 64, pp. 3871-7.

Strathdee, G., MacKean, M.J., Illand, M. and Brown, R., 1999. A role for methylation of the hMLH1 promoter in loss of hMLH1 expression and drug resistance in ovarian cancer. *Oncogene*, 18, pp. 2335-41.

Su, G.H., Sohn, T.A., Ryu, B. and Kern, S.E., 2000. A Novel Histone Deacetylase Inhibitor Identified by High-Throughput Transcriptional Screening of a Compound Library. *Cancer Research*, 60, pp. 3137-42.

Subramaniam, S., Bates, S.E., Wright, J.J., Espinoza-Delgado I. and Piekarz R.L., 2010. Clinical Toxicities of Histone Deacetylase Inhibitors. *Pharmaceuticals*, 3(9), pp. 2751-67.

Sullivan, S., Sink, D.W., Trout, K.L., Makalowska, I., Taylor, P.M., Baxevanis, A.D. and Landsman, D., 2002. The Histone Database. *Nucleic Acids Research,* 30 (1), pp. 341-2.

Takai, D. and Jones, P.A., 2003. The CpG island searcher: a new WWW resource. *In Silico Biology*, 3 (3), pp. 235-40.

Tan, J., Cang, S., Ma, Y., Petrillo, R.L. and Liu, D., 2010. Novel histone deacetylase inhibitors in clinical trials as anti-cancer agents. *Journal of Hematology & Oncology*, 3, 5.

Taniguchi, T., Tischkowitz, M., Ameziane, N., Hodgson, S.V., Mathew, C.G., Joenje, H., Mok, S.C. and D'Andrea, A.D., 2003. Disruption of the Fanconi anemia-BRCA pathway in cisplatin-sensitive ovarian tumors. *Nature Medicine*, 9, pp. 568-74.

Teodoridis, J.M., Strathdee, G., Plumb, J.A. and Brown, R., 2004. CpG-island methylation and epigenetic control of resistance to chemotherapy. *Biochemistry of Society Transactions*, 32, pp. 916-7.

Toedling, J., Skylar, O., Krueger, T., Fischer, J.J., Sperling, S. and Huber, W., 2007. Ringo – an R/Bioconductor package for analyzing ChIP-chip readouts. *BMC Bioinformatics*, 8, pp. 443.

Toft, N.J., Winton, D.J., Kelly, J., Howard, L.A., Dekker, M., te Riele, H., Arends, M.J., Wyllie, A.H., Margison, G.P. and Clarke, A.R., 1999. Msh2 status modulates both apoptosis and mutation frequency in the murine small intestine. *Proceedings of the National Academy of Sciences of USA*, 96, pp. 3911-4.

Tost, J., Schatz, P., Schuster, M., Berlin, K. and Gut, I.G., 2003. Analysis and accurate quantification of CpG methylation by MALDI mass spectrometry. *Nucleic Acids Research*, 31 (9), e50.

Toyota, M. and Issa, J.P., 2005. Epigenetic changes in solid and hematopoietic tumors. *Seminars in Oncology*, 32 (5), pp. 521-30.

Villar-Garea, A., Fraga, M.F., Espada, J. and Esteller, M., 2003. Procaine is a DNA-demethylating agent with growth-inhibitory effects in human cancer cells. *Cancer Research*, 63, pp. 4984-9.

Vu T.H., Chuyen N.V., Li T., Hoffman A.R. 2003. Loss of imprinting of IGF2 sense and antisense transcripts in Wilms' tumor. *Cancer Research*, 63, pp. 1900-1905

Wang, D.F., Helquist, P., Wiech, N.L. and Wiest, O., 2005. Toward selective histone deacetylase inhibitor design: homology modeling, docking studies, and molecular dynamics simulations of human class I histone deacetylases. *Journal of Medical Chemistry*, 48 (22), pp. 6936-47.

Wang, Y.S., Xiong, X.R., An, Z.X., Wang, L.J., Liu, J., Quan, F.S., Hua, S., and Zhang, Y., 2010. Production of cloned calves by combination treatment of both donor cells and early cloned embryos with 5-aza-2'-deoxycytidine and trichostatin A. *Theriogenology*, Vol. 75 (5), pp. 819-25.

Weng, S., Wu, E., Kulp, S.K., Wang, D., Chen, C., Yee, L.D., 2009. The antitumor effects of OSU-HDAC42, a novel histone deacetylase inhibitor, in HER-2-positive breast cancer. *Journal of Clinical Oncology*, Vol. 27, e14587, pp. 4792-8.

Wilhelm, M., O'Brien, S., Rios, M.B., Estey, E., Keating, M.J., Plunkett, W., Sorenson, M. and Kantarjian, H.M., 1999. Phase I study of arabinosyl-5-azacytidine (fazarabine) in adult acute leukemia and chronic myelogenous leukemia in blastic phase. *Leukemia and Lymphoma*, 3, pp. 511-8.

Won, K.J., Chepelev, I., Ren, B. and Wang, W., 2008. Prediction of regulatory elements in mammalian genomes using chromatin signatures. *BMC Bioinformatics*, 9, pp. 547.

Xu, H., Wei, C.L., Lin, F. and Sung, W.K., 2008. An HMM approach to genome-wide identification of differential histone modification sites from ChIP-seq data. *Bioinformatics*, 24 (20), pp. 2344-9.

Yoo, C.B., Cheng, J.C. and Jones, P.A., 2004. Zebularine: a new drug for epigenetic therapy. *Biochemical Society Transactions*, 32 (6), pp. 910-2.

Yoshida, M., Kijima, M., Akita, M. and Beppu, T., 1990. Potent and specific inhibition of mammalian histone deacetylase both *in vivo* and *in vitro*. *Journal of Biological Chemistry*, 265, pp. 17174-9.

Zhang, Y., Lv, J., Liu, H., Zhu, J., Su, J., Wu, Q., Qi, Y., Wang, F. and Li, X., 2010. HHMD: the human histone modification database. *Nucleic Acids Research*, 38, pp. D149-54.

Zhang, Z., 2001. Technology evaluation: MG-98, MethylGene. *Current Opinion in Molecular Therapeutics*, 3, 599-604.

Send Orders for Reprints to reprints@benthamscience.net
Cutting Edge Therapies for Cancer in the 21st Century, 2014, 81-110

CHAPTER 3

Radiation in Cancer Therapy

Ana L. Romero-Weaver[1,*] and Candace M. Howard[2,3]

[1]Department of Radiation Oncology, University of Pennsylvania School of Medicine, Philadelphia, PA, USA; [2]Tri-State Radiology, Dept. of Radiology, King's Daughters Medical Center, Ashland, KY and [3]Department of Orthopedic Surgery, and Department of Biochemistry and Microbiology, Joan C. Edwards School of Medicine, Marshall University, Huntington, WV, USA

Abstract: The discovery of x-rays by Wilhelm Conrad Roentgen and natural radiation by Henry Becquerel and Marie and Pierre Curie at the end of the 19th century was the cornerstone for the development of a new discipline: Radiology. Soon after the discovery of radiation, its diagnostic and therapeutic applications became evident and for more than 100 years it has been utilized in the diagnosis and treatment of cancer. During the last three decades the invention of computerized tomography, magnetic resonance and the development of fractionated therapy have improved planning and provided more accurate dosing. The current radiation techniques are capable of delivering more individualized treatment with less harm to normal adjacent tissue; therefore, more patients are treated with some form of radiation. Current radiation treatment planning modalities include three-dimensional conformational radiation therapy (3D-CRT), which accounts for tumor volume to approximate the radiation beam to the shape of the tumor; intensity-modulated radiation therapy (IMRT), a more advanced form of 3D-CRT, which utilizes varying intensities of radiation beams to produce dosage distributions that are more precise than with 3D-CRT; and four-dimensional radiation therapy (4D-RT) which not only accounts for volume and tumor shape but also considers patient and organ motion. Radiation treatment modalities can be divided into external beam radiation treatment, brachytherapy, and targeted radiotherapy. This chapter will focus on the historical events that have led to the current progress in radiation therapy, the generation of therapeutic radiation, mode of action, current radiation planning and treatment modalities, and side effects.

Keywords: Cancer, radiation therapy, ionizing radiation, x-rays, three-dimensional conformational radiation therapy (3D-CRT), intensity-modulated radiation therapy (IMRT), four-dimensional radiation therapy (4D-RT),

***Address correspondence to Ana L. Romero-Weaver:** Department of Radiation Oncology, University of Pennsylvania School of Medicine, Philadelphia, PA 19104, USA; Tel: (215) 898-0270; Fax: (215) 898-1411; E-mail: ana.romero-weaver@uphs.upenn.edu

brachytherapy, external beam radiation treatment, targeted radiotherapy, radium, nuclear reactors, particle accelerators, cycle accelerators, linear accelerator, conformal radiotherapy, stereotactic radiotherapy, gamma knife, neutron beam therapy, proton beam therapy, Bragg peak.

I. HISTORICAL OVERVIEW

The discovery of radiation at the end of the 19th century is closely associated with "cathode rays" research. During the 1920s Michael Faraday, an English chemist and physicist, observed that when a current was applied to electrodes contained in a glass tube, a luminescent light was emitted (Dahl PF 1997, Thompson 1938, AGN 1931). Physicists of the 1800s were interested in determining the nature of that luminescent light. Around 1857 Julius Plücker evacuated the air from the tube utilizing a pump designed by the German physicist and glassblower Johann Heinrich Wilhelm Geissler and observed that application of a magnetic force changed the direction of the luminescence (Dahl PF 1997, Rossi and Kellerer 1995). In 1869 Johann Wilhelm Hittorf, a German physicist, was the first to observe that the luminescence was traveling in a straight line from the cathode (Muller 2011, Dahl PF 1997). In 1871 Cromwell Fleetwood Varley, an English engineer published a paper suggesting that the luminescence emanated from the cathode was caused by the collision of particles, and since it can be deflected by a magnetic field, the particles must be electrically charged (Lee 1932). In 1875, the English physicist William Crookes improved the glass tubes and designed his own pump with which almost all the air could be evacuated (Dahl PF 1997). The "Crookes tube" soon replaced the "Geissler tubes". Crookes concluded that the rays were particles from the residual air that became electrically charged and were repelled at the cathode (Rossi and Kellerer 1995, Dahl PF 1997). In 1876 another German physicist, Eugene Goldstein, gave the name of "cathode rays" to the luminescence traveling from the cathode to the anode (Dahl PF 1997, Rossi and Kellerer 1995). In 1886 Goldstein also demonstrated that in addition to cathode rays there were other rays traveling in the opposite direction, and he named them canal rays (Dahl PF 1997).

In the early 1890s, the German physicist Heinrich Hertz, observed that the cathode rays were able to penetrate thin metal foil placed in the path of the rays, and the glass still glowed, as though the rays slipped through the foil (Peh 1995). His assistant, Philipp Lenard, continued with Hertz experiments. Finding it difficult to study cathode rays inside a sealed glass tube, he introduced a thin aluminum window. This was enough to maintain the vacuum inside the tube, but yet thin enough to allow the cathode rays to pass out (Peh 1995). In 1895 Wilhem Conrad Roentgen, a professor at the Wuerzburd University, Germany (Haas 2001), was working with the cathode rays introducing a thin aluminum window in a similar way as Philipp Lenard (Peh 1995, Eisenberg 1992, Frankel 1996), Roentgen also covered the tube with cardboard and observed that when a high voltage was applied to the tube a fluorescent light was emitted, which was captured by a nearby piece of paper painted with barium platinocyanide (Rossi and Kellerer 1995, Frankel 1996). He concluded that the rays were emitted from the tube and were capable of passing through a heavy opaque paper which was impenetrable to ordinary light (Mould 1995a), he found that the new rays could pass through most substances including human tissue, but they were unable to penetrate bones or metal objects (Mould 1995a). He could not detect any appreciable reflection or refraction of the rays, and, contrary to cathode rays, these new rays were not deflected with a magnetic field (Turner 2007, Mould 1995a). He called them x-rays, with the "x" representing the unknown. In 1901 he was awarded the first Nobel Prize in Physics for his discovery (Mould 1995a).

Roentgen's findings created a great sensation and inspired several scientists to initiate investigations in this new field. Shortly after Roentgen's discovery of x-rays, the French scientist and member of the French Academy of Sciences (Blaufox 1996), Antoine Henri Becquerel found another form of radiation, natural radiation. He was working with the phenomenon of fluorescence and decided to investigate whether there was a connection between x-rays and fluorescence (Allisy 1996). He initiated his studies with a supply of uranium salts he inherited from his father (Blaufox 1996). These salts phosphoresced upon exposure to light (Blaufox 1996). He placed sheets of double sulphate of uranium and potassium on photographic plates enveloped in black paper or protected by a sheet of aluminum. After he exposed them to light for several hours, the plates were found to be fogged. He repeated this experiment, but because the day was cloudy, he put the covered plate in a drawer (Dutreix and Dutreix 1995). Later when he developed the plate, he found that the images were very intense (Myers 1976). Thus, the uranium salt emitted rays capable of penetrating black paper, whether or not it had been previously exposed to sunlight (Becquerel and Crowther 1948). Becquerel stated in his Nobel Prize reception speech "…the emission was independent of any familiar source of excitation, such as light, electricity or heat; this was a spontaneous phenomenon of a new order…" (Nobel lectures 1967). Later, Becquerel also showed that the rays emitted by uranium caused gases to ionize (Allisy 1996).

Pierre and Marie Sklodowska Curie continued studies on the Becquerel's rays. Marie repeated the Becquerel's experiments and confirmed that the intensity of uranium radiation emission was proportional to the amount of uranium in the compound and independent of its chemical state (de Hevesy 1984, Coppes-Zantinga and Coppes 1998a). Marie and Pierre Curie examined all the elements they knew and found that only thorium emitted rays similar to uranium (Mould 1998). This led them to investigate natural ores and found that the radioactivity of the ores was greater than could be accounted for by only the uranium and thorium content (Diamantis *et al*., 2008). They isolated the strong activity to fractions containing bismuth or barium. By the end of June 1898 a substance with an activity about 900 times stronger than uranium was purified from the bismuth fraction and it was concluded that this was a new element, which they named polonium in honor of Marie's native country Poland (Coppes-Zantinga and Coppes 1998b, Diamantis *et al.,* 2008). They also separated radioactivity from the barium fraction and found a new compound more radioactive than polonium, which they called radium (Mazeron and Gerbaulet 1998, Diamantis *et al.,* 2008). Marie proposed the word "radioactivity" to describe the phenomenon of spontaneous radiation (Mould 1998). For their discoveries of spontaneous radiation Becquerel and Pierre and Marie Curie were awarded with the Nobel Prize in Physics in 1903 (Mould 1998).

The discovery of x-ray and spontaneous radioactivity created a lot of interest among the scientific community and paved the way for other important discoveries that produced several Nobel Prize laureates and led to the development of current radiation technologies and many other improvements in science and medicine (Rosenow 1995), some of which are described here. With the possibility of visualizing not only bones but also soft tissues and some of their abnormalities without pain, the potential diagnostic and therapeutic applications of x-rays were soon apparent. Months after the discovery of the x-rays the first fluoroscopes to obtain images of the inner body were designed (Frankel 1996). These fluoroscopes consisted of cardboard coated with barium platinocyanide; however the images obtained were faint. In 1896, the American scientist Thomas A. Edison designed the first commercially available fluoroscopes in which barium platinocyanide was substituted by calcium tungstate producing brighter images (Tselos 1995, Frankel 1996). Later in 1916, William Coolidge designed the hot cathode tube, which utilized a tungsten filament allowing for the controling of the quality and quantity of radiation independently (Benier *et al.,* 2004, Frankel 1996). The first therapeutic treatment with x-rays was performed in Vienna in October 1896 by the dermatologist Leopold Freund on a 5 year-old patient suffering from hirsutism, a condition characterized by excessive hair growth in several parts of the body (Mould 2007, Feund 1897). The first verifiable x-ray treatment of cancer was in Stockholm on December 1899 where two general practitioners; Tage Sjogren and Tor Stenbeck, simultaneously reported two successful cancer treatments, one of a basal cell carcinoma of the nose and the other of a squamous cell carcinoma of the cheek (Mould 1995b). In 1903 the first case of cancer of the cervix cured by x-rays was reported by Dr. Margaret Cleaves (Bernier *et al.,* 2004). The therapeutic applications of natural radioactivity were also initiated. The Curies loaned some radium to Henri Danlos in Paris, to treat patients at the St. Louis hospital where he, in 1901, performed the first local application of a sealed radium source to treat a patient with the non-malignant skin condition lupus erythematous (Mazeron and Gerbaulet 1998). The first successful radium treatment for cancer was in 1903 in St Petersburg, Russia, by Goldberg and London who treated two patients suffering from basal cell carcinoma of the face utilizing a similar technique of that utilized by Danlos in Paris (Mazeron and Gerbaulet 1998, Mould 1995b).

During these early years the danger of radiation exposure in patients and medical personnel began to emerge. Patients that were exposed for long periods to fluoroscopy and radiography developed dermatitis, lost hair and manifested deep tissue damage. One of the most dramatic cases was that of Edison's assistant,

Clearance Dally, who suffered from severe radio dermatitis resulting in the amputation of his arm and his subsequent death in 1904 (Brown 1995). Henry Becquerel also noted skin ulceration in the lower abdomen close to the pocket in which he was carrying a tube with radium salts (Myers 1976). Doctors and medical personnel also experienced radiation complications. However, it was difficult for the scientific community to accept that something that could not be seen was the cause of those complications. During 1920s there were several reports supporting the restriction of radiation exposure, which led to the establishment of the International x-ray and Radium Protection Committee (XRPC) in 1928 (Coppes-Zantinga and Coppes 1998a), which was later established as the International Committee of Radiological Protection (ICRP) (Taylor 1958). The radiation field continued evolving and many important discoveries occurred such as the discovery of the electron by Joseph John Thompson in 1897 (Thomas 2006). At about the same time Ernest Rutherford discovered the alpha rays (Hall and Giaccia 2011).

In 1900 Paul Villard discovered gamma-rays (Gerward 1999). In 1932 James Chadwick discovered the neutron (Hall and Giaccia 2011) and in the same year Irene Joliot-Curie, Pierre and Marie Curie's daughter and her husband Frederick Joliot discovered artificial radioactivity (Mazeron and Gerbaulet 1998). In 1934, the United States XRPC proposed the first standard for individual radiation protection (Jones 2005). Also in 1934 Ernest Laurence invented the cyclotron, a device to accelerate nuclear particles (Podgorsak 2010). After his discovery other particle accelerators were developed. During World War II, advances were made in the production of magnetrons in radar systems, which allowed the use of microwave generators for electron acceleration, and in 1946 D. W. Fry demonstrated the first traveling-wave linear accelerator (Fry *et al.,* 1947, Fry *et al.,* 1948). After World War II, the effects of radiation in the atomic bomb survivors of Hiroshima and Nagasaki were more evident and decisive for the establishment of legislation for radiation protection, which has been adopted by many countries (Clarke and Valentin 2005). The development of computed tomography (CT), magnetic resonance imaging (MRI) and positron emission tomography (PET) during the 1970's (Lauterbur 1980, Mansfield and Maudsley 1977, Ak 2000) revolutionized not only diagnostic medicine but also radiation treatment and planning allowing the development of three-dimensional (3D) and four-dimensional (4D) planning techniques which are capable of providing a more precise treatment of tumors with less harm to normal tissue (Smith *et al.,* 2006). More recently in 2008, the first hybrid PET/MRI system for use in humans was developed which represents the next generation of instruments for radiation treatment planning (Pichler *et al.,* 2008). This field is continuously evolving, and many more exciting discoveries are expected.

II. TYPES OF THERAPEUTIC RADIATION

The spectrum of radiation can be divided into two major types of radiation: non-ionizing radiation and ionizing radiation. In this section only ionizing radiation will be considered, since it is the type of radiation utilized in cancer treatment. Ionization is the process by which a neutral atom becomes negatively or positively charged (Khan 2010). Acquisition of one or more electrons by a neutral atom leaves the atom negatively charged, while removal of one or more orbital electrons from a neutral atom leaves it positively charged (Khan 2010). This process requires a lot of energy. Ionizing radiation has enough energy to ionize adjacent atoms (Khan 2010). Ionizing radiation can be subdivided into the following categories, also summarized in Table **1**:

A. According to Their Nature

Ionizing radiation can be divided according to its nature in electromagnetic radiation or particulate radiation (Hall & Giaccia 2011). Electromagnetic radiation is a wave and a packet of energy also known as photon radiation. There are two forms of electromagnetic radiation: x-rays which are produced extranuclearly by electrical machines such as linear accelerators (Hall & Giaccia 2011) and gamma-rays, produced intranuclearly, most commonly by decay of radioactive isotopes such as cobalt-60 (Hall & Giaccia 2011). Particulate radiation possesses mass and comes primarily from radioactive materials, outer space, or machines that accelerate particles to very high velocities (Silari 2011).

B. According to the Mode of Ionization

Ionizing radiation can be divided into directly ionizing radiation and indirectly ionizing radiation. Directly ionizing radiation comprises charged particles such as electrons, protons, alpha particles and heavy ions (Podgorsak 2010). This type of radiation directly ionizes cellular components, usually DNA, causing critical damage to the cell. Indirectly ionizing particles comprise neutral particles, such as x-rays, gamma-rays, and neutrons (Hall and Giaccia 2011, Podgorsak 2010). In this case the radiation does not have a direct interaction with cellular components, but with other molecules in the cell, usually water, produces highly reactive free radicals that then can damage critical cell components (Hall and Giaccia 2011).

C. According to Their Linear Energy Transfer

Ionizing radiation can also be classified according to the energy it deposits over a given length of the track it crosses which is known as linear energy transfer (LET), in low LET radiation and high LET radiation. Low LET radiation creates ion pairs separated by relatively large distances while high LET radiation creates ion pairs that are of relatively short range. Gamma-rays and x-rays emit low LET radiation while neutrons and heavy ions emit high LET. The LET of electrons and protons varies according to their energy (Table **1**) (Yang 1999, Cucinotta *et al.,* 1991, Podgorsak 2010).

Table 1: Classification of ionizing radiation.

Radiation	Nature	Mode of Action	LET
x-rays	Electromagnetic	Indirect	Low
Gamma-rays	Electromagnetic	Indirect	Low
Electrons (10 MeV, 1 MeV)	Particulate	Direct	Low
Electrons (1 KeV)	Particulate	Direct	High
Neutrons	Particulate	Indirect	High
Protons (9000 to 10 MeV)	Particulate	Direct	Low
Protons (>1 GeV, 2 MeV)	Particulate	Direct	High

III. UNITS OF THERAPEUTIC RADIATION

Only radiation units utilized in this chapter will be defined, these include the following:

A. Energy Unit

The smallest energy unit is the electron volt (eV). Therapeutic radiation is expressed in eV multiples such as kiloelectron volts (keV) and megaelectron volts (MeV) (Jayaraman and Lanzl 2004, Huda 2003).

B. Absorbed Dose Unit

Dose is defined as the energy absorbed per mass of the absorbing matter. Its international system (SI) unit is the gray (Gy), which is defined as 1 Joule of energy absorbed per kilogram of matter (Jayaraman and Lanzl 2004, Huda and Slone 2003).

C. Frequency Unit

The SI unit of frequency is the Hertz (Hz) it describes the number of cycles per second. In radiation, the radiofrequency is measured in megahertz (MHz) (Jayaraman and Lanzl 2004, Huda and Slone 2003).

IV. GENERATION OF THERAPEUTIC RADIATION

Radiation for therapeutic purposes can be produced in nuclear reactors or in particle accelerators.

A. Nuclear Reactors

Gamma-rays and radioactive isotopes are generated in nuclear reactors. Activation of cobalt-59 is the main source of gamma-rays. In this process stable cobalt-59 atoms are bombarded with an excess of thermal neutrons in a nuclear reactor (Podgorsak 2010). The bombarded atoms absorb some of the neutrons causing an increase of one in the atomic weight to produce the radioisotope cobalt-60, which emits radioactive energy through the process of radioactive decay, in which the unstable parent nucleus of cobalt-60 loses energy as it transforms into one or several more stable daughter nuclei (1953 Radio-Cobalt). Cobalt-60 has a half-life of 5.3 years; it decays to the stable atom nickel-60 with the emission of beta particles and gamma-rays with energies of 1.17 MeV and 1.33 MeV per each disintegration (Podgorsak 2010). Beta emitter radioisotopes utilized in brachytherapy and radioimmunotherapy are produced in nuclear reactors by thermal neutrons bombarded in a similar way as for the production of cobalt-60 (Volkert *et al.,* 1991, Cantone and Hoeschen 2011).

B. Particle Accelerators

Particle accelerators can be divided into electrostatic accelerators and cyclic accelerators. The use of electrostatic accelerators has decreased considerably as cyclic accelerators are becoming the standard for the production of conventional radiation, x-rays and electrons, as well as for the production of non-conventional radiation such as neutrons and protons.

B. 1. Cyclic Accelerators

Cyclic accelerators can be divided according to the trajectory of the particle during its acceleration in circular and linear accelerators. There are several types of circular accelerators used in medicine, which include cyclotron, betatron and synchrotron (Podgorsak 2010).

Cyclotron

This accelerator was developed by Ernest Lawrence in 1934 (Bridge 1940) for the acceleration of ions to a kinetic energy of a few MeV (Podgorsak 2010). It is utilized for the production of radionuclides for nuclear medicine as well as in the production of proton and neutron beams for radiotherapy (Herbert 1968). A cyclotron consists of two evacuated half-cylindrical electrodes with a D-shape known as Ds separated by a gap. In each D there is a magnetic field perpendicular to the electric field. A radiofrequency voltage with a constant frequency between 10 MHz and 30MHz is applied between the two Ds to produce an electric field (Podgorsak 2010). The charged particle is accelerated while crossing the gap between the two electrodes. The magnetic field bends the path of the particle into a semicircle (Podgorsak 2010). The accelerating electric field reverses just as the particles finish their half cycle to accelerate them across the gap with a higher speed, and they move into a larger semicircle. After repeating this process several times, particles are accelerated to a very high speed (Strijckmans 2001, Foster 1938). For the production of neutrons, cyclotron accelerated protons are bent by a series of magnets that aim the proton beam to strike a beryllium target which produces neutrons as a result of the interaction (Wakabayashi *et al.,* 1986).

Betatron

This accelerator was developed by Donald W. Krest in 1940 as a cyclic electron accelerator (Podgorsak 2010). In the 1950s betatrons played a major role in the production of megavoltage x-rays and electron beams (Hogstrom and Almond 2006, Podgorsak 2010). A betatron consists of a doughnut shaped evacuated tube between the poles of a laminated silicon-steel magnet that is fed by an alternating current of frequencies between 50 Hz and 200 Hz (Jayaraman and Lanzl 2004). A hot filament produces electrons (Podgorsak 2010). A strong burst of positive charge moves them into the evacuated tube where they are accelerated by a magnetic field. As electrons accelerate, the magnetic field increases to maintain the electrons in a circular movement. At each rotation the electrons gain speed. Electrons can circle the evacuated tube thousands of times becoming highly accelerated (Khan 2010). To maintain electrons in a constant circular radius, half of the average of the magnetic field within the circle has to be equal to the magnetic field at the orbit (Jayaraman and Lanzl 2004). Once accelerated to a relativistic speed, electrons are deflected about 1½ inches to strike a metal target producing high energy x-rays which are concentrated into a narrow beam at a known position (Khan 2010).

Synchrotron

It was described in 1948 by Frank Elder, Robert Langmuir, and Herb Pollock (Elder *et al.*, 1948). The synchrotron is the most recent and most powerful member of the circular accelerator family (Podgorsak 2010). Although both electrons and protons can be accelerated, most medical synchrotrons are utilized for the acceleration of protons (Podgorsak 2010). In the synchrotron, like in a betatron, the particles follow a large circular orbit of constant radius inside a circular vacuum chamber. In the case of electrons, an electric shotgun injects them into the evacuated circular chamber (Vylet and Liu 2001). In the case of protons, they are first produced and accelerated in a proton linear accelerator, and then injected into the synchrotron system. Microwave frequency fields accelerate the particles, electrons or protons. A booster ring imparts higher energy to the particles and accelerates them close to the speed of light. Two types of magnets are placed below the buster ring to provide a guiding magnetic field. One type directs the particles around the booster ring, while the other type forces the particles into a fine beam within the evacuated chamber (Margaritondo and Meuli 2003).

B. 2. Linear Accelerators

Medical linear accelerators (Linacs) have become the primary machines for the production of electrons and x-rays for cancer treatment. A typical Linac is composed of an electron gun, a magnetron for the generation of microwaves, an evacuated accelerator tube called an accelerated waveguide, a bending magnet, a metal target, and movable and fixed collimators (Podgorsak 2010). In a Linac electrons are accelerated following straight linear trajectories. Electrons are injected from the electron gun into the waveguide (Vylet and Liu 2001), this waveguide contains several electrically charged chambers. The electrons possessing a negative electric charge move to the next positive charged chamber which then changes from positive to negative charge pushing the electrons forward to the next positively charged chamber (Jayaraman and Lanzl 2004). The microwave radiofrequency of the magnetron in synchrony with the change in magnetic field within the chambers accelerates electrons close to the speed of light (Podgorsak 2010). As the electrons leave the electrically charged chambers, the bending magnets bend the electron beam to a perpendicular direction to strike them with the heavy metal target, which results in the production of x-rays. Then movable and fixed collimators align and shape the x-ray beam (Brown *et al.,* 1999). Electrons can be accelerated to kinetic energies from 4 MeV to 25 MeV (Podgorsak 2010).

V. MODE OF ACTION OF THERAPEUTIC RADIATION

Ionizing radiation targets critical cellular structures. DNA is the main target of ionizing radiation (Willers *et al.,* 2006). DNA damage can be introduced by direct ionization within the DNA molecule produced mainly by high LET radiation or indirectly by the action of free radicals formed as a result of the ionization of water molecules, mainly by low LET radiation (Matsumoto *et al.,* 2009). Different types of DNA damage can be produced which include base damage, DNA-protein cross-links, single strand breaks (SSB) and double strand breaks (DSB) (Belli *et al.,* 2002). Normal cells have mechanisms to repair the majority of ionizing radiation-induced damage (Willers *et al.,* 2004). DSBs are the most difficult to repair, and the most toxic DNA lesions. Unrepaired or misrepaired DSBs can cause mutations or chromosomal aberrations that can lead to cell death or cell transformation (Willers *et al.,* 2006). Unrepaired SSBs can produce DBSs if another hit of ionizing radiation causes a second SSB in close proximity with the previous one (Peoples *et al.,* 2010) or when a replication fork encounters an SSB on the leading strand of the template DNA, causing the fork to collapse with a consequent production of a DSB (Saleh-Gohari *et al.,* 2005). Ionizing radiation cell killing can also occur through the process of apoptosis when, as a consequence of radiation damage at a specific phase of the cell cycle, progression into the cell cycle is delayed to allow the cell repair mechanisms to correct the damage, but due to irreparable damage the cell undergoes programmed cell death (Willers *et al.,* 2006, Harms-Ringdahl 1996, Lichter *et al.,* 1995) or when ionizing radiation damages the cell membrane and/or the mitochondria (Somosy 2000). Lymphocytes, small intestinal crypt cells, germ cells and salivary-gland cells die from apoptosis after a small dose of radiation (Lichter *et al.,* 1995). Other cellular components that are targets of ionizing radiation and contribute to the overall damage include proteins, enzymes, carbohydrates and lipids (Edwards *et al.,* 1984). Recently it has been recognized that ionizing radiation can also affect cells that have not been damaged directly by the radiation. These can be cells that were near or that shared medium with the irradiated cells and this phenomenon is known as the bystander effect (Snyder 2004). This effect is more pronounced when the cells are in gap-junction communication with the irradiated cells (Azzam *et al.,* 2001) than in cells that are separated by several hundred micrometers from the irradiated cells. In the latter case the effect is presumably due to the release of soluble cytotoxic molecules by the irradiated cells (Ramesh *et al.,* 1996). Several factors influence the response of the cell to ionizing radiation, including the cell cycle stage, oxygen concentration, type of LET, radiation dose rate and fractionation. The effects of ionizing radiation appear to be more pronounced during M (mitosis) and G_2 (Gap-2) phases of the cell cycle (Hogle 2006, Kassis 2008). It is believed that oxygen reacts with free radicals formed during ionization of water producing more toxic byproducts that cause cells to be more sensitive to ionizing radiation (Kassis 2008). Solid tumors contain regions with lower blood supply where oxygen concentration is reduced (hypoxia); therefore, these regions are more resistant to the effects of ionizing radiation than well-oxygenated cells (Willers and Held 2006). Low LET radiation produces few direct hits within the nucleus (Feinendegen *et al.,* 2004). High LET radiation is more likely to produce more hits within the nucleus, therefore causing more damage (Goodhead 1999, Hada and Georgakilas 2008). The rate in which a radiation dose is administered affects the effectiveness of radiation treatment. Low dose rates are less effective in producing lethal cell damage than high dose rates. Also fractionation affects the effectiveness of the treatment (Hogle 2006). A fractionated dose of radiation is less effective than a single dose, but it is less toxic to healthy surrounding tissue. Therefore, higher total doses are necessary during fractionation to produce the same effect than with a single dose (Hogle 2006). Some of these parameters may be modified to increase the biological effect of ionizing radiation.

VI. RADIATION TREATMENT MODALITIES

The main objective in cancer radiation therapy is to treat malignant tumor(s) while causing the least amount of damage possible to adjacent normal tissues. This section describes the most current modalities of radiation utilized in cancer therapy, which can be divided into three main groups: external beam radiotherapy, sealed radiotherapy (brachytherapy) and targeted radiotherapy.

A. External Beam Radiotherapy

This form of radiation is utilized for almost all types of tumors. It can be divided into conventional external beam radiotherapy, conformal therapy, stereotactic radiation, intraoperative radiation and charged particle treatment.

A.1. Conventional External Beam Radiotherapy

It is also known as teletherapy and consists of a single beam delivered from one to four directions. In this modality the healthy tissue that is in close proximity to the target tumor may receive toxic doses of radiation, limiting the dose that can be delivered to the tumor. For this reason, this modality is being substituted by conformal radiotherapy, which is becoming the standard treatment for a number of tumor sites (Gerber and Chan 2008).

A.2. Conformal Radiotherapy

It is a linear accelerator-based treatment. In this form of therapy, radiation treatment planning is very important to shape the dose as close as possible to the desired target tumor while minimizing the exposure to the adjacent normal tissue. Radiation planning involves several modalities, including: three-dimensional conformal radiotherapy (3D-CRT), intensity modulated radiation therapy (IMRT), and four dimensional radiation therapy (4D-RT). The use of specialized CT and

MRI scanners as well as specialized three dimensional (3D) planning software has allowed better planning and delivery of the radiation treatment to the target tumor while toxicity to the surrounding normal tissue is reduced (Gerber and Chan 2008). The current radiation planning modalities are described below:

Three- Dimensional Conformal Radiotherapy (3D-CRT)

In this modality the radiation therapy is delivered by medical linear accelerators. Tumor target, target volume and organ risk contours are delineated using a volumetric CT database (Gerber and Chan 2008). The 3D images are linked to a treatment planning software that possesses a beam's eye view (BEV) display that allows to visualize critical structure volumes and target volumes (Stephenson and Wiley 1995) thus shielding blocks and multileaf collimators, that contain multiple pairs of thin leaves, can be moved independently from each other to create and to determine beam direction and intensity. Then the dose can be calculated using a rectilinear coordinate system attached to the patient's 3D-CT. The treatment plan is then evaluated and, if necessary, it can be modified until an accepted plan is approved. This modality is known as forward planning (Smith *et al.,* 2006, Bucci *et al.,* 2005, Hogle 2006).

Intensity-Modulated-Radiation Therapy (IMRT)

This modality is an advanced form of 3D-CRT planning. It is a linear accelerator based radiation treatment (Gerber and Chan 2008). Contrary to 3D-CRT which is a forward treatment planning, IMRT is an inverse treatment planning (Smith *et al.,* 2006), meaning that dose distribution for both the target and avoidance structures is established first, then computer optimization proceeds to adjust beam intensities in order to achieve the determined dose distribution (Smith *et al.,* 2006). It also has the advantage over 3D-CRT that can conform the treatment volume to concave shaped tumors. As the name implies, IMRT allows the modulation of the intensity of each beam of radiation producing areas of low-intensity radiation among the surrounding normal tissue and high-intensity radiation near the gross tumor volume and in this way each patient's treatment can be customized (Bucci *et al.,* 2005, Hogle 2006). IMRT can be delivered using linear accelerators with static multi-leaf collimators (MLC, step and shoot IMRT) or dynamic leaf MLCs, tomotherapy machines or volumetric arc modulated therapy (VMAT) (Hong *et al.,* 2005). In IMRT planning the verification of the radiation dose is more time consuming than with 3D-CRT (Smith *et al.,* 2006). In both 3D-CRT and IMRT planning, organ movement produced by breathing should be considered. Organ movement can increase the apparent size of a tumor causing the actual dose delivered to be different than the calculated dose, which may result in overdosing adjacent critical organs or under dosing the target tumor; therefore, it may be necessary to increase normal tissue irradiation to ensure that the target tumor is not missed as a result of movement (Smith *et al.,* 2006). Also, as daily treatment times increase, the volume of normal tissue receiving some radiation dose increases. In this regard, consideration of physiologic organ motion is crucial for radiation therapy planning, especially for tumors in the thorax and abdomen, which are particularly affected by respiratory movement (Ikushima 2010). Recently, 4D-CT scanners have been developed to account for organ motion.

Four-Dimensional Radiation Therapy (4D-RT)

This technique was developed to account for tumor and normal tissue movement as a result of respiration. It can provide a more accurate treatment by reducing acute complications resulting from dose delivered to critical normal organs. In this technique a 4D-CT scan or 4D-MRI take constant images that are utilized to produce a 3D image showing the body's movement, and the time that the target tumor remains in each phase of the breathing cycle (inhalation and exhalation) is determined (Biederer *et al.,* 2010, Li *et al.,* 2008, Ikushima 2010). Then the radiation dose is delivered to the tumor within a certain interval in the breathing cycle, this reduces toxicity to adjacent normal tissue and allows the dose to the target tumor to be increased (Verellen *et al.,* 2010). However, not all the breathing cycles are regular, and some dose can be delivered to the normal tissue.

A.3. Stereotactic Radiotherapy

This form of external beam radiation therapy was developed by Lars Leksell, a Swedish neurosurgeon in 1951 (Leksell 1951). It was originally developed for intracranial lesions, but it has been extended to treat other sites. It utilizes 3D planning imagery and a precise dose determination and treatment set-up to deliver conformed high dose radiation with extreme accuracy and improves tumor control while limiting toxicity to the normal tissue (Ikushima 2010). Two current stereotactic techniques are the gamma knife and the ciberknife.

Gamma Knife

It utilizes gamma-rays produced from cobalt-60 sources (Leksell 1968) or neutrons and protons produced from a cyclotron. It is most often used for the treatment of small and medium tumors and other lesions in the brain (Koga *et al.,* 2010). It can also be utilized when the brain lesion cannot be reached by conventional surgical techniques or patient condition do not allow a surgical procedure. The precise location of the lesion to be treated is determined using CT scans and MRI imaging (Gerber and Chan 2008). Once the images are obtained the radiation team determines the dose and treatment plan. Several beams of radiation are very precisely focused to reach the area being treated while reducing exposure of the surrounding normal tissue (Gerber and Chan 2008). It is important to prevent head movement during treatment. This is accomplished by attaching a box-shaped frame to the head, which also helps guide and focus the gamma-rays beams to the exact area of treatment (Gerber and Chan 2008). During gamma knife treatment the equipment remains static.

Ciberknife

The current cyberknife technology utilizes image-guided lightweight linear accelerators attached to a very versatile robotic arm (Adler *et al.,* 1997, Hogle 2006). An advanced software imaging system localizes the tumor while real-time images allow compensating for breathing and patient movement (Gibbs 2006, Sarfaraz 2007). The dose is calculated, and a robotic arm delivery system conveys multiple beams of high radiation dose from different angles that converge in the target tumor. Because corrections from movement can be made and the robotic arm is not static; there is no need to immobilize the patient (Kilby *et al.,* 2010). The treatment is not restricted to intracranial lesions, but it can be expended to virtually all lesions in the body. However, when extracranial lesions are treated, interstitial fiducial markers may be necessary to guide the CT scan, so the image-guided software can precisely focus on the target (Pop *et al.,* 2010).

A.4. Particle Radiation Therapy (Hadrontherapy)

Conventional external beam radiation therapy uses high-energy x-rays and electron beams to deliver the radiation dose. Non-conventional external radiation treatment involves the use of particle radiation instead of x-rays or electrons. Particle radiation has the advantage that it allows precise dose localization and better depth dose distribution (Rong and Welsh 2010). It is useful to treat tumors located in or near critical body parts or to treat hypoxic tumors which are usually more resistant to conventional radiation therapy, but respond better to particle radiation (Shahri *et al.,* 2011).

Neutron Therapy

It was initiated in the late 1930's in an attempt to increase killing of hypoxic cells, which are more radioresistant to photon therapy (Stone 1948). Neutrons are high LET radiation; therefore, they cause more damage to the cells they hit than x-rays or gamma-rays (Shahri *et al.,* 2011). Some sites that may be appropriated for neutron radiation therapy include: salivary glands, tongue, pharynx, oral cavity, nasopharinx, prostate, bladder, uterus, rectosigmoid, soft tissue, bone, cartilage, pancreas, colon, bile duct, ampulla vater, peritoneum, localized tumors of lung, mediastinum, pleura, and pericardium (Cohen and Hendrickson 1989). A promising approach utilizing neutrons is the boron neutron capture therapy (BNCT). In this technique patients are injected with boron-10, a stable compound, which preferentially binds to tumor cells. Then patients are irradiated with low energy thermal neutrons from a nuclear reactor causing the production of the unstable boron-11 isotope, which then undergoes instantaneous nuclear fission producing high-energy alpha particles and recoiling lithium-7 nuclei (Coderre and Morris 1999, Noda *et al.,* 2009). These particles have pathlengths of approximately one cell diameter (5-9 μm) and deposit most of their energy within the boron containing cells sparing the normal adjacent cells (Barth *et al.,* 2005). Clinical interest in BNCT has focused primarily on the treatment of high-grade gliomas, cutaneous melanomas or cerebral metastases of melanoma, head and neck and liver cancer (Barth *et al.,* 2005).

Proton Therapy

Protons are produced in cyclotron and synchrotron accelerators. Protons achieve most of their advantage over photons in their physical dose distribution (Smith *et al.,* 2006, MacDonald *et al.,* 2006). Photons deliver the largest dose immediately after penetration into the body, while when protons pass through tissue, the dose they deposit increases slowly with depth, reaching a sharp dose increase at its maximum depth of penetration known as the Bragg peak (Fig. **1**), and then falls off rapidly to virtually zero (Smith *et al.,* 2006, Levin *et al.,* 2005), therefore, the tumor can be irradiated more precisely. The maximum depth of penetration may be adjusted by varying the energy of the proton beam. It is possible to deposit a homogenous 3 D-dose in the target tumor by spreading out the Bragg peak depth using specialized filters that help to achieve the dose deposition pattern desired, thereby sparing the surrounding normal tissue (Cella *et al.,* 2001). Usually proton therapy has been utilized for tumors in close proximity to critical structures or tumors with previously poor cure and control rates (Smith *et al.,* 2006), but recently its use has been extended to other locations. Tumors treated with protons include chordomas, chondrosarcomas, glioblastoma multiforme, uveal melanoma, tumors of the paranasal sinuses, meningioma, prostate cancer, hepatocellular carcinoma, and non–small cell lung cancer (Smith *et al.,* 2006, Levin *et al.,* 2005). Protons have also been used in stereotactic radiosurgery (Levy *et al.,* 1999, Chen *et al.,* 2007). Proton therapy is one of the most promising modalities; however the high cost of proton facility installation has been an obstacle for the generalization of this radiation treatment technique.

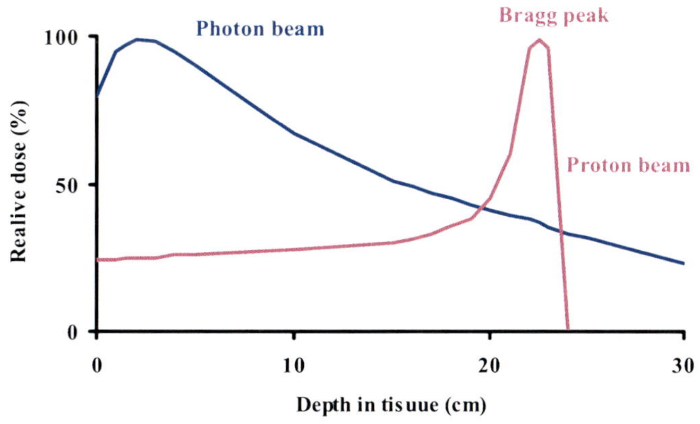

Figure 1: Depth dose distribution of a photon beam and a proton beam showing the proton's Bragg peak.

B. Brachytherapy

In this radiation treatment modality beta emitter radioinuclides produced in nuclear reactors are precisely placed temporarily or permanently in close proximity to the tumor. It can be placed directly into a body cavity (intracavity) (Brenner 1997), into the tissue (interstitial) (Kolotas and Zamboglou 2001), onto a tissue surface (plaque) (Wen and McCannel 2009), into a body lumen (intraluminal) (Murakami 2011), into the lungs (endobronchial) (Gejerman *et al.,* 2002), and into blood vessels (endovascular) (Balter 1998). Precise placement of the radiation sources allows the delivery of high doses of radiation to the specific tumor while the radiation dose drops off within the adjacent normal tissue reducing toxicity in this area. CT and MRI have been utilized to determine the exact location where the radioactive source will be inserted (Williamson 2006, Erickson 2005). New developments in 3D ultrasound imaging have allowed for a more accurate planning and a more precise placement of the radiation source (Wei *et al.,* 2005). Some of the most common radionuclides utilized in brachytherapy include Cesium-137, Cobalt-60, Iridium-192, Iodine-125, Palladium-103, Gold-198, Strontium-90 and Ruthenium-106 (Welsh 2007, Brady and Hernandez 1992). Special applicators, depending on tumor location, are utilized to place the radiation source (Perea and Brady's 2008). Both high dose rate (HDR) and low dose rate (LDR) brachytherapy can be utilized (Crownover *et al.,* 1999). HDR brachyhterapy is usually an outpatient procedure (Nag 2004), while LDR brachytherapy often requires hospitalization (Watkins *et al.,* 2011). Locations were brachytherapy sources can be placed include: head and neck, prostate gland, central nervous system, breast, lungs, cervix, uterus, bladder, soft tissue, and the vascular system.

C. Targeted Radiotherapy

In this form of radiotherapy the tissue to be treated can be targeted utilizing the chemical properties of a radionuclide which can be specifically absorbed by a specific tissue, for example the radionuclide Iodine-131 is absorbed by the thyroid gland with a much higher affinity than any other organ, and is utilized to treat malignancies in this specific tissue (Gerber and Chan 2008). Targeting can also be achieved by attaching the radioisotope to other molecules such as monoclonal antibodies resulting in a more localized target-specific irradiation (Brechbiel

2007). This type of treatment is referred as radioimmunotherapy (RIT) (Britton *et al.* 1991). Beta-emitters produced in nuclear reactors are the most commonly used radionuclides for targeted radiotherapy; however, some alpha-emitters and auger-electron emitters can be utilized (Kassis 2008, Ng 2006). High-energy beta-emitters such as Yttrium-90 can be utilized for large tumors; however, due to the high percent of radiation energy they can deposit outside a small tumor, they are not utilized in tumors measuring a few mm in diameter (O'Donoghue *et al.,* 1995, Koppe *et al.,* 2005). For these types of tumors, medium-beta emitter radionuclide such as Iodine-131 and Lutetium-177 are preferred (Cardillo *et al.,* 2001, O'Donoghue *et al.,* 1995, Koppe *et al.,* 2005). Two radioactive monoclonal antibodies approved by the United Stated Food and Drug Administration (FDA) during the early 2000's have shown promising results for the treatment of follicular, non-Hodgkin's lymphoma. These are Yttrium-90-Ibritumomab (Zevalin) which is a monoclonal antibody anti-CD-20 conjugated to Yttrium-90 and Tositumomab Iodine-131 (Bexxar) in which the monoclonal antibody anti-CD20 has been conjugated to Iodine-131 (Emmanouilides 2007). In the case of solid tumors, RIT has not been very efficient, perhaps due to the lower sensitivity of this type of tumors to radiation (Hanaoka *et al.,* 2009) and/or limited penetration of antibodies into solid tumors (Mattes 2002).

VII. RADIATION TREATMENT SIDE EFFECTS

Although the current radiation treatment modalities are capable of focusing the radiation dose to the target tumor with minimum exposure to the normal tissue, side effects are expected during radiation treatment. The nature, severity and duration of the side effects depend on the tissue treated, the type of radiation, dose, fractionation and the patient co-morbidities. They can be divided in early or acute effects and late or long-term effects.

A. Acute Side Effects

These effects occur during the course of the therapy and can last for several weeks. Some general acute effects include fatigue (Jereczek-Fossa *et al.,* 2002), radiodermatitis (Markouizou *et al.,* 2007) and myelosuppression (Kulkarn *et al.,* 2010) while others correlate with the site being treated. Site specific acute effects include:

A.1. Brain

Treatment of this area may cause erythema on the forehead, irritation of the external auditory canal, cerebral inflammation, headaches, nausea and vomiting, dizziness, and obstruction of lumen (Hogle 2006, Gerber and Chan 2008).

A.2. Head and Neck

When head and neck are treated the symptoms may include erythema of the skin area around the neck, ulceration of the mouth and throat that can affect swallowing, xerostomia, dysphagia, odynophagia, xerostamia, dysgeusia, and ageusia (Hogle 2006, Gerber and Chan 2008).

A.3. Lungs

Radiation treatment of the lungs may cause skin erythema, esophagitis, gastric reflux, acute pericarditis, shortness of breath, pneumonitis, and cardiac complications (Hogle 2006, Gerber and Chan 2008).

A.4. Abdomen

Symptoms caused by radiation treatment of the abdominal area include skin erythema, dyspepsia, nausea and vomiting, diarrhea, anorexia, symptoms of proctitis and cystitis, vaginal dryness, decreased libido, and perianal mucositis. If the gonads are exposed, infertility may result (Hogle 2006, Gerber and Chan 2008).

B. Long-Term Side Effects

These effects appear several months after treatment and include:

B. 1. Fibrosis and Scaring

The symptoms are associated with atrophy of accessory tissues. The tissue becomes less elastic, with a less suppleness and less resistance to injury (Yarnold and Brotons 2010).

B. 2. Hair Loss

Radiation-induced hair lose occurs only in the exposed area. The loss may or may not be reversible (Imanishi *et al.,* 2005).

B. 3. Radiation-Induced Malignancies

Secondary cancer may result as consequence of radiation treatment (Newhauser and Durante 2011).

B. 4. Psychological Effects

Patients who have received radiation therapy may experience depression, post-treatment anxiety, and sleep disturbances (Brans *et al.,* 2003, Andersen and Tewfik 1985).

CONCLUSIONS

Since the discovery of radiation at the end of the 19th century, significant advances in radiation treatment planning and delivery have taken place allowing the advent of several therapy modalities to treat nearly all types of cancer. Current therapeutic techniques can target malignant tumors with high precision; however, no technique can completely avoid the delivery of some dose of radiation to the surrounding normal tissue. This field will continue progressing as the search for techniques that strive to minimize normal tissue radiation-induced toxicity while maximizing the effects to the target cancerous tumor remains.

ACKNOWLEDGEMENT

We thank Daniel R. Weaver for his helpful comments and critical reading of this manuscript.

CONFLICT OF INTEREST

The authors confirm that this chapter content has no conflict of interest.

REFERENCES

1953. Radio-Cobalt beam therapy, *Br Med J* 1, 666.

A, G. N., 1931. Michael Faraday, *Can Med Assoc J* 25, 601-603.

Adler, J. R., Jr., S. D. Chang, M. J. Murphy, J. Doty, P. Geis, and S. L. Hancock, 1997. The Cyberknife: a frameless robotic system for radiosurgery, *Stereotact Funct Neurosurg* 69, 124-128.

Ak, I., M. P. Stokkel, and E. K. Pauwels, 2000. Positron emission tomography with 2-[18F]fluoro-2-deoxy-D-glucose in oncology. Part II. The clinical value in detecting and staging primary tumours, *J Cancer Res Clin Oncol* 126, 560-574.

Allisy A. 1996. Henri Becquerel: The Discovery of Radioactivity. *Radiation Protection Dosimetry*. 68:3-10.

Andersen, B. L., and H. H. Tewfik, 1985. Psychological reactions to radiation therapy: reconsideration of the adaptive aspects of anxiety, *J Pers Soc Psychol* 48, 1024-1032.

Azzam, E. I., S. M. de Toledo, and J. B. Little, 2001. Direct evidence for the participation of gap junction-mediated intercellular communication in the transmission of damage signals from alpha -particle irradiated to nonirradiated cells, *Proc Natl Acad Sci U S A* 98, 473-478.

Balter, S., 1998. Endovascular brachytherapy: physics and technology, *Cathet Cardiovasc Diagn* 45, 292-298.

Barth, R. F., J. A. Coderre, M. G. Vicente, and T. E. Blue, 2005. Boron neutron capture therapy of cancer: current status and future prospects, *Clin Cancer Res* 11, 3987-4002.

Becquerel, J., and J. A. Crowther, 1948. Discovery of radioactivity, *Nature* 161, 609.

Belli, M., O. Sapora, and M. A. Tabocchini, 2002. Molecular targets in cellular response to ionizing radiation and implications in space radiation protection, *J Radiat Res (Tokyo)* 43 Suppl, S13-19.

Bernier, J., E. J. Hall, and A. Giaccia, 2004. Radiation oncology: a century of achievements, *Nat Rev Cancer* 4, 737-747.

Biederer, J., C. Hintze, M. Fabel, and J. Dinkel, 2010. Magnetic resonance imaging and computed tomography of respiratory mechanics, *J Magn Reson Imaging* 32, 1388-1397.

Birge, R. T., 1940. Presentation of the Nobel Prize to Professor Ernest O. Lawrence, *Science* 91, 323-329.

Blaufox, M. D., 1996. Becquerel and the discovery of radioactivity: early concepts, *Semin Nucl Med* 26, 145-154.

Brady, L. W., and J. C. Hernandez, 1992. Brachytherapy of choroidal melanomas, *Strahlenther Onkol* 168, 61-65.

Brans, B., F. van den Eynde, K. Audenaert, M. Vervaet, K. van Daele, C. van Heeringen, and R. A. Dierckx, 2003. Depression and anxiety during isolation and radionuclide therapy, *Nucl Med Commun* 24, 881-886.

Brechbiel, M. W., 2007. Targeted alpha-therapy: past, present, future?, *Dalton Trans*, 4918-4928.

Britton, K. E., S. J. Mather, and M. Granowska, 1991. Radiolabelled monoclonal antibodies in oncology. III. Radioimmunotherapy, *Nucl Med Commun* 12, 333-347.

Brown BH, Smallwood RH, Barber DC, Lawford PV and Hose DR (1999), *Medical Physics and Biomedical Engineering, IOP, London, UK.*

Brown, P., 1995. American martyrs to radiology. Clarence Madison Dally (1865-1904). 1936, *AJR Am J Roentgenol* 164, 237-239.

Bucci, M. K., A. Bevan, and M. Roach, 3rd, 2005. Advances in radiation therapy: conventional to 3D, to IMRT, to 4D, and beyond, *CA Cancer J Clin* 55, 117-134.

Cantone MC and Hoeschen C (2011), Radiation physics for nuclear medicine, 1st ed, Springer. New York.

Cardillo, T. M., Z. Ying, and D. V. Gold, 2001. Therapeutic advantage of (90)yttrium- *versus* (131)iodine-labeled PAM4 antibody in experimental pancreatic cancer, *Clin Cancer Res* 7, 3186-3192.

Cella, L., A. Lomax, and R. Miralbell, 2001. New techniques in hadrontherapy: intensity modulated proton beams, *Phys Med* 17 Suppl 1, 100-102.

Chen, C. C., P. Chapman, J. Petit, and J. Loeffler, 2007. Proton radiosurgery in neurosurgery, *Neurosurg Focus* 23, E5.

Clarke, R., and J. Valentin, 2005. A history of the international commission on radiological protection, *Health Phys* 88, 717-732.

Coderre, J. A., and G. M. Morris, 1999. The radiation biology of boron neutron capture therapy, *Radiat Res* 151, 1-18.

Cohen, L., and F. R. Hendrickson, 1989. Neutron therapy for nonresectable radioresistant tumors, *Arch Surg* 124, 294-300.

Coppes-Zantinga, A. R., and M. J. Coppes, 1998a. The early years of radiation protection: a tribute to Madame Curie, *CMAJ* 159, 1389-1391.

Coppes-Zantinga, A. R., and M. J. Coppes, 1998b. Madame Marie Curie (1867-1934): a giant connecting two centuries, *AJR Am J Roentgenol* 171, 1453-1457.

Crownover, R. L., D. A. Wilkinson, and M. S. Weinhous, 1999. The radiobiology and physics of brachytherapy, *Hematol Oncol Clin North Am* 13, 477-487.

Cucinotta, F. A., R. Katz, J. W. Wilson, L. W. Townsend, J. Shinn, and F. Hajnal, 1991. Biological effectiveness of high-energy protons: target fragmentation, *Radiat Res* 127, 130-137.

Dahl PF (1997), *Flash of the cathode rays*, IOP publishing Ltd.

de Hevesy, G. C., 1984. Marie Curie and her contemporaries. The Becquerel-Curie memorial lecture, *J Nucl Med* 25, 116-131.

Diamantis, A., E. Magiorkinis, A. Papadimitriou, and G. Androutsos, 2008. The contribution of Maria Sklodowska-Curie and Pierre Curie to Nuclear and Medical Physics. A hundred and ten years after the discovery of radium, *Hell J Nucl Med* 11, 33-38.

Dutreix, J., and A. Dutreix, 1995. Henri Becquerel (1852-1908), *Med Phys* 22, 1869-1875.

Edwards, J. C., D. Chapman, W. A. Cramp, and M. B. Yatvin, 1984. The effects of ionizing radiation on biomembrane structure and function, *Prog Biophys Mol Biol* 43, 71-93.

Eisenberg, R. L., 1992. Cathode rays and controversy, *AJR Am J Roentgenol* 159, 996.

Elder, F. R., R. V. Langmuir, and H. C. Pollock, 1948. Effect of vacuum-tube size on x-ray output of a synchrotron, *Rev Sci Instrum* 19, 121.

Emmanouilides, C., 2007. Radioimmunotherapy for non-hodgkin lymphoma : historical perspective and current status, *J Clin Exp Hematop* 47, 43-60.

Erickson, B., 2005. Image-based brachytherapy: a forum for collaboration between radiation oncologists and diagnostic radiologists, *J Am Coll Radiol* 2, 753-758.

Feinendegen, L. E., M. Pollycove, and C. A. Sondhaus, 2004. Responses to low doses of ionizing radiation in biological systems, *Nonlinearity Biol Toxicol Med* 2, 143-171.

Foster, J. S., 1938. The Cyclotron and Its Contacts with x-ray and Radium Therapy, *Can Med Assoc J* 38, 222-226.

Frankel, R. I., 1996. Centennial of Rontgen's discovery of x-rays, *West J Med* 164, 497-501.

Fry, D. W., R. B. R-Shersby-Harvie, and *et al.*, 1948. A traveling-wave linear accelerator for 4-MeV. electrons, *Nature* 162, 859-861.

Gejerman, G., E. A. Mullokandov, E. Bagiella, A. Blaivas, and J. J. Beitler, 2002. Endobronchial brachytherapy and external-beam radiotherapy in patients with endobronchial obstruction and extrabronchial extension, *Brachytherapy* 1, 204-210.

Gerber, D. E., and T. A. Chan, 2008. Recent advances in radiation therapy, *Am Fam Physician* 78, 1254-1262.

Geward L. 1999. Paul Villard and his Discovery of Gamma-Rays. *Physics in Perspective*, 1, 367-383.

Gibbs, I. C., 2006. Frameless image-guided intracranial and extracranial radiosurgery using the Cyberknife robotic system, *Cancer Radiother* 10, 283-287.

Goldman, M., 1982. Ionizing radiation and its risks, *West J Med* 137, 540-547.

Goodhead, D. T., 1999. Mechanisms for the biological effectiveness of high-LET radiations, *J Radiat Res (Tokyo)* 40 Suppl, 1-13.

Haas, L. F., 2001. Wilhelm Conrad Von Rontgen (1845-1923), *J Neurol Neurosurg Psychiatry* 70, 126.

Hada, M., and A. G. Georgakilas, 2008. Formation of clustered DNA damage after high-LET irradiation: a review, *J Radiat Res (Tokyo)* 49, 203-210.

Hall EJ & Giaccia AJ, (2011), *Radiobiology for the radiologist*, 7th ed. Lippicott Williams & Wilkins, Philadelphia, PA.

Hanaoka, H., T. Katagiri, C. Fukukawa, H. Yoshioka, S. Yamamoto, Y. Iida, T. Higuchi, N. Oriuchi, B. Paudyal, P. Paudyal, Y. Nakamura, and K. Endo, 2009. Radioimmunotherapy of solid tumors targeting a cell-surface protein, FZD10: therapeutic efficacy largely depends on radiosensitivity, *Ann Nucl Med* 23, 479-485.

Harms-Ringdahl, M., P. Nicotera, and I. R. Radford, 1996. Radiation induced apoptosis, *Mutat Res* 366, 171-179.

Herbert C. (1968) *An American Genius: The life of Ernest Orlando Lawrence, father of the cyclotron.* E.P. Dutton & Co., Inc. New York, NY.

Hogle, W. P., 2006. The state of the art in radiation therapy, *Semin Oncol Nurs* 22, 212-220.

Hogstrom, K. R., and P. R. Almond, 2006. Review of electron beam therapy physics, *Phys Med Biol* 51, R455-489.

Hong, T. S., M. A. Ritter, W. A. Tome, and P. M. Harari, 2005. Intensity-modulated radiation therapy: emerging cancer treatment technology, *Br J Cancer* 92, 1819-1824.

Huda W (2003). *Review of radiologic physics.* 3rd ed. Lippicott Williams and Wilkins. Philadelphia, PA.

Ikushima, H., 2010. Radiation therapy: state of the art and the future, *J Med Invest* 57, 1-11.

Imanishi, Y., A. Fukui, H. Niimi, D. Itoh, K. Nozaki, S. Nakaji, K. Ishizuka, H. Tabata, Y. Furuya, M. Uzura, H. Takahama, S. Hashizume, S. Arima, and Y. Nakajima, 2005. Radiation-induced temporary hair loss as a radiation damage only occurring in patients who had the combination of MDCT and DSA, *Eur Radiol* 15, 41-46.

Jayaraman S and Lanzl LH (2004), *Clinical raditherapy physiscs*, 2nd ed, Springer, Chicago, IL.

Jereczek-Fossa, B. A., H. R. Marsiglia, and R. Orecchia, 2002. Radiotherapy-related fatigue, *Crit Rev Oncol Hematol* 41, 317-325.

Jones, C. G., 2005. A review of the history of U.S. radiation protection regulations, recommendations, and standards, *Health Phys* 88, 105-124.

Kassis, A. I., 2008. Therapeutic radionuclides: biophysical and radiobiologic principles, *Semin Nucl Med* 38, 358-366.

Khan FM, (2010), The physics of radiation therapy, 4th ed, Lippincott Williams & Wilkin, Philadelphia, PA.

Kilby, W., J. R. Dooley, G. Kuduvalli, S. Sayeh, and C. R. Maurer, Jr., 2010. The CyberKnife Robotic Radiosurgery System in 2010, *Technol Cancer Res Treat* 9, 433-452.

Koga, T., M. Shin, and N. Saito, 2010. Role of gamma knife radiosurgery in neurosurgery: past and future perspectives, *Neurol Med Chir (Tokyo)* 50, 737-748.

Kolotas, C., and N. Zamboglou, 2001. Role of interstitial brachytherapy in the treatment of malignant disease, *Onkologie* 24, 222-228.

Koppe, M. J., E. J. Postema, F. Aarts, W. J. Oyen, R. P. Bleichrodt, and O. C. Boerman, 2005. Antibody-guided radiation therapy of cancer, *Cancer Metastasis Rev* 24, 539-567.

Kulkarni, S., S. P. Ghosh, M. Hauer-Jensen, and K. S. Kumar, 2010. Hematological targets of radiation damage, *Curr Drug Targets* 11, 1375-1385.

Lauterbur, P. C., 1980. Progress in n.m.r. zeugmatography imaging, *Philos Trans R Soc Lond B Biol Sci* 289, 483-487.

Lee AG. 1932. The Varley brothers: Cromwell Fleetwood Varley and Samuel Alfred Varley. *J Inst Elect Eng* 71:958-964.

Leksell, L., 1951. The stereotaxic method and radiosurgery of the brain, *Acta Chir Scand* 102, 316-319.

Leksell, L., 1968. Cerebral radiosurgery. I. Gammathalanotomy in two cases of intractable pain, *Acta Chir Scand* 134, 585-595.

Levin, W. P., H. Kooy, J. S. Loeffler, and T. F. DeLaney, 2005. Proton beam therapy, *Br J Cancer* 93, 849-854.

Levy, R. P., R. W. Schulte, J. D. Slater, D. W. Miller, and J. M. Slater, 1999. Stereotactic radiosurgery--the role of charged particles, *Acta Oncol* 38, 165-169.

Li, G., D. Citrin, K. Camphausen, B. Mueller, C. Burman, B. Mychalczak, R. W. Miller, and Y. Song, 2008. Advances in 4D medical imaging and 4D radiation therapy, *Technol Cancer Res Treat* 7, 67-81.

Lichter, A. S., and T. S. Lawrence, 1995. Recent advances in radiation oncology, *N Engl J Med* 332, 371-379.

MacDonald, S. M., T. F. DeLaney, and J. S. Loeffler, 2006. Proton beam radiation therapy, *Cancer Invest* 24, 199-208.

Mansfield, P., and A. A. Maudsley, 1977. Medical imaging by NMR, *Br J Radiol* 50, 188-194.

Margaritondo, G., and R. Meuli, 2003. Synchrotron radiation in radiology: novel x-ray sources, *Eur Radiol* 13, 2633-2641.

Markouizou, A., N. Koliarakis, M. Paraskevaidis, G. Tsakiris, A. Karageorgis, and P. Karageorgis, 2007. Radiation dermatitis: implicated factors, clinical aspects, possible prevention, and medical care, *J BUON* 12, 463-470.

Matsumoto, K., A. Okajo, K. Nagata, W. G. Degraff, M. Nyui, M. Ueno, I. Nakanishi, T. Ozawa, J. B. Mitchell, M. C. Krishna, H. Yamamoto, K. Endo, and K. Anzai, 2009. Detection of free radical reactions in an aqueous sample induced by low linear-energy-transfer irradiation, *Biol Pharm Bull* 32, 542-547.

Mattes, M. J., 2002. Radionuclide-antibody conjugates for single-cell cytotoxicity, *Cancer* 94, 1215-1223.

Mazeron, J. J., and A. Gerbaulet, 1998. The centenary of discovery of radium, *Radiother Oncol* 49, 205-216.

Mould, R. F., 1995a. Invited review: Rontgen and the discovery of x-rays, *Br J Radiol* 68, 1145-1176.

Mould, R. F., 1995b. Invited review: the early years of radiotherapy with emphasis on x-ray and radium apparatus, *Br J Radiol* 68, 567-582.

Mould, R. F., 1998. The discovery of radium in 1898 by Maria Sklodowska-Curie (1867-1934) and Pierre Curie (1859-1906) with commentary on their life and times, *Br J Radiol* 71, 1229-1254.

Mould, R. F., 2007. Priority for radium therapy of benign conditions and cancer, *Curr Oncol* 14, 118-122.

Muller, F., 2011. Johann Wilhelm Hittorf and the material culture of nineteenth-century gas discharge research, *Br J Hist Sci* 44, 211-244.

Murakami, Y., Y. Nagata, I. Nishibuchi, T. Kimura, M. Kenjo, Y. Kaneyasu, T. Okabe, Y. Hashimoto, and Y. Akagi, 2011. Long-term outcomes of intraluminal brachytherapy in combination with external beam radiotherapy for superficial esophageal cancer, *Int J Clin Oncol.*

Myers, W. G., 1976. Becquerel's discovery of radioactivity in 1896, *J Nucl Med* 17, 579-582.

Nag, S., 2004. High dose rate brachytherapy: its clinical applications and treatment guidelines, *Technol Cancer Res Treat* 3, 269-287.

Newhauser, W. D., and M. Durante, 2011. Assessing the risk of second malignancies after modern radiotherapy, *Nat Rev Cancer* 11, 438-448.

Ng, D., 2006. Radioimmunotherapy: a brief overview, *Biomed Imaging Interv J* 2, e23.

Nobel lectures: including presentation speeches and laureates' biographies. 1901-1921, Physics (1967), Elsevier, New York. NY

Noda, S. E., T. Lautenschlaeger, M. R. Siedow, D. R. Patel, A. El-Jawahri, Y. Suzuki, J. S. Loeffler, M. R. Bussiere, and A. Chakravarti, 2009. Technological advances in radiation oncology for central nervous system tumors, *Semin Radiat Oncol* 19, 179-186.

O'Donoghue, J. A., M. Bardies, and T. E. Wheldon, 1995. Relationships between tumor size and curability for uniformly targeted therapy with beta-emitting radionuclides, *J Nucl Med* 36, 1902-1909.

Peh, W. C., 1995. Part II--controversies surrounding and following Rontgen's discovery, *Singapore Med J* 36, 554-558.

Peoples, A. R., K. R. Mercer, and W. A. Bernhard, 2010. What fraction of DNA double-strand breaks produced by the direct effect is accounted for by radical pairs?, *J Phys Chem B* 114, 9283-9288.

Perea and Brady's (2008), *Principles and practice of radiation oncology*, 5th ed, Lippincott Williams & Wilkins, Philadelphia, PA.

Pichler, B. J., M. S. Judenhofer, and H. F. Wehrl, 2008. PET/MRI hybrid imaging: devices and initial results, *Eur Radiol* 18, 1077-1086.

Podgorsak EB (2010), *Radiation Physics for medical physicists*, 2nd ed. Springer. Montreal, Canada.

Pop, D., N. Venissac, P. Y. Bondiau, and J. Mouroux, 2010. Peroperative fiducial placement for postoperative stereotactic Cyberknife radiosurgery, *Interact Cardiovasc Thorac Surg* 10, 1034-1036.

Ramesh, R., A. J. Marrogi, A. Munshi, C. N. Abboud, and S. M. Freeman, 1996. *In vivo* analysis of the 'bystander effect': a cytokine cascade, *Exp Hematol* 24, 829-838.

Ramesh, R., A. J. Marrogi, A. Munshi, C. N. Abboud, and S. M. Freeman, 1996. *In vivo* analysis of the 'bystander effect': a cytokine cascade, *Exp Hematol* 24, 829-838.

Rong, Y., and J. Welsh, 2010. Basics of particle therapy II biologic and dosimetric aspects of clinical hadron therapy, *Am J Clin Oncol* 33, 646-649.

Rosenow, U. F., 1995. Notes on the legacy of the Rontgen rays, *Med Phys* 22, 1855-1867.

Rossi, H. H., and A. M. Kellerer, 1995. Roentgen, *Radiat Res* 144, 124-128.

Saleh-Gohari, N., H. E. Bryant, N. Schultz, K. M. Parker, T. N. Cassel, and T. Helleday, 2005. Spontaneous homologous recombination is induced by collapsed replication forks that are caused by endogenous DNA single-strand breaks, *Mol Cell Biol* 25, 7158-7169.

Sarfaraz, M., 2007. CyberKnife robotic arm stereotactic radiosurgery, *J Am Coll Radiol* 4, 563-565.

Shahri, K. K., L. R. Motavalli, and H. M. Hakimabad, 2011. Neutrons applications in cancer treatment and in specific diagnostics, *Hell J Nucl Med* 14, 110-113.

Silari, M., 2011. Applications of particle accelerators in medicine, *Radiat Prot Dosimetry* 146, 440-450.

Smith, R. P., D. E. Heron, M. S. Huq, and N. J. Yue, 2006. Modern radiation treatment planning and delivery--from Rontgen to real time, *Hematol Oncol Clin North Am* 20, 45-62.

Snyder, A. R., 2004. Review of radiation-induced bystander effects, *Hum Exp Toxicol* 23, 87-89.

Somosy, Z., 2000. Radiation response of cell organelles, *Micron* 31, 165-181.

Stephenson, J. A., and A. L. Wiley, Jr., 1995. Current techniques in three-dimensional CT simulation and radiation treatment planning, *Oncology (Williston Park)* 9, 1225-1232, 1235; discussion 1235-1240.

Stone, R. S., 1948. Neutron therapy and specific ionization, *Am J Roentgenol Radium Ther* 59, 771-785.

Strijckmans, K., 2001. The isochronous cyclotron: principles and recent developments, *Comput Med Imaging Graph* 25, 69-78.

Taylor, L. S., 1958. History of the International Commission on Radiological Protection (ICRP), *Health Phys* 1, 97-104.

Thomas, J. M., 2006. J. J. Thomson: winner of the Nobel Prize for Physics 1906, *Angew Chem Int Ed Engl* 45, 6797-6800.

Thompson SP (1938), *Michael Faraday. His life and work.* Henry Roscoe Editor. Cassell and Company.

Tselos, G. D., 1995. New Jersey's Thomas Edison and the fluoroscope, *N J Med* 92, 731-733.

Turner JE. (2007), *Atoms, radiation, and radiation protection.* Wyley, Weinheim, Germany.

Verellen, D., T. Depuydt, T. Gevaert, N. Linthout, K. Tournel, M. Duchateau, T. Reynders, G. Storme, and M. De Ridder, 2010. Gating and tracking, 4D in thoracic tumours, *Cancer Radiother* 14, 446-454.

Volkert, W. A., W. F. Goeckeler, G. J. Ehrhardt, and A. R. Ketring, 1991. Therapeutic radionuclides: production and decay property considerations, *J Nucl Med* 32, 174-185.

Vylet, V., and J. C. Liu, 2001. Radiation protection at high energy electron accelerators, *Radiat Prot Dosimetry* 96, 333-343.

Wakabayashi, H., S. Suzuki, and A. Ito, 1983. Measurement of relative biological effectiveness (RBE) for the radiation beam from neutron source reactor YAYOI--comparisons with cyclotron neutron and 60Co gamma ray, *J Radiat Res (Tokyo)* 24, 305-316.

Watkins, J. M., P. L. Kearney, K. J. Opfermann, S. J. Ackerman, J. M. Jenrette, and M. F. Kohler, 2011. Ultrasound-guided tandem placement for low-dose-rate brachytherapy in advanced cervical cancer minimizes risk of intraoperative uterine perforation, *Ultrasound Obstet Gynecol* 37, 241-244.

Wei, Z., M. Ding, D. Downey, and A. Fenster, 2005. Dynamic Intraoperative Prostate Brachytherapy Using 3D TRUS Guidance with Robot Assistance, *Conf Proc IEEE Eng Med Biol Soc* 7, 7429-7432.

Welsh, J. S., 2007. Beta decay in science and medicine, *Am J Clin Oncol* 30, 437-439.

Wen, J. C., and T. A. McCannel, 2009. Treatment of radiation retinopathy following plaque brachytherapy for choroidal melanoma, *Curr Opin Ophthalmol* 20, 200-204.

Willers, H., J. Dahm-Daphi, and S. N. Powell, 2004. Repair of radiation damage to DNA, *Br J Cancer* 90, 1297-1301.

Willers, H., and K. D. Held, 2006. Introduction to clinical radiation biology, *Hematol Oncol Clin North Am* 20, 1-24.

Williamson, J. F., 2006. Brachytherapy technology and physics practice since 1950: a half-century of progress, *Phys Med Biol* 51, R303-325.

Yang, T. C., 1999. Proton radiobiology and uncertainties, *Radiat Meas* 30, 383-392.

Yarnold, J., and M. C. Brotons, 2010. Pathogenetic mechanisms in radiation fibrosis, *Radiother Oncol* 97, 149-161.

Send Orders for Reprints to reprints@benthamscience.net
Cutting Edge Therapies for Cancer in the 21st Century, 2014, 111-155

CHAPTER 4

Interferons: Production, Signaling and Uses in Cancer Treatment

Ana L. Romero-Weaver*

Department of Radiation Oncology, University of Pennsylvania School of Medicine, Philadelphia, PA, USA

Abstract: Interferons (IFNs) are a family of cytokines with several biological functions. Currently, IFNs are classified in three groups: Type I, Type II and Type III. Type I IFNs include a family of several related proteins produced by essentially all eukaryotic cells. Type II IFN has only one member, IFN-γ, is mainly produced by T cells, NK cells and NKT cells. Type III IFNs include 3 related proteins, IFN-λ1/IL-29, IFN-λ2/IL-28A and IFN-λ3/IL28B, which are produced by several cells types. IFNs exhibit antiviral, anti-proliferative, immune-modulatory and anti-angiogenic properties. Their potent anti-proliferative effects make them good candidates for cancer therapy. Type II and type III IFNs have been investigated mainly in cancer cell lines and in animal models. Several clinical trials have been conducted with type I IFNs; the results of some of them have led to the approval and use of this type of IFN for the treatment of some malignancies. However, many patients develop toxicity and this has limited their use as anticancer agents, making it necessary to find a way to determine the patients who would most likely benefit from IFN treatment to avoid exposing non responsive patients to its toxic effects. In this chapter the mechanism of IFN production and signaling and their use in different types of cancer will be addressed.

Keywords: Interferon, cancer, leukemia, chronic myelogenous leukemia, hairy cell leukemia, osteosarcoma, kaposi sarcoma, melanoma, renal cell carcinoma, follicular lymphoma, head and neck squamous cell carcinomas, breast cancer, ovarian cancer, cervical cancer, lung cancer, bladder cancer, brain tumors, hepatocellular carcinoma, multiple myeloma.

I. HISTORICAL OVERVIEW

Two groups working independently identified interferon activity. In the first group, two Japanese virologists, Yasuichi Nagano and Yasuhiko Kohima,

***Address correspondence to Ana L. Romero-Weaver:** Department of Radiation Oncology, University of Pennsylvania School of Medicine, Philadelphia, PA 19104, USA; Tel: (215) 898-0270; Fax: (215) 898-1411; E-mail: ana.romero-weaver@uphs.upenn.edu

working to develop a chicken pox vaccine at the Institute of Infectious Diseases of the University of Tokyo, found a natural protein with viral inhibitory activity in rabbits inoculated with UV inactivated virus and challenged with live virus, they called this protein "virus inhibitory factor" and published their findings in 1954 (Nagano and Kojima 1954). Their experiments were complex and they did not receive much credit from the scientific community. In another group, the British virologist Alick Isaacs and the Swiss researcher Jean Lindenmann, working at the National Institute for Medical Research in London, found that cells from chicken embryos injected with heat-inactivated influenza virus produced a protein that interferes with the growth of influenza viruses and also inhibits the growth of other viruses, they called this protein interferon (IFN) and published their results in 1957 (Isaac and Lindenmann 1957), their work created more interest than the work of Nagano and Kojima, therefore Issacs and Lindenmann were credited with the discovery of IFN (type I IFN). The antiviral activities of this new protein created big expectations for the development of new antiviral agents; however, the research on IFN was slow due to limited quantities available at the time. In 1965 another antiviral agent was identified (Kleinschmid and Murphy 1965), it was determined to be different than type I IFN and it was originally named "immune" IFN since it was believed that it was only expressed by leukocytes (Falcoff 1972), later in 1980 it was named IFN-γ. During the early 1970s, Kari Cantell and collaborators developed a method to obtain useful amounts of IFN from human white blood cells (Cantell and Tovell 1971, Tovell and Cantell 1971), but it was not until 1978 that human leukocyte interferon was purified to homogeneity (Rubinstein *et al.,* 1978), allowing for the conduction of the first clinical trials (Borden 1979). During the 1980s two of the first human genes to be cloned were those of IFN-α and IFN-β (Nagata *et al.,* 1980, Masucci *et al.,* 1980, Taniguchi *et al.,* 1980), later in 1982 the gene of IFN-γ was cloned (Devos *et al.,* 1982). Clinical trials performed with partially purified type I IFN demonstrated anti-tumor effects in some malignancies. These results were later confirmed with recombinant IFN. In 1986, the United Stated Food and Drug Administration (FDA) approved the therapeutic use of type I IFNs for the treatment of hairy cell leukemia (Dianzani 1992). In 1988 type I IFNs were FDA approved for the treatment of Kaposi's sarcoma. Further studies demonstrated that type I IFNs were effective in other malignancies and were also approved for the treatment of chronic myelogenous leukemia (CML), melanomas, and renal cell carcinoma (Weiss 1998, Chelbi-Alix and Wietzerbin 2007). In 2003 two groups working independently identified the most recent members of the IFN family which were classified as type III IFNs (Kotenko *et al.,* 2003, Sheppard *et al.,* 2003), they comprise 3 associated proteins: IFN-λ1/IL-29, IFN-λ2/IL-28A and IFN-λ3 /IL-28B with promising potential applications. Despite the approval of type I IFNs for the treatment of many types of cancer, their current use in cancer therapy is limited due to the frequent development of toxic side effects, the development of resistance to IFN therapy, and the advent of new drugs with fewer side effects. Despite the approval of type I IFNs for the treatment of many types of cancer, their current use in cancer therapy is limited due to the frequent development of toxic side effects, the development of resistance to IFN therapy, and the advent of new drugs with fewer side effects. However, advances in the understanding of IFN anti-tumor mechanisms, the development of long-lasting pegylated forms of IFN (Kozlowski and Harris 2001), and new methods of IFN administration with fewer side effects has led to a re-evaluation of the role of IFN in cancer therapy. Several clinical trials have been conducted and many more are currently ongoing to determine new doses, administration routes and combinations with other drugs for the treatment of several malignancies. In this chapter some of the most current studies of IFNs in cancer therapy are presented.

II. CLASSIFICATION OF IFNs

IFNs are small cytokine with antiviral anti-proliferative, immune-modulatory and anti-angiogenic properties (Pestka 1987). In 1980, the United States National Institute of Allergy and Infectious Diseases and the World Health Organization introduced the current nomenclature of IFNs which classifies them into three types according to their gene sequence, chromosomal location and cell surface receptor binding (Interferon nomenclature 1980). Table **1** shows the current classification of human IFNs. Type I IFNs are produced by almost all nucleated cells but mainly by plasmacytoid dendritic cells (Fitzgerald-Bocarsly and Feng 2007). Several forms of type I IFN exist, in humans there are 13 forms of IFN-α, one form of IFN-β, one form of IFN-e, one form of IFN-κ and one form of IFN-ω (Cheng *et al.,* 2004). These molecules signal through a ubiquitously expressed receptor which is composed of an IFN-αR1 chain, also known as IFNAR1 and an IFN-αR2 chain, also known as IFNAR2 (de Weerd *et al.,* 2007). The genes of type I IFNs are located on the short arm of chromosome 9 (Diaz *et al.,* 1994). Type II IFN is composed only by IFN-γ which is expressed mainly by T cells, NK cells and NKT cells (Young 1996, Carnaud *et al.,* 1999). IFN-γ signals *via* a ubiquitously expressed hetero-oligomeric receptor composed of two IFN-γR1 chains and two IFN-γR2 chains (Pestka 1997). There genes are located on chromosome 12 (Zimonjic *et al.,* 1995). Type III IFNs comprise three members: IFN-λ1 also known as interleukin-29 (IL-29), IFN-λ2 (IL-28A), and IFN-λ3 (IL-28B) (Sheppard *et al.,* 2003, Kotenko *et al.,* 2003). Type III IFNs signal through a receptor composed of two subunits, an IFN-λ-specific receptor chain, IFN-λR1 (IL28Rα), which is selectively expressed in certain cell types and a ubiquitously expressed IL-10Rβ chain (Uze and Monneron 2007). Their genes are located in chromosome 19 (Sheppard *et al.,* 2003, Kotenko *et al.,* 2003).

Table 1: Classification of human IFNs.

Type	Forms	Gene Location	Receptor
Type I	IFN-α, IFN-β, IFN-δ, IFN-κ, IFN-ω	Chromosome 9	IFN-αR1 (one chain) IFN-αR2 (one chain)
Type II	IFN-γ	Chromosome 12	IFN-γR1 (two chains) IFN-λR2 (two chains)
Type III	IFN-λ1 (IL-19), IFN-λ2 (IL28A), IFN-λ3 (IL-28B)	Chromosome 19	IL-28Rα (one chain) IL-10β (one chain)

III. PRODUCTION AND SIGNALING OF IFNs

IFNs are produced directly or indirectly after microbial infections and/or stress. Once produced, they are secreted and exert their biological function in an autocrine or a paracrine manner. Signaling of IFNs involves binding to a specific receptor. IFN receptors belong to the class II cytokine receptor family which lacks intrinsic phosphatase and kinase activity (Schroder *et al.,* 2004); therefore, members of the Janus kinase (JAK) proteins are associated to the receptor to phosphorylate key proteins involved in IFN signaling. This section describes how IFNs are produced and once produced, how they exert their biological functions.

A. Type I IFNs

Cells identify microbial invaders and cellular stress through specific pathogen recognition receptors (PRR) (Akira *et al.,* 2006) which detect specific components that are essential for microbial survival such as double-stranded RNA (dsRNA) (Field *et al.,* 1967), single-stranded (ssRNA) (Lund *et al.,* 2004) unmethylated CpG DNA (Hemmi *et al.,* 2000, Krieg 2002), dsDNA (Ablasser *et al.,* 2009, Chiu *et al.,* 2009) and glycolipids (Hoshino *et al.,* 1999), these components can induce the production of type I IFN through different pathways (Pietras *et al.,* 2006). Two RNA helicases: retinoic acid–inducible gene I (RIG-I) and melanoma differentiation–associated gene 5 (Mda5), are PRRs that act as intracellular sensors for the detection of cytosolic dsRNA (Yoneyama *et al.,* 2004, Kato *et al.,* 2006), once activated RIG-I and Mad5 initiate a series of signaling events that activate the IFN transcription factors IRF3 and IRF7 (Yoneyama *et al.,* 2005) which then homodimerize, translocate to the nucleus and induce the transcription of IFN-α and IFN-β genes. Toll-like receptor 3 (TLR3) is another PRR present in endosomas that recognizes dsRNA (Alexopoulou *et al.,* 2001). TLR3 associates with the TRI-domain-containing adaptor inducing IFN-β (TRIF) (Yamamoto *et al.* 2003) and induces activation of TANK-binding kinase-1 (TBK1) (Fitzgerald *et al.,* 2003) and other downstream steps leading to the activation of IRF3 and IRF7 which then translocate to the nucleus and induce the transcription of type I IFN genes (Sharma *et al.,* 2003). TLR4 localized in the plasma membrane, recognizes microbial glycolipids (Hoshino *et al.,* 1999) and signals through TRIF and TRIF-related adaptor molecule (TRAM) (Fitzgerald *et al.,* 2003b) which induce a cascade of events that activate IRF3 and IRF9 which in turn induce the transcription of type I IFN genes (Yamamoto *et al.,* 2003). TLR7/8 and TLR9 are other endosome PRRs which recognize ssRNA and unmethylated CpG DNA, respectively (Lund *et al.,* 2004, Heil *et al.,* 2004, Diebol *et al.,* 2004, Alexopoulou *et al.,* 2001). These receptors recruit MyD88 which then recruits and activates interleukin-1-associated kinase 1 (IRAK1), IRAK4, and necrosis factor receptor-associated factor 6 (TRAF6) forming a tertiary complex that binds to and phosphorylates IRF5 and IRF7 (Kawai *et al.,* 2004, Honda *et al.,* 2004) these phosphorylated proteins then translocate to the nucleus and induce the transcription of type I IFN genes (Hemmi *et al.,* 2002, Kawai *et al.,* 2004). Recently, it has been discovered that cytosolic RNA polymerase III can sense and transcribe microbial dsDNA into 5'triphosphate (5'-ppp) dsRNA (Ablasser *et al.,* 2009, Chiu *et al.,* 2009) which is recognized by the RIG-I-Mda-5 pathway as previously described. Once produced type I IFNs are secreted and can act in an autocrine or a paracrine manner. Binding of Type I IFN's to their receptor activates the receptor associated proteins kinases Jak1 and Tyk2; which in turn phosphorylate the receptor at a specific tyrosine position (Colamonici *et al.,* 1994, Gauzzi *et al.,* 1996, Platanias and Fish 1999). Activated Jak kinases then phosphorylate several members of the signal transducers and activators of transcription (STAT) protein family (Fu 1992, Schindler *et al.,* 1992). Activated STAT1 forms homodimers and heterodimers with STAT2. Additionally, the STAT1/STAT2 heterodimer binds to IRF9 forming the IFN-stimulated gene factor-3 (ISGF3) complex. Both STAT1 homodimer and ISGF3 complex translocate to the nucleus, STAT1 homodimes bind to a gamma activated sequence (GAS) and ISGF3 binds to an IFN-stimulated response element (ISRE) region located in the promoter of IFN stimulated genes inducing their transcription (Stark *et al.,* 1998) (Fig. **1**).

B. Type II IFN

IFN-γ is expressed mainly by T cells, NK cells and NKT cells (Miller *et al.,* 2009). Contrary to type I IFNs, its production is not directly induced by PRRs but by effector molecules such as interleukins (ILs) which are produced in response to microbial stimulation. IL-2 and IL-18 are the main inducers of IFN-γ production (Trinchieri 1995, Micallef *et al.,* 1996). Microbial stimulation induces IL-12 production in macrophages and dendritic cells (Trincheri 1995). Binding of IL-12 to its receptor activates the receptor associated protein kinases Jak2 and Tyk2, which in turn phosphorylate STAT3 and STAT4 at a specific tyrosine residue (Jacobson *et al.,* 1995) causing the formation of STAT3/STAT4 heterodimers and STAT4 homodimers which then translocate to the nucleus, bind to a GAS sequence and induce the transcription of the IFN-γ gene (Watford *et al.,* 2005) and other genes with stimulatory effect on the production of IFN-γ, such as Ets variant gene 5 (ERM) which has a modest stimulatory effect (Ouyang *et al.,* 1999) and T-box 21 (T-bet) which is a key transcription factor for the expression of IFN-γ in CD4+ cells and NK cells (Yang *et al.,* 2007, Szabo *et al.,* 2000). IL-18 in concert with IL-12 exerts a synergistic effect in the production of IFN-γ either in a T-cell receptor (TCR) dependent or TCR independent manner (Okamura *et al.,* 1998, Tominaga *et al.,* 2000). IL-12, IL-18 and TCR signaling induces the transcription of growth arrest and DNA-damage-inducible, beta and gamma (GADD45β,

GADD45γ) proteins (Lu 2001) which then activate mitogen-activated protein kinase kinase 4 (MEKK4 or MAP3K4) (Chi *et al.,* 2004). Activated MEKK4 initiates a cascade of phosphorylation events leading to the activation of mitogen-activated protein kinase 14 (p38α or MAPK14) and mitogen-activated protein kinase 8-10 (MAPK8-10 or JNK) (Takekawa and Saito 1998, Lu *et al.,* 2001). Then, p38 phosphorylates STAT4 at a serine residue necessary for maximal transcriptional activity (Morinobu *et al.,* 2002, Visconti *et al.,* 2000) it also phosphorylates transcription factor 2 (ATF-2) which can regulate the production of IFN-γ (Raingeaud *et al.,* 1996, Nakayama *et al.,* 2001). JNK phosphorylates Jun oncogene (c-Jun) (Halfter *et al.,* 2005), then STAT4 in cooperation with c-jun induces IFN-γ promoter activation (Nakahira *et al.,* 2002). Additionally, IL-18 induces the activator protein 1 (AP-1) which is then recruited to the IFN-γ promoter by IL-12 induced STAT4 (Nakahira *et al.,* 2002). After production and secretion, IFN-γ forms a dimer and binds to two IFN-γR1 chains causing oligomeriztion and rearrangement of the receptor (Sakatsume *et al.,* 1995, Kotenko *et al.,* 1995), and then the associated kinases, Jak1 and Jak2 phosphorylate the receptor at a specific site where STAT1 is recruited and phosphorylated by Jak1 (Igarashi *et al.,* 1994, Bach *et al.,* 1997). Phosphorylated STAT1 homodimerizes and along with IFN-γ and IFNγR1 are transported into the nucleus as a STAT1:IFN-γ:IFN-γR1 complex (Sadir *et al.,* 2000). Once in the nucleus, the STAT1 homodimer dissociates from the complex, binds to a GAS promoter sequence and induces the transcription of IFN-γ genes (Farrar and Schreiber 1993) (Fig. **1**).

C. Type III IFNs

Although Type I and type III IFNs bind to different receptors, their production and signaling are regulated in a similar way which has suggested overlapping functions. As in the case of type I IFNs, TLRs 3,4,7,8 and 9 as well as RIG-1 and Mda5 helicases can also regulate the production of type III IFNs (Onoguchi *et al.,* 2007, Osterlund *et al.,* 2007). Recently, a cytosolic DNA sensor that induces the production of type III IFN but not type I IFN has been described (Zhang *et al.,* 2011). Binding of type III IFNs to their receptor results in activation of the Jak/STAT pathway, formation of the ISFG3 complex and transcription of ISGs in a similar way as for type I IFNs (Zhou *et al.,* 2007, Dumoutier *et al.,* 2004, Kotenko *et al.,* 2003) (Fig. **1**).

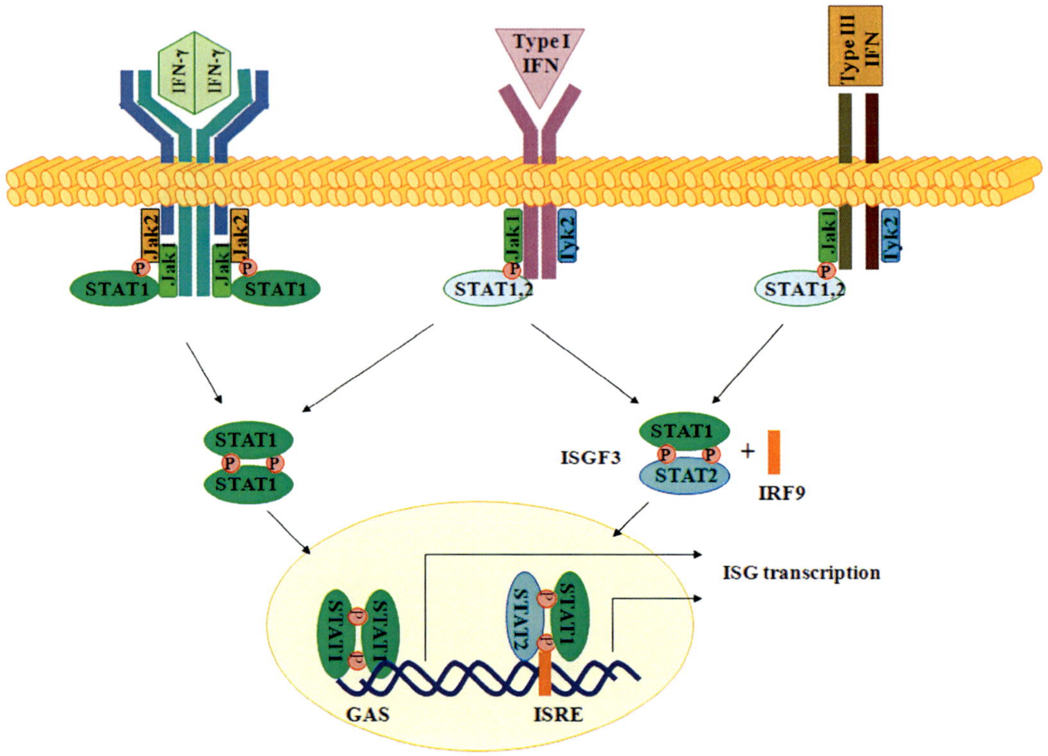

Figure 1: IFN signaling. Type I IFN (middle), type II IFN (left) and type III IFN (right) activate the Jak/STAT pathway leading to the transcription of interferon stimulated genes (ISG), (see text for details).

IV. INTERFERONS IN CANCER TREATMENT

In vitro studies with cell lines and *in vivo* studies with animal models have shown that all types of IFNs posses anti-tumor effects in different types of cancers. The majority of the IFN clinical trials in cancer treatment have been conducted with type I IFNs, few have been conducted with type II IFN and so far no clinical trials in cancer treatment have been conducted with type III IFNs. The initial clinical trials with type I IFN demonstrated its efficacy in the treatment of certain malignancies. Once recombinant IFNs were produced, the results of the initial clinical trials were confirmed, thus type I IFNs were approved for the treatment of hairy cell leukemia, chronic myelogenous leukemia, Kaposi's sarcoma, melanoma and renal cell carcinoma. Table **2** shows the current IFN preparations that are commercially available from which only IFN-α-2a and IFN-α-2b are approved in cancer treatment. This section describes current clinical trials of the use of IFNs in cancer treatment.

Hairy Cell Leukemia

This condition is a rare B-cell non-Hodgkin lymphoma first described in 1958 (Bouroncle *et al.,* 1958, Golde *et al.,* 1977), it courses with splenomegaly, pancytopenia, and morphologically typical neoplastic mononuclear cells in the blood and bone marrow and several opportunistic infections (Anderson *et al.,* 1985, Golomb and Hanauer 1981); the only treatment available during the early 1980s was splenectomy (Golde 1982, Mintz and Golomb 1979, Golomb and Vardiman 1983). Early clinical trials with partially purified IFN-α resulted in complete remission in some patients for whom the incidence of opportunistic infections disappeared and blood cells returned to normal levels (Quesada *et al.,* 1984, Lepe-Zuniga *et al.,* 1987). These results were later confirmed with recombinant IFN-α (Jacobs *et al.,* 1985, Quesada *et al.,* 1987), leading to the approval of this therapy by the FDA in 1986 (Ratain *et al.*1985, Quesada *et al.,* 1986, Dianzani 1992). However, some patients relapsed after cessation of IFN treatment (Ratain *et al.,* 1988). Purine analogues such as pentostatin and clabridine have been found to be more effective that IFN in the treatment of HCL, thus since 1990, these analogues have substituted IFN as a first line treatment for this condition (Ahmed and Rai 2003, Dillman 2004). It has recently been reported that, at a reduced dosage, IFN is well tolerated as a maintenance treatment and is associated with long-term survival and good quality of life (Damasio *et al.,* 2000, Benz *et al.,* 2009).Today, the use of IFN in the treatment of HCL is limited and reserved for patients who are unable to undergo purine analogue treatment or patients who have failed or become resistant to prior therapy with purine analogues (Ramakrishna and Manoharan 2010). It has also been suggested that IFN-α should still be considered for patients that do not respond to purine analogue treatment and patients with early relapses in order to diminish the risk of secondary cancers that can develop several years after purine analogue treatment (Benz 2010, Hoffman 2010).

Table 2: Preparations of IFNs commercially available.

Type	Trade Name
Human leukocyte IFN-α	Multiferon
IFN-α-2a	Roferon-A
IFN-α-2b	IntronA
IFN-alfacon-1	Infergen
IFN-α-n3	Alferon
Combination of IFN-α-2b and ribavirin	Rebetron
Pegylated IFN-α-2a	Pegasys
Pegylated IFN-α-2b	Pegintron
IFN-β-1a	Rebif
	Avonex
IFN-β-1b	Betaseron
	Extravia
IFN-γ-1b	Actimmune

Chronic Myelogenous Leukemia (CML)

This disease is an uncommon type of cancer characterized by the presence of a cytogenetic aberration commonly known as the Philadelphia chromosome (Kurzrock *et al.,* 1988, Clarkson and Strife 1993, Nowell 2007, Erikson *et al.,* 1986) which consists of a reciprocal translocation between the long arms of chromosomes 22 and chromosome 9 (Rowley 1973, Kurzrock *et al.,* 1988) with relocation of the oncogene *abl* from chromosome 9 to the BCR region of chromosome 22 (Groffen *et al.,* 1984), resulting in a *BCR/ABL* fusion gene which encodes a 210 KDa chimeric protein with stronger tyrosine kinase activity than the normal c-abl protein (Deininger *et al.,* 2000), which leads to the development of the CML phenotype of the chronic phase (Melo 1996) characterized by an increase in peripheral granulocytes and spleen enlargement (Zhang and Ren 1998). CML progresses from a chronic phase to an accelerated phase characterized by the presence of undifferentiated myeloid and lymphoid blast cells in peripheral blood (Faderl *et al.,* 1999). The disease can advance to a blast crisis which progresses rapidly leading to a shortened survival (Sawyers 1999). Some CML patients can be cured with bone marrow transplantation (Gale *et al.,* 1998). Early studies with partially purified IFN-α have showed normalization of blood counts in 75% of patients and suppression of the Philadelphia chromosome in about 25% of patients in the chronic phase (Gutterman 1994, Talpaz *et al.,* 1989). These studies were confirmed with recombinant IFN-α (Talpaz 1986, Talpaz 1989). Therefore IFN-α was used as a first-line treatment for CML until 2001. Imatinib, a tyrosine kinase inhibitor that specifically targets the BCR/ABL fusion, has replaced the use of IFN for this condition and is now the first-line treatment for CML. However, this treatment is rarely curative, only about 30% of treated patients show a 5 year survival rate. Most patients ultimately relapse with the development of imatinib resistance (Guilhot *et al.,* 2009, Jabbour *et al.,* 2009). It has been shown that maintenance treatment with IFN-α enables discontinuation of imatinib in patients after prior IFN/Imatinib therapy, leading to a sustained molecular response (Burchert *et al.,* 2010). Also, patients initially treated with IFN-α and then switched to an imatinib treatment demonstrated long term remission at a high rate, leading to the proposal that pre-treatment with IFN-α sensitizes CML stem cells to imatinib (Essers *et al.,* 2009). New information on the anti-leukemic mechanisms of IFN as well as the development of longer-acting pegylated forms of IFN (Platanias 2005, Benjamin *et al.,* 2007) have led to suggest a re-evaluation of the value of IFN in the treatment of myeloid leukemias (Anguille *et al.,* 2011). Two large randomized studies have demonstrated that pegylated IFN-α-2a in combination with imatinib can significantly increase cytogenetic and molecular responses in patients with chronic CML (Nicolini *et al.,* 2011, Preudhomme *et al.,* 2010). Also, new data suggests that this combination produces a response that is more rapid than that of imatinib alone. Therefore, IFN in combination with tyrosine inhibitors could be utilized to increase molecular and curative responses (Palandri *et al.,* 2010).

Osteosarcoma

This condition is a very aggressive form of bone cancer with a significant risk of fatal systemic relapse (Kirkwood and Ernstoff 1984). Approximately 20% to 25% of patients present a metastatic disease at the time of diagnosis. The main site of metastasis is the lung (Kager *et al.,* 2003). Animal studies demonstrated that IFN-α delays or inhibits the development of metastatic tumors (Whelan *et al.,* 2010). Also, *in vitro* studies have shown that both IFN-α and IFN-β are effective in the treatment of multi-drug resistant osteosarcoma cells (Manara *et al.,* 2004) The Karolinska hospital in Sweden conducted an analysis on osteosarcoma patients that were treated from 1971 to 1990 at this institution and concluded that IFN-α has activity as an adjuvant treatment in high grade osteosarcoma (Muller *et al.,* 2005). Currently a phase I trial, the EURAMOS I, is being conducted by the European and American osteosarcoma study group. In one arm of this study, pegylated recombinant IFN-α-2b is administered to postoprerative patients that have received chemotherapy with *cis*-platin, doxorubicin and high dose methotrexate, free survival is the end point evaluated (Whelan *et al.,* 2010).

Kaposi Sarcoma (KS)

This condition is the most common human immunodeficiency virus (HIV)-associated neoplasm. KS is worldwide the fourth most common cancer caused by an infectious agent, the human herpes virus 8 (Martin 2007). On November of 1988 the FDA approved the use of IFN-α-2b for the treatment of KS. The use of low doses of IFN has been evaluated. A randomized phase II clinical study was conducted to evaluate the efficacy of a low dose or an intermediate dose of IFN-α-2b in combination with the nucleoside reverse reductase inhibitor didanosine in patients with AIDS-associated KS. The response rate was 40% with the low dose and 55% with the intermediate dose; however patients in the intermediate dose experienced more toxic effects (Krown *et al.,* 2002). A more recent phase I study of the combination of IFN-α-2b with protease inhibitor-based highly active antiretroviral therapy in patients with AIDS-associated KS determined the maximum tolerable dose which increased CD4+ cells, almost 43% of the patients experienced a significant decrease in the median HIV RNA level and in 35% of the patients, tumor regression was observed (Krown *et al.,* 2006).

Metastatic Melanoma

This condition is a serious malignancy that develops in the cells that produce the skin pigment known as melanocytes (Slominski *et al.,* 2005). During early stages it can be cured with surgery however the metastatic form of the disease is one of the most resistant malignancies to chemotherapy and has a very poor prognosis

(Blesa *el at.* 2011). Early clinical trials showed activity of IFN-α-2b in patients with high risk melanoma. One in particular, the E1684 trial conducted in 1995 showed that high-doses of IFN-α-2b improved overall survival and extended relapse-free survival in high risk resected melanoma patients (Kirkwood *et al.,* 1996). Based on these results the FDA approved the use of IFN-α-2b as adjuvant treatment in post-surgical high risk melanoma patients. Since then, several clinical trials and meta-analyses have been conducted to evaluate the role of type I IFN as adjuvant in the treatment of advanced melanoma. The results of some of them revealed that high doses of IFN-α increased recurrence-free survival but have no impact on overall survival (Lens and Dawes 2002, Wheatley *et al.,* 2003, Pirard *et al.* 2004, Kirkwood *et al.,* 2004) while more recent trials and meta-analyses have shown that high doses of IFN-α increased recurrence-free survival as well as overall survival (Richtig *et al.,* 2004, Verma *et al.,* 2006, Kirkwood *et al.,* 2008, Mocellin *et al.,* 2010). Low-doses of IFN-α-2a have shown improved disease-free survival and overall survival in patients with metastatic melanoma that has spread to regional lymph nodes (Garbe *et al.,* 2008). It has been shown that the combination of low doses of IFN-α-2b with low doses of thalidomide is a safe palliative treatment for metastatic melanoma patients that have not responded to prior therapy (Solti *et al.,* 2007). A study of the combination of IFN-α-2b in combination with temozolomide in patients with metastatic melanoma stage IV showed and overall survival response of 27.6 %, toxicity was observed in 10.6% of the patients and the longest overall survival was observed in patients with total remission after 3 cycles (Richtig *et al.,* 2004). A recent randomized study showed that 83 % of the treated patients with metastatic melanoma experienced increased overall survival with the combination of IFN-α, thymosin alpha and decarbazine (Maio *et al.,* 2010). The use of pegylated IFN in metastatic melanoma has also been investigated. A study conducted to evaluate the effects on health-related quality of life in stage III melanoma patients treated with pegylated IFN-α-2b revealed improvement in recurrence-free survival, however, the treatment was associated with a negative effect on health-related quality of life (Bottomley *et al.,* 2009). A phase II study conducted in patients with stage IV melanoma without brain metastasis showed that pegylated IFN-α-2a in combination with dacabazine produced partial response in 16% of the patients, 2 of 28 patients showed long lasting responses and the response rate was 24%, this regimen was well tolerated.

(Hauschild *et al.,* 2008). Another more recent study showed that the combination of pegylated IFN-α-2b with temozolomide was well tolerated, 31 % of the patients showed objective tumor response with 8.5% complete responses (Hwu *et al.* 2006). It has also been shown that IFN is effective in the treatment of advanced non-melanoma skin cancer. In patients with recurrent advanced basal cell skin carcinomas and squamous cell skin carcinomas that have been resistant to other treatments, the combination of IFN-α and IFN-γ peri- and intralesionally produced complete tumor elimination in 28 of 60 patients and 24 of 60 patients showed more than 30% tumor reduction, the therapy was well tolerated. (Anasagasti-Angulo *et al.,* 2009). *In vitro* studies have shown that type III IFNs have anti-tumor activities in B16 melanoma cells (Lasfar *et al.,* 2006).

Renal Cell Cancercinoma (RCC)

This condition originates in the lining of the small kidney tubes; it is the most common malignancy of the kidneys (Banumathy and Cairns 2010). If diagnosed while the tumor is still localized in the kidney it can be cured with surgery, however when it metastasizes it becomes resistant to most chemotherapeutic agents (Oudard *et al.,* 2007). For many years the standard treatment for metastatic RCC was therapy with either IFN-α or IL-2 but only few patients showed beneficial effects from these therapies (Negrier *et al.,* 1998, McDermott *et al.,* 2005). New therapies have emerged, multikinase inhibitors such as sunitinib, have provided longer progression-free survival than IFN (Motzer *et al.,* 2007) and since 2006 is FDA approved as the first line treatment for RCC in patients with favorable to intermediate prognosis. Another kinase inhibitor, temsirolimus has shown moderate prolongation of survival in patients with poor prognosis compared to IFN-α (Hudes *et al.,* 2007) and was FDA approved in 2007 as first line treatment for these patients. Sorafenib is another tyrosine kinase inhibitor that has shown efficacy in the treatment of advanced renal carcinoma in patients previously treated with IFN-α or IL-2 (Escudier *et al.,* 2009) and was therefore FDA approved since 2005 as a second-line treatment of RCC in patients previously treated with biological therapy. Due to the high cost of these drugs only a limited amount of patients have access to this form of therapy. A review of clinical trials, meta-analyses, systematic reviews and practice guidelines of IFN-α treatment in patients with inoperable advanced or metastatic RCC concluded that

IFN-α has anti-tumor activity against this malignancy with a modest survival benefit and it should be considered as an option for those patients that do not have access to the costly treatment with kinase inhibitors (Canil *et al*., 2010) The use of IFN in combination with kinase inhibitors has been explored. A phase II trial in patients with metastatic or unresectable renal carcinoma who have not received previous systemic therapy showed a better response with the combination of IFN-α and sorafenib than with each drug alone (Ryan *et al.,* 2007). Another phase II study with the combination of IFN-α-2b and sorafenib in the treatment of naïve and IL-2 treated patients with metastatic RCC demonstrated high activity of the combination treatment, in more than half of the patients the dose had to be adjusted due to toxicity but then the therapy was successfully continued (Gollob *et al.,* 2007) A recent phase I trial of the combined therapy of IFN-α2-and sorafenib demonstrated partial response in 61% of the patients and was generally well tolerated (Niwakawa *et al.,* 2011). Another form of therapy involves the use of antibodies directed against vascular endothelial growth factor (VEGF) which is usually overexpressed in RCC. Bevacizumab a humanized monoclonal antibody against VEGF-A has been utilized in combination with IFN-α-2a. A randomized, double-blind phase III study (Escudier 2010) and a recent phase III trial (Melichar 2008) have demonstrated that the combination of IFN-α-2a and bevacizumab as a first-line treatment in patients with metastatic RCC increases median overall survival compared with that of patients receiving a combination of IFN-α and a placebo or IFN-α alone. This combination was approved by the FDA in July 2009 for the treatment of metastatic RCC. Several trials have also evaluated the use pegylated IFN-α-2a in RCC patients and have shown similar responses and toxicity than those obtained with the standard no pegylated IFN (Bex *et al.,* 2005, Feldman *et al.,* 2008, George *et al.,* 2008, Lyrdal *et al.,* 2009).

Follicular Lymphoma

Follicular lymphoma is the second most common lymphoma in adults (De Jong 2005), it mainly affects lymph nodes, in the early stages it can be treated with radiation but in more advanced stages a combination of chemoimunotherapy is often utilized (Griffiths *et al.,* 2010). Immunotherapy with IFN has been extensively studied for the treatment of this condition. A randomized study evaluated the combination of the anti-CD20 monoclonal antibody rituximab, chemotherapy and IFN-α-2a in the first-line treatment of follicular lymphoma patients who have a high tumor burden. This combination improved the outcome and provided superior disease control (Salles 2008). A meta-analysis of 1,922 newly diagnosed patients with follicular lymphoma treated with high doses of IFN-α-2 given in combination with relatively intensive initial chemotherapy showed prolongation of survival and remission duration (Rohatiner *et al.,* 2005). More recently, the evaluation of 8 clinical trials, 6 with IFN-α-2b and two with IFN-α-2a, demonstrated that IFN, in combination with chemotherapy, was effective in prolonging progression-free survival, although high toxicity was observed (Baldo *et al.,* 2010). A randomized study concluded that IFN-α-2b at a low dose in combination with cyclophosphamide did not significantly increase the response rate, duration of response, event-free, or overall survival in naïve patients with follicular lymphoma. (Smith *et al.,* 2009). A more recent randomized controlled study compared the combination of IFN-α and IL-2 in patients with non-Hodgkin's lymphoma (NHL) or Hodgkin's lymphoma (HL). A significant increase in disease free survival was observed only in NHL patients treated with IFN-IL-2 combination with no serious toxicity events. (Nagler *et al.,* 2010).

Head and Neck Squamous Cell Carcinomas (HNSCC)

These carcinomas originate from the upper-respiratory-digestive tract. HNSCC represent about 90% of all head and neck cancers (Forastiere *et al.,* 2003). It is a malignant tumor of epithelial origin. Head and neck cancer is a prevalent condition in the United States and the sixth leading site of new cancer cases among men (Leemans *et al.,* 2011). IFNs have been evaluated as therapeutic agents in this condition. In human esophageal cancer cells, IFN-β gene entrapped in cationic multilamellar liposomes in combination with 5-fluorouracil (5-FU) showed higher growth inhibition than either 5-FU or hIFN-β gene entrapped in liposomes alone (Tsunoo *et al.,* 2002). A pilot study evaluating the combination of IFN-*α*, cisplatin, and 5-FU in patients with advanced esophageal cancer showed that this combination was associated with an overall response rate of 55%, however this response was accompanied by considerable toxicity (Bazarbashi *et al.* 2002). A more recent phase II trial by the same group demonstrated a high response rate of the adjuvant combination therapy with IFN-α, cisplatin and 5FU in patients with resectable HNSCC (Bazarbashi *et al.,* 2008). A phase II study of IFN-*α* plus isotretinoin and vitamin E in patients with locally advanced HNSCC showed an increase in the 5-year survival rate and overall survival rate and prevented recurrence (Seixas-Silva *et al.,* 2005). A combination treatment with a low dose of recombinant IL-2 and interferon alpha-2a has also produced significant clinical tumor regressions in 2 of 11 patients. It has also been shown that IFN-α-2b can be used as an effective adjuvant to overcome the suppression of immune functions that occur in patients with tobacco-related HNSCC (Bose *et al.,* 2006). Recombinant human IFN-γ has shown a potent antitumor effect in human nasopharyngeal carcinoma cell lines (Wu *et al.,* 2006). HCNN patients are at high risk of developing a second primary tumor which is often localized in the head and neck, esophagus, or lung. Recently, it has been reported that IFN-λ in combination with cisplatin has anti-tumor effects in esophageal carcinoma cell lines and constitutes a promising therapy for this condition (Li *et al.,* 2010).

Breast Cancer

Worldwide this condition is the most commonly diagnosed type of cancer and the leading cause of cancer deaths among females (Jemel *et al.,* 2011). In 2008 there were about 1.38 million new breast cancer cases and 458,400 breast cancer related deaths (Jemal *et al.,* 2011). Although rare, breast cancer can also occur in men, it accounts for about 1% of all breast cancers (Niveditha *et al.,* 2004, Di Benedetto *et al.* 1998). There are two main types of breast cancers; one that originates in the lobules that produce milk known as lobular carcinoma (Venkitaraman 2010) and another that originates in the tubes that conduct milk known as ductal carcinoma, the later is the most common type of breast cancer (Allred 2010). Localized breast cancer is treated with surgery, radiation, chemotherapy and/or hormonal replacement (Shenkier *et al.,* 2004). Distant metastases from breast cancer have no cure and the treatment concentrates in alleviate the symptoms. Antiestrogens are usually administered as first and second line treatment in endocrine-responsive patients (Rugo 2008). However, many of them become resistant to this treatment. Studies in mice have shown that IFN-α and IFN-β inhibited the growth of breast carcinomas (Balkwill *et al.,* 1980, Kimoto *et al.,* 1987). A recent exploratory trial demonstrated that the combination of IFN-β and IL-2 with antiestrogens in breast cancer endocrine-dependant patients with distant metastasis was well tolerated and increased survival (Nicolini and Carpi 2005). A more recent pilot phase II study of the combined therapy with IFN-β, retinoids and tamoxifen in metastatic breast cancer patients showed that this regimen was well tolerated and prolonged survival (Recchia *et al.,* 2009). Fulvestrant is a drug prescribed for the treatment of hormone receptor-positive metastatic breast cancer in post menopausal patients whose disease had progressed after treatment with anti-estrogens such as tamoxifen, however fulvestrant resistance can occur (McKeage *et al.,* 2004). It has been shown that IFN-γ is capable of restoring sensitivity of fulvestrant in anti-estrogen resistant human breast cancer cell lines, making this type of IFN a potential treatment for this group of patients (Ning *et al.,* 2010).

Ovarian Cancer

Ovarian cancer is the fifth most common malignancy in women (Jemal *et al.,* 2011). The majority of patients present an advanced-stage disease at the time of diagnosis. More than 90% of ovarian cancers originate from the epithelium which is a highly lethal form of cancer (Scully 1995). It has been recently reported that high-grade carcinomas may arise from the fallopian tubes rather that the ovaries (Diniz *et al.,* 2011). The 5-year survival rate for all stages is less than 40% (Cannistra 2004). The standard treatment includes surgery and chemotherapy (Pignata *et al.,* 2011); however relapses are common (Markman *et al.,* 2006). Therefore, alternative therapies have been investigated. It has been shown that IFN-α is well tolerated and increased response rate in platinum sensitive patients with minimal residual epithelial ovarian cancer but not in platinum resistant patients (Berek *et al.,* 1999). A recent study reports that the anti-proliferative and anti-tumor effects of IFN-α in epithelial ovarian cancer cultures correlates with the presence of side populations which are present in 37% of patients with epithelial ovarian cancer tumors, indicating that side populations can be utilized as markers for IFN sensitivity in ovarian cancer patients (Moserle *et al.,* 2008). Administration of pegylated IFN-α in combination with paclitaxel showed a significant synergistic decreasing effect in angiogenesis and progressive growth of human ovarian carcinoma cells (Tedjarati *et al.,* 2002). A phase I/II study with IFN-γ-1b in combination with carboplatin and paxlitaxel in patients with stage III/IV ovarian cancer determined that this combination was safe and increased overall response rate suggesting that it could be used as a first-line treatment for patients with advanced ovarian cancer (Marth *et al.,* 2006). However, a more recent randomized phase III trial has evaluated the same combination in naïve advanced ovarian cancer and primary peritoneal cancer patients and showed significantly shorter overall survival with this combination than chemotherapy alone and was associated with high toxicity therefore this combination was not recommended as a first-line treatment in advanced ovarian cancer (Alberts *et al.,* 2008). A phase II study evaluated the efficacy and toxicity of the combination of IFN-γ, granulocyte macrophage colony stimulating factor (GM-CFS) and carboplatin in the treatment of recurrent, platinum-sensitive ovarian, fallopian tube and primary peritoneal cancer, demonstrating a reasonable response with improved quality of life in the responders (Schemeler *et al.,* 2009).

Cervical Cancer

Cancer of uterine cervix or cervical cancer is the third most common cancer among women worldwide and is the second leading cause of cancer-related deaths among women in the developing countries (Jemal *et al.,* 2011). If treated during the early stages it can be cured. Treatment involves surgery, radiation and chemotherapy (Powell 2010, Colombo and Peiretti 2010). However in advanced stages treatment becomes more difficult. It has been shown that the combination of IFN-α and retinoic acid have synergistic effects against squamous cell carcinoma cell lines, especially when combined with radiation (Blase *et al.,* 1999, Ryu *et al.,* 1998). A phase II trial evaluated the combination of IFN-α, retinoic acid and cisplatin in patients that have previously received treatment for metastatic cervical squamous cell carcinoma, although a consistent response rate was observed, 52% of the patients stopped or reduced treatment due to toxicity or progression (Braud *et al.,* 2002). A recent study in patients with high-grade cervical intraepithelial neoplasia treated with IFN-α-2b demonstrated a satisfactory response in 60% of the patients and higher expression of Th1 cytokines such as IFN-γ, TNF-α and IL-2, with a reduction in detectable human papilloma virus were observed (Ramos *et al.,* 2010).

Lung Cancer

This condition is the leading cause of cancer-related deaths in men in the second leading cause of cancer-related deaths in women worldwide (Jemal *et al.,* 2011).

Few patients survive more than 2 years. Surgery has been the main treatment in the early stages. However, this therapy is not effective in the advanced form of the disease. The majority of the patients show advanced lung cancer at the time of diagnosis which makes treatment more challenging. It has been reported that a maintenance treatment with IFN-α-2a and 13-*cis*-retinoic was well tolerated and increased median survival progression in patients with small cell lung cancer (Ruotsalainen *et al.,* 2000). Malignant mesothelioma is a very aggressive neoplasma that develops in the pleura and peritoneum associated with exposure to asbestos (Robinson *et al.,* 2005). It has been shown that IFN-β but not IFN-α has an anti-proliferative effect in a human microvascular lung endothelial cancer cell line (Erdmann 2011). Studies in murine models have shown that an adenoviral vector expressing IFN-β was highly effective in eradicating mesothelioma tumors and Bronchogenic Adenocarcinoma of the Lung (Odaka *et al.,* 2001, Wilderman *et al.* 2005). A phase I trial was conducted to determine safety, toxicity and efficacy of two doses of adenoviral-mediated IFN-β gene transfer in patients with malignant pleural mesothelioma and metastatic pleural effusions. Minimal toxicity and an increase in median survival were observed. However the second dose showed no evidence of increased duration of IFN-β gene expression and resulted in the development of neutralizing antibodies (Sterman *et al.,* 2010).

Bladder Cancer

This type of cancer is the fourth most common malignant disease among men in the US where the most common type of bladder cancer is urothelial carcinoma (Jemal *et al.,* 2011). This condition is less common in women. Intravesical Bacillus Calmette-Gurin (BCG) is the mainstay of superficial bladder cancer treatment (Kapoor *et al.,* 2008). Disease-free has been reported in patients treated with intravesical therapy with BCG and IFN-α-2b even in patients that have previously failed BCG therapy. (O'Donnell *et al.* 2001, Lam *et al.,* 2003). It has been reported a synergistic apoptotic and anti-growth effect of IFN-α-2a in combination with retinoids in human bladder cells lines (Zou *et al.,* 2005). A data base has been created with several parameters that affect the outcome of patients treated with BCG and IFN combination and constitutes a source of information for a more individualized IFN therapy for patients with bladder cancer (Shah *et al.,* 2006).

Pancreatic Cancer

Pancreatic cancer is the fourth leading cause of cancer related mortality in the U.S with a 5-year survival rate of 5% (Jemal *et al.,* 2010). Approximately 90% of pancreatic cancers originate from ductal cells (Adsay *et al.,* 2005). Treatment depends on the advance of the disease. The localized stage is treated with surgery. Radiation and chemotherapy are utilized in the treatment of the locally advanced stage. In the mestatatic stage of the disease the treatment is mainly palliative. A study to evaluate external radiation in combination with 5-FU, cisplatin and IFN-α in patients with adenocarcinomas in the pancreatic head showed increased overall survival (Picozzi *et al.,* 2003). Studies in an orthotopic mice model have shown that IFN-α restitutes the sensitivity of pancreatic cancer cells to chemotherapy (Hoffmann *et al.,* 2008), this is a significant finding considering that multidrug resistance is a major problem in treatment this type of cancer. Another pancreatic cancer orthotopic study in a mouse model showed that the combination of IFN-α, 5-FU, cisplatin and radiation increased survival and showed less metastasis (Zhu *et al.,* 2008). Analysis of the concomitant administration of IFN-α, radiation, chemotherapy and 5-FU in 7 patients with localized carcinoma of the pancreas or 4 periampullary patients showed a 4 year overall survival of 55%, demonstrating that this combination is a possible new treatment of pancreatic cancer in resected patients (Nitsche *et al.,* 2008). A phase II study evaluated IFN-α as adjuvant therapy of patients with resectable adenocarcinoma treated with radiation and gemcitabine showed that the combination increased media overall survival compared to historical controls, 13% of the patients did not complete the adjuvant therapy due to toxicities (Linehan *et al.,* 2008). A recent study in pancreatic cell lines demonstrated that IFN-β in combination with gemcitabine produced a more potent synergistic growth inhibitory effect than the combination of IFN-α and gemcitabine, the effect was also observed in pancreatic cells with a weak expression of IFN-α-R2 (Tomimaru *et al.,* 2011). In patients with neuroendocrine carcinomas of the gastroenteropancreatic system, pegylated IFN-α induced inhibition of tumor growth and was better tolerated than IFN-α, providing a good alternative treatment for patients that do not tolerate conventional treatment with IFN-α (Pavel *et al.,* 2006). A multicenter, randomized phase III trial to study the use of IFN-α-2a in combination with chemotherapy and radiation in patients with resected pancreatic adenocarcinoma showed an increase in median survival and reduction in local recurrence with this combination compared with patients treated with 5FU/FA, especially in high risk patients. (Marten *et al.,* 2009). In this trial a significantly longer survival was observed in patients who responded to single IFN-α challenge with a decrease in T helper cells and regulatory T cells or with a pronounced increase in NK cell mediated cytotoxicity, this observation has been previously described (Schnmidt *et al.,* 2006). IFN-λ1 and IFN-λ2 showed anti-proliferative and apoptotic properties in the human pancreatic neuroendocrine tumor cells, BON1, indicating a potential therapeutic use of these types of IFN in neuroendocrine tumors (Zitzmann *et al.,* 2006).

Brain Tumors

Malignant gliomas are the most common primary central nervous system tumors in adults (Schneider *et al.,* 2010). Despite the advances in radiation therapy and chemotherapy administered after the surgical resection of the tumor, the prognosis of malignant glioma remains poor, with a median survival of less than one year (Hentschel and Sawaya 2003, Stieber 2001). A phase I trial conducted in 11 patients with malignant glioma showed that injections with adenovirus vector expressing the human IFN-β gene directly into the tumor and surrounding areas was feasible and associated with induction of apoptosis (Chiocca *et al.,* 2008). Two phase II trials have shown that the combination of pegylated or non-pegylated IFN-α-2b with temozolomide showed improved efficacy in patients with glioblastoma multiforme compared with patients receiving only temozolomide or with historical controls (Groves *et al.,* 2009). Patients with high-grade gliomas exhibit decreased peripheral T-cell responsiveness as well as an overall decrease in immune function (Morford *et al.,* 1997). *In vivo* intracranial injections of glioma cells inoculated with adenovirus bearing the murine IFN-γ gene in mouse showed prolonged survival, decreased tumor size and increased intratumoral expression of MHC and enhanced $CD4^+$ and $CD8^+$ T-cell infiltration compared with control mice receiving intracranial inoculations of glioma cells inoculated with saline (Ehtesham *et al.,* 2002). A recent study revealed a significant increase in median survival time in patients with newly diagnosed primary glioblastoma treated with a combination of IFN-β with temozolomine compared to those who received temozolomine alone, especially in patients with unmethylated MGMT promoter who usually have a poor response to alkylating agents such as temozolomine (Motomura *et al.,* 2011). Brainstem gliomas are tumors which occur in the posterior part of the brain known as the brainstem and are more common in children who died within 2 years of diagnosis. A study of 15 patients with newly diagnosed brainstem tumors and treated with IFN-β, ranimustine and radiotherapy showed that the therapy was well tolerated and in five patients partial response and stable disease was observed indicating that this combination constitutes a promising therapy for this condition (Ohno *et al.,* 2009). Intratumoral injections of IFN-α has shown efficacy in the treatment of cranioprangyomas which are brain tumors derived from the pituitary gland and occur more commonly in children and adolescents, partial tumor reduction and complete disappearance of the lesions have been reported in some patients (Cavalheiro *et al.,* 2005, Cavalheiro *et al.,* 2010).

Hepatocellular Carcinoma (HCC)

This condition is the fifth most common cancer worldwide (Jemal *et al.,* 2011). Liver transplantation can be curative; however it is not a feasible option for the majority of the patients due to cost and availability. Liver resection is the first-line curative treatment for most HCC patients; tumor ablation is another curative option (Clavien 2007). However, about half of the patients present recurrence at 3 years after resection or ablation (Mazzaferro *et al.,* 2006). A randomized controlled trial of the use of IFN-α-2b as an adjuvant therapy in HCC patients after hepatic resection showed increased survival rate (Lo *et al.,* 2007). A randomized controlled trial showed that IFN-α did not suppress carcinoma but it decreased incidence of recurrence after resection of HCV-related HCC (Kubo *et al.,* 2001). A prospective randomized clinical trial showed that IFN-α increased the cumulative survival rate in HCC patients after resection; however 13% of IFN treated patients showed recurrence (Kubo *et al.,* 2002). Another randomized trial showed that IFN-α reduced the late recurrence rate in cirrhotic HCC patients after liver resection but it had no effect on the overall prevention of tumor recurrence after resection (Mazzaferro *et al.,* 2006). A randomized trial showed an increase in the survival rate in HCC patients that had been successfully treated with ablation and further treated with IFN-α. Toxicity was observed in some patients (Lin *et al.,* 2004). A randomized study of HCC male patients showed a cumulative survival rate increase after resection in patients treated with IFN-α

(Nishiguchi *et al.,* 2005). Another study showed that IFN-α increased overall survival in HCC patients after resection, but no significant effect in recurrence or disease free survival after curative resection was observed (Sun *et al.,* 2006). Three systematic reviews and meta-analyses have concluded that IFN-α prevents tumor recurrence and improves survival after curative resection or ablation of HCC patients with viral-related hepatitis (Breitenstein *et al.,* 2009, Yang *et al.,* 2009, Zhang *et al.,* 2009). Moreover, one of these meta-analysis has shown that IFN-α reduces the risk of HCC and cirrhosis in patients with chronic hepatitis B (Yang *et al.,* 2009) While another meta-analysis concluded that treatment with IFN-α in hepatitis C virus-related cirrhosis reduces the risk of HCC only in patients with sustained virological response (Singal *et al.,* 2010). The already poor prognosis of advanced HCC can be complicated by the development of portal vein tumor thrombosis (PVTT) which decreases blood supply to the normal liver parenchyma causing deterioration of the liver function. Recently intra-arterial 5-FU/IFN combination therapy with or without radiotherapy in patients with HCC and PVTT resulted in complete response of PVTT in 19% of the patients, 56% partial responses and 25 % stable disease (Katamura *et al.,* 2009). Another possible therapy for HCC patients is the combination of IFN-α-2a with TS-1 which has been reported to be a feasible and effective method to treat this disease (Ueshima *et al.,* 2008). *In vivo* studies showed anti-tumor activities of type III IFNs in mice inoculated with a hepatoma cell line expressing IFN-λ, indicating its potential use in this type of cancer (Abushahba *et al.,* 2010).

Multiple Myeloma

This malignancy affects a specific type of blood cells known as plasma cells (Palumbo 2011). It is a relatively uncommon condition, it is estimated that 20,000 new cases occur in the US each year; the majority of the diagnosed patients are 60 years old or older (Jemal *et al.,* 2010). Patients with stable multiple myeloma may need no treatment, patients with non-stable multiple myeloma are usually treated with chemotherapy and bone marrow transplant (Palumbo 2011). The use of IFN in this condition has been evaluated. A meta-analysis of 30 randomized trials, 17 of which were conducted in patients who received IFN-chemotherapy induction treatment or chemotherapy alone and 13 were conducted in patients who received IFN maintenance therapy or no treatment, demonstrated that cumulative relapse-free and overall survival were always significantly higher in the IFN trial arms (Fritz and Ludwig 2000). A recent randomized, controlled phase II study comparing pegylated IFN-α-2b and non-pegylated IFN-α-2b in patients with multiple myeloma showed that patients have a better quality of life when treated with pegylated IFN-α-2b (Sirohi *et al.,* 2007).

V. CONCLUSIONS

Many clinical trials have been conducted for the use of IFNs in cancer therapy, some of them led to the approval of type I IFN in the treatment of some malignancies. The toxicity associated with IFN treatment and the development of more effective drugs with fewer side effects has limited the use of IFNs in cancer therapy. However, the current clinical trials and meta-analysis described in this chapter have demonstrated that IFNs, especially type I IFNs, are effective therapeutic anti-cancer agents but only for a particular group of patients. Therefore, it is critical to identify this selected group of patients that can benefit from IFN therapy to avoid exposing non-responsive patients to its toxic side effects. Some indicators of the response to IFN therapy have been identified for certain conditions, for example, in high-risk melanoma patients treated with IFN-α-2b, the pretreatment serum levels of the pro-inflammatory proteins IL-1β, IL-1α, IL-6, TNF-α, and the chemokines MIP-1α and MIP-1β were significantly higher in patients with longer relapse-free survival than in patients with shorter relapse-free survival (Yurkovetsky *et al.,* 2007). The presence of unmethylated MGMT seems to provide a more favorable outcome in patients with primary glioblastoma treated with the combination of IFN-β and temozolomide (Motomura *et al.,* 2011). Patients with hepatitis C virus-related cirrhosis who exhibited a sustained virological response showed a reduced risk of developing hepatocellular carcinoma (Singal *et al.,* 2010). *In vitro* studies have demonstrated that methylthioadenosine phosphorylase (mtap) is expressed in some melanoma cell lines, loss of expression of mtap is associated with inhibition of the STAT signaling regulated by IFN, therefore patients with primary tumors lacking mtap expression are unlikely to respond to IFN therapy (Wild *et al.,* 2007, Meyer *et al.,* 2010). The monitoring of IFN treatment may be possible in some conditions. For instance, in patients with stage IIB/III melanoma treated with high dose of IFN the presence of auto-antibodies is associated with significant improvement in relapse-free survival and overall survival (Gogas *et al.,* 2006, Bouwhuis *et al.,* 2009). Therefore development of autoimmunity can be considered a prognostic marked during IFN therapy. It is important to determine the factors that predispose patients to develop autoimmunity upon IFN treatment, since these factors can identify the melanoma patients who are most likely to respond to IFN therapy. As we acquire more knowledge about the anti-tumor mechanisms of IFNs more predictors of IFN therapy response will be indentified. The toxicity associated with IFN treatment can be reduced utilizing new forms of IFN administration, such as direct administration of IFN or adenovirus expressing IFN into the tumor site (Choicca *et al.,* 2008, Sterman *et al.,* 2010, Cavalheiro 2005). In summary identification of patients who respond to IFN therapy along with administration techniques with fewer side effects can warrant the use of IFNs as effective anti-cancer agents for the treatment of several types of cancer.

ACKNOWLEDGEMENT

I thank Daniel R. Weaver for his helpful comments and critical reading of this manuscript.

CONFLICT OF INTEREST

The authors confirm that this chapter content has no conflict of interest.

REFERENCES

Ablasser A., Bauernfeind F., Hartmann G., Latz E., Fitzgerald K.A. & Hornung V. (2009) RIG-I-dependent sensing of poly(dA:dT) through the induction of an RNA polymerase III-transcribed RNA intermediate. *Nat Immunol,* 10, 1065-1072.

Abushahba W., Balan M., Castaneda I., Yuan Y., Reuhl K., Raveche E., de la Torre A., Lasfar A. & Kotenko S.V. (2010) Antitumor activity of type I and type III interferons in BNL hepatoma model. *Cancer Immunol Immunother,* 59, 1059-1071.

Adsay N.V., Basturk O., Cheng J.D. & Andea A.A. (2005) Ductal neoplasia of the pancreas: nosologic, clinicopathologic, and biologic aspects. *Semin Radiat Oncol,* 15, 254-264.

Ahmed S. & Rai K.R. (2003) Interferon in the treatment of hairy-cell leukemia. *Best Pract Res Clin Haematol*, 16, 69-81.

Akira S., Uematsu S. & Takeuchi O. (2006) Pathogen recognition and innate immunity. *Cell,* 124, 783-801.

Alberts D.S., Marth C., Alvarez R.D., Johnson G., Bidzinski M., Kardatzke D.R., Bradford W.Z., Loutit J., Kirn D.H., Clouser M.C. & Markman M. (2008) Randomized phase 3 trial of interferon gamma-1b plus standard carboplatin/paclitaxel *versus* carboplatin/paclitaxel alone for first-line treatment of advanced ovarian and primary peritoneal carcinomas: results from a prospectively designed analysis of progression-free survival. *Gynecol Oncol,* 109, 174-181.

Alexopoulou L., Holt A.C., Medzhitov R. & Flavell R.A. (2001) Recognition of double-stranded RNA and activation of NF-kappaB by Toll-like receptor 3. *Nature,* 413, 732-738.

Allred D.C. (2010) Ductal carcinoma *in situ*: terminology, classification, and natural history. *J Natl Cancer Inst Monogr*,2010, 134-138.

Anasagasti-Angulo L., Garcia-Vega Y., Barcelona-Perez S., Lopez-Saura P. & Bello-Rivero I. (2009) Treatment of advanced, recurrent, resistant to previous treatments basal and squamous cell skin carcinomas with a synergistic formulation of interferons. Open, prospective study. *BMC Cancer,* 9, 262.

Anderson K.C., Boyd A.W., Fisher D.C., Leslie D., Schlossman S.F. & Nadler L.M. (1985) Hairy cell leukemia: a tumor of pre-plasma cells. *Blood,* 65, 620-629.

Anguille S., Lion E., Willemen Y., Van Tendeloo V.F., Berneman Z.N. & Smits E.L. (2011) Interferon-alpha in acute myeloid leukemia: an old drug revisited. *Leukemia.*

Ank N., West H. & Paludan S.R. (2006) IFN-lambda: novel antiviral cytokines. *J Interferon Cytokine Res,* 26, 373-379.

Bach E.A., Aguet M. & Schreiber R.D. (1997) The IFN gamma receptor: a paradigm for cytokine receptor signaling. *Annu Rev Immunol,* 15, 563-591.

Baldo P., Rupolo M., Compagnoni A., Lazzarini R., Bearz A., Cannizzaro R., Spazzapan S., Truccolo I. & Moja L. (2010) Interferon-alpha for maintenance of follicular lymphoma. *Cochrane Database Syst Rev*, CD004629.

Balkwill F., Taylor-Papadimitriou J., Fantes K.H. & Sebesteny A. (1980) Human lymphoblastoid interferon can inhibit the growth of human breast cancer xenografts in athymic (nude) mice. *Eur J Cancer,* 16, 569-573.

Banumathy G. & Cairns P. (2010) Signaling pathways in renal cell carcinoma. *Cancer Biol Ther,* 10, 658-664.

Bazarbashi S., Abdelsalam M., Amin T., El-Bassiouni M., Soudy H., Elweshi A., Alhusseiny H., Rehman K., Memon M. & Ajarim D. (2008) Phase II trial of neoadjuvant cisplatin, 5-fluorouracil and interferon-alpha in operable squamous cell carcinoma of the esophagus. *Chemotherapy,* 54, 315-322.

Bazarbashi S., Rahal M., Raja M.A., El Weshi A., Pai C., Ezzat A., Ajarim D., Memon M. & Al Fadda M. (2002) A pilot trial of combination cisplatin, 5-fluorouracil and interferon-alpha in the treatment of advanced esophageal carcinoma. *Chemotherapy,* 48, 211-216.

Benjamin R., Khwaja A., Singh N., McIntosh J., Meager A., Wadhwa M., Streck C., Ng C., Davidoff A.M. & Nathwani A.C. (2007) Continuous delivery of human type I interferons (alpha/beta) has significant activity against acute myeloid leukemia cells *in vitro* and in a xenograft model. *Blood,* 109, 1244-1247.

Benz R., Siciliano R.D., Stussi G. & Fehr J. (2009) Long-term follow-up of interferon-alpha induction and low-dose maintenance therapy in hairy cell leukemia. *Eur J Haematol* 82, 194-200.

Benz R., Stussi G. & Fehr J. (2010) Interferon as an alternative to purine analogues in the treatment of hairy cell leukaemia. *Br J Haematol,* 148, 664-665; author reply 665-666.

Berek J.S., Markman M., Stonebraker B., Lentz S.S., Adelson M.D., DeGeest K. & Moore D. (1999) Intraperitoneal interferon-alpha in residual ovarian carcinoma: a phase II gynecologic oncology group study. *Gynecol Oncol,* 75, 10-14.

Bex A., Mallo H., Kerst M., Haanen J., Horenblas S. & de Gast G.C. (2005) A phase-II study of pegylated interferon alfa-2b for patients with metastatic renal cell carcinoma and removal of the primary tumor. *Cancer Immunol Immunother,* 54, 713-719.

Blase M., Zaruba M.M., Santo-Hoeltje L., Bamberg M., Hoffmann W. & Rodemann H.P. (1999) 13-*cis* retinoic acid in combination with interferon-alpha enhances radiation sensitivity of human squamous cell carcinoma cells of the oral cavity. *Strahlenther Onkol,* 175, 563-568.

Blesa J.M., Pulido *E.G.*, Candel V.A. & Pulla M.P. Melanoma: from darkness to promise. *Am J Clin Oncol,* 34, 179-187.

Borden E.C. (1979) Interferons: rationale for clinical trials in neoplastic disease. *Ann Intern Med,* 91, 472-479.

Bose A., Ghosh D., Pal S., Mukherjee K.K., Biswas J. & Baral R. (2006) Interferon alpha2b augments suppressed immune functions in tobacco-related head and neck squamous cell carcinoma patients by modulating cytokine signaling. *Oral Oncol,* 42, 161-171.

Bottomley A., Coens C., Suciu S., Santinami M., Kruit W., Testori A., Marsden J., Punt C., Sales F., Gore M., Mackie R., Kusic Z., Dummer R., Patel P., Schadendorf D., Spatz A., Keilholz U. & Eggermont A. (2009) Adjuvant therapy with pegylated interferon alfa-2b *versus* observation in resected stage III melanoma: a phase III randomized controlled trial of health-related quality of life and symptoms by the European Organisation for Research and Treatment of Cancer Melanoma Group. *J Clin Oncol,* 27, 2916-2923.

Bouroncle B.A., Wiseman B.K. & Doan C.A. (1958) Leukemic reticuloendotheliosis. *Blood,* 13, 609-630.

Bouwhuis M.G., Suciu S., Collette S., Aamdal S., Kruit W.H., Bastholt L., Stierner U., Sales F., Patel P., Punt C.J., Hernberg M., Spatz A., ten Hagen T.L., Hansson J. & Eggermont A.M. (2009) Autoimmune antibodies and recurrence-free interval in melanoma patients treated with adjuvant interferon. *J Natl Cancer Inst,* 101, 869-877.

Braud A.C., Gonzague L., Bertucci F., Genre D., Camerlo J., Gravis G., Goncalves A., Moutardier V., Viret F., Maraninchi D. & Viens P. (2002) Retinoids, cisplatin and interferon-alpha in recurrent or metastatic cervical squamous cell carcinoma: clinical results of 2 phase II trials. *Eur Cytokine Netw,* 13, 115-120.

Breitenstein S., Dimitroulis D., Petrowsky H., Puhan M.A., Mullhaupt B. & Clavien P.A. (2009) Systematic review and meta-analysis of interferon after curative treatment of hepatocellular carcinoma in patients with viral hepatitis. *Br J Surg,* 96, 975-981.

Brenner D.J. (1997) Radiation biology in brachytherapy. *J Surg Oncol,* 65, 66-70.

Burchert A., Muller M.C., Kostrewa P., Erben P., Bostel T., Liebler S., Hehlmann R., Neubauer A. & Hochhaus A. (2010) Sustained molecular response with interferon alfa maintenance after induction therapy with imatinib plus interferon alfa in patients with chronic myeloid leukemia. *J Clin Oncol,* 28, 1429-1435.

Canil C., Hotte S., Mayhew L.A., Waldron T.S. & Winquist E. (2010) Interferon-alfa in the treatment of patients with inoperable locally advanced or metastatic renal cell carcinoma: a systematic review. *Can Urol Assoc, J* 4, 201-208.

Cannistra S.A. (2004) Cancer of the ovary. *N Engl J Med* 351, 2519-2529.

Cantell K. & Tovell D.R. (1971) Substitution of milk for serum in the production fo human leukocyte interferon. *Appl Microbiol,* 22, 625-628.

Carnaud C., Lee D., Donnars O., Park S.H., Beavis A., Koezuka Y. & Bendelac A. (1999) Cutting edge: Cross-talk between cells of the innate immune system: NKT cells rapidly activate NK cells. *J Immunol,* 163, 4647-4650.

Catovsky D., Quesada J.R. & Golomb H.M. (1987) Guidelines for the treatment of hairy cell leukemia. *Leukemia,* 1, 405-406.

Cavalheiro S., Dastoli P.A., Silva N.S., Toledo S., Lederman H. & da Silva M.C. (2005) Use of interferon alpha in intratumoral chemotherapy for cystic craniopharyngioma. *Childs Nerv Syst,* 21, 719-724.

Cavalheiro S., Di Rocco C., Valenzuela S., Dastoli P.A., Tamburrini G., Massimi L., Nicacio J.M., Faquini I.V., Ierardi D.F., Silva N.S., Pettorini B.L. & Toledo S.R. (2010) Craniopharyngiomas: intratumoral chemotherapy with interferon-alpha: a multicenter preliminary study with 60 cases. *Neurosurg Focus,* 28, E12.

Chelbi-Alix M.K. & Wietzerbin J. (2007) Interferon, a growing cytokine family: 50 years of interferon research. *Biochimie,* 89, 713-718.

Chen J., Baig E. & Fish E.N. (2004) Diversity and relatedness among the type I interferons. *J Interferon Cytokine Res,* 24, 687-698.

Chi H., Lu B., Takekawa M., Davis R.J. & Flavell R.A. (2004) GADD45beta/GADD45gamma and MEKK4 comprise a genetic pathway mediating STAT4-independent IFNgamma production in T cells. *EMBO J,* 23, 1576-1586.

Chiocca E.A., Smith K.M., McKinney B., Palmer C.A., Rosenfeld S., Lillehei K., Hamilton A., DeMasters B.K., Judy K. & Kirn D. (2008) A phase I trial of Ad.hIFN-beta gene therapy for glioma. *Mol Ther,* 16, 618-626.

Chiu Y.H., Macmillan J.B. & Chen Z.J. (2009) RNA polymerase III detects cytosolic DNA and induces type I interferons through the RIG-I pathway. *Cell,* 138, 576-591.

Clarkson B. & Strife A. (1993) Linkage of proliferative and maturational abnormalities in chronic myelogenous leukemia and relevance to treatment. *Leukemia,* 7, 1683-1721.

Clavien P.A. (2007) Interferon: the magic bullet to prevent hepatocellular carcinoma recurrence after resection? *Ann Surg,* 245, 843-845.

Colamonici O., Yan H., Domanski P., Handa R., Smalley D., Mullersman J., Witte M., Krishnan K. & Krolewski J. (1994) Direct binding to and tyrosine phosphorylation of the alpha subunit of the type I interferon receptor by p135tyk2 tyrosine kinase. *Mol Cell Biol,* 14, 8133-8142.

Colombo N. & Peiretti M. (2010) Critical review of neoadjuvant chemotherapy followed by surgery for locally advanced cervical cancer. *Int J Gynecol Cancer,* 20, S47-48.

Damasio E.E., Clavio M., Masoudi B., Isaza A., Spriano M., Rossi E., Casciaro S., Cerri R., Risso M., Nati S., Siccardi M., Truini M. & Gobbi M. (2000) Alpha-interferon as induction and maintenance therapy in hairy cell leukemia: a long-term follow-up analysis. *Eur J Haematol,* 64, 47-52.

de Jong D. (2005) Molecular pathogenesis of follicular lymphoma: a cross talk of genetic and immunologic factors. *J Clin Oncol,* 23, 6358-6363.

de Weerd N.A., Samarajiwa S.A. & Hertzog P.J. (2007) Type I interferon receptors: biochemistry and biological functions. *J Biol Chem,* 282, 20053-20057.

Deininger M.W., Goldman J.M. & Melo J.V. (2000) The molecular biology of chronic myeloid leukemia. *Blood,* 96, 3343-3356.

Devos R., Cheroutre H., Taya Y., Degrave W., Van Heuverswyn H. & Fiers W. (1982) Molecular cloning of human immune interferon cDNA and its expression in eukaryotic cells. *Nucleic Acids Res,* 10, 2487-2501.

Di Benedetto G., Pierangeli M. & Bertani A. (1998) Carcinoma of the male breast: an underestimated killer. *Plast Reconstr Surg,* 102, 696-700.

Dianzani F. (1992) Interferon treatments: how to use an endogenous system as a therapeutic agent. *J Interferon Res,* Spec No, 109-118.

Diaz M.O., Pomykala H.M., Bohlander S.K., Maltepe E., Malik K., Brownstein B. & Olopade O.I. (1994) Structure of the human type-I interferon gene cluster determined from a YAC clone contig. *Genomics,* 22, 540-552.

Diebold S.S., Kaisho T., Hemmi H., Akira S. & Reis e Sousa C. (2004) Innate antiviral responses by means of TLR7-mediated recognition of single-stranded RNA. *Science,* 303, 1529-1531.

Dillman R.O. (2004) Pentostatin (Nipent) in the treatment of chronic lymphocyte leukemia and hairy cell leukemia. *Expert Rev Anticancer Ther,* 4, 27-36.

Diniz P.M., Carvalho J.P., Baracat E.C. & Carvalho F.M. (2011) Fallopian tube origin of supposed ovarian high-grade serous carcinomas. *Clinics (Sao Paulo),* 66, 73-76.

Dumoutier L., Tounsi A., Michiels T., Sommereyns C., Kotenko S.V. & Renauld J.C. (2004) Role of the interleukin (IL)-28 receptor tyrosine residues for antiviral and antiproliferative activity of IL-29/interferon-lambda 1: similarities with type I interferon signaling. *J Biol Chem,* 279, 32269-32274.

Ehtesham M., Samoto K., Kabos P., Acosta F.L., Gutierrez M.A., Black K.L. & Yu J.S. (2002) Treatment of intracranial glioma with *in situ* interferon-gamma and tumor necrosis factor-alpha gene transfer. *Cancer Gene Ther,* 9, 925-934.

Erdmann J., Vitale G., van Koetsveld P.M., Croze E., Sprij-Mooij D.M., Hofland L.J. & van Eijck C.H. (2011) Effects of Interferons alpha/beta on the Proliferation of Human Micro- and Macrovascular Endothelial Cells. *J Interferon Cytokine Res.*

Erikson J., Griffin C.A., ar-Rushdi A., Valtieri M., Hoxie J., Finan J., Emanuel B.S., Rovera G., Nowell P.C. & Croce C.M. (1986) Heterogeneity of chromosome 22 breakpoint in Philadelphia-positive (Ph+) acute lymphocytic leukemia. *Proc Natl Acad Sci U S A,* 83, 1807-1811.

Escudier B., Bellmunt J., Negrier S., Bajetta E., Melichar B., Bracarda S., Ravaud A., Golding S., Jethwa S. & Sneller V. (2007) Phase III trial of bevacizumab plus interferon alfa-2a in patients with metastatic renal cell carcinoma (AVOREN): final analysis of overall survival. *J Clin Oncol,* 28, 2144-2150.

Escudier B., Eisen T., Stadler W.M., Szczylik C., Oudard S., Staehler M., Negrier S., Chevreau C., Desai A.A., Rolland F., Demkow T., Hutson T.E., Gore M., Anderson S., Hofilena G., Shan M., Pena C., Lathia C. & Bukowski R.M. (2009) Sorafenib for treatment of renal cell carcinoma: Final efficacy and safety results of the phase III treatment approaches in renal cancer global evaluation trial. *J Clin Oncol,* 27, 3312-3318.

Essers M.A., Offner S., Blanco-Bose W.E., Waibler Z., Kalinke U., Duchosal M.A. & Trumpp A. (2009) IFNalpha activates dormant haematopoietic stem cells *in vivo*. *Nature,* 458, 904-908.

Faderl S., Talpaz M., Estrov Z. & Kantarjian H.M. (1999) Chronic myelogenous leukemia: biology and therapy. *Ann Intern Med,* 131, 207-219.

Falcoff R. (1972) Some properties of virus and immune-induced human lymphocyte interferons. *J Gen Virol,* 16, 251-253.

Farrar M.A. & Schreiber R.D. (1993) The molecular cell biology of interferon-gamma and its receptor. *Annu Rev Immunol,* 11, 571-611.

Feldman D.R., Kondagunta G.V., Schwartz L., Patil S., Ishill N., DeLuca J., Russo P. & Motzer R.J. (2008) Phase II trial of pegylated interferon-alpha 2b in patients with advanced renal cell carcinoma. *Clin Genitourin Cancer,* 6, 25-30.

Field A.K., Lampson G.P., Tytell A.A., Nemes M.M. & Hilleman M.R. (1967) Inducers of interferon and host resistance, IV. Double-stranded replicative form RNA (MS2-Ff-RNA) from *E. coli* infected with MS2 coliphage. *Proc Natl Acad Sci U S A,* 58, 2102-2108.

Fitzgerald K.A., McWhirter S.M., Faia K.L., Rowe D.C., Latz E., Golenbock D.T., Coyle A.J., Liao S.M. & Maniatis T. (2003) IKKepsilon and TBK1 are essential components of the IRF3 signaling pathway. *Nat Immunol,* 4, 491-496.

Fitzgerald-Bocarsly P. & Feng D. (2007) The role of type I interferon production by dendritic cells in host defense. *Biochimie,* 89, 843-855.

Forastiere A.A., Goepfert H., Maor M., Pajak T.F., Weber R., Morrison W., Glisson B., Trotti A., Ridge J.A., Chao C., Peters G., Lee D.J., Leaf A., Ensley J. & Cooper J. (2003) Concurrent chemotherapy and radiotherapy for organ preservation in advanced laryngeal cancer. *N Engl J Med,* 349, 2091-2098.

Fritz E. & Ludwig H. (2000) Interferon-alpha treatment in multiple myeloma: meta-analysis of 30 randomised trials among 3948 patients. *Ann Oncol,* 11, 1427-1436.

Fu X.Y. (1992) A transcription factor with SH2 and SH3 domains is directly activated by an interferon alpha-induced cytoplasmic protein tyrosine kinase(s). *Cell,* 70, 323-335.

Gale R.P., Hehlmann R., Zhang M.J., Hasford J., Goldman J.M., Heimpel H., Hochhaus A., Klein J.P., Kolb H.J., McGlave P.B., Passweg J.R., Rowlings P.A., Sobocinski K.A. & Horowitz M.M. (1998) Survival with bone marrow transplantation *versus* hydroxyurea or interferon for chronic myelogenous leukemia. The German CML Study Group. *Blood,* 91, 1810-1819.

Garbe C., Radny P., Linse R., Dummer R., Gutzmer R., Ulrich J., Stadler R., Weichenthal M., Eigentler T., Ellwanger U. & Hauschild A. (2008) Adjuvant low-dose interferon (alpha)2a with or without dacarbazine compared with surgery alone: a prospective-randomized phase III DeCOG trial in melanoma patients with regional lymph node metastasis. *Ann Oncol,* 19, 1195-1201.

Gauzzi M.C., Velazquez L., McKendry R., Mogensen K.E., Fellous M. & Pellegrini S. (1996) Interferon-alpha-dependent activation of Tyk2 requires phosphorylation of positive regulatory tyrosines by another kinase. *J Biol Chem,* 271, 20494-20500.

George S., Hutson T.E., Mekhail T., Wood L., Finke J., Elson P., Dreicer R. & Bukowski R.M. (2008) Phase I trial of PEG-interferon and recombinant IL-2 in patients with metastatic renal cell carcinoma. *Cancer Chemother Pharmacol,* 62, 347-354.

Gogas H., Ioannovich J., Dafni U., Stavropoulou-Giokas C., Frangia K., Tsoutsos D., Panagiotou P., Polyzos A., Papadopoulos O., Stratigos A., Markopoulos C., Bafaloukos D., Pectasides D., Fountzilas G. & Kirkwood J.M. (2006) Prognostic significance of autoimmunity during treatment of melanoma with interferon. *N Engl J Med,* 354, 709-718.

Golde D.W. (1982) Therapy of hairy-cell leukemia. *N Engl J Med,* 307, 495-496.

Golde D.W., Stevens R.H., Quan S.G. & Saxon A. (1977) Immunoglobulin synthesis in hairy cell leukaemia. *Br J Haematol,* 35, 359-365.

Gollob J.A., Rathmell W.K., Richmond T.M., Marino C.B., Miller E.K., Grigson G., Watkins C., Gu L., Peterson B.L. & Wright J.J. (2007) Phase II trial of sorafenib plus interferon alfa-2b as first- or second-line therapy in patients with metastatic renal cell cancer. *J Clin Oncol,* 25, 3288-3295.

Golomb H.M. & Hanauer S.B. (1981) Infectious complications associated with hairy cell leukemia. *J Infect Dis,* 143, 639-643.

Golomb H.M. & Vardiman J.W. (1983) Response to splenectomy in 65 patients with hairy cell leukemia: an evaluation of spleen weight and bone marrow involvement. *Blood,* 61, 349-352.

Griffiths R., Gleeson M., Reyes C., Knopf K. & Danese M. (2010) Survival in elderly follicular lymphoma patients who receive frontline chemo-immunotherapy. *Am J Hematol,* 85, 963-967.

Groffen J., Stephenson J.R., Heisterkamp N., de Klein A., Bartram C.R. & Grosveld G. (1984) Philadelphia chromosomal breakpoints are clustered within a limited region, bcr, on chromosome 22. *Cell,* 36, 93-99.

Groves M.D., Puduvalli V.K., Gilbert M.R., Levin V.A., Conrad C.A., Liu V.H., Hunter K., Meyers C., Hess K.R. & Alfred Yung W.K. (2009) Two phase II trials of temozolomide with interferon-alpha2b (pegylated and non-pegylated) in patients with recurrent glioblastoma multiforme. *Br J Cancer,* 101, 615-620.

Guilhot F., Roy L., Saulnier P.J. & Guilhot J. (2009) Interferon in chronic myeloid leukaemia: past and future. *Best Pract Res Clin Haematol,* 22, 315-329.

Gutterman J.U. (1994) Cytokine therapeutics: lessons from interferon alpha. *Proc Natl Acad Sci U S A,* 91, 1198-1205.

Halfter U.M., Derbyshire Z.E. & Vaillancourt R.R. (2005) Interferon-gamma-dependent tyrosine phosphorylation of MEKK4 *via* Pyk2 is regulated by annexin II and SHP2 in keratinocytes. *Biochem J,* 388, 17-28.

Hauschild A., Dummer R., Ugurel S., Kaehler K.C., Egberts F., Fink W., Both-Skalsky J., Laetsch B. & Schadendorf D. (2008) Combined treatment with pegylated interferon-alpha-2a and dacarbazine in patients with advanced metastatic melanoma: a phase 2 study. *Cancer,* 113, 1404-1411.

Heil F., Hemmi H., Hochrein H., Ampenberger F., Kirschning C., Akira S., Lipford G., Wagner H. & Bauer S. (2004) Species-specific recognition of single-stranded RNA *via* toll-like receptor 7 and 8. *Science,* 303, 1526-1529.

Hemmi H., Kaisho T., Takeuchi O., Sato S., Sanjo H., Hoshino K., Horiuchi T., Tomizawa H., Takeda K. & Akira S. (2002) Small anti-viral compounds activate immune cells *via* the TLR7 MyD88-dependent signaling pathway. *Nat Immunol,* 3, 196-200.

Hentschel S.J. & Sawaya R. (2003) Optimizing outcomes with maximal surgical resection of malignant gliomas. *Cancer Control,* **10**, 109-114.

Hoffman M.A. (2010) Interferon-alpha is a very effective salvage therapy for patients with hairy cell leukemia relapsing after cladribine: a report of three cases. *Med Oncol.*

Hoffmann K., Mehrle S., Schmidt J., Buchler M.W. & Marten A. (2008) Interferon-alpha restitutes the chemosensitivity in pancreatic cancer. *Anticancer Res,* 28, 1499-1507.

Hogle W.P. (2006) The state of the art in radiation therapy. *Semin Oncol Nurs,* 22, 212-220.

Honda K., Yanai H., Mizutani T., Negishi H., Shimada N., Suzuki N., Ohba Y., Takaoka A., Yeh W.C. & Taniguchi T. (2004) Role of a transductional-transcriptional processor complex involving MyD88 and IRF-7 in Toll-like receptor signaling. *Proc Natl Acad Sci U S A,* 101, 15416-15421.

Hoshino K., Takeuchi O., Kawai T., Sanjo H., Ogawa T., Takeda Y., Takeda K. & Akira S. (1999) Cutting edge: Toll-like receptor 4 (TLR4)-deficient mice are hyporesponsive to lipopolysaccharide: evidence for TLR4 as the Lps gene product. *J Immunol,* 162, 3749-3752.

Hudes G., Carducci M., Tomczak P., Dutcher J., Figlin R., Kapoor A., Staroslawska E., Sosman J., McDermott D., Bodrogi I., Kovacevic Z., Lesovoy V., Schmidt-Wolf I.G., Barbarash O., Gokmen E., O'Toole T., Lustgarten S., Moore L. & Motzer R.J. (2007) Temsirolimus, interferon alfa, or both for advanced renal-cell carcinoma. *N Engl J Med,* 356, 2271-2281.

Hwu W.J., Panageas K.S., Menell J.H., Lamb L.A., Aird S., Krown S.E., Williams L.J., Chapman P.B., Livingston P.O., Wolchok J.D. & Houghton A.N. (2006) Phase II study of temozolomide plus pegylated interferon-alpha-2b for metastatic melanoma. *Cancer,* 106, 2445-2451.

Igarashi K., Garotta G., Ozmen L., Ziemiecki A., Wilks A.F., Harpur A.G., Larner A.C. & Finbloom D.S. (1994) Interferon-gamma induces tyrosine phosphorylation of interferon-gamma receptor and regulated association of protein tyrosine kinases, Jak1 and Jak2, with its receptor. *J Biol Chem,* 269, 14333-14336.

Interferon nomenclature (1980). *Nature* 286, 110.

Isaacs A. & Lindenmann J. (1987) Virus interference. I. The interferon. By A. Isaacs and J. Lindenmann, 1957. *J Interferon Res,* **7**, 429-438.Jabbour E., Cortes J. & Kantarjian H. (2009) Treatment selection after imatinib resistance in chronic myeloid leukemia. *Target Oncol,* 4, 3-10.

Jacobs A.D., Champlin R.E. & Golde D.W. (1985) Recombinant alpha-2-interferon for hairy cell leukemia. *Blood,* 65, 1017-1020.

Jacobson N.G., Szabo S.J., Weber-Nordt R.M., Zhong Z., Schreiber R.D., Darnell J.E., Jr. & Murphy K.M. (1995) Interleukin 12 signaling in T helper type 1 (Th1) cells involves tyrosine phosphorylation of signal transducer and activator of transcription (Stat)3 and Stat4. *J Exp Med,* 181, 1755-1762.

Jemal A., Bray F., Center M.M., Ferlay J., Ward E. & Forman D. (2011) Global cancer statistics. *CA Cancer J Clin,* 61, 69-90.

Jemal A., Siegel R., Xu J. & Ward E. (2010) Cancer statistics, 2010. *CA Cancer J Clin,* 60, 277-300.

Kager L., Zoubek A., Potschger U., Kastner U., Flege S., Kempf-Bielack B., Branscheid D., Kotz R., Salzer-Kuntschik M., Winkelmann W., Jundt G., Kabisch H., Reichardt P., Jurgens H., Gadner H. & Bielack S.S. (2003) Primary metastatic osteosarcoma: presentation and outcome of patients treated on neoadjuvant Cooperative Osteosarcoma Study Group protocols. *J Clin Oncol,* 21, 2011-2018.

Kapoor R., Vijjan V. & Singh P. (2008) Bacillus Calmette-Guerin in the management of superficial bladder cancer. *Indian J Urol,* 24, 72-76.

Katamura Y., Aikata H., Takaki S., Azakami T., Kawaoka T., Waki K., Hiramatsu A., Kawakami Y., Takahashi S., Kenjo M., Toyota N., Ito K. & Chayama K. (2009) Intra-arterial 5-fluorouracil/interferon combination therapy for advanced hepatocellular carcinoma with or without three-dimensional conformal radiotherapy for portal vein tumor thrombosis. *J Gastroenterol,* 44, 492-502.

Kato H., Takeuchi O., Sato S., Yoneyama M., Yamamoto M., Matsui K., Uematsu S., Jung A., Kawai T., Ishii K.J., Yamaguchi O., Otsu K., Tsujimura T., Koh C.S., Reis e Sousa C.,

Matsuura Y., Fujita T. & Akira S. (2006) Differential roles of MDA5 and RIG-I helicases in the recognition of RNA viruses. *Nature,* 441, 101-105.

Kawai T., Sato S., Ishii K.J., Coban C., Hemmi H., Yamamoto M., Terai K., Matsuda M., Inoue J., Uematsu S., Takeuchi O. & Akira S. (2004) Interferon-alpha induction through Toll-like receptors involves a direct interaction of IRF7 with MyD88 and TRAF6. *Nat Immunol,* 5, 1061-1068.

Kimoto Y., Fujita M. & Taguchi T. (1987) Interferon treatment of human stomach and breast carcinoma xenografts in nude mice. *J Interferon Res,* 7, 345-356.

Kirkwood J.M. & Ernstoff M.S. (1984) Interferons in the treatment of human cancer. *J Clin Oncol,* 2, 336-352.

Kirkwood J.M., Manola J., Ibrahim J., Sondak V., Ernstoff M.S. & Rao U. (2004) A pooled analysis of eastern cooperative oncology group and intergroup trials of adjuvant high-dose interferon for melanoma. *Clin Cancer Res,* 10, 1670-1677.

Kirkwood J.M., Strawderman M.H., Ernstoff M.S., Smith T.J., Borden E.C. & Blum R.H. (1996) Interferon alfa-2b adjuvant therapy of high-risk resected cutaneous melanoma: the Eastern Cooperative Oncology Group Trial EST 1684. *J Clin Oncol,* 14, 7-17.

Kirkwood J.M., Tarhini A.A., Moschos S.J. & Panelli M.C. (2008) Adjuvant therapy with high-dose interferon alpha 2b in patients with high-risk stage IIB/III melanoma. *Nat Clin Pract Oncol,* 5, 2-3.

Kleinert S., Kurzai O., Elias J., Marten K., Engelke C., Feuchtenberger M., Sandstede J., Frosch M., Tony H.P. & Kneitz C. (2010) Comparison of two interferon-gamma release assays and tuberculin skin test for detecting latent tuberculosis in patients with immune-mediated inflammatory diseases. *Ann Rheum Dis,* 69, 782-784.

Kleinschmidt W.J. & Murphy E.B. (1965) Investigations on interferon induced by statolon. *Virology,* 27, 484-489.

Kotenko S.V., Gallagher G., Baurin V.V., Lewis-Antes A., Shen M., Shah N.K., Langer J.A., Sheikh F., Dickensheets H. & Donnelly R.P. (2003) IFN-lambdas mediate antiviral protection through a distinct class II cytokine receptor complex. *Nat Immunol,* 4, 69-77.

Kotenko S.V., Izotova L.S., Pollack B.P., Mariano T.M., Donnelly R.J., Muthukumaran G., Cook J.R., Garotta G., Silvennoinen O., Ihle J.N. & *et al.,* (1995) Interaction between the components of the interferon gamma receptor complex. *J Biol Chem,* 270, 20915-20921.

Kozlowski A. & Harris J.M. (2001) Improvements in protein PEGylation: pegylated interferons for treatment of hepatitis C. *J Control Release,* 72, 217-224.

Krieg A.M. (2002) CpG motifs in bacterial DNA and their immune effects. *Annu Rev Immunol,* 20, 709-760.

Krown S.E., Lee J.Y., Lin L., Fischl M.A., Ambinder R. & Von Roenn J.H. (2006) Interferon-alpha2b with protease inhibitor-based antiretroviral therapy in patients with AIDS-associated Kaposi sarcoma: an AIDS malignancy consortium phase I trial. *J Acquir Immune Defic Syndr,* 41, 149-153.

Krown S.E., Li P., Von Roenn J.H., Paredes J., Huang J. & Testa M.A. (2002) Efficacy of low-dose interferon with antiretroviral therapy in Kaposi's sarcoma: a randomized phase II AIDS clinical trials group study. *J Interferon Cytokine Res,* 22, 295-303.

Kubo S., Nishiguchi S., Hirohashi K., Tanaka H., Shuto T. & Kinoshita H. (2002) Randomized clinical trial of long-term outcome after resection of hepatitis C virus-related hepatocellular carcinoma by postoperative interferon therapy. *Br J Surg,* 89, 418-422.

Kubo S., Nishiguchi S., Hirohashi K., Tanaka H., Shuto T., Yamazaki O., Shiomi S., Tamori A., Oka H., Igawa S., Kuroki T. & Kinoshita H. (2001) Effects of long-term postoperative interferon-alpha therapy on intrahepatic recurrence after resection of hepatitis C virus-related hepatocellular carcinoma. A randomized, controlled trial. *Ann Intern Med,* 134, 963-967.

Kurzrock R., Gutterman J.U. & Talpaz M. (1988) The molecular genetics of Philadelphia chromosome-positive leukemias. *N Engl J Med,* 319, 990-998.

Lam J.S., Benson M.C., O'Donnell M.A., Sawczuk A., Gavazzi A., Wechsler M.H. & Sawczuk I.S. (2003) Bacillus Calmete-Guerin plus interferon-alpha2B intravesical therapy maintains an extended treatment plan for superficial bladder cancer with minimal toxicity. *Urol Oncol,* 21, 354-360.

Landolfo S., Guarini A., Riera L., Gariglio M., Gribaudo G., Cignetti A., Cordone I., Montefusco E., Mandelli F. & Foa R. (2000) Chronic myeloid leukemia cells resistant to interferon-alpha lack STAT1 expression. *Hematol J,* 1, 7-14.

Lasfar A., Lewis-Antes A., Smirnov S.V., Anantha S., Abushahba W., Tian B., Reuhl K., Dickensheets H., Sheikh F., Donnelly R.P., Raveche E. & Kotenko S.V. (2006)

Characterization of the mouse IFN-lambda ligand-receptor system: IFN-lambdas exhibit antitumor activity against B16 melanoma. *Cancer Res,* 66, 4468-4477.

Leemans C.R., Braakhuis B.J. & Brakenhoff R.H. (2011) The molecular biology of head and neck cancer. *Nat Rev Cancer,* 11, 9-22.

Lens M.B. & Dawes M. (2002) Interferon alfa therapy for malignant melanoma: a systematic review of randomized controlled trials. *J Clin Oncol,* 20, 1818-1825.

Lepe-Zuniga J.L., Quesada J.R., Baron S., Reuben J. & Gutterman J.U. (1987) Alpha interferon production in patients with hairy cell leukemia: correlations with disease activity and remission status. *Hematol Pathol,* 1, 157-165.

Li Q., Kawamura K., Ma G., Iwata F., Numasaki M., Suzuki N., Shimada H. & Tagawa M. (2010) Interferon-lambda induces G1 phase arrest or apoptosis in oesophageal carcinoma cells and produces anti-tumour effects in combination with anti-cancer agents. *Eur J Cancer,* 46, 180-190.

Lin S.M., Lin C.J., Hsu C.W., Tai D.I., Sheen I.S., Lin D.Y. & Liaw Y.F. (2004) Prospective randomized controlled study of interferon-alpha in preventing hepatocellular carcinoma recurrence after medical ablation therapy for primary tumors. *Cancer,* 100, 376-382.

Linehan D.C., Tan M.C., Strasberg S.M., Drebin J.A., Hawkins W.G., Picus J., Myerson R.J., Malyapa R.S., Hull M., Trinkaus K. & Tan B.R., Jr. (2008) Adjuvant interferon-based chemoradiation followed by gemcitabine for resected pancreatic adenocarcinoma: a single-institution phase II study. *Ann Surg,* 248, 145-151.

Lo C.M., Liu C.L., Chan S.C., Lam C.M., Poon R.T., Ng I.O., Fan S.T. & Wong J. (2007) A randomized, controlled trial of postoperative adjuvant interferon therapy after resection of hepatocellular carcinoma. *Ann Surg,* 245, 831-842.

Lu B., Yu H., Chow C., Li B., Zheng W., Davis R.J. & Flavell R.A. (2001) GADD45gamma mediates the activation of the p38 and JNK MAP kinase pathways and cytokine production in effector TH1 cells. *Immunity,* 14, 583-590.

Lund J.M., Alexopoulou L., Sato A., Karow M., Adams N.C., Gale N.W., Iwasaki A. & Flavell R.A. (2004) Recognition of single-stranded RNA viruses by Toll-like receptor 7. *Proc Natl Acad Sci U S A,* 101, 5598-5603.

Lyrdal D., Stierner U. & Lundstam S. (2009) Metastatic renal cell carcinoma treated with Peg-interferon alfa-2b. *Acta Oncol,* 48, 901-908.

Maio M., Mackiewicz A., Testori A., Trefzer U., Ferraresi V., Jassem J., Garbe C., Lesimple T., Guillot B., Gascon P., Gilde K., Camerini R. & Cognetti F. (2010) Large randomized study of thymosin alpha 1, interferon alfa, or both in combination with dacarbazine in patients with metastatic melanoma. *J Clin Oncol,* 28, 1780-1787.

Manara M.C., Serra M., Benini S., Picci P. & Scotlandi K. (2004) Effectiveness of Type I interferons in the treatment of multidrug resistant osteosarcoma cells. *Int J Oncol,* 24, 365-372.

Markman M., Liu P.Y., Rothenberg M.L., Monk B.J., Brady M. & Alberts D.S. (2006) Pretreatment CA-125 and risk of relapse in advanced ovarian cancer. *J Clin Oncol,* 24, 1454-1458.

Marten A., Schmidt J., Debus J., Harig S., Lindel K., Klein J., Bartsch D.K., Capussotti L., Zülke C. and Buchler M. (2010), CapRI: Final results of the open-label, multicenter, randomized phase III trial of adjuvant chemoradiation plus interferon-α2b (CRI) *versus* 5-FU alone for patients with resected pancreatic adenocarcinoma (PAC). *Journal of Clinical Oncology*, 18, suppl.

Marten A., Wente M.N., Ose J., Buchler M.W., Rotzer I., Decker-Baumann C., Karapanagiotou-Schenkel I., Harig S., Schmidt J. & Jager D. (2009) An open label randomized multicentre phase IIIb trial comparing parenteral substitution *versus* best supportive nutritional care in subjects with pancreatic adenocarcinoma receiving 5-FU plus oxaliplatin as 2nd or higher line chemotherapy regarding clinical benefit - PANUSCO. *BMC Cancer,* 9, 412.

Marth C., Windbichler G.H., Hausmaninger H., Petru E., Estermann K., Pelzer A. & Mueller-Holzner E. (2006) Interferon-gamma in combination with carboplatin and paclitaxel as a safe and effective first-line treatment option for advanced ovarian cancer: results of a phase I/II study. *Int J Gynecol Cancer,* 16, 1522-1528.

Martin J.N. (2007) 'The epidemiology of KSHV and its association with malignant disease'. In: A. Arvin, G Campadelli-Fiume, E Mocarski, PS Moore, B Roizman, R Whitley, K Yamanishi, (Eds), *Human Herpesviruses: Biology, Therapy, and Immunoprophylaxis*, Cambridge University Press. London

Masucci M.G., Szigeti R., Klein E., Klein G., Gruest J., Montagnier L., Taira H., Hall A., Nagata S. & Weissmann C. (1980) Effect of interferon-alpha 1 from *E. coli* on some cell functions. *Science,* 209, 1431-1435.

Mazzaferro V., Romito R., Schiavo M., Mariani L., Camerini T., Bhoori S., Capussotti L., Calise F., Pellicci R., Belli G., Tagger A., Colombo M., Bonino F., Majno P. & Llovet J.M. (2006) Prevention of hepatocellular carcinoma recurrence with alpha-interferon after liver resection in HCV cirrhosis. *Hepatology,* 44, 1543-1554.

McDermott D.F., Regan M.M., Clark J.I., Flaherty L.E., Weiss G.R., Logan T.F., Kirkwood J.M., Gordon M.S., Sosman J.A., Ernstoff M.S., Tretter C.P., Urba W.J., Smith J.W., Margolin K.A., Mier J.W., Gollob J.A., Dutcher J.P. & Atkins M.B. (2005) Randomized phase III trial of high-dose interleukin-2 *versus* subcutaneous interleukin-2 and interferon in patients with metastatic renal cell carcinoma. *J Clin Oncol,* 23, 133-141.

McKeage K., Curran M.P. & Plosker G.L. (2004) Fulvestrant: a review of its use in hormone receptor-positive metastatic breast cancer in postmenopausal women with disease progression following antiestrogen therapy. *Drugs,* 64, 633-648.

Melichar B., Koralewski P., Ravaud A., Pluzanska A., Bracarda S., Szczylik C., Chevreau C., Filipek M., Delva R., Sevin E., Negrier S., McKendrick J., Santoro A., Pisa P. & Escudier B. (2008) First-line bevacizumab combined with reduced dose interferon-alpha2a is active in patients with metastatic renal cell carcinoma. *Ann Oncol,* 19, 1470-1476.

Melo J.V. (1996) The diversity of BCR-ABL fusion proteins and their relationship to leukemia phenotype. *Blood,* 88, 2375-2384.

Meyer S., Wild P.J., Vogt T., Bataille F., Ehret C., Gantner S., Landthaler M., Klinkhammer-Schalke M., Hofstaedter F. & Bosserhoff A.K. (2010) Methylthioadenosine phosphorylase represents a predictive marker for response to adjuvant interferon therapy in patients with malignant melanoma. *Exp Dermatol,* 19, e251-257.

Micallef M.J., Ohtsuki T., Kohno K., Tanabe F., Ushio S., Namba M., Tanimoto T., Torigoe K., Fujii M., Ikeda M., Fukuda S. & Kurimoto M. (1996) Interferon-gamma-inducing factor enhances T helper 1 cytokine production by stimulated human T cells: synergism with interleukin-12 for interferon-gamma production. *Eur J Immunol,* 26, 1647-1651.

Miller C.H., Maher S.G. & Young H.A. (2009) Clinical Use of Interferon-gamma. *Ann N Y Acad Sci,* 1182, 69-79.

Mintz U. & Golomb H.M. (1979) Splenectomy as initial therapy in twenty-six patients with leukemic reticuloendotheliosis (hairy cell leukemia). *Cancer Res,* 39, 2366-2370.

Mocellin S., Pasquali S., Rossi C.R. & Nitti D. (2010) Interferon alpha adjuvant therapy in patients with high-risk melanoma: a systematic review and meta-analysis. *J Natl Cancer Inst,* 102, 493-501.

Morford L.A., Elliott L.H., Carlson S.L., Brooks W.H. & Roszman T.L. (1997) T cell receptor-mediated signaling is defective in T cells obtained from patients with primary intracranial tumors. *J Immunol,* 159, 4415-4425.

Moserle L., Indraccolo S., Ghisi M., Frasson C., Fortunato E., Canevari S., Miotti S., Tosello V., Zamarchi R., Corradin A., Minuzzo S., Rossi E., Basso G. & Amadori A. (2008) The side population of ovarian cancer cells is a primary target of IFN-alpha antitumor effects. *Cancer Res,* 68, 5658-5668.

Motomura K., Natsume A., Kishida Y., Higashi H., Kondo Y., Nakasu Y., Abe T., Namba H., Wakai K. & Wakabayashi T. (2011) Benefits of interferon-beta and temozolomide combination therapy for newly diagnosed primary glioblastoma with the unmethylated MGMT promoter: A multicenter study. *Cancer,* 117, 1721-30.

Motzer R.J., Hutson T.E., Tomczak P., Michaelson M.D., Bukowski R.M., Rixe O., Oudard S., Negrier S., Szczylik C., Kim S.T., Chen I., Bycott P.W., Baum C.M. & Figlin R.A. (2007) Sunitinib *versus* interferon alfa in metastatic renal-cell carcinoma. *N Engl J Med,* 356, 115-124.

Muller C.R., Smeland S., Bauer H.C., Saeter G. & Strander H. (2005) Interferon-alpha as the only adjuvant treatment in high-grade osteosarcoma: long term results of the Karolinska Hospital series. *Acta Oncol,* 44, 475-480.

Nagano Y, Kojima Y (1954). "Pouvoir immunisant du virus vaccinal inactivé par des rayons ultraviolets" (in French). *C R Seances Soc Biol Fil,* 148, 1700–1702.

Nagata S., Mantei N. & Weissmann C. (1980) The structure of one of the eight or more distinct chromosomal genes for human interferon-alpha. *Nature,* 287, 401-408.

Nagler A., Berger R., Ackerstein A., Czyz J.A., Diez-Martin J.L., Naparstek E., Or R., Gan S., Shimoni A. & Slavin S. (2010) A randomized controlled multicenter study comparing recombinant interleukin 2 (rIL-2) in conjunction with recombinant interferon alpha (IFN-alpha) *versus* no immunotherapy for patients with malignant lymphoma postautologous stem cell transplantation. *J Immunother,* 33, 326-333.

Nakahira M., Ahn H.J., Park W.R., Gao P., Tomura M., Park C.S., Hamaoka T., Ohta T., Kurimoto M. & Fujiwara H. (2002) Synergy of IL-12 and IL-18 for IFN-gamma gene expression: IL-12-induced STAT4 contributes to IFN-gamma promoter activation by up-regulating the binding activity of IL-18-induced activator protein 1. *J Immunol,* 168, 1146-1153.

Nakayama A., Kawasaki H., Jin C., Munekata E., Taira K. & Yokoyama K.K. (2001) Transcriptional regulation of interferon gamma gene by p300 co-activator. *Nucleic Acids Res Suppl*, 89-90.

Negrier S., Escudier B., Lasset C., Douillard J.Y., Savary J., Chevreau C., Ravaud A., Mercatello A., Peny J., Mousseau M., Philip T. & Tursz T. (1998) Recombinant human interleukin-2, recombinant human interferon alfa-2a, or both in metastatic renal-cell carcinoma. Groupe Francais d'Immunotherapie. *N Engl J Med,* 338, 1272-1278.

Nicolini A. & Carpi A. (2005) Beta-interferon and interleukin-2 prolong more than three times the survival of 26 consecutive endocrine dependent breast cancer patients with distant metastases: an exploratory trial. *Biomed Pharmacother,* 59, 253-263.

Nicolini F.E., Hayette S., Legros L., Rousselot P., Maloisel F., Tulliez M., Guerci A., Charbonnier A., Prebet T., Rigal-Huguet F., Chabane K., Magaud J.P., Paillet C., Pivot C. & Michallet M. (2011) Pegylated IFN-alpha2a combined to imatinib mesylate 600mg daily can induce complete cytogenetic and molecular responses in a subset of chronic phase CML patients refractory to IFN alone or to imatinib 600mg daily alone. *Leuk Res,* 35, 80-86.

Ning Y., Riggins R.B., Mulla J.E., Chung H., Zwart A. & Clarke R. (2010) IFNgamma restores breast cancer sensitivity to fulvestrant by regulating STAT1, IFN regulatory factor 1, NF-kappaB, BCL2 family members, and signaling to caspase-dependent apoptosis. *Mol Cancer Ther,* 9, 1274-1285.

Nishiguchi S., Tamori A. & Kubo S. (2005) Effect of long-term postoperative interferon therapy on intrahepatic recurrence and survival rate after resection of hepatitis C virus-related hepatocellular carcinoma. *Intervirology,* 48, 71-75.

Nitsche M., Horstmann O., Christiansen H., Hermann R.M., Hess C.F., Becker H., Pradier O. & Schmidberger H. (2008) Chemoradioimmunotherapy with 5-fluorouracil, cisplatin and interferon-alpha in pancreatic and periampullary cancer: results of a feasibility study. *Cancer Radiother,* 12, 817-821.

Niveditha S.R., Bajaj P. & Nangia A. (2004) Secretory carcinoma of the male breast. *J Clin Pathol,* 57, 894.

Niwakawa M., Hashine K., Yamaguchi R., Fujii H., Hamamoto Y., Fukino K., Tanigawa T. & Sumiyoshi Y. (2011) Phase I trial of sorafenib in combination with interferon-alpha in Japanese patients with unresectable or metastatic renal cell carcinoma. *Invest New Drugs.*

Normanno N., Di Maio M., De Maio E., De Luca A., de Matteis A., Giordano A. & Perrone F. (2005) Mechanisms of endocrine resistance and novel therapeutic strategies in breast cancer. *Endocr Relat Cancer,* 12, 721-747.

Nowell P.C. (2007) Discovery of the Philadelphia chromosome: a personal perspective. *J Clin Invest,* 117, 2033-2035.

Odaka M., Sterman D.H., Wiewrodt R., Zhang Y., Kiefer M., Amin K.M., Gao G.P., Wilson J.M., Barsoum J., Kaiser L.R. & Albelda S.M. (2001) Eradication of intraperitoneal and distant tumor by adenovirus-mediated interferon-beta gene therapy is attributable to induction of systemic immunity. *Cancer Res,* 61, 6201-6212.

O'Donnell M.A., Krohn J. & DeWolf W.C. (2001) Salvage intravesical therapy with interferon-alpha 2b plus low dose bacillus Calmette-Guerin is effective in patients with superficial bladder cancer in whom bacillus Calmette-Guerin alone previously failed. *J Urol,* 166, 1300-1304, discussion 1304-1305.

Ohno M., Natsume A., Fujii M., Ito M. & Wakabayashi T. (2009) Interferon-beta, MCNU, and conventional radiotherapy for pediatric patients with brainstem glioma. *Pediatr Blood Cancer,* 53, 37-41.

Okamura H., Kashiwamura S., Tsutsui H., Yoshimoto T. & Nakanishi K. (1998) Regulation of interferon-gamma production by IL-12 and IL-18. *Curr Opin Immunol,* 10, 259-264.

Onoguchi K., Yoneyama M., Takemura A., Akira S., Taniguchi T., Namiki H. & Fujita T. (2007) Viral infections activate types I and III interferon genes through a common mechanism. *J Biol Chem,* 282, 7576-7581.

Osterlund P.I., Pietila T.E., Veckman V., Kotenko S.V. & Julkunen I. (2007) IFN regulatory factor family members differentially regulate the expression of type III IFN (IFN-lambda) genes. *J Immunol,* 179, 3434-3442.

Oudard S., George D., Medioni J. & Motzer R. (2007) Treatment options in renal cell carcinoma: past, present and future. *Ann Oncol,* 18 Suppl 10, x25-31.

Ouyang W., Jacobson N.G., Bhattacharya D., Gorham J.D., Fenoglio D., Sha W.C., Murphy T.L. & Murphy K.M. (1999) The Ets transcription factor ERM is Th1-specific and induced by IL-12 through a Stat4-dependent pathway. *Proc Natl Acad Sci U S A,* 96, 3888-3893.

Ouyang W., Jacobson N.G., Bhattacharya D., Gorham J.D., Fenoglio D., Sha W.C., Murphy T.L. & Murphy K.M. (1999) The Ets transcription factor ERM is Th1-specific and induced by IL-12 through a Stat4-dependent pathway. *Proc Natl Acad Sci U S A,* 96, 3888-3893.

Palandri F., Castagnetti F., Iacobucci I., Martinelli G., Amabile M., Gugliotta G., Poerio A., Testoni N., Breccia M., Bocchia M., Crugnola M., Rege-Cambrin G., Martino B., Pierri I., Radaelli F., Specchia G., Pane F., Saglio G., Rosti G. & Baccarani M. (2010) The response to imatinib and interferon-alpha is more rapid than the response to imatinib alone: a retrospective analysis of 495 Philadelphia-positive chronic myeloid leukemia patients in early chronic phase. *Haematologica,* 95, 1415-1419.

Palumbo A. & Anderson K. (2011) Multiple myeloma. *N Engl J Med,* 364, 1046-1060.

Pavel M.E., Baum U., Hahn *E.G.*, Schuppan D. & Lohmann T. (2006) Efficacy and tolerability of pegylated IFN-alpha in patients with neuroendocrine gastroenteropancreatic carcinomas. *J Interferon Cytokine Res,* 26, 8-13.

Pestka S. (1997) The interferon receptors. *Semin Oncol,* 24, S9-18-S19-40.

Pestka S., Kotenko S.V., Muthukumaran G., Izotova L.S., Cook J.R. & Garotta G. (1997) The interferon gamma (IFN-gamma) receptor: a paradigm for the multichain cytokine receptor. *Cytokine Growth Factor Rev,* 8, 189-206.

Picozzi V.J., Kozarek R.A. & Traverso L.W. (2003) Interferon-based adjuvant chemoradiation therapy after pancreaticoduodenectomy for pancreatic adenocarcinoma. *Am J Surg,* 185, 476-480.

Pietras E.M., Saha S.K. & Cheng G. (2006) The interferon response to bacterial and viral infections. *J Endotoxin Res,* 12, 246-250.

Pignata S., Cannella L., Leopardo D., Pisano C., Bruni G.S. & Facchini G. (2011) Chemotherapy in epithelial ovarian cancer. *Cancer Lett,* 303, 73-83.

Pirard D., Heenen M., Melot C. & Vereecken P. (2004) Interferon alpha as adjuvant postsurgical treatment of melanoma: a meta-analysis. *Dermatology,* 208, 43-48.

Platanias L.C. (2005) Mechanisms of type-I- and type-II-interferon-mediated signalling. *Nat Rev Immunol,* 5, 375-386.

Platanias L.C. & Fish E.N. (1999) Signaling pathways activated by interferons. *Exp Hematol,* 27, 1583-1592.

Powell M.E. (2010) Modern radiotherapy and cervical cancer. *Int J Gynecol Cancer,* 20, S49-51.

Preudhomme C., Guilhot J., Nicolini F.E., Guerci-Bresler A., Rigal-Huguet F., Maloisel F., Coiteux V., Gardembas M., Berthou C., Vekhoff A., Rea D., Jourdan E., Allard C., Delmer A., Rousselot P., Legros L., Berger M., Corm S., Etienne G., Roche-Lestienne C., Eclache V., Mahon F.X. & Guilhot F. (2010) Imatinib plus peginterferon alfa-2a in chronic myeloid leukemia. *N Engl J Med,* 363, 2511-2521.

Quesada J.R., Hersh E.M., Manning J., Reuben J., Keating M., Schnipper E., Itri L. & Gutterman J.U. (1986) Treatment of hairy cell leukemia with recombinant alpha-interferon. *Blood,* 68, 493-497.

Quesada J.R., Lepe-Zuniga J.L. & Gutterman J.U. (1987) Mid-term observations on the efficacy of alpha-interferon in hairy cell leukemia and status of the interferon system of patients in remission. *Leukemia,* 1, 317-319.

Quesada J.R., Reuben J., Manning J.T., Hersh E.M. & Gutterman J.U. (1984) Alpha interferon for induction of remission in hairy-cell leukemia. *N Engl J Med,* 310, 15-18.

Raingeaud J., Whitmarsh A.J., Barrett T., Derijard B. & Davis R.J. (1996) MKK3- and MKK6-regulated gene expression is mediated by the p38 mitogen-activated protein kinase signal transduction pathway. *Mol Cell Biol,* 16, 1247-1255.

Ramakrishna R. & Manoharan A. (2010) Sustained long-term remissions with weekly interferon maintenance therapy in hairy cell leukemia. *Asia Pac J Clin Oncol,* 6, 210-212.

Ramos M.C., Mardegan M.C., Peghini B.C., Adad S.J., Michelin M.A. & Murta E.F. (2010) Expression of cytokines in cervical stroma in patients with high-grade cervical intraepithelial neoplasia after treatment with intralesional interferon alpha-2b. *Eur J Gynaecol Oncol,* 31, 522-529.

Ratain M.J., Golomb H.M., Vardiman J.W., Vokes E.E., Jacobs R.H. & Daly K. (1985) Treatment of hairy cell leukemia with recombinant alpha 2 interferon. *Blood,* 65, 644-648.

Ratain M.J., Golomb H.M., Vardiman J.W., Westbrook C.A., Barker C., Hooberman A., Bitter M.A. & Daly K. (1988) Relapse after interferon alfa-2b therapy for hairy-cell leukemia: analysis of prognostic variables. *J Clin Oncol,* 6, 1714-1721.

Recchia F., Sica G., Candeloro G., Necozione S., Bisegna R., Bratta M. & Rea S. (2009) Beta-interferon, retinoids and tamoxifen in metastatic breast cancer: long-term follow-up of a phase II study. *Oncol Rep,* 21, 1011-1016.

Richtig E., Hofmann-Wellenhof R., Pehamberger H., Forstinger C., Wolff K., Mischer P., Raml J., Fritsch P., Zelger B., Ratzinger G., Koller J., Lang A., Konrad K., Kindermann-Glebowski E., Seeber A., Steiner A., Fialla R., Pachinger W., Kos C., Klein G., Kehrer H., Kerl H., Ulmer H. & Smolle J. (2004) Temozolomide and interferon alpha 2b in metastatic melanoma stage IV. *Br J Dermatol,* 151, 91-98.

Robinson B.W. & Lake R.A. (2005) Advances in malignant mesothelioma. *N Engl J Med,* 353, 1591-1603.

Rohatiner A.Z., Gregory W.M., Peterson B., Borden E., Solal-Celigny P., Hagenbeek A., Fisher R.I., Unterhalt M., Arranz R., Chisesi T., Aviles A. & Lister T.A. (2005) Meta-analysis to evaluate the role of interferon in follicular lymphoma. *J Clin Oncol,* 23, 2215-2223.

Rowley J.D. (1973) Letter: A new consistent chromosomal abnormality in chronic myelogenous leukaemia identified by quinacrine fluorescence and Giemsa staining. *Nature,* 243, 290-293.

Rubinstein M., Rubinstein S., Familletti P.C., Gross M.S., Miller R.S., Waldman A.A. & Pestka S. (1978) Human leukocyte interferon purified to homogeneity. *Science,* 202, 1289-1290.

Rugo H.S. (2008) The breast cancer continuum in hormone-receptor-positive breast cancer in postmenopausal women: evolving management options focusing on aromatase inhibitors. *Ann Oncol,* 19, 16-27.

Ruotsalainen T., Halme M., Isokangas O.P., Pyrhonen S., Mantyla M., Pekonen M., Sarna S., Joensuu H. & Mattson K. (2000) Interferon-alpha and 13-*cis*-retinoic acid as maintenance therapy after high-dose combination chemotherapy with growth factor support for small cell lung cancer--a feasibility study. *Anticancer Drugs,* 11, 101-108.

Ryan C.W., Goldman B.H., Lara P.N., Jr., Mack P.C., Beer T.M., Tangen C.M., Lemmon D., Pan C.X., Drabkin H.A. & Crawford E.D. (2007) Sorafenib with interferon alfa-2b as first-line treatment of advanced renal carcinoma: a phase II study of the Southwest Oncology Group. *J Clin Oncol,* 25, 3296-3301.

Ryu S., Kim O.B., Kim S.H., He S.Q. & Kim J.H. (1998) *In vitro* radiosensitization of human cervical carcinoma cells by combined use of 13-*cis*-retinoic acid and interferon-alpha2a. *Int J Radiat Oncol Biol Phys,* 41, 869-873.

Sadir R., Lortat-Jacob H. & Morel G. (2000) Internalization and nuclear translocation of IFN-gamma and IFN-gammaR: an ultrastructural approach. *Cytokine,* 12, 711-714.

Sakatsume M., Igarashi K., Winestock K.D., Garotta G., Larner A.C. & Finbloom D.S. (1995) The Jak kinases differentially associate with the alpha and beta (accessory factor) chains of the interferon gamma receptor to form a functional receptor unit capable of activating STAT transcription factors. *J Biol Chem,* 270, 17528-17534.

Salles G., Mounier N., de Guibert S., Morschhauser F., Doyen C., Rossi J.F., Haioun C., Brice P., Mahe B., Bouabdallah R., Audhuy B., Ferme C., Dartigeas C., Feugier P., Sebban C., Xerri L. & Foussard C. (2008) Rituximab combined with chemotherapy and interferon in follicular lymphoma patients: results of the GELA-GOELAMS FL2000 study. *Blood,* 112, 4824-4831.

Sawyers C.L. (1999) Chronic myeloid leukemia. *N Engl J Med,* 340, 1330-1340.

Schillinger M. & Minar E. (2004) Advances in vascular brachytherapy over the last 10 years: focus on femoropopliteal applications. *J Endovasc Ther,* 11 Suppl 2, II180-191.

Schindler C., Shuai K., Prezioso V.R. & Darnell J.E., Jr. (1992) Interferon-dependent tyrosine phosphorylation of a latent cytoplasmic transcription factor. *Science,* 257, 809-813.

Schmeler K.M., Vadhan-Raj S., Ramirez P.T., Apte S.M., Cohen L., Bassett R.L., Iyer R.B., Wolf J.K., Levenback C.L., Gershenson D.M. & Freedman R.S. (2009) A phase II study of GM-CSF and rIFN-gamma1b plus carboplatin for the treatment of recurrent, platinum-sensitive ovarian, fallopian tube and primary peritoneal cancer. *Gynecol Oncol,* 113, 210-215.

Schmidt J., Patrut E.M., Ma J., Jager D., Knaebel H.P., Buchler M.W. & Marten A. (2006) Immunomodulatory impact of interferon-alpha in combination with chemoradiation of pancreatic adenocarcinoma (CapRI). *Cancer Immunol Immunother,* 55, 1396-1405.

Schroder K., Hertzog P.J., Ravasi T. & Hume D.A. (2004) Interferon-gamma: an overview of signals, mechanisms and functions. *J Leukoc Biol,* 75, 163-189.

Scully R.E. (1995) Pathology of ovarian cancer precursors. *J Cell Biochem Suppl,* 23, 208-218.

Seixas-Silva J.A., Jr., Richards T., Khuri F.R., Wieand H.S., Kim E., Murphy B., Francisco M., Hong W.K. & Shin D.M. (2005) Phase 2 bioadjuvant study of interferon alfa-2a, isotretinoin, and vitamin E in locally advanced squamous cell carcinoma of the head and neck: long-term follow-up. *Arch Otolaryngol Head Neck Surg,* 131, 304-307.

Shah S.C., Kusiak A. & O'Donnell M.A. (2006) Patient-recognition data-mining model for BCG-plus interferon immunotherapy bladder cancer treatment. *Comput Biol Med,* 36, 634-655.

Sharma S., tenOever B.R., Grandvaux N., Zhou G.P., Lin R. & Hiscott J. (2003) Triggering the interferon antiviral response through an IKK-related pathway. *Science,* 300, 1148-1151.

Shenkier T., Weir L., Levine M., Olivotto I., Whelan T. & Reyno L. (2004) Clinical practice guidelines for the care and treatment of breast cancer: 15. Treatment for women with stage III or locally advanced breast cancer. *CMAJ,* 170, 983-994.

Sheppard P., Kindsvogel W., Xu W., Henderson K., Schlutsmeyer S., Whitmore T.E., Kuestner R., Garrigues U., Birks C., Roraback J., Ostrander C., Dong D., Shin J., Presnell S., Fox B., Haldeman B., Cooper E., Taft D., Gilbert T., Grant F.J., Tackett M., Krivan W., McKnight G., Clegg C., Foster D. & Klucher K.M. (2003) IL-28, IL-29 and their class II cytokine receptor IL-28R. *Nat Immunol,* 4, 63-68.

Singal A.K., Singh A., Jaganmohan S., Guturu P., Mummadi R., Kuo Y.F. & Sood G.K. (2010) Antiviral therapy reduces risk of hepatocellular carcinoma in patients with hepatitis C virus-related cirrhosis. *Clin Gastroenterol Hepatol,* 8, 192-199.

Sirohi B., Powles R., Lawrence D., Treleaven J., Kulkarni S., Leary A., Rudin C., Horton C. & Morgan G. (2007) An open, randomized, controlled, phase II, single centre, two-period cross-over study to compare the quality of life and toxicity experienced on PEG interferon with interferon-alpha2b in patients with multiple myeloma maintained on a steady dose of interferon-alpha2b. *Ann Oncol,* 18, 1388-1394.

Slominski A., Fischer T.W., Zmijewski M.A., Wortsman J., Semak I., Zbytek B., Slominski R.M. & Tobin D.J. (2005) On the role of melatonin in skin physiology and pathology. *Endocrine,* 27, 137-148.

Smith S.M., Johnson J., Cheson B.D., Canellos G., Petroni G., Oken M., Duggan D., Hurd D., Gockerman J.P., Parker B., Prchal J. & Peterson B.A. (2009) Recombinant interferon-alpha2b added to oral cyclophosphamide either as induction or maintenance in treatment-naive follicular lymphoma: final analysis of CALGB 8691. *Leuk Lymphoma,* 50, 1606-1617.

Solti M., Berd D., Mastrangelo M.J. & Sato T. (2007) A pilot study of low-dose thalidomide and interferon alpha-2b in patients with metastatic melanoma who failed prior treatment. *Melanoma Res,* 17, 225-231.

Stark G.R., Kerr I.M., Williams B.R., Silverman R.H. & Schreiber R.D. (1998) How cells respond to interferons. *Annu Rev Biochem,* 67, 227-264.

Steen H.C. & Gamero A.M. (2010) Interferon-lambda as a potential therapeutic agent in cancer treatment. *J Interferon Cytokine Res,* 30, 597-602.

Sterman D.H., Recio A., Haas A.R., Vachani A., Katz S.I., Gillespie C.T., Cheng G., Sun J., Moon E., Pereira L., Wang X., Heitjan D.F., Litzky L., June C.H., Vonderheide R.H., Carroll R.G. & Albelda S.M. (2010) A phase I trial of repeated intrapleural adenoviral-mediated interferon-beta gene transfer for mesothelioma and metastatic pleural effusions. *Mol Ther,* 18, 852-860.

Stieber V.W. (2001) Low-grade gliomas. *Curr Treat Options Oncol,* 2, 495-506.

Sun H.C., Tang Z.Y., Wang L., Qin L.X., Ma Z.C., Ye Q.H., Zhang B.H., Qian Y.B., Wu Z.Q., Fan J., Zhou X.D., Zhou J., Qiu S.J. & Shen Y.F. (2006) Postoperative interferon alpha treatment postponed recurrence and improved overall survival in patients after curative resection of HBV-related hepatocellular carcinoma: a randomized clinical trial. *J Cancer Res Clin Oncol,* 132, 458-465.

Sun W.H., Pabon C., Alsayed Y., Huang P.P., Jandeska S., Uddin S., Platanias L.C. & Rosen S.T. (1998) Interferon-alpha resistance in a cutaneous T-cell lymphoma cell line is associated with lack of STAT1 expression. *Blood,* 91, 570-576.

Szabo S.J., Kim S.T., Costa G.L., Zhang X., Fathman C.G. & Glimcher L.H. (2000) A novel transcription factor, T-bet, directs Th1 lineage commitment. *Cell,* 100, 655-669.

Takekawa M. & Saito H. (1998) A family of stress-inducible GADD45-like proteins mediate activation of the stress-responsive MTK1/MEKK4 MAPKKK. *Cell,* 95, 521-530.

Talpaz M., Kantarjian H., Kurzrock R. & Gutterman J.U. (1989) Clinical studies with interferons in Philadelphia positive chronic myelogenous leukemia. *Bone Marrow Transplant,* 4 Suppl 1, 63.

Talpaz M., Kurzrock R., Kantarjian H., O'Brien S. & Gutterman J.U. (1989) Recombinant interferon-alpha therapy of Philadelphia chromosome-negative myeloproliferative disorders with thrombocytosis. *Am J Med,* 86, 554-558.

Talpaz M., McCredie K., Kantarjian H., Trujillo J., Keating M. & Gutterman J. (1986) Chronic myelogenous leukaemia: haematological remissions with alpha interferon. *Br J Haematol,* 64, 87-95.

Taniguchi T., Fujii-Kuriyama Y. & Muramatsu M. (1980) Molecular cloning of human interferon cDNA. *Proc Natl Acad Sci U S A,* 77, 4003-4006.

Tedjarati S., Baker C.H., Apte S., Huang S., Wolf J.K., Killion J.J. & Fidler I.J. (2002) Synergistic therapy of human ovarian carcinoma implanted orthotopically in nude mice by optimal biological dose of pegylated interferon alpha combined with paclitaxel. *Clin Cancer Res,* 8, 2413-2422.

Tomimaru Y., Eguchi H., Wada H., Tomokuni A., Kobayashi S., Marubashi S., Takeda Y., Tanemura M., Umeshita K., Mori M., Doki Y. & Nagano H. (2011) Synergistic antitumor effect of interferon-ss with gemcitabine in interferon-alpha-non-responsive pancreatic cancer cells. *Int J Oncol,* 38, 1237-1243.

Tominaga K., Yoshimoto T., Torigoe K., Kurimoto M., Matsui K., Hada T., Okamura H. & Nakanishi K. (2000) IL-12 synergizes with IL-18 or IL-1beta for IFN-gamma production from human T cells. *Int Immunol,* 12, 151-160.

Tovell D. & Cantell K. (1971) Kinetics of interferon production in human leukocyte suspensions. *J Gen Virol,* 13, 485-489.

Trinchieri G. (1995) Interleukin-12: a proinflammatory cytokine with immunoregulatory functions that bridge innate resistance and antigen-specific adaptive immunity. *Annu Rev Immunol,* 13, 251-276.

Tsunoo H., Komura S., Ohishi N., Yajima H., Akiyama S., Kasai Y., Ito K., Nakao A. & Yagi K. (2002) Effect of transfection with human interferon-beta gene entrapped in cationic multilamellar liposomes in combination with 5-fluorouracil on the growth of human esophageal cancer cells *in vitro*. *Anticancer Res,* 22, 1537-1543.

Ueshima K., Kudo M., Nagai T., Tatsumi C., Ueda T., Takahashi S., Hatanaka K., Kitai S., Ishikawa E., Inoue T., Hagiwara S., Minami Y. & Chung H. (2008) Combination therapy with S-1 and pegylated interferon alpha for advanced hepatocellular carcinoma. *Oncology,* 75 Suppl 1, 106-113.

Uze G. & Monneron D. (2007) IL-28 and IL-29: newcomers to the interferon family. *Biochimie,* 89, 729-734.

Venkitaraman R. (2010) Lobular neoplasia of the breast. *Breast J,* 16, 519-528.

Verma S., Quirt I., McCready D., Bak K., Charette M. & Iscoe N. (2006) Systematic review of systemic adjuvant therapy for patients at high risk for recurrent melanoma. *Cancer,* 106, 1431-1442.

Vestergaard A.L., Knudsen U.B., Munk T., Rosbach H. & Martensen P.M. (2011) Transcriptional expression of type-I interferon response genes and stability of housekeeping genes in the human endometrium and endometriosis. *Mol Hum Reprod,* 17, 243-254.

Visconti R., Gadina M., Chiariello M., Chen E.H., Stancato L.F., Gutkind J.S. & O'Shea J.J. (2000) Importance of the MKK6/p38 pathway for interleukin-12-induced STAT4 serine phosphorylation and transcriptional activity. *Blood,* 96, 1844-1852.

Watford W.T., Hissong B.D., Bream J.H., Kanno Y., Muul L. & O'Shea J.J. (2004) Signaling by IL-12 and IL-23 and the immunoregulatory roles of STAT4. *Immunol Rev,* 202, 139-156.

Weiss K. (1998) Safety profile of interferon-alpha therapy. *Semin Oncol,* 25, 9-13.

Wheatley K., Ives N., Hancock B., Gore M., Eggermont A. & Suciu S. (2003) Does adjuvant interferon-alpha for high-risk melanoma provide a worthwhile benefit? A meta-analysis of the randomised trials. *Cancer Treat Rev,* 29, 241-252.

Whelan J., Patterson D., Perisoglou M., Bielack S., Marina N., Smeland S. & Bernstein M. (2010) The role of interferons in the treatment of osteosarcoma. *Pediatr Blood Cancer,* 54, 350-354.

Wild P.J., Meyer S., Landthaler M., Hofstaedter F. & Bosserhoff A.K. (2007) A potential predictive marker for response to interferon in malignant melanoma. *J Dtsch Dermatol Ges,* 5, 456-459.

Wilderman M.J., Sun J., Jassar A.S., Kapoor V., Khan M., Vachani A., Suzuki E., Kinniry P.A., Sterman D.H., Kaiser L.R. & Albelda S.M. (2005) Intrapulmonary IFN-beta gene therapy using an adenoviral vector is highly effective in a murine orthotopic model of bronchogenic adenocarcinoma of the lung. *Cancer Res,* 65, 8379-8387.

Wu J., Xiao X., Zhao P., Xue G., Zhu Y., Zhu X., Zheng L., Zeng Y. & Huang W. (2006) Minicircle-IFNgamma induces antiproliferative and antitumoral effects in human nasopharyngeal carcinoma. *Clin Cancer Res,* 12, 4702-4713.

Yamamoto M., Sato S., Hemmi H., Hoshino K., Kaisho T., Sanjo H., Takeuchi O., Sugiyama M., Okabe M., Takeda K. & Akira S. (2003) Role of adaptor TRIF in the MyD88-independent toll-like receptor signaling pathway. *Science,* 301, 640-643.

Yang J., Zhu H., Murphy T.L., Ouyang W. & Murphy K.M. (2001) IL-18-stimulated GADD45 beta required in cytokine-induced, but not TCR-induced, IFN-gamma production. *Nat Immunol,* 2, 157-164.

Yang Y., Ochando J.C., Bromberg J.S. & Ding Y. (2007) Identification of a distant T-bet enhancer responsive to IL-12/Stat4 and IFNgamma/Stat1 signals. *Blood,* 110, 2494-2500.

Yang Y.F., Zhao W., Zhong Y.D., Xia H.M., Shen L. & Zhang N. (2009) Interferon therapy in chronic hepatitis B reduces progression to cirrhosis and hepatocellular carcinoma: a meta-analysis. *J Viral Hepat,* 16, 265-271.

Yoneyama M., Kikuchi M., Matsumoto K., Imaizumi T., Miyagishi M., Taira K., Foy E., Loo Y.M., Gale M., Jr., Akira S., Yonehara S., Kato A. & Fujita T. (2005) Shared and unique functions of the DExD/H-box helicases RIG-I, MDA5, and LGP2 in antiviral innate immunity. *J Immunol,* 175, 2851-2858.

Yoneyama M., Kikuchi M., Natsukawa T., Shinobu N., Imaizumi T., Miyagishi M., Taira K., Akira S. & Fujita T. (2004) The RNA helicase RIG-I has an essential function in double-stranded RNA-induced innate antiviral responses. *Nat Immunol,* 5, 730-737.

Young H.A. (1996) Regulation of interferon-gamma gene expression. *J Interferon Cytokine Res,* 16, 563-568.

Yurkovetsky Z.R., Kirkwood J.M., Edington H.D., Marrangoni A.M., Velikokhatnaya L., Winans M.T., Gorelik E. & Lokshin A.E. (2007) Multiplex analysis of serum cytokines in melanoma patients treated with interferon-alpha2b. *Clin Cancer Res,* 13, 2422-2428.

Zhang C.H., Xu G.L., Jia W.D. & Ge Y.S. (2009) Effects of interferon alpha treatment on recurrence and survival after complete resection or ablation of hepatocellular carcinoma: a meta-analysis of randomized controlled trials. *Int J Cancer,* 124, 2982-2988.

Zhang X., Brann T.W., Zhou M., Yang J., Oguariri R.M., Lidie K.B., Imamichi H., Huang D.W., Lempicki R.A., Baseler M.W., Veenstra T.D., Young H.A., Lane H.C. & Imamichi T. (2011) Cutting edge: Ku70 is a novel cytosolic DNA sensor that induces type III rather than type I IFN. *J Immunol,* 186, 4541-4545.

Zhang X. & Ren R. (1998) Bcr-Abl efficiently induces a myeloproliferative disease and production of excess interleukin-3 and granulocyte-macrophage colony-stimulating factor in mice: a novel model for chronic myelogenous leukemia. *Blood,* 92, 3829-3840.

Zhao Y.O., Konen-Waisman S., Taylor G.A., Martens S. & Howard J.C. (2010) Localisation and mislocalisation of the interferon-inducible immunity-related GTPase, Irgm1 (LRG-47) in mouse cells. *PLoS One,* 5, e8648.

Zhou Z., Hamming O.J., Ank N., Paludan S.R., Nielsen A.L. & Hartmann R. (2007) Type III interferon (IFN) induces a type I IFN-like response in a restricted subset of cells through signaling pathways involving both the Jak-STAT pathway and the mitogen-activated protein kinases. *J Virol,* 81, 7749-7758.

Zhu Y., Tibensky I., Schmidt J., Ryschich E. & Marten A. (2008) Interferon-alpha enhances antitumor effect of chemotherapy in an orthotopic mouse model for pancreatic adenocarcinoma. *J Immunother,* 31, 599-606.

Zimonjic D.B., Rezanka L.J., Evans C.H., Polymeropoulos M.H., Trent J.M. & Popescu N.C. (1995) Mapping of the immune interferon gamma gene (IFNG) to chromosome band 12q14 by fluorescence *in situ* hybridization. *Cytogenet Cell Genet,* 71, 247-248.

Zitzmann K., Brand S., Baehs S., Goke B., Meinecke J., Spottl G., Meyer H. & Auernhammer C.J. (2006) Novel interferon-lambdas induce antiproliferative effects in neuroendocrine tumor cells. *Biochem Biophys Res Commun,* 344, 1334-1341.

Zou C., Ramakumar S., Qian L., Zang R., Wang J., Grossman H.B., Lotan R. & Liebert M. (2005) Effect of retinoic acid and interferon alpha-2a on transitional cell carcinoma of bladder. *J Urol,* 173, 247-251.

Send Orders for Reprints to reprints@benthamscience.net

CHAPTER 5

Use of Energetic Charged Particles in Radiotherapy

Marco Durante[1,*] and Daniela Trani[2,3]

[1]GSI Helmholtzzentrum für Schwerionenforschung, Biophysics Department – Director, Planckstraße 1, 64291 Darmstadt – Germany; Technische Universität Darmstadt, Institut für Festkörperphysik, Hochschulstraße 6, 64289 Darmstadt, Germany; [2]Department of Biochemistry and Molecular & Cellular Biology, Lombardi Comprehensive Cancer Center, Georgetown University, Room E504 Research Building, 3970 Reservoir Rd., NW, Washington, DC 20057-1468, USA and [3]Department of Radiation Oncology (MaastRO Lab/Maastro Clinic), GROW-School for Oncology and Developmental Biology, Maastricht University Medical Centre, 6200 MD Maastricht, The Netherlands

Abstract: Radiation therapy is among the most common and effective therapies employed in both curative and palliative management of cancer patients. About 50% of all patients diagnosed with localized malignant tumors are treated with radiation, usually high-energy X-rays, as a part of the initial cancer therapy. Many years ago, it was proposed that high-energy ions might be successfully employed in the treatment of localized tumors, owing their physical and biological advantages toward X-rays. Indeed, high-energy charged particles are characterized by a more favorable tissue depth-dose distribution and higher relative biological effectiveness (RBE) compared with X-rays. Currently, many facilities in the U.S.A., Europe, and Japan use high-energy protons and carbon ions for the treatment of solid tumors and several new centers are under construction. These types of therapies present very high costs due to the expensive technologies used in building accelerators and for beam delivery. Therefore, the debate on cost: benefit ratio of these techniques is ongoing, although strong evidence suggests that charged particle therapy provides an important clinical advantage in treatment of localized tumors. In this chapter, we will describe clinical applications and results of charged particle radiotherapy compared to X-rays, and identify and discuss important questions that need to be addressed in this field.

Keywords: Radiation therapy, x-rays, γ-rays, high-energy photons, argon, carbon, Ion, biological effective dose (BED), relative biological effectiveness (RBE), ionizing radiation, radium, nuclear reactors, particle accelerators, cycle

***Address correspondence to Marco Durante:** GSI Helmholtzzentrum für Schwerionenforschung, Biophysics Department, Planckstraße 1 – 64291 Darmstadt – Germany; Tel: +49 (0)6159 71 2009; Fax: +49 (0)6159 71 2106; E-mail: M.Durante@gsi.de

Pier Paolo Claudio and Paraskevi Vogiatzi (Eds)

accelerators, linear accelerator, conformal radiotherapy, stereotactic radiotherapy, gamma knife, neutron beam therapy, proton beam therapy.

1. INTRODUCTION

Radiotherapy remains an important and effective therapy used in the curative and palliative management of patients with cancer. Approximately 50% of all patients with localized malignant tumors are treated with radiation, normally high-energy X-rays as part of their initial therapy. The success of the radiation therapy treatment strongly depends on the total radiation dose delivered to the tumor: in theory, any tumor can be controlled if a tumoricidal dose can be delivered. Unfortunately, the tolerance of the normal tissues surrounding or within the tumor limits the dose. There is also significant inter-individual variation in the severity of toxicity following a given dose of radiotherapy, depending on genetic or physiological factors that often can not be predicted before treatment.

While the potential of X-rays for treating cancer was recognized soon after their discovery, Dr. Robert R. Wilson in 1946 proposed energetic protons for therapy, based on their favorable depth-dose distribution (for an historical review of the development of particle therapy (Halperin, 2006)). In fact, contrary to X- or γ rays that are absorbed in the tissue leading to an exponential decay of the dose by increasing depth, charged particles deposit little energy at the entrance, when their velocity is high, while most of the energy is delivered at the end of their range in the tissue (Bragg peak, Fig. **1**). Since for each mono-energetic proton beam the Bragg peak is very narrow, beams of different energies have to be superimposed using either passive range shifters or active energy variation to produce a spread-out-Bragg-peak (SOBP), which covers the whole tumor. The Bragg curve clearly indicates that particle therapy can provide excellent dose distributions in the patients, even compared to the most advanced X-ray methods, such as intensity-modulated radiation therapy (IMRT) (Fig. **2**).

2. PHYSICAL BASES OF PARTICLE THERAPY

The main advantage of ion beams compared to conventional photon irradiation (x-rays, γ rays, high-energy photons) is the different depth dose distribution (Durante and Loeffler, 2010).

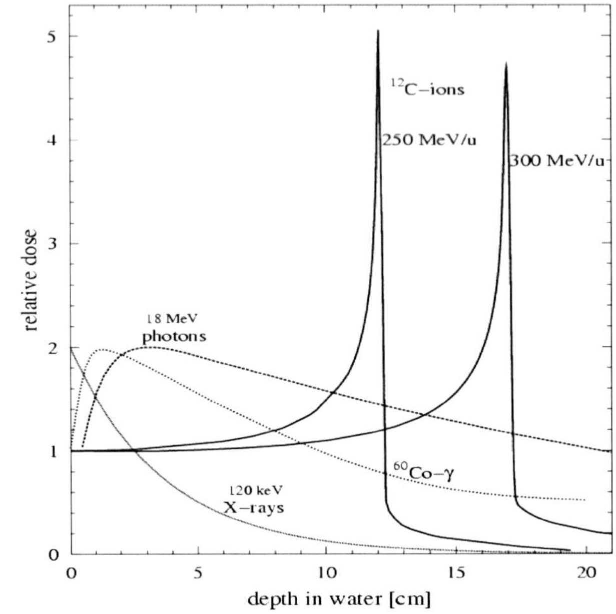

Figure 1: Depth-dose distribution of photons and particle beams. In the case of photons the dose decreases exponentially after a maximum in the beginning. In contrast, particle beams (^{12}C-ions) have a dose maximum at the end of the range. This maximum can be guided over the tumor in order to achieve the best tumor dose distribution.

For photons, the dose decreases exponentially after initial maximum yielding a maximum located a few centimeters below the skin. Hence, for a single field irradiation of a deep-seated tumor the dose before the tumor would be larger than the dose in the target volume. In order to reach a high dose in the tumor without too much damage in the normal tissue many entrance channels are used to irradiate the tumor in a "crossfire" technique. Using this technique, the undesired integral dose to the normal tissues is not reduced but is distributed over a larger volume.

In general, IMRT produces excellent dose distribution over the target volume but on the costs of a high integral dose to the normal tissue. Energetic ions are characterized by both a different physical interaction with the target and a more favorable depth dose distribution in the tissue compared to photons (Fig. **2**).

At present, light hydrogen ions (protons) or the heavier carbon ions (C-ions) are used in therapy (Weber and Kraft, 2009). Because ions are charged particles, they mainly interact with the electrons of the penetrated tissue. At the high initial speed this interaction is small and only little energy is transferred to the tissue. With increasing depth the ions are slowed down, the local interaction becomes greater and a higher dose is transferred to the tissue. Then, at the end of the ion-range, the dose increases to very high values. After the Bragg peak (Fig. **1**) the dose decreases to zero when the ions come to rest. The described process yields an ideal depth-dose distribution and is optimal for cancer therapy: a low dose at the entrance channel in the normal tissue and the large dose at the end of the penetration path, in the tumor volume.

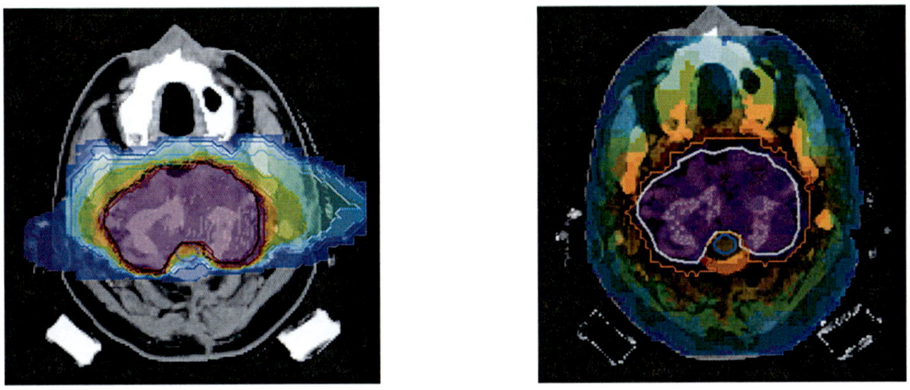

Figure 2: Comparison of carbon irradiation (left) and photon irradiation (right). For photon IMRT nine channels are used to distribute the dose to the normal tissue. For carbon scanning therapy the dose in the only two entrance channels is much smaller than for IMRT. (Image courtesy of Dr. Oliver Jäkel, DKFZ, Heidelberg).

Ions are charged particles and can be deflected with magnetic fields. Therefore, it is possible to replace the initially used passive modulation systems by active systems (Fig. **3**) where the beam is laterally deflected by magnets and modulated in depth by an energy variation in the accelerators. For the irradiation, the target volume is dissected in slices of equal ion energy and the beam is scanned in lines over each slice (Weber *et al.*, 2000).

When irradiating some deeper, more distal layers with the Bragg maximum, the more proximal layers are partly pre-irradiated. This has to be corrected for and yields in general to an inhomogeneous dose distribution for all individual layers.

In addition, the variation of the relative biological effectiveness (RBE) has to be taken into account in treatment planning which yields in an even larger variation in particle covering per slice. This is necessary in order to reach a homogenous distribution of the biological effect over the complete tumor volume.

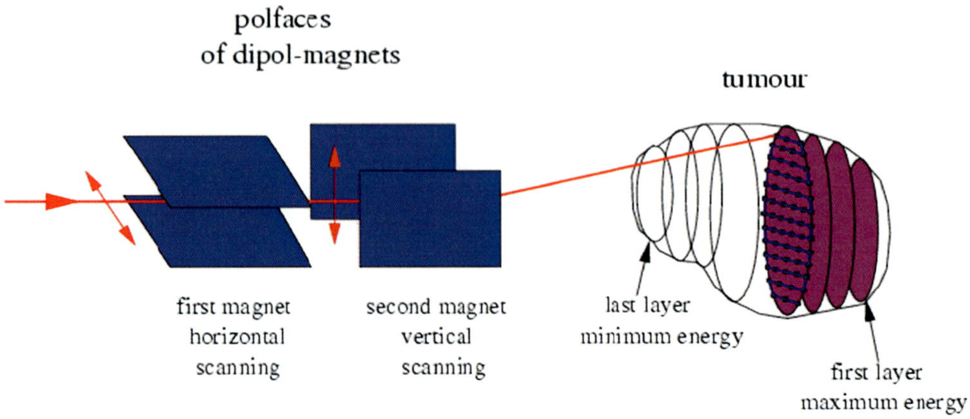

Figure 3: Principle of active 3D dose shaping with the raster scanner. Lateral deflection is obtained by two dipole magnets, depth coverage by energy variation of the beam. The tumor is dissected in slices. Each iso-energy slice is covered by a net of pixels for which the number of particles has been calculated before. Then the beam is guided by the magnetic system in a raster-like pattern from pixel to pixel.

Another important parameter for treatment planning is in many cases the dose gradient between the target volume and critical organs.

In Fig. **4** the same patient is planned for carbon therapy (which was indeed applied later on) and for a proton treatment using the same treatment planning system. Carbon ions have a 3 times steeper gradient compared to energetic protons. This ratio between protons and heavy ion gradients holds approximately for all penetration depths. Therefore, tumors close to critical organs can be treated with high carbon doses and the recurrence of tumors is very rare.

3. BIOLOGICAL BASES OF ION THERAPY

The essential advantage of a carbon beam is the higher biological effectiveness at the end of the range of the tumor compared to the entrance channel where the RBE is only slightly elevated (Durante and Loeffler, 2010). This means that the low dose in the entrance channels induces less biological damage, which is more reparable than in the target tumor volume. An essential goal of the development of the heavy ion therapy at the newer therapies was to maximize the difference in the biological effectiveness between entrance channel and tumor area.

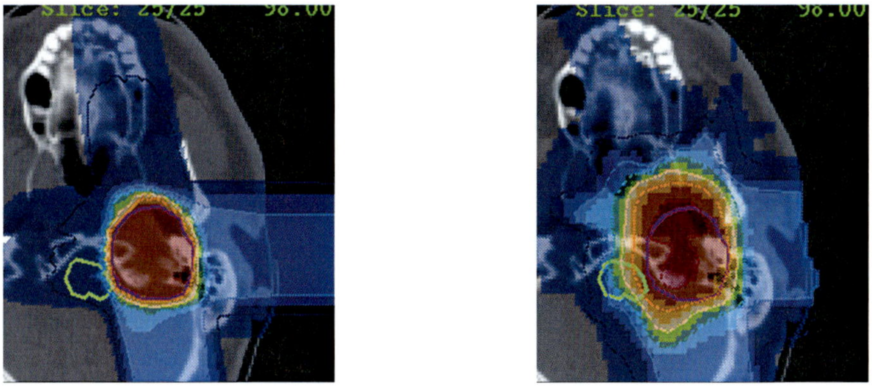

Figure 4: Comparison of a treatment plan with carbon ion at the left side and a proton plan at the right side. The carbon plan shows a very steep dose gradient. With such a steep dose gradient the irradiation can be closer to the brain steam which is a critical structure shown in green at the left side. In addition, the proton plan was performed being a passive beam application system, which allows only a less precise covering of the target volume (courtesy to Oliver Jäkel, DKFZ Heidelberg).

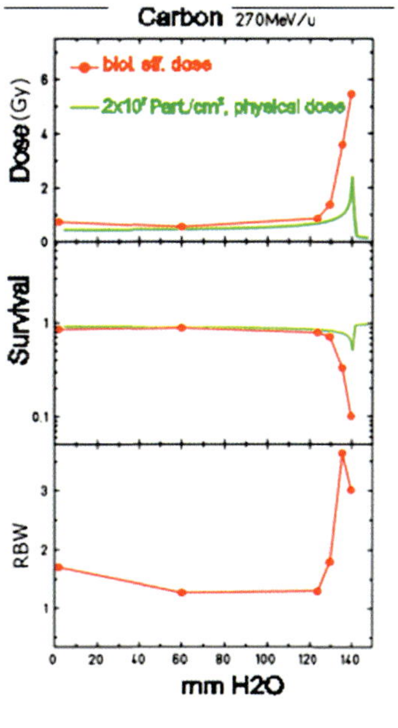

Figure 5: As a function of penetration depth dose, survival and RBE are compared for a carbon beam. In the top panel the physical dose *i.e.* the Bragg curve is compared as the lower curve with the biological effective dose (BED). BED yields from the dose multiplied by the RBE (lower panel). RBB is determined from the expected survival based on photon sensitivity with the measured survival (Tsujii *et al.*, 2004).

The goal of the older heavy ion therapy at Berkeley was to maximize the absolute effects in the tumor area while taking into account higher side effects in the normal tissue. Therefore Argon ions have been used first and later on neon ions. Both ions produce an extreme high tumor control rate, but also many late effects in the normal tissues are found. This clinical response can be explained with cell experiments (Weyrather *et al.*, 1999). Cells are irradiated in a water tank as a tissue equivalent in different depth of the ion beam and the measured cell survival does not correspond to sparsely ionizing radiation like photons (Fig. **5**, green curve in the middle). For carbon ions the experimentally measured cell survival in the entrance channel is close to the calculated survival rate based on photons. But in the range of the Bragg maximum the survival (red curve, Fig. **5**) is very much reduced and corresponds to that generated by about 3 times higher photon dose than that measured in the ion Bragg peak. Therefore, comparing the doses, the relative biological effectiveness in this case is RBE = 3.

A similar behavior of the RBE is found for all ions. But for protons the range of an elevated RBE is restricted to the last fractions of a millimeter of the ion range, *i.e.* elevated RBE values are only found on the very distal part of the dose maximum. Consequently, in the clinical application the slightly elevated RBE values of protons are not important for therapy and are taken into account with the global factor of 10–20%, (RBE = 1.15 to 1.20). For very heavy ions, like argon, the increase of RBE starts very early in the entrance channel of the normal tissue. This leads to the undesired side effects mentioned above. For carbon ions, however, the increase in RBE is restricted to the last 2 cm of the ion range. This range can be used clinically in an optimal way, in order to destroy the tumor cells in the target volume very effectively, while minimizing the normal tissue toxicity.

4. CLINICAL RESULTS AND INTERNATIONAL SITUATION

In 1994 the National Institute for Radiological Science (NIRS) in Chiba, Japan, was the first to start carbon ion therapy. There, up to now about 5,000 patients have been treated very successfully (Schulz-Ertner and Tsujii, 2007). In 1997 carbon therapy started also at the Gesellschaft für Schwerionenforschung (GSI) in Darmstadt, Germany, in collaboration with the radiology of the Deutsches Krebsforschungszentrum (DKFZ), Heidelberg, as well as the Forschungs Zentrum

Rossendorf (FZR), Dresden. Between December 1997 until the Summer of 2008 more than 400 patients have been treated with carbon ions at GSI. A typical result of these treatments is given in Fig. **6**.

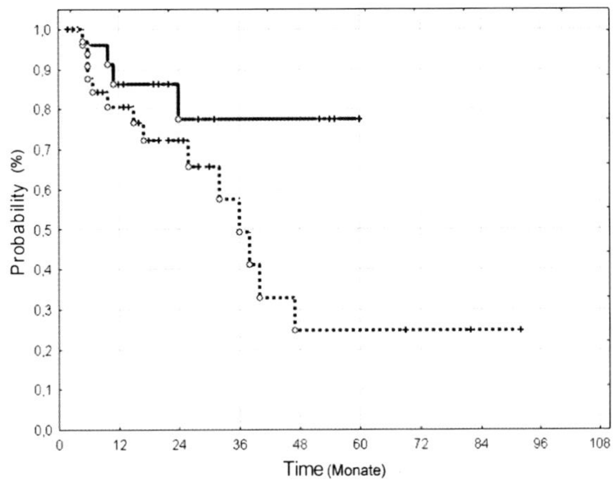

Figure 6: Local tumor control rate of patients presenting with advanced adenoidcystical carcinoma. The upper curve shows the local tumor control rate in a cohort of 29 patients treated at GSI with photon IMRT combined with a carbon boost. The lower curve shows the result for 35 patients which were treated with IMRT only. The carbon ions boost significantly increased the local control rate after 60 months from about 25% to 80% percent (Weber *et al.,* 2000).

For the patients treated at GSI the very precise irradiation technique using the raster scan system yielded in addition to the good tumor control a much smaller incidence of side effects as this would be possible with conventional therapy. A tumor control rate of 80% is a typical figure for all radioresistant tumors at GSI.

The good tumor control rate at Chiba (Tsujii *et al.*, 2004) together with the low rate of side effects at Darmstadt was the rationale to start other carbon therapy projects. In Japan, at Hyogo a unit for carbons and protons started in 2002. The construction of a third Japanese unit in Gunma prefecture is under way.

In 1992 an initiative for hadron therapy (TERA) was founded in Italy which first propagated a center for all hadrons, such as protons, neutrons, pions and heavy ions. After a short time, this proposal was reduced to proton and carbon therapy only. In 2004 the construction of a therapy unit was financed by the government and the Centro Nazionale Adroterapia Oncologica (CNAO) was founded to operate this project.

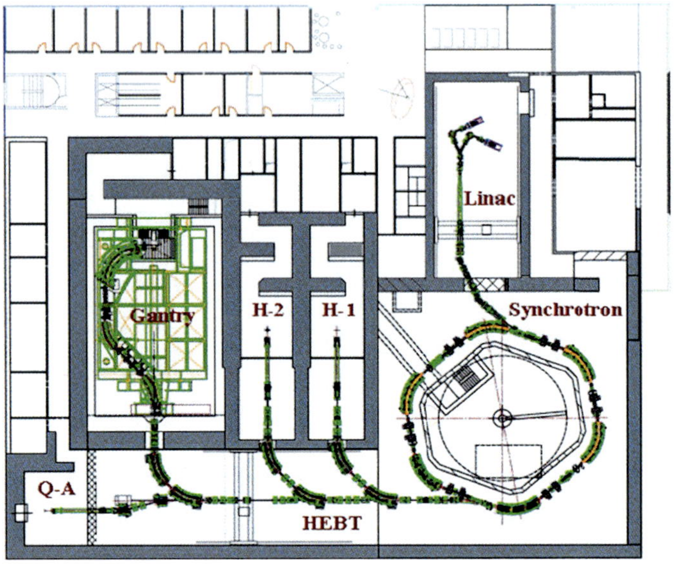

Figure 7: Layout of the Heidelberg Heavy Ion Therapy HIT. Ion source and the synchrotron at the right side produce the beam for two irradiation places having a fixed horizontal beam similar to GSI and for one beam that can be rotated around the patient (Gantry) is shown at the left side (Weyrather *et al.,* 1999).

In 1994, Med-AUSTRON, a project for the construction of a carbon-proton therapy, started in Austria. In the beginning, this project was combined with a spallation-neutron source, using the same synchrotron. However, after a short time it became evident that different accelerators, one for therapy and another neutron production would be more effective and, as a consequence, Med-AUSTRON designed its own dedicated therapy system for. After the termination of the spallation project the construction of the therapy unit was decided by the government in January of 2005.

In 2003, the construction of the heavy ion therapy facility (HIT) at the Heidelberg clinic was started (Fig. 7). The first patient was treated there in November 2009. HIT is at present on of the few European facilities providing treatment with C-ions (Haberer *et al.*, 2004).

In 2005 in Pavia, Italy, the foundation stone for the Italian C-ion therapy unit was laid and the Center opened at the beginning of 2010. At the beginning of 2005 the Med-AUSTRON project was funded by the Austrian government and in May 2005 money was given by the French government for the ETOILE-project in Lyon. These projects are presently under completion and the ground breaking is expected for both in the near future.

Meanwhile in Germany a second project at Marburg was also started by the Rhoen Klinikum AG (RKA) a private hospital supplier and patient treatments are expected to start in late summer of 2011. According to this in the next two years 5 units will be active in Europe. For an estimated need of about 1 unit per 10 Millions Inhabitants, these first 5 units are not sufficient for Germany. Foe the European Union, approximately 30 units are necessary to provide a good care for all patients. How many additional heavy ion therapies will be constructed at the end will essentially depend on the clinical success, especially in comparison to the proton units, which require an initial investment 25% cheaper. At the end, as for any big medical investments, the success will determine the number of units. In the European market, Siemens Medical Solutions has taken over the GSI know-how and patents. In addition, the Belgian company Ion Beam Application (IBA) and the Japanese Hitatchi Company, as well as the German company ACCEL are offering heavy ion therapy units.

The large interest of these companies shows that an important market for heavy ion therapy is expected in the forthcoming years for the benefit of many cancer patients that will witness a higher chance to be cured.

ACKNOWLEDGEMENTS

D. Trani was supported by the National Space Biomedical Research Institute (NSBRI) through NCC 9-58.

CONFLICT OF INTEREST

The authors confirm that this chapter content has no conflict of interest.

REFERENCES

Durante, M. & Loeffler, J.S. (2010) Charged particles in radiation oncology. *Nat Rev Clin Oncol*, 7, 37-43.

Haberer, T. *et al.,* (2004) The Heidelberg Ion Therapy Center. *Radiother Oncol*, 73 Suppl 2, S186-90.

Halperin, E.C. (2006) Particle therapy and treatment of cancer. *Lancet Oncol*, 7, 676-685.

Schulz-Ertner, D. & Tsujii, H. (2007) Particle radiation therapy using proton and heavier ion beams. *J Clin Oncol*, 25, 953-964.

Tsujii, H. *et al.,* (2004) Overview of clinical experiences on carbon ion radiotherapy at NIRS. *Radiother Oncol*, 73 Suppl 2, S41-9.

Weber, U., Becher, W. & Kraft, G. (2000) Depth scanning for a conformal ion beam treatment of deep seated tumours. *Phys Med Biol*, 45, 3627-3641.

Weber, U. & Kraft, G. (2009) Comparison of carbon ions *versus* protons. *Cancer J*, 15, 325-332.

Weyrather, W.K. *et al.,* (1999) RBE for carbon track-segment irradiation in cell lines of differing repair capacity. *Int J Radiat Biol*, 75, 1357-1364.

Send Orders for Reprints to reprints@benthamscience.net
Cutting Edge Therapies for Cancer in the 21st Century, 2014, 167-183

CHAPTER 6

Agonist and Antagonist Acting on The Leptin-Leptin Receptor Interface: Present and Future

Laszlo Otvos*

OLPE, LLC., Inc., 801 Mockingbird Lane, Audubon, PA 19403, USA

Abstract: In this chapter, the impact of lipid molecules on hematopoiesis will be reviewed in a format friendly to those outside the field. The focus of the review is on how dietary fatty acids impact hematopoiesis through changes in differentiation. We begin with a discussion of general hematopoiesis including the concepts of stem and progenitor cells that drive hematopoiesis and the various cell types they produce. We then will discuss the principles of epigenetic gene regulation and differentiation pertinent to hematopoietic stem and progenitor cells. Once these principles have been introduced, we will examine how dietary lipids can impact hematopoietic differentiation. The relationship of epigenetics and dietary lipids to leukemic and preleukemic states will also be explored. We will conclude with a look at how WNT signaling can impact hematopoiesis through epigenetic gene regulation, dietary lipids, and differentiation.

Keywords: Cancer, Leptin, Leptin Receptor, Adipokine receptor, PI-3K, JAK/STAT3, Obesity, Breast Cancer, Adipokine Receptor, WNT, NF (nuclear factor)-κB, TNF-alpha, Blood Brain Barrier (BBB), Adiponectin, Adiponectin receptor, ERK-1/2, Ras, central nervous system (CNS).

1. LEPTIN AND LEPTIN SIGNAL

Leptin is a 167 amino acid-containing cytokine-like hormone secreted by adipose tissue in direct proportion to amount of body fat (Considine *et al.*, 1996). Circulating leptin levels reflect the amount of stored energy with a result of leptin controlling the regulation of energy homeostasis, neuroendocrine function, and metabolism (Kelesidis *et al.*, 2010). The absence of leptin induces morbid obesity, hyperphagia, neuroendocrine dysfunction as well as hyperglycemia and insulin resistance (Friedman and Halaas, 1998).

***Address correspondence to Laszlo Otvos:** OLPE, LLC., Inc., 801 Mockingbird Lane, Audubon, PA 19403, USA; Tel: 1-(610)-666-7110; Fax: +1 215 204 6646; E-mail: lotvos@comcast.net

In normal conditions, leptin acts on the central nervous system (CNS), mainly in the hypothalamus, to activate its cognate receptor ObR (Bjoerbaek, 2009). A long form of ObR mediates signal transduction and is strongly expressed in the hypothalamus where the control of energy homeostasis and neuroendocrine functions reside (Fei *et al.*, 1997). A shorter form of ObR is found in the blood-brain barrier (BBB) and promotes the transport of leptin into the CNS without clear signaling functions (Bjoerbaek *et al.*, 1998). Superimposition of leptin's sequence with other cytokines reveals three potential dual-chain receptor binding sites labeled as I-III (Peelman *et al.*, 2004).

The signaling pathways activated by ObR include the classic cytokine JAK2/STAT3 (Janus kinase 2/signal transducer and activator of transcription 3) pathway; the Ras/ERK1/2 (Ras/extracellular signal-regulated kinases 1/2) signaling cascade; and the PI-3K/Akt/GSK3 (phosphoinositide 3 kinase/protein kinase B/glycogen synthase kinase 3) growth/antiapoptotic pathway (Sweeney, 2002). From these, PI-3K and STAT are crucial to energy homeostasis, and yet another signaling series involved, the mitogen-activated protein kinase pathway may play a role in the regulation of linear growth and reproductive function (Bates *et al.*, 2003; Banks *et al.*, 2000). Importantly, the PI-3K pathway is also the major intracellular pathway activated by insulin receptor signaling, making this a crucial stage at which leptin and insulin may coordinately act to control energy homeostasis (Oswal and Yeo, 2010). The fourth major signaling target of ObR is the transcription factor NF (nuclear factor)-κB driving pro-inflammatory gene expression (Rose *et al.*, 2002).

From less discussed leptin signaling events, leptin may also regulate the hedonic component of satiety by determining the perception of reward associated with feeding. This action of leptin probably occurs at the level of the mesolimbic dopaminergic system, explaining the weight gain commonly induced by antipsychotic drugs, which act as mixed dopamine receptor antagonists (Bergman and Ader, 2005). ObR is expressed on dopaminergic neurons within the ventral tegmental area of the brainstem as well as other extra-hypothalamic areas including brainstem nuclei such as the nucleus *tractus solitari* (Coll *et al.*, 2007).

It is probably fair to assume that receptor activation by the 3 independent ObR binding sites contribute to somewhat different signaling pathways. Interestingly a leptin fragment with weight reduction promoting activity neither binds ObR nor induces its characteristic signaling pathways (Grasso *et al.*, 1999), forcing a hypothesis that this particular leptin fragment binds the melanocortin-4 receptor instead (Grasso *et al.*, 2007). In addition, leptin induces hypertrophy through the activation of the peroxisome proliferator-activated receptor α pathway in cultured neonatal rat cardiomyocytes (Hou *et al.*, 2010).

The multiple binding sites to its cognate receptor together with the fact that the protein may also initiate ObR-independent signal transduction processes suggest that for potential pharmaceutical use peptides representing single binding sites offer pharmacologically more accepted models than the full protein.

2. MIXED CLINICAL DATA

When in 1995 Amgen paid $20 million for the commercializing rights of the patent on leptin for the clinical treatment of obesity, it was one of the largest academical licensing deals in history (Neill, 2010). In the first set of clinical trials with recombinant methionyl human leptin (r-metHuLeptin), a subset of obese patients lost significant amounts of weight, but the average magnitude of the effect was minimal (Heymsfield *et al.*, 1999). Likewise, treatment with pegylated human leptin results in a 3 kg weight loss compared to placebo-treated overweight male patients, but the 2 treatment groups do not differ significantly in changes in body composition, energy expenditure, and metabolic variables (Hukshorn *et al.*, 2003). R-metHuLeptin replacement at a subcutaneous dose of 0.04 mg/kg/day in human immunodeficiency virus positive leptin-deficient patients with Highly Active Antiretroviral Therapy (HAART)-induced lipoatrophy improves insulin resistance, high-density lipoprotein, and truncal fat mass (Lee *et al.*, 2006). It needs to be mentioned that the study included only 7 men. In general, while leptin has been successfully used in the treatment of leptin-deficient obese patients, trials in hyperleptinemic obese patients, who constitute far the greater percentage of obese and overweight, have yielded variable results (Bell-Anderson and Bryson, 2004).

Long-acting leptins have been tried but with no greater success. Pharmacokinetic study of r-metHuLeptin measured the available leptin in the serum, but did not include any estimate for the amount of the protein in the brain, where the targeted physiological effects are manifested (Chan *et al.*, 2008). The reason for the lack of improvements is potentially that engineered leptin conjugates intend to increase the circulation time to overcome the clinical failures rather than improving penetration across the BBB (Lo *et al.*, 2005).

A single Arg → Gln amino acid change in the third ObR-binding site (site III) yields a protein analog that retains leptin-like efficacy in a genetically obese mouse model, but *in vitro* the protein mutant acts like an ObR antagonist (Brunner *et al.*, 1999) suggesting that the design of ObR agonists and antagonists based on full-sized leptin protein is more complex than it meets the eye.

The lack of clear clinical efficacy after peripheral leptin administration is probably connected to the inactivity of the elevated levels of leptin in obese individuals (Munzberg, 2010). Central resistance to leptin in obesity with associated peripheral hyperleptinemia is attributable to decreased efficiency of leptin transport into the brain and not to intra-hypothalamic leptin insensitivity as others suggested (Myers *et al.*, 2008). The jury is still out whether the central leptin resistance is reversible or not after weight reduction (Banks and Farrel, 2003; Adam and Findlay, 2010).

As for the mechanism of leptin resistance, several studies point to a saturable leptin transporter (Banks *et al.*, 2002; Banks, 2008). However, in rats the BBB-resident form of ObR can easily be saturated (Burguera *et al.*, 2000). Saturation of the BBB-resident short ObR form in obese individuals would explain the defect in leptin transport into the brain (Burguera and Couce, 2001). Several attempts have been made to improve the BBB penetration of leptin. These approaches include co-synthesis of leptin with the Tat protein-derived transduction domain and passive transport *via* the negatively charged cell surface (Zhang *et al.*, 2009), conjugation to amphiphilic polyethylene-based copolymers known to improve brain transport (Price *et al.*, 2010) or the use of BBB activators prior or concomitant with leptin administration (Banks, 2001). ObR-binding leptin fragments themselves can be used to deliver other drugs into the CNS (Barret *et al.*, 2009), although BBB-resident ObR saturation can limit the applicability of this approach. Perhaps the most promising method is to bypass BBB restrictions altogether by intranasally administered leptin (Schulz *et al.*, 2004). Intranasally administered drugs can be taken up directly by olfactory neurons (Charlton *et al.*, 2008).

3. OVERCOMING LEPTIN RESISTANCE WITH SINGLE SITE PEPTIDES AND CARBOHYDRATE-MEDIATED BRAIN PENETRATION

We synthesized leptin fragments corresponding to all 3 ObR-binding regions. To assess the pharmacological utility of leptin fragments, we studied the peptides' ability to stimulate the growth of ObR-positive and ObR-negative cells (Otvos *et al.*, 2008). From these peptides, a designer site III analog termed E1Free, featuring non-natural amino acids at terminal positions to decrease proteolysis and a BBB penetration-enhancing carbohydrate moiety, proved to be a full agonist to ObR. The peptide induces the proliferation of different ObR-positive but not ObR-negative cells in the presence or absence of leptin. This glycopeptide binds ObR in a direct binding assay and activates ERK-1/2 signaling at 100 – 500 nM concentrations. Importantly for future drug development, the glycopeptide is stable in mouse serum, readily crosses endothelial/astrocyte cell layers in a cellular BBB model, and is distributed into the brain of Balb/c mice after intraperitoneal administration better than a similarly labeled full-sized and carbohydrate-lacking leptin protein (Knappe *et al.*, 2008). These characteristics suggest a potential pharmaceutical utility of E1Free in leptin-deficient diseases. To provide proof-of-concept *in vivo*, the efficacy of E1Free was tested on typical leptin functions in sheep. The glycopeptide reduces voluntary food intake of program-fed animals by 25% and central infusion increases post-prandial thermogenesis in muscle by 3°C (Otvos *et al.*, 2009). While this is not the first peptide fragment that reduces appetite *in vivo* this is the first one that does it through activation of ObR.

Later the peptide was further improved for ObR binding stronger than leptin protein itself. Leptin stimulates the proliferation of ObR-positive cells around 6 nM concentration (Garofalo *et al.*, 2004). The second generation ObR agonist glycopeptide, containing altered non-natural residues at the termini and a threonine-linked N-acetyl galactosamine (instead of a serine-linked glucose such as in E1Free) carbohydrate moiety, is termed E1/Aca. E1/Aca induces leptin effects in ObR-positive cell lines at picomolar concentrations (Kovalszky *et al.*, 2010) and can be classified as a superagonist. The glycopeptide readily crosses the blood-brain barrier following intraperitoneal administration and initiates typical leptin-dependent signal transduction pathways both in the presence and absence of leptin protein. In a diet-induced obese mouse model, mice receiving peptide E1/Aca lose weight in a dose-dependent manner. At 0.5 mg/kg/day the weight loss corresponds to a net 6.5% total body weight after 11 days of treatment. Similar mice treated with 0.1 mg/kg/day leptin protein lose weight only until the fifth day when they become resistant to treatment in perfect analogy to the human clinical trials. Upon cessation of the weight loss treatment, the abnormal metabolic profile and liver histology are normalized in peptide-, but not leptin-treated, mice. Remarkably, E1/Aca restores the fertility of the mice that was lost due to obesity. E1/Aca administered intranasally to growing normal rats also decelerates normal weight gain corresponding to a net 6.8% net total body weight loss. Significantly, no resistance induction to peptide E1/Aca or toxicity in either obese or healthy rodents is observed, indicating the potential for widespread utility of the peptidomimetic in the treatment of leptin-deficiency disorders.

4. LEPTIN AS A LINK OF OBESITY TO OTHER HEALTH CONDITIONS

An estimated 300,000 deaths per year and significant morbidity are directly attributable to obesity, mainly due to heart disease, diabetes, cancer, asthma, sleep apnea, arthritis, reproductive complications and psychological disturbances (Gale *et al.*, 2004). In 2003, it was estimated that overweight and obesity were responsible for 14% and 20% of cancer cases among men and women, respectively, in the United States (Calle *et al.,* 2003). Increasing body mass index is associated with a significant increase in the risk of for endometrial cancer and adenocarcinoma of the esophagus where as much as half of all cases in postmenopausal women are attributable to overweight or obesity (Reeves *et al.*, 2007). Recent studies have demonstrated that the impaired immune response in the obese host leads to increased susceptibility to infection with a number of different pathogens such as community-acquired tuberculosis, influenza, *Mycobacterium tuberculosis*, coxsackievirus, *Helicobacter pylori* and encephalomyocarditis virus (Karlsson and Beck, 2010).

Obesity-associated disturbances of adipose tissue function are believed to play a crucial role in the development of insulin resistance, type 2 diabetes, and obesity-related cardiovascular disease (van Kruijsdijk *et al.*, 2009). Adipokines circulating in the blood can exert their biological actions on target cells by classical endocrine mechanisms, but in addition, like the inflammatory cytokines, they also operate at the local level through paracrine pathways (Vona-Davis and Rose, 2007). In addition to its role as a neurohormone, leptin can modulate immune response, fertility, and hematopoiesis, acting as a mitogen, metabolic regulator, or pro-angiogenic factor (Wauters *et al.*, 2000). Leptin is a mitogen for various cell types, including myelocytic and primitive hematopoietic progenitor cells (Bennett *et al.*, 1996) normal and transformed breast epithelial cells (Hu *et al.*, 2002; Somasundar *et al.*, 2003) and vascular endothelial cells (Park *et al.*, 2001). Leptin stimulates breast cancer cell growth (Dieudonne *et al.*, 2002), interferes with the action of antiestrogens (Garofalo *et al.*, 2004), and may be involved in metastasis (Hu *et al.*, 2002). In hormone-dependent tumor types, such as breast and colorectal cancer, both leptin and ObR are overexpressed (Ishikawa *et al.*, 2004; Koda *et al.*, 2007) and the leptin/ObR system has been proposed to serve as a novel prognostic marker (Tessitore *et al.*, 2004). It has been repeatedly argued that leptin is a novel pharmaceutical target, and leptin antagonists may represent a new family of cancer drugs (Surmacz, 2007).

5. FULL-SIZED LEPTIN RECEPTOR ANTAGONISTS

Recombinant rat and mouse leptins contain a triple Leu39, Asp40 and Phe41 to Ala change in ObR-binding site I resulting in L39A/D40A/F41A mutants. These were developed in order to block the biological effects of leptin in a series of *in vivo* and *in vitro* studies (Gertler, 2006). Leptin versions containing the same mutation but corresponding to various species are commercially available, and the mutant protein has been prepared in large scale (Salomon *et al.*, 2006). In detailed later assays this protein analog turned out to be an antagonist for the central effects of leptin on food intake and body weight but an agonist at sites where leptin induces acute neuronal activation (Peters *et al.*, 2007, Abdemmeni-Najar *et al.*, 2011). While the authors suggested the activation of multiple and in certain applications different receptor subtypes, potentially activation by different or multiple binding sites provokes non-canonical receptor responses. This triply mutated protein variant attenuates leptin-induced liver fibrosis but it does not influence body weight (Elinav *et al.*, 2009a), confirming the suggestion that it has ObR antagonistic activity only in a subset of leptin functions. Indeed, intracerebroventricular administration of the leptin mutant has profound orexigenic responses in rats, without influencing the STAT3 signal transduction pathway (Scarpace *et al.*, 2007). An additional Asp23 → Leu change is reported to increase both the ObR affinity and antagonistic selectivity (Shpilman *et al.*, 2010). Even further adding to the puzzle, a pegylated analog of this protein mutant shows both peripheral and central ObR antagonistic effects although it is shown not to penetrate the BBB (Elinav *et al.*, 2009b).

No protein mutant has been made corresponding to ObR-binding site II. Single-point mutations in full-sized leptin at binding site III drastically attenuate the agonistic activity and convert those mutants into both partial antagonists and weak agonists (Niv-Spector *et al.*, 2005). For example, mutation of Tyr119 to alanine yields a ligand with 95% antagonistic activity without affecting the binding strength to the receptor. Recombinant leptin featuring a Ser120 → Ala, Thr121 → Ala double mutation at ObR binding site III avidly binds to the CRH2 domain of the receptor where activation by leptin may take place (Iserentant *et al.*, 2005) but fails to induce proper downstream signaling (Peelman *et al.*, 2004). Human leptin containing a glutamine in position 128 (instead of the natural arginine) loses its cell proliferating activity and becomes a weak antagonist, whereas the activities of similar mutated ovine and chicken leptins are reduced 25- and 80-fold (Raver *et al.*, 2002). As it was found for site I mutant proteins and peptides covering the entire leptin protein (Otvos *et al.*, 2008), the emergence of both partial antagonists and weak agonists as listed above may indicate that depending on individual cell context as well as the presence or absence of native, unmodified leptin, the same mutant protein or large subunit can trigger different downstream signaling responses.

An anti-ObR monoclonal antibody termed 9F8, inhibits leptin induced TNF-alpha production from human monocytes and anti-CD3 mAb induced proliferation of human T cells in a peripheral blood mononuclear cell culture (Fazeli *et al.*, 2006). On the flip side of the coin, an anti-leptin antiserum reverses lipopolysaccharide-induced reduction of food intake and body weight (Sachot *et al.*, 2004). With this limited information on antibody activities it remains to be seen whether anti-ObR or anti-leptin antibodies are as useful in potential human therapy as antibodies to other proteins.

6. PEPTIDE-BASED LEPTIN RECEPTOR ANTAGONISTS

A peptide comprising residues 70-95 of leptin (ObR binding site II) binds specifically and with high affinity ($K_i \sim 60$ pM) to ObR and inhibits its functions in rabbit endometrial cells and mouse mammary cancer cells (Gonzalez and Leavis, 2003; Gonzalez *et al*., 2006). Intraperitoneal injection of a pegylated analog of the 70-95 peptide impairs the establishment of endometriosis-like lesions and results in a reduction of mitotic activity (Styer *et al.,* 2008). This pegylated peptide more effectively reduces the expression of pro-angiogenic and pro-proliferative molecules as well as the growth of estrogen receptor positive (>40-fold) than estrogen receptor negative breast cancer xenografts (Gonzalez *et al*., 2009). However, this peptide cannot be considered as a full antagonist, as an extended analog of the same peptide shows strong agonistic activities in cell cultures when leptin protein is not present (Otvos *et al*., 2008).

We developed 9-amino acid-long, pharmacologically advantageous peptide analogs of ObR-binding site III of leptin that act as selective ObR inhibitors without any partial agonistic activity (Otvos *et al*., 2011a). These peptides reduce leptin-dependent growth and signaling in cancer cell lines at picomolar and low nanomolar concentrations. In severe immunocompromised mice the lead peptide termed Allo-aca suppresses the growth of rapidly proliferating hormone receptor positive orthotopic human breast cancer xenografts by 50% when administered either intraperitoneally or subcutaneously at a 0.1 mg/kg/day dose. The peptides are distributed to the brain, and when added to growing C57BL/6 normal mice intraperitoneally, subcutaneously or even or orally, the tested antagonist accelerates normal weight increase without producing any toxic effects. Weight gain increases cannot be observed after 10-12 days of treatment indicating that the mice become resistant to the CNS activity of leptin antagonists. However, in normal growing rats intranasal administration at 0.1 mg/kg/day result in a 2% net total body weight gain without signs of resistance induction. In addition to the potential of these peptides in drug development against primary and metastatic tumors and cachexia, these data confirm that resistance to leptin resides at the blood-brain barrier.

7. BEST CHANCE FOR SUCCESS: EFFICACY IN A MOUSE MODEL OF TRIPLE NEGATIVE BREAST CANCER

Triple-negative breast cancers (expressing no receptors for estrogen, progesterone or HER-2), which represent 10-20% of all mammary tumors, are characterized by the aggressive phenotype, are often found in younger women and have been associated with poor prognosis (Rodriguez-Pinila *et al.*, 2006; Vona-Davis and Rose 2009). Obesity increases the risk for triple-negative breast cancer development (Phipps *et al.*, 2008). Because triple-negative breast cancer patients are unresponsive to current targeted therapies and other treatment options are only partially effective, new pharmacological modalities are urgently needed. In human triple-negative breast cancer tissues, the leptin receptor is expressed in 92% (64/69) and leptin in 86% (59/69) of cases (Otvos *et al.*, 2011b). In a model triple-negative breast cancer cell line MDA-MB-231, the leptin receptor antagonist peptide Allo-aca inhibits leptin-induced proliferation at 50 pM concentration. In an MDA-MB-231 orthotopic mouse xenograft model, Allo-aca administered subcutaneously significantly extends the average survival time from 15.4 days (untreated controls) to 28.1 days at a 1 mg/kg/day dose. In the same model, conventional treatment with 1 mg/kg/day intraperitoneal cisplatin, the current method of choice for triple negative breast cancer therapy (Pal and Mortimer, 2009) prolongs the average survival time to 18.6 days. In normal CD-1 mice, Allo-aca does not exhibit any signs of systemic toxicity up to the highest studied subcutaneous bolus dose of 50 mg/kg. As expected from an ObR antagonist, Allo-aca induces a modest body weight increase. These most recent results indicate that true ObR antagonists have the potential to become attractive options for triple-negative breast cancer treatment, especially in the obese patient population.

8. ADIPOKINE RECEPTORS ARE MAJOR TARGETS IN FUTURE DRUG DEVELOPMENT

When discussing the role of inhibition of the leptin/ObR signaling in cancer research, experts frequently point to another adipokine: adiponectin. Many factors appear to be important in the mechanism of the obesity-related increased risk for cancer development, including estrogen, estrogen receptors, and both adipokines leptin and adiponectin (Cleary *et al.*, 2010). On one hand, blood levels of adiponectin are inversely correlated with breast cancer risk (Barb *et al*., 2007). On the other, metabolic syndrome is a cardiovascular risk factor that is related to underlying insulin resistance and adiponectin has anti-atherogenic effects and augments the metabolic effects of insulin (Takeuchi *et al*., 2007). Adiponectin is a 247 amino acid-long protein which, in animal models, has been shown to have beneficial effects against obesity-related vascular diseases. Adiponectin actions are clearly beneficial against breast cancer development as it was shown *in vitro* and in clinical samples and this is exactly opposite to the influence of leptin on breast cancer progression (Jarde *et al*., 2009). Up to this point, two adiponectin receptors have been identified, AdipoR1 and AdipoR2 (Yamauchi *et al*., 2003). While the precise receptor regions that bind the ligand are not known, the active adiponectin active site has been identified between residues 149 and 166 (Otvos *et al.,* 2011c). Future research will focus on identifying adiponectin receptor agonists for cancer treatment.

For now, we will focus on the clinical development of ObR peptide antagonists against triple-negative breast cancer and other malignant modalities. Peptide Allo-aca extends the average survival time of mice carrying triple negative breast cancer xenografts by 80%. If developed as a drug, the peptide with its advantageous administration route and safety profile can be a useful addition to the existing oncology drug repertoire against various forms of cancers characterized by ObR overexpression such as breast, brain, prostate and colon cancers. Even better, an ObR antagonist exhibiting peripheral activity only might become an attractive addition to current treatment protocols of these aggressive tumors.

ACKNOWLEDGEMENT

Declared None.

CONFLICT OF INTEREST

The author declare no conflict of interest.

REFERENCES

Abdennebi-Najar, L, Desai, M, Han, G, Casillas, E, Jean, D, Arieh, G, & Ross MG (2011), 'Basal, endogenous leptin is metabolically active in newborn rat pups', *Journal of Maternal- Fetal Neonatal Medicine*, 24, p. 1486-1491.

Adam, CL, & Findlay PA (2010), 'Decreased blood-brain barrier leptin transfer in an ovine model of obesity and weight loss: resolving the cause of leptin resistance', *International Journal of Obesity*, no 34, p. 980-988

Banks, AS, Davis, SM, Bates, SH & Myers, MG, Jr (2000), 'Activation of downstream signals by the long form of the leptin receptor', *Journal of Biological Chemistry*, no 275, p 14563-14572

Banks, WA (2001), 'Enhanced leptin transport across the blood-brain barrier by alpha 1-adrenergic agents', *Brain Research* no 899, p. 209-217

Banks, WA, Niehoff, ML, Martin, D, & Farrell CL (2002), 'Leptin transport across the blood-brain barrier of the Koletsky rat is not mediated by a product of the leptin receptor gene', *Brain Research*, no 950, p. 130-136.

Banks, WA, & Ferrell, CL (2003), 'Impaired transport of leptin across the blood-brain barrier in obesity is acquired and reversible', *American Journal of Physiology, Endocrinology and Metabolism*, no 285, p. E10-15

Banks, WA (2008), 'The blood-brain barrier as a cause of obesity', *Current Pharmaceutical Design* no 14, p 1606-1614

Barb, D, Williams, CJ, Neuwirth AK, & Mantzoros, CS (2007), 'Adiponectin in relation to malignancies: a review of existing basic research and clinical evidence', *American Journal of Clinical Nutrition* no 86, p. 858S-866S

Barret, GL, Trieu, J, & Naim T (2009), 'The identification of leptin-derived peptides that are taken up by the brain', *Regulatory Peptides* no 155, p. 55-61

Bates, SH, Steams, WH, Dunson, TA, Schubert, M, Tsao, ZW, Wang, Y, Banks, AS, Lavery, HJ, Haq, AK, Maratos-Flier, E, Neel, BG, Schwatrz, MW, Myers, MG, Jr (2003), 'STAT3 signalling is required for leptin regulation of energy balance but not reproduction', *Nature*, no 421, p. 856-859

Bell-Anderson, KS, & Bryson, JM (2004), 'Leptin as a potential treatment for obesity: progress to date', *Treatments in Endocrinology*, no 3, p. 11-18

Bennett, BD, Solar, GP, Yuan, JQ, Mathias, J, Thomas, GR, & Matthews, W (1996), 'A role for leptin and its cognate receptor in hematopoiesis', *Current Biology*, no 6, p. 1170-1180

Bergman, RN, & Ader, M (2005), 'Atypical antiphychotics and glucose homeostasis', *Journal of Clinical Psychiatry*, no 66, p 504-514

Bjoerbaek, C, Elmquist, JK, Michl, P, Ahima, RS, van Bueren A, McCall, AL, & Flier, JS (1998), 'Expression of leptin receptor isoforms in rat brain microvessels', *Endocrinology*, no 139, p. 3485-3491

Bjoerbaek, C (2009), 'Central leptin receptor action and resistance in obesity', *Journal of Investigational Medicine*, no 57, p. 789-794

Brunner, L, Whitebread, S, Leconte, I, Stricker-Krongrad, A, Cumin, F, Chiesi, M, Levens, N (1999), 'A peptide leptin antagonist reduces food intake in rodents', *International Journal of Obesisty and Related Metabolic Disorders*, no 23, p. 463-469

Burguera, B, Couce, ME, Curran, GL, Jensen, MD, Lloyd, RV, Cleary, MP, & Poduslo, JF (2000), 'Obesity is associated with a decreased leptin transport across the blood-brain barrier in rats', *Diabetes*, no 49, p 1219-1223

Burguera, B, & Couce, ME (2001), 'Leptin access into the brain: a saturated transport mechanism in obesity', *Physiology and Behavior*, no 74, p. 717-720

Calle, EE, Rodriguez, C, Walker-Thurmond, K, & Thun MJ (2003), 'Overweight, obesity, and mortality from cancer in a prospectively studied cohort of U.S. adults', *New England Journal of Medicine*, no 358, p. 1625-1638

Chan, JL, Wong, SL, & Mantzoros, CS (2008), 'Pharmacokinetics of subcutaneous recombinant methionyl human leptin administration in healthy subjects in the fed and fasting states: regulation by gender and adiposity', *Clinical Pharmacokinetics*, no 47, p. 753-764

Charlton, ST, Whetstone, J, Fayinka, ST, Read, KD, Illum, L, & Davis SS (2008), 'Evaluation of direct transport pathways of glycine receptor antagonists and an angiotensin antagonist from the nasal cavity to the central nervous system in the rat model', *Pharmaceutical Research* no 25, p. 1531-1543

Cleary MP, Grossmann ME, & Ray, A (2010), 'Effect of obesity on breast cancer development' *Veterinary Pathology*, no 47, p. 202-213

Coll, AP, Farooqi, IS & O'Rahilly, S (2007), 'The hormonal control of food intake', *Cell*, no 129, p 251-262

Considine, RV, Sinha, MK, Heiman, ML, Kriauciunas, A, Stephens, TW, Nyce, MR, Ohannesian, JP, Marco, CC, McKee LJ, Bauer TL, & Caro, JF (1996), 'Serum immunoreactive-leptin concentrations in normal-weight and obese humans', *New England Journal of Medicine*, no 334, p. 292-295.

Dieudonne, MN, Machinal-Quelin, F, Serazin-Leroy, V, Leneveu, MC, Pecquery, R, & Giudicelli, Y (2002), 'Leptin mediates a proliferative response in human MCF-7 breast cancer cells', *Biochemical and Biophysical Research Communications* no 293, 622-628

Elinav, E, Ali, M, Bruck, R, Brazowski, E, Phillips, A, Shapira, Y, Katz, M, Solomon, G, Halpern, Z, & Gertler A (2009a), 'Competitive inhibition of leptin signaling results in amelioration of liver fibrosis through modulation of stellate cell function', *Hepatology*, no 49, p. 278-286

Elinav, E, Niv-Spector, L, Katz, M, Price, TO, Ali, M, Yacobovitz, M, Solomon, G, Reicher, S, Lynch, JL, Halpern, Z, Banks, WA, & Gertler A (2009b), 'Pegylated leptin antagonist is a potent orixenic agent: preparation and mechanism of activity', *Endocrinology* no 150, p. 3083-3091

Fazeli, M, Zarkesh-Esfahani, H, Wu, Z, Maamra, M, Bidlingmaier, M, Pockley, AG, Watson, P, Matarese, G, Strasburger, CJ, & Ross RJ. (2006), 'Identification of a monoclonal antibody against the leptin receptor that acts as an antagonist and blocks human monocyte and T cell activation', *Journal of Immunological Methods* no 312, p. 190-200

Fei, H, Okano, HJ, Le, C, Lee, GH, Zhao, C, Darnell, R, & Friedman, JM (1997), 'Anatomic localization of alternatively spliced leptin receptors (Ob-R) in mouse brain and other tissues', *Proceedings of the National Academy of Sciences of the United States of America*, no 94, p. 7001-7005

Friedman, JM, & Halaas, JL (1998), 'Leptin and the regulation of body weight in mammals', *Nature*, no 395, p. 763-770

Gale, SM, Castracane, VD, & Mantzoros CS (2004), 'Energy homeostasis, obesity and eating disorders: recent advances in endocrinology', *Journal of Nutrition*, no 134, p 295-298

Garofalo, C, Sisci, D, & Surmacz, E, (2004), 'Leptin interferes with the effects of the antiestrogen ICI 182,780 in MCF-7 breast cancer cells', *Clinical Cancer Research* no 10, p. 6466-6475

Gertler, A (2006), 'Development of leptin antagonists and their potential use in experimental biology and medicine', *Trends in Endocrinology and Metabolism*, no 17, p. 372-378

Gonzalez, R.R., & Leavis, PC (2003), 'A peptide derived from the human leptin molecule is a potent inhibitor of the leptin receptor function in rabbit endometrial cells', *Endocrine* no 21, p. 185-195

Gonzalez, GG, Cherfils, S, Escobar, M, Yoo, JH, Carino, C, Styer, AK, Sullivan, BT, Sakamoto, H, Olawaiye, A, Serikawa, T, Lynch, MP, & Rueda, BR (2006), 'Leptin signaling promotes the growth of mammary tumors and increases the expression of vascular endothelial growth factor (VEGF) and its receptor type two (VEGF-R2)', *Journal of Biological Chemistry* no 281, p. 26320-26328

Gonzalez, R, Watters, A, Xu, Y, Singh, UP, Mann, DR, Rueda, BR, & Penichet, ML (2009), 'Leptin-signaling inhibition results in efficient anti-tumor activity in estrogen receptor positive or negative breast cancer', *Breast Cancer Research,* no 11, p. R36

Grasso, P, White, DW, Tartaglia, LA, Leinung, MC, & Lee, DW (1999), 'Inhibitory effects of leptin-related synthetic peptide 116-130 on food intake and body weight gain in female C57BL/6J ob/ob mice may not be mediated by peptide activation of the long isoform of the leptin receptor', *Diabetes*, no 48, p. 2204-2209

Grasso, P, Lee, DW, & Leinung, MC (2007), *Leptin-related peptides*, US Patent 7,208,572

Heymsfield, SB, Greenberg, AS, Fujioka, K, Dixon, RM, Kushner, R, Hunt, T, Lubina, JA, Patane, J, Self, B, Hunt, P, & McCamish M. (1999), 'Recombinant leptin for weight loss in obese and lean adults: a randomized, controlled, dose-escalation trial', *Journal of the American Medical Association*, no 282, p. 1568-1575

Hou, N, Luo, MS, Liu, SM, Zhang, HN, Xiao, Q, Sun, P, Zhang, GS, Luo, JD, & Chen MS (2010), 'Leptin induces hypertrophy through activating the peroxisome proliferator-activated receptor α pathway in cultured neonatal rat cardiomyocytes', *Clinical and Experimental Pharmacology and Physiology*, no 37, p. 1087-1095

Hu, X, Juneja, SC, Maihle, MJ, & Cleary, MP (2002), 'Leptin-a growth factor in normal and malignant breast cells and for normal mammary gland development', *Journal of the National Cancer Institute* no 94, p. 1704-1711

Hukshorn, CJ, Westerterp-Plantenga, MS, & Saris, WH (2003), 'Pegylated human recombinant leptin (PEG-OB) causes additional weight loss in severely energy-restricted, overweight men', *American Journal of Clinical Nutrition*, no 77, p. 771-776

Iserentant, H, Peelman, F, Defeau, D, Vandekerckhove, J, Zabeau, L, & Tavernier, J (2005), 'Mapping the interface between leptin and the leptin receptor CHR2 domain', *Journal of Cell Sciences*, no 118, p. 2519-2527

Ishikawa, M, Kitayama, J, & Nagawa, H (2004), 'Enhanced expression of leptin and leptin receptor (OB-R) in human breast cancer', *Clinical Cancer Research* no 10, p. 4325-4331

Jarde, T, Caldefie-Chézet, F, Goncalves-Mendes, N, Mishellany, F, Buechler, C, Penault-Llorca, F, & Vasson, MP (2009), 'Involvement of adiponectin and leptin in breast cancer: clinical and *in vitro* studies', *Endocrinology Related Cancer* no 16, p. 1197-1210

Karlsson, EA & Beck MA (2010), 'The burden of obesity on infectious disease', *Experimental Biology and Medicine*, no 235, p 1412-1424

Kelesidis, T, Kelesidis, I, Chou, S, & Mantzoros, CS (2010), 'Narrative review: the role of leptin in human physiology: emerging clinical applications', *Annals of Internal Medicine*, no 152, p 93-100

Knappe, D., Otvos, L., Jr., De Pascali, F., Cassone, M., Scolaro, L., Abbadessa, G., Carrillo-Infante, C., Kiani, M.F., Donelson, F., Hoffmann, R., & Surmacz, E (2008), 'Drug development-targeted screening of leptin agonist glycopeptides', *International Journal of Peptide Research and Therapeutics*, no 14, p. 247-254

Koda, M, Sulkowska, M, Kanczuga-Koda, L, Cascio, S, Colucci, G, Russo, A, Surmacz, E, & Sulkowski, S (2007), 'Expression of the obesity hormone leptin and its receptor correlates with hypoxia-inducible factor-1α in human colorectal cancer', *Annals of Oncology* no 18, p. vi116-vi119

Kovalszky, I, Surmacz, E, Scolaro, L, Cassone, M, Sztodola, A, Olah, J, Hatfield, MPD, Lovas, S, & Otvos, L, Jr (2010), 'Leptin-based glycopeptide induces weight loss and simultaneously restores fertility in animal models', *Diabetes Obesity and Metabolism* no 12, p. 393-402

Lee, JH, Chan, JL, Sourlas, E, Raptopoulos, V, & Mantzoros, CS (2006), 'Recombinant methionyl human leptin therapy in replacement doses improves insulin resistance and metabolic profile in patients with lipoatrophy and metabolic syndrome induced by the highly active antiretroviral therapy', *Journal of Clinical Endocrinology and Metabolism*, no 91, p. 2605-2611

Lo, KM, Zhang, J, Sun, Y, Morelli, B, Lan, Y, Lauder, S, Brunkhorst, B, Webster, G, Hallakou-Bozec, S, Doaré, L, & Gillies SD (2005), 'Engineering a pharmacologically superior form of leptin for the treatment of obesity', *Protein Engineering, Design and Selection*, no 18, p. 1-10

Munzberg, H (2010), 'Leptin-signaling pathways and leptin resistance', *Forum of Nutrition*, no 63, p. 123-132

Myers, MG, Cowley, MA & Munzberg, H. (2008), 'Mechanisms of leptin action and leptin resistance', *Annual Reviews of Physiology*, no 70, p. 537-556

Neill, U. (2010), 'Leaping for leptin: the 2010 Albert Lasker basic medical research award goes to Douglas Coleman and Jeffrey M. Friedman', *Journal of Clinical Investigation*, no 120, p 3413-3418

Niv-Spector, L, Gonen-Berger, D, Gourdou, L, Biener, E, Gussakovsky, EE, Benomar, Y, Ramunajan, KV, Taouis, M, Herman, B, Callebaut, I, Djiane, J, Gertler, A (2005), 'Identification of the hydrophobic strand in the A-B loop of leptin as major binding site III: implications for large-scale preparation of potent recombinant human and ovine leptin antagonists', *Biochemical Journal*, no 391, p. 221-230

Oswal, A, & Yeo G (2010), Leptin and control of body weight: a review of its diverse central targets, signaling mechanisms, and role in the pathogenesis of obesity', *Obesity*, no 18, p 221-229

Otvos, L., Jr., Terrasi, M., Cascio, S., Cassone, M., Abbadessa, G., di Pascali, F., Scolaro, L., Knappe, D., Stawikowski, M., Cudic, P., Wade, J.D., Hoffmann, R., & Surmacz, E (2008), 'Development of a pharmacologically improved peptide agonist of the leptin receptor', *Biochimica et Biophysica Acta*, no 1783, p. 1745-1754

Otvos, L., Jr., Cassone, M., Wade, J., Knappe, D., Hoffmann, R., Henry, B., Clarke, I., &Surmacz, E (2009), 'Leptin receptor agonist glycopeptide for leptin replacement therapy' In: H. Lankinen, (Ed.), *Peptides 2008. Proceedings of the 30th European Peptide Symposium,* Finnish Peptide Society, Helsinki, pp 498-499

Otvos, L, Jr, Kovalszky, I, Scolaro, L, Sztodola, A, Olah, J, Cassone, M, Knappe, D, Hoffmann, R, Lovas, S, Hatfield, MP, Beko, G, Zhang, S, Wade, JD, & Surmacz, E (2011a), 'Peptide-based receptor antagonists for cancer treatment and appetite regulation', *Biopolymers Peptide Science* 96, p.117-125

Otvos, L., Kovalszky, I, Riolfi, M, Ferla, R, Olah, J, Sztodola, A, Nama, K, Molina, A, Piobello, Q, Wade, JD, & Surmacz E (2011b), 'Efficacy of a leptin receptor antagonist peptide in a mouse model of triple-negative breast cancer', *European Journal of Cancer* 47, p. 1578-1584

Otvos L. Jr, Haspinger E., La Russa F., Maspero F., Graziano P., Kovalszky, I., Lovas S., Nama K., Hoffmann R. , Knappe D., Cassone M., Wade JD.,& Surmacz, E (2011c), 'Design and development of a peptide-based adiponectin receptor agonist for cancer treatment', BMC Biotechnology, no 11, p. 90

Pal, SK, & Mortimer, J (2009), 'Triple-negative breast cancer: Novel therapies and new directions', *Mauritas* no 63, p. 269-274

Park, HY, Kwon, HM, Lim, HJ, Hong, BK, Lee, JY, Park, BE, Jang, Y, Cho, SY, Kim, HS (2001), 'Potential role of leptin in angiogenesis: leptin induces endothelial cell proliferation and expression of matrix metalloproteinases *in vivo* and *in vitro*', *Experimental and Molecular Medicine* , no 33, p. 95-102

Peelman, F, Van Beneden, K, Zabeau, L, Iserentant, H, Ulrichts, P, Defeau, D, Verhee, A, Catteeuw, D, Elewaut, D, & Tavernier, J (2004), 'Mapping of the leptin binding sites and design of a leptin antagonist', *Journal of Biological Chemistry,* no 279, p. 41038-41046

Peters, JH, Simasko, SM, & Ritter RC (2007), 'Leptin analog antagonizes leptin effects on food intake and body weight but mimics leptin-induced vagal afferent activation', *Endocrinology*, no 148, p. 2878-2885

Phipps, AI, Malone, KE, Porter PL, Daling, JR, & Li, CI (2008), 'Body size and risk of luminal, HER2-overexpressing, and triple-negative breast cancer in postmenopausal women', *Cancer Epidemiology and Biomarkers Prevention* no 17, p. 2076-2086

Price, TO, Farr, SA, Yi, X, Vinogradov, S, Batrakova, E, Banks, WA, & Kabanov AV (2010), 'Transport across the blood-brain barrier of pluronic leptin', *Journal of Pharmacology and Experimental Therapeutics*, no 333, p. 253-263

Raver, N, Vardy, E, Livnah, O, Devos, R,& Gertler, A (2002), 'Comparison of R128Q mutations in human, ovine, and chicken leptins', *General and Comparative Endocrinology*, no 126, p. 52-58

Reeves, GK, Pirie, K, Beral, V, Green, J, Spencer E, Bull, D (2007), 'Cancer incidence and mortality in relation to body mass index in the Million Women Study: cohort study', *British Medical Journal*, no 335, p 1134

Rodriguez-Pinilla, SM, Sarrio, D, Honrado, E, Hardisson, D, Calero, F, Benitez, J, & Palacios, J *(2006), 'Prognostic significance of basal-like phenotype and fascin expression in node-negative invasive breast carcinomas', Clinical Cancer Research no* 12, *p.* 1533-*39*

Rose, DP, Gilhooly EM & Nixon DW (2002), 'Adverse effects of obesity on breast cancer prognosis, and the biological actions of leptin (review)', *International Journal of Oncology*, no 21, p 1285-1292

Sachot, C, Poole, S, & Luheshi, GN (2004), 'Circulating leptin mediates lipopolysaccharide-induced anorexia and fever in rats', *Journal of Physiology* no 561, p. 263-272.

Salomon, G, Niv-Spector, L, Gussakovsky, EE, & Gertler A (2006), 'Large-scale preparation of biologically active mouse and rat leptins and their L39A/D40A/F41A muteins which act as potent antagonists', *Protein Expression and Purification*, no 47, p. 128-136

Scarpace, PJ, Matheny, M, Zhang, Y, Cheng, KY, & Tümer N (2007), 'Leptin antagonist reveals an uncoupling between leptin receptor signal transducer and activator of transcription 3 signaling and metabolic responses with central leptin resistance', *Journal of Pharmacology and Experimental Therapeutics*, no 320, p. 706-712

Schulz, C, Paulus K, & Lehnert, H (2004), 'Central nervous and metabolic effects of intranasally applied leptin', *Endocrinology*, no 145, p. 2696-2701

Shpilman, M, Niv-Spector, L, Katz, M, Varol, C, Solomon, G, Ayalon-Soffer, M, Boder, E, Halpern, Z, Elinav, E, & Gertler, A (2011), 'Development and characterization of high-affinity leptins and leptin antagonists', *Journal of Biological Chemistry,* no 286, p. 4429-4442

Somasundar, P, Yu, AK, Vona-Davis, L, & McFadden DW (2003), 'Differential effects of leptin on cancer *in vitro*', *Journal of Surgical Research*, no 113, p. 50-55

Styer, AK, Sullivan, BT, Puder, M, Arsenault, D, Petrozza, JC, Serikawa, T, Chang, S, Hasan, T, Gonzalez, RR, & Rueda BR (2008), 'Ablation of leptin signaling disrupts the establishment, development, and maintenance of endometriosis-like lesions in a murine model', *Endocrinology,* no 149, p. 506-514

Surmacz, E (2007), 'Obesity hormone leptin-a new target in breast cancer?', *Breast Cancer Research* no 9, p. 301

Sweeney, G (2002), 'Leptin signalling', *Cellular Signalling*, no 14, p. 655-663.

Takeuchi, T, Adachi, Y, Ohtsuki, Y, & Furihata, M (2007), 'Adiponectin receptors, with special focus on the role of the third receptor, T-cadherin, in vascular disease', *Medical Molecular Morphology* no 40, p. 115-120

Tessitore, L, Vizio, B, Pesola, D, Cecchini, F, Mussa, A, Argiles, JM, & Bendetto, C (2004), 'Adipocyte expression and circulating levels of leptin increase in both gynaecological and breast cancer patients', *International Journal of Oncology* no 24, p. 1529-1535.

van Kruijsdijk, RC, van der Wall E, & Visseren FL (2009), 'Obesity and cancer: the role of dysfunctional adipose tissue Cancer Epidemiology', *Biomarkers and Prevention*, no. 18, p. 2569-2578

Vona-Davis, L, & Rose DP (2007), 'Adipokines as endocrine, paracrine and autocrine factors in breast cancer risk and progression', *Endocrine-related Cancer*, no 14, p. 189-206

Vona-Davis L, & Rose, DP (2009), 'The influence of socioeconomic disparities on breast cancer tumor biology and prognosis: a review', *Journal of Women's Health (Larchmont)* no 18, p. 883-893

Wauters, M, Considine, RW, & Van Gaal, LF (2000), 'Human leptin: from an adipocyte hormone to an endocrine mediator', *European Journal of Endocrinology* no 143, p. 293-311

Yamauchi, T, Kamon, J, Ito, Y, Tsuchida, A, Yokomizo, T., Kita, S. Sugiyama, T, Miyagishi, M, Hara, K, Tsunoda, M, Murakami, K, Ohteki, T, Uchida, S, Takekawa, S, Waki, H, Tsuno, NH, Shibata, Y, Terauchi, Y, Froguel, P, Tobe, K, Koyasu, S, Taira, K, Kitamura, T, Shimizu, T, Nagai, R, & Kadowaki T (2003), 'Cloning of adiponectin receptors that mediate antidiabetic effects', *Nature* no 423, p. 762-769

Zhang, C, Su, Z, Zhao, B, Qu, Q, Tan, Y, Cai, L, & Li, X (2009), 'Tat-modified leptin is more accessible to hypothalamus through brain-blood barrier with a significant inhibition of body weight gain in high fat diet-fed mice', *Experimental Clinical Endocrinology and Diabetes*, no 118, p 31-37

Send Orders for Reprints to reprints@benthamscience.net

CHAPTER 7

Jak2/Stat5a/b Signaling Axis and Novel Therapeutic Strategies in Prostate Cancer

Shilpa Gupta[1,2,#], Paraskevi Vogiatzi[3,4,#], David T. Hoang[3] and Marja T. Nevalainen[1,3,5,*]

[1]Department of Medical Oncology, Thomas Jefferson University, Philadelphia, PA, USA; [2]The H. Lee Moffitt Cancer Center and Research Institute, Tampa, FL, USA; [3]Department of Cancer Biology, Kimmel Cancer Center, Thomas Jefferson University, Philadelphia, PA., USA; [4]Department of Pathology, University of Michigan Medical School, Ann Arbor, MI, USA and [5]Department of Urology, Thomas Jefferson University, Philadelphia, PA, USA

Abstract: Prostate cancer (PCa) is the third leading cause of cancer death in the US. It is a heterogeneous disease with clinical course ranging from indolent disease to rapidly progressing, often fatal disease. Complex molecular mechanisms lead to development of metastatic castrate-resistant prostate cancer (CRPC) for which no curative therapies exist. There is an urgent need to develop rational biomarkers and therapeutic targets that will help expedite discovery of curative therapies. This chapter describes the treatment options for localized and metastatic PCa and provides an in-depth review of the Jak2/Stat5a/b signaling pathway in PCa, which is critical in prostate cancer progression, development of castrate-resistance and metastases. Target validation of Jak2/Stat5a/b pathway is discussed in detail, including the role of pharmacological inhibitors of Jak2 and Stat5a/b, providing a strong rationale for targeting this pathway to improve outcomes in PCa. Furthermore, the prognostic and predictive significance of Stat5a/b in providing personalized therapy in PCa is reviewed as well.

Keywords: Stat5a/b, Jak2, Stat3, survival, proliferation, prostate cancer, therapy development, surgery, radiation therapy, metastasis, caveolin, prolactin, placental lactogen, estrogen, androgen, androgen deprivation therapy.

***Address correspondence to Marja T. Nevalainen:** Department of Cancer Biology, Kimmel Cancer Center, Thomas Jefferson University, 233 S. 10th St., BLSB 309, 19107 Philadelphia, PA, USA; E-mail: Marja.Nevalainen@jefferson.edu

#These authors equally contributed.

Pier Paolo Claudio and Paraskevi Vogiatzi (Eds)

1. INTRODUCTION

Prostate cancer (PCa) is the most common non-cutaneous malignancy and the second leading cause of cancer death in American men. There were 238,590 new cases and 29,720 deaths from PCa in 2013 in the US (American Cancer Society 2013). Despite aggressive therapy for localized disease, a significant number of patients develop disseminated castrate-resistant PCa (CRPC), for which there is no cure and hence an unmet need to develop novel targeted therapeutic agents to improve survival. The Jak2/Stat5a/b signaling pathway is one such potential therapeutic target in PCa; this chapter summarizes the importance of this pathway in growth and survival of PCa cells and the molecular basis of inhibitors of Jak2/Stat5a/b signaling as a therapeutic strategy for PCa.

2. CURRENT STANDARD TREATMENT OF PROSTATE CANCER

2.1. Localized Prostate Cancer

Standard therapeutic options for patients with clinically localized PCa include surgery, radiation therapy or active surveillance.

Surgery

Radical prostatectomy involves removal of the entire prostate gland. It has the highest potential for cure when the cancer is confined to the prostate gland, with the 15-year prostate-cancer specific mortality rate being less than 2% for organ-confined cancer (Eggener *et al.,* 2011). The complications of radical prostatectomy include urinary and fecal incontinence, urethral strictures, impotence and the morbidity associated with general anesthesia and a major surgical procedure (Catalona *et al.,* 1990, Sanda *et al.,* 2008). Given the morbidity and the potential negative impact of the surgery on the quality of life of patients, this approach is usually recommended for patients with a life expectancy of 10 years or more (National Comprehensive Cancer Network).

Radiation Therapy

Definitive radiation therapy is used to treat PCa confined to the prostate and/or surrounding tissues, and the two widely used techniques for delivering therapeutic radiation to the prostate gland are external beam radiation therapy and brachytherapy.

Complications of external-beam radiation therapy include acute cystitis, urinary complications, proctitis, erectile dysfunction, and enteritis (Fowler *et al.,* 1996, Lim *et al.,* 1995). Some of the advantages of external beam radiation therapy over surgery are the non-invasive nature of the procedure, avoidance of peri-operative complications and a lower rate of urinary incontinence; it can also be used in combination with androgen deprivation therapy for patients with locally advanced PCa. However, the disadvantages are a risk of protracted rectal symptoms and erectile dysfunction, which increases with time (Sanda *et al.,* 2008, Potosky *et al.,* 2004). Also, in case of cancer recurrence, salvage surgery is associated with higher risk of complications as compared to primary surgery. Brachytherapy is an internal radiation technique which involves placing a radioactive source within the prostate tissue and may be considered for patients with low-risk PCa. Its disadvantages include the need for general anesthesia and the risk of acute urinary retention (Blasko *et al.,* 1991, Wallner *et al.,* 1996). Although there are no data from randomized clinical trials comparing the treatment outcomes of surgery and radiation, observational data suggest that long-term disease control achieved with radiation therapy is similar to that achieved with surgery.

Active Surveillance

Active surveillance is defined as the postponement of immediate therapy and institution of curative therapy at the time of disease progression (Dall'Era *et al.,* 2008). Active surveillance avoids unnecessary therapy-related complications for patients at low risk for recurrence, who are amenable to cure in case of progression. There are no data from randomized clinical trials that have compared active surveillance to surgery or radiation therapy for disease recurrence or PCa-specific death. Clinical trials are ongoing to compare active surveillance with other treatment strategies and better define the role of active surveillance as a therapeutic option for PCa.

2.2. Locally Advanced Prostate Cancer

The treatment options for locally advanced PCa are external beam radiation therapy combined with androgen deprivation therapy or radical prostatectomy.

Various randomized trials have shown that addition of androgen deprivation therapy to definitive radiation therapy improves PCa outcomes and survival in locally advanced PCa (Bria *et al.,* 2009, Lawton *et al.,* 1997, Lawton *et al.,* 2005, Lawton *et al.,* 2001, Pilepich *et al.,* 1997, Pilepich *et al.,* 2005, Roach *et al.,* 2008). However, there are conflicting data on the optimal duration of androgen deprivation therapy when combined with radiation (D'Amico *et al.,* 2004, Denham *et al.,* 2005).

Drugs Targeting the Androgen Pathway

Androgen deprivation therapy (ADT) utilizes either surgical castration (bilateral orchiectomy) or medical castration with gonadotropin releasing hormone (GnRH) agonists. Surgical castration is used rarely in situations where an urgent decrease in testosterone is necessary or when patient compliance might be an issue. Medical castration involves use of GnRH agonists with or without an anti-androgen (Ginzburg & Albertsen 2011). GnRH agonists suppress luteinizing hormone (LH) production and thus inhibit synthesis of testicular androgens (Loblaw *et al.,* 2004). A number of GnRH agonists are commercially available (leuprolide, goserelin, buserelin and triptorelin). More recently, Degarelix, a GnRH antagonist, has become available (Klotz *et al.,* 2008), which has the advantage of not causing an initial LH surge and "flare up" symptoms seen with GnRH agonists. Many patients report a negative impact on their quality of life with these agents due to side effects including, but not limited to, erectile dysfunction, loss of libido, gynecomastia, hot flashes, loss of body mass, increased body fat, osteoporosis, bone fractures and cardiovascular disease (Alibhai *et al.,* 2010). In addition, patients can experience disabling fatigue and behavioral side effects as well (Basaria *et al.,* 2002).

Despite castrate levels of testosterone, androgen receptor (AR) signaling continues to remain active through a variety of mechanisms (Feldman & Feldman 2001). Anti-androgens or AR antagonists like flutamide, bicalutamide and nilutamide inhibit AR activation, thus providing the rationale for combined androgen blockade (CAB) where these agents are combined with medical or surgical castration. Enzalutamide (formerly known as MDV-3100) is a novel AR antagonist that blocks androgens from binding to the AR and prevents nuclear translocation and co-activator recruitment to the ligand-receptor complex; it lacks any partial AR agonist activity unlike other anti-androgens (Tran *et al.,* 2009). It has been recently approved by the US Food and Drug Administration (FDA) for treatment of metastatic CRPC patients who progress on docetaxel chemotherapy, based on the pivotal AFFIRM trial, a phase III placebo-controlled trial of around 1200 men. Enzalutamide significantly prolonged overall survival as compared to placebo (Scher *et al.,* 2012).

Ketoconazole is a conventional antifungal agent, which causes non-specific inhibition of cytochrome P450 17A1 (CYP14A1), an enzyme implicated in androgen biosynthesis (*Trachtenberg et al., 1983).* Variable response rates of 30-60% are sometimes achieved, but are seldom durable or long-standing; there are many side effects, including nausea, anorexia, nail atrophy and hepatic dysfunction (Small & Vogelzang 1997). Abiraterone is a newer, more potent inhibitor of CYP17A1 as compared to ketoconazole, and inhibits both the 17α-hydroxylase and 17,20-lyase activities of the CYP17A1 enzyme (O'Donnell *et al.,* 2004).

2.3. Metastatic Prostate Cancer

Selection and timing of systemic therapy for metastatic PCa depends upon the extent of disease and history of prior treatment. There is no curative therapy for metastatic PCa and the goal of treatment is control of disease and symptoms while maintaining quality of life (Omlin & de Bono 2012). CAB is employed as the initial approach, but the majority of patients receiving CAB progress to CRPC. These patients may be considered for secondary hormonal manipulations; however, durable responses are infrequent and most patients eventually require systemic chemotherapy.

The only first-line systemic chemotherapy for metastatic PCa is docetaxel, offering a median survival of only 21 months (Berthold *et al.,* 2008). Until recently, there was no second-line systemic therapy that prolonged survival in metastatic CRPC cancer patients who were previously treated with docetaxel. Cabazitaxel was the first agent to be approved by the FDA as second-line chemotherapy, based on the TROPIC trial which demonstrated an overall survival improvement of 2.4 months over mitoxantrone and prednisone, a regimen commonly used in this setting despite conferring no survival advantage (De Bono *et al.,* 2010). However, safety may be an issue with cabazitaxel as it caused severe grade 3-4 neutropenia in 82% patients, febrile neutropenia in 7.5% patients, diarrhea in 6% of patients and fatal events related to adverse events in 5% of patients (De Bono *et al.,* 2010). These side effects make it a somewhat difficult drug to offer to elderly patients with compromised marrow function after docetaxel therapy (Omlin & de Bono 2012). Abiraterone, an androgen synthesis inhibitor, is now FDA-approved for metastatic CRPC patients who experience disease progression on docetaxel. In a pivotal phase III trial, treatment with abiraterone led to an improvement in overall survival when compared to placebo (de Bono *et al.,* 2011). However, no therapy is currently approved for patients who do not respond to or undergo disease progression while receiving abiraterone.

Sipuleucel-T is an autologous active cellular immunotherapy which was recently approved by the FDA for treatment of asymptomatic or minimally symptomatic metastatic CRPC, based on the IMPACT study which demonstrated that median survival was 4.1 months longer in the group treated with sipuleucel-T *vs.* placebo (25.8 *versus* 21.7 months) (Kantoff *et al.,* 2010). However, patients need to be very carefully selected for this treatment, as they cannot have any visceral metastases or be dependent on narcotics for pain control, making the option of immunotherapy available to only a fraction of patients (National Comprehensive Cancer Network). Moreover, it is difficult to predict which patients would benefit most from this therapy.

Radium 223-chloride is an alpha pharmaceutical which showed improvement in survival when compared to placebo for metastatic CRPC patients with bone metastases only in the ALSYMPCA trial (Parker *et al.,* 2012). It is currently under FDA consideration for approval.

While many drugs have been recently approved for PCa and research for more effective therapies is ongoing, there are no established criteria for choosing the best therapy for each patient, which is the essence of personalized treatment. Moreover, it is not established as to which drug to use first following progression of patients on docetaxel, or even whether the sequence matters at all (Omlin & de Bono 2012). There is an urgent, unmet need to identify new targeted therapies for CRPC based on overexpression or activation of potential therapeutic target proteins. Finally, there are several variants of PCa described as the "anaplastic variety", which behave more aggressively than expected, (Humphrey 2012, Schwartz *et al.,* 1998) based on their Gleason score. These cancers do not respond to hormonal therapy and are associated with poor outcomes (Omlin & de Bono 2012). It is likely that there may be underlying molecular pathways which lead to the rapid progression of such PCas. Research over the last two decades has shed more light on understanding the biologic basis of CRPC development as well as various mechanisms which may be responsible for sustaining the growth, survival and invasive behavior of PCa cells, culminating in metastasis. This has led to the identification of new therapeutic targets in PCa and the development of novel targeted agents, some of which are currently in clinical trials. The identification and validation of the Jak2/Stat5a/b signaling pathway as the regulator of a pro-survival, pro-metastatic cell program in PCa provides novel therapeutic targets for drug development.

3. JAK2/STAT5A/B SIGNALING PATHWAY

3.1. Stat5a/b Protein Structure

Stat5 refers to two highly homologous, yet distinct, protein isoforms: Stat5a (794 aa, 94 kD) and Stat5b (788 aa, 92 kD). Stat5a/b belongs to the STAT (Signal Transducer and Activator of Transcription) gene family of transcription factors and signaling proteins, which consists of seven members: STAT1, STAT2, STAT3, STAT4, STAT5A, STAT5B and STAT6. STAT1 is currently the most fully characterized member of the family (Darnell, Kerr and Stark, 1994, Zhong, Wen and Darnell, 1994).

STAT genes are localized to three chromosomal regions: STAT1 and STAT4 map to human chromosome 2q12-q33 (Haddad, Pabon-Pena, Young and Sun, 1998, Yamamoto, Kobayashi, Arai *et al.*, 1997); STAT2 and STAT6 map to 12q13-q14.1 (Goureau, Garrigues, Tosser-Klopp *et al.*, 2001, Leek, Hamlin, Bell and Lench, 1997); and STAT3, STAT5A, and STAT5B map to 17q11.2-q22 (Copeland, Gilbert, Schindler *et al.*, 1995, Lin *et al.,* 1996). Stat5a was initially identified as a prolactin (PRL)-inducible, mammary-gland specific transcription factor (MGF) in mice (Schmitt-Ney, Doppler, Ball and Groner, 1991, Schmitt-Ney, Happ, Ball and Groner, 1992, Schmitt-Ney, Happ, Hofer, Hynes and Groner, 1992, Wakao, Schmitt-Ney and Groner, 1992) and later sheep (Gouilleux, Wakao, Mundt and Groner, 1994, Wakao, Gouilleux and Groner, 1994). The mouse STAT5A gene is segmented into 20 exons, arranged with a single upstream promoter, a translation initiation codon located in exon 3 and a stop codon located in exon 20 (Miyoshi *et al.*, 2001). Stat5b was later discovered to be encoded by a separate gene in mouse mammary gland tissue (Lin, Mietz, Modi, John and Leonard, 1996, Liu, Mietz, Modi, John and Leonard, 1996, Liu, Robinson, Gouilleux, Groner and Hennighausen, 1995). The mouse STAT5B gene is segmented into 20 exons; however, in contrast to STAT5A, it is arranged with two upstream promoters (I and II), an initiation codon in exon 2 and a stop codon in exon 19. This arrangement is similar to the human STAT5B gene, which also contains 19 exons and possesses two alternative first exons, 1a and 1b, driven by alternative promoters I and II, respectively. RT-PCR demonstrated the existence of two distinct STAT5B transcripts: one set of transcripts, driven by promoter I, was ubiquitously expressed in all tissues, whereas those transcripts driven by promoter II were selectively expressed in a tissue-specific manner, with high expression levels evident only in the placenta and lower levels present in spleen, brain and heart (Ambrosio *et al.,* 2002).

Structural and functional protein domains are almost completely conserved between Stat5a and Stat5b, with the exception of several C-terminal amino acids unique to each protein (20 and 8 residues for Stat5a and Stat5b, respectively). Stat5a and Stat5b are activated through phosphorylation on tyrosine 694 (pY694) and 699 (pY699), respectively (Gouilleux, Wakao, Mundt and Groner, 1994, Liu, Mietz, Modi, John and Leonard, 1996, Liu, Robinson, Gouilleux, Groner and Hennighausen, 1995). Stat5a is activated primarily *via* upstream signaling initiated by PRL binding to the prolactin receptor (PRLR), while Stat5b activation occurs predominantly through upstream signaling initiated by growth hormone (GH) binding to the growth hormone receptor (GHR). Other ligands are capable of activating Stat5a/b upon binding to their cognate receptors, including erythropoietin (EPO) (Gouilleux, Pallard, Dusanter-Fourt *et al.*, 1995, Pallard,

Gouilleux, Charon *et al.*, 1995, Wakao, Gouilleux and Groner, 1994), granulocyte-macrophage colony-stimulating factor (GM-CSF) (Barahmand-pour, Meinke, Eilers *et al.*, 1995, Mui, Wakao, O'Farrell, Harada and Miyajima, 1995), insulin (Wartmann, Cella, Hofer *et al.*, 1996) and interleukins (IL)-2, 3, 5 and 7 (Hou, Schindler, Henzel, Wong and McKnight, 1995, Mui, Wakao, Harada, O'Farrell and Miyajima, 1995) (Foxwell, Beadling, Guschin, Kerr and Cantrell, 1995), and thrombopoietin (TPO) (Pallard, Gouilleux, Benit *et al.*, 1995).

All Stats, including Stat5a/b, display a common multi-domain structural organization with distinct functional properties. These conserved protein domains include: **(1) N-Terminal**, **(2) Coiled-Coil**, **(3) DNA-Binding**, **(4) Linker**, **(5) Src Homology 2 (SH2)** and **(6) Transcriptional Activation** (Schindler and Darnell, 1995).

Tetramerization of Stat5a/b dimers is enabled by the **N-Terminal Domain (NTD; aa 1-126)**. The activity of weak Stat5a/b-driven promoters may be potentiated by Stat5a/b tetramer formation, which allows Stat5a/b binding to tandemly-linked γ (gamma)-interferon activation sequence (GAS) elements, one of which may display an imperfect (non-consensus) sequence (Horvath, Wen and Darnell, 1995, John, Vinkemeier, Soldaini, Darnell and Leonard, 1999, Meyer, Reichenbach, Schindler, Soldaini and Nabholz, 1997, Soldaini, John, Moro *et al.*, 2000). Glycosylation of Stat5a/b on threonine 92 within the NTD is indispensable for productive interaction of Stat5a/b with p300/cAMP Response Element-Binding (CREB) protein (Gewinner, Hart, Zachara *et al.*, 2004). Interestingly, a recent finding demonstrates the existence of a short form of Stat5a/b which lacks the NTD domain in human PCa cells (Dagvadorj *et al.*, 2010).

The **Coiled-Coil Domain (CCD; aa 138-330)** interacts with chaperone proteins (Xu, Yu, Yan *et al.*, 2004), recruits co-activators (Zhu, John, Berg and Leonard, 1999) and co-repressors (Maurer, Wichmann, Gross *et al.*, 2002, Nakajima, Brindle, Handa and Ihle, 2001) and participates in protein-protein interactions required for transcriptional regulation.

The central **DNA-Binding Domain (DBD; aa 332-583)** is responsible for Stat5a/b binding to consensus GAS elements located within the regulatory elements (promoters/enhancers) of target genes (Decker, Lew, Mirkovitch and Darnell, 1991, Horvath, Wen and Darnell, 1995, Soldaini, John, Moro *et al.*, 2000). The nuclear localization signal required for nuclear import spans the DNA-binding and N-terminal domains in some Stats (McBride, Banninger, McDonald and Reich, 2002, McBride, McDonald and Reich, 2000, Melen, Kinnunen and Julkunen, 2001, Meyer, Gavenis and Vinkemeier, 2002, Vinkemeier, Moarefi, Darnell and Kuriyan, 1998), while export of Stats from the nuclear compartment is believed to be dependent on the coiled-coil and DNA-binding domains (Begitt *et al.,* 2000, McBride *et al.,* 2000). MgcRacGAP, a chaperone protein, binds to the phosphorylated Stat5a/b dimer *via* its DNA-binding domain and is responsible for trafficking of phosphorylated Stat5a/b dimers between the nucleus and cytoplasm (Kawashima *et al.,* 2009).

Crystallographic investigations led to identification of the **Linker Domain (LD; aa 475-592)**, a highly conserved region located between the DNA-binding and SH2 domains, but were unable to attribute a function to this region. However, site-directed mutagenesis of the Stat1 linker region resulted in a mutant dimer that binds and dissociates from DNA more rapidly than the wild-type protein. This finding suggests a temporal effect on DNA binding is conferred by the linker region, which may function as a critical contact point during the formation of a STAT1-driven transcriptional complex (Yang, Henriksen, Schaefer, Zakharova and Darnell, 2002).

The **Src Homology 2 domain (SH2; aa 593-670)**, a highly conserved motif found in Src family kinases and numerous intracellular signal-transducing proteins, mediates Stat5a/b recruitment and docking to phosphorylated tyrosine residues on the PRLR, as well as the phosphotyrosine-SH2 interaction required for Stat5a/b dimerization (Stocklin, Wissler, Gouilleux and Groner, 1996). Jak2-mediated phosphorylation of Stat5a and Stat5b on tyrosine residues Y694 and Y699, respectively, induces Stat5a/b homo- or heterodimerization and produces a transcriptionally active dimer (Becker, Groner and Muller, 1998, Chen, Vinkemeier, Zhao *et al.*, 1998). The dimer interface is formed following the binding of the Stat5a/b monomer SH2 domain to the phosphorylated C-terminal tyrosine residue (Stat5a: pY694, Stat5b: pY699) of another Stat5a/b monomer

(Wakao, Gouilleux and Groner, 1994, Welte, Garimorth, Philipp and Doppler, 1994).

The C-terminal variable domain is known as the **Transcriptional Activation Domain (TAD; STAT5A, aa 722-794; STAT5B, aa 727-787)**. The TAD interacts with critical co-activator and co-repressor proteins, including centrosomal P4.1-associated protein (CPAP) (Peng, Sutherland, Sum *et al.*, 2002), EBNA2 coactivator P100 (Paukku, Yang and Silvennoinen, 2003), octamer-binding transcription factor 1 (Oct-1) (Litterst, Kliem, Lodrini and Pfitzner, 2005, Magne, Caron, Charon, Rouyez and Dusanter-Fourt, 2003) and p300/CREB-binding protein (CBP)-associated co-activator NcoA-1 (Litterst, Kliem, Marilley and Pfitzner, 2003), and is therefore directly involved in transcriptional activity. Phosphorylation of serine residues S726 and S731 may inhibit transcriptional activity of Stat5a and Stat5b, respectively (Beuvink, Hess, Flotow *et al.*, 2000 Decker *et al.*, 1991, Decker, Lew, Mirkovitch and Darnell, 1991, Horvath, Wen and Darnell, 1995, Soldaini, John, Moro *et al.*, 2000).

3.2. Activation of the Jak2/Stat5a/b Pathway

Prolactin (PRL), a member of the PRL/GH/placental lactogen (PL) family, is a peptide hormone which was first characterized in the 1930's (Riddle *et al.,* 1933, Stricker & Grueter 1928) and is primarily associated with lactation (Friesen & Astwood 1965). PRL-secreting cells, known as lactotrophs, make up about 20% of cells in the anterior pituitary gland and produce PRL in response to various stimulatory hormone signals including estrogens, progesterone and thyrotropin-releasing hormone. PRL is also produced in other tissues including the mammary glands, ovaries, heart, lung, thymus, spleen, liver, pancreas, kidney, adrenal gland, uterus, skeletal muscle, skin and sites within the central nervous system. Hypothalamic neuroendocrine cells, such as the tuberoinfundibular dopamine (TIDA) neurons of the arcuate nucleus, inhibit PRL secretion through release of dopamine, which suppresses the high intrinsic secretory activity of pituitary lactotrophs. Binding of PRL to the PRL Receptor (PRLR) is the first step of a signaling cascade which ultimately results in activation of the downstream Jak2 kinase and Stat5a/b transcription factor. The repertoire of genes activated by PRL therefore largely depends on Stat5a/b binding to DNA.

Studies of interferon-induced signaling in the 1990s led to the discovery of the Janus Kinases (Jaks), a unique subfamily of cytoplasmic tyrosine kinases, which link membrane receptors such as the PRLR to the activation of nuclear genes. The binding of cytokines, growth factors and hormones to their cognate receptors activate receptor-associated Jaks, which phosphorylate the cytoplasmic domains of the receptor at key tyrosine residues, allowing for recruitment of signaling molecules to these same residues (Darnell, 1997, Ihle, 2001, Schindler, 2002). Jaks then activate the receptor-bound signaling molecules by phosphorylation, leading to their dissociation from the receptor, nuclear translocation and, finally, regulation of gene expression. In mammals, four Jaks are known: Jak1, Jak2, Jak3, and Tyk2. All four kinases consist of seven highly homologous domains (Aaronson and Horvath, 2002, Darnell, 1997, Ihle, 2001, Levy and Darnell, 2002) and are ubiquitously expressed (Leonard and O'Shea, 1998) with the exception of JAK3, which is restricted mainly to hematopoietic cells. Jak3 is known to associate with the common gamma chain (y6) of receptors for IL-2, 4, 7, 9 and 15, and is activated by these cytokines. Disruption of the Jak3-4c interaction is implicated in several different types of immunodeficiency disorders; (Candotti *et al.,* 1997, Russell *et al.,* 1994, Thomis *et al.,* 1997) for instance, severe combined immunodeficiency syndrome (SCID) is associated with inactivating JAK3 gene mutations (Ghoreschi K *et al.,* 2009).

Once phosphorylated by Jak2, active Stat5a/b dimers translocate from cytosol to nucleus in an active, energy-dependent process (Reich and Liu, 2006, Vinkemeier, 2004) utilizing components of Ran-dependent nuclear import machinery (Sekimoto, Imamoto, Nakajima, Hirano and Yoneda, 1997, Sekimoto, Nakajima, Tachibana, Hirano and Yoneda, 1996). The chaperone protein MgcRacGAP cooperates with Rac1, a small G protein, and karyophe in (importin) β1 a carrier protein, to form a nuclear shuttling complex capable of transporting the Stat5a/b dimer (Kawashima, *et al.,* 2009). In contrast, unphosphorylated Stat proteins, which exist as monomers, can freely shuttle between distinct nuclear and cytoplasmic pools at a high exchange rate, even in the absence of upstream cytokine and hormone signals (Marg, Shan, Meyer *et al.*, 2004, Meyer, Gavenis and Vinkemeier, 2002, Reich and Liu, 2006, Vinkemeier, 2004, Zeng, Yellaturu, Neeli and Rao, 2002).

Within the nucleus, Stat5a/b dimers bind palindromic DNA consensus sequences (TTC(C/T)N(G/A)GAA) known as GAS elements and regulate transcription of Stat5a/b-driven genes (Decker, Lew, Mirkovitch and Darnell, 1991, Horvath, Wen and Darnell, 1995, Soldaini, John, Moro *et al.*, 2000). Stat5a and Stat5b homodimers have equal binding specificity for palindromes that are spaced 3 base pairs apart (Ehret, Reichenbach, Schindler *et al.*, 2001, Soldaini, John, Moro *et al.*, 2000), whereas Stat5a/b tetramers are capable of binding tandem consensus and non-consensus GAS motifs that are 6 base pairs apart (Soldaini, John, Moro *et al.*, 2000). Stat5a/b exhibits non-redundant functions during development, arising not from differences in Stat5a/b binding specificity, but rather differential recruitment of co-regulators in a cell-type specific manner (Ehret, Reichenbach, Schindler *et al.*, 2001). Interestingly, a few reports suggest that unphosphorylated Stats may be able to bind to DNA in association with other transcription factors (Chatterjee-Kishore, Wright, Ting and Stark, 2000, Yang, Chatterjee-Kishore, Staugaitis *et al.*, 2005, Yang, Liao, Agarwal *et al.*, 2007).

3.3. Switching Stat5a/b On and Off: Positive and Negative Regulators of Stat5a/b Signaling

Although the Stat5a/b signaling cascade remains an area of active research, the exact mechanisms responsible for Stat5a/b activation in primary and advanced prostate tumors are not yet precisely known. Stat5a/b activity can be modulated by both positive and negative regulatory molecules. Here, we briefly summarize the current understanding of Stat5a/b activation and inhibition in PCa.

3.3.1. Major Positive Regulators of Stat5a/b in Prostate Cancer

The autocrine/paracrine mechanism of PRL provides an explanation for constitutive activation of Stat5a/b in human PCa (Li, Ahonen, Alanen *et al.*, 2004, Nevalainen, Valve, Ahonen *et al.*, 1997, Nevalainen, Valve, Ingleton *et al.*, 1997). It is possible that such locally produced PRL, secreted directly into the extracellular space surrounding PCa cells, is capable of achieving elevated local concentrations which saturate the PRLRs (Goffin *et al.,* 2011). PRL is produced by normal prostate tissue as well as prostate carcinoma and plays a critical role in sustaining cell proliferation and survival (Ahonen, Harkonen, Laine *et al.*, 1999, Dagvadorj, Collins, Jomain *et al.*, 2007, Kindblom, Dillner, Ling, Tornell and

Wennbo, 2002, Kindblom, Dillner, Sahlin *et al.*, 2003, Nevalainen, Valve, Ahonen *et al.*, 1997, Nevalainen, Valve, Ingleton and Harkonen, 1996, Nevalainen, Valve, Ingleton *et al.*, 1997, Nevalainen, Valve, Makela *et al.*, 1991, Wennbo, Kindblom, Isaksson and Tornell, 1997). Increased PRL and PRLR expression significantly correlate with high histological grade of human PCa (Li, Ahonen, Alanen *et al.*, 2004).

It is currently known that PRL activates Jak2-Stat5a/b signaling in normal and malignant prostate (Ahonen, Harkonen, Rui and Nevalainen, 2002, Dagvadorj, Collins, Jomain *et al.*, 2007, Li, Ahonen, Alanen *et al.*, 2004). In prostate, Jak2 is the predominant kinase which activates Stat5a/b (Li, Ahonen, Alanen *et al.*, 2004).

GH, a known activator of Stat5b signaling, is another molecule with the potential to trigger Stat5a/b activation in PCa. However, GH has not thus far been demonstrated to have a direct effect on growth of PCa cells (Chopin, Veveris-Lowe, Philipps and Herington, 2002, Halmos, Schally, Czompoly *et al.*, 2002, Letsch, Schally, Busto, Bajo and Varga, 2003, Stangelberger, Schally, Varga *et al.*, 2005, Wang, Prins, Coschigano *et al.*, 2005, Weiss-Messer, Merom, Adi *et al.*, 2004).

3.3.2. Negative Regulators of Stat5a/b in Prostate Cancer

A possible mechanism for suppression of Stat5a/b signaling is provided by the actions of the cytosolic protein tyrosine phosphatase **PTP1B** and the nuclear phosphatase **TC-PTP**, which may counteract Stat5a/b activation by Jak2-mediated phosphorylation (Aoki & Matsuda, 2000).

The Suppressors of Cytokine Signaling (**SOCS**) are another group of proteins involved in the negative regulation of Jak2-Stat5a/b signaling. SOCS proteins comprise eight members, SOCS1-7 and CIS (cytokine-inducible SH2 domain protein), of known structure with a central SH2 domain and a conserved C-terminal SOCS box motif (Alexander and Hilton, 2004). SOCS target Stats for proteasomal degradation (Kamizono, Hanada, Yasukawa *et al.*, 2001, Ungureanu, Saharinen, Junttila, Hilton and Silvennoinen, 2002, Zhang, Farley, Nicholson *et al.*, 1999) and are rapidly induced by activated Stats. SOCS may suppress upstream signaling by multiple mechanisms, as evidenced by the ability of SOCS1 to directly inhibit Jaks and competitively bind phosphorylated tyrosine residues on receptors which serve as Stat docking sites (Alexander and Hilton, 2004, Ram and Waxman, 1999).

The CAVEOLIN-1 gene, a member of the caveolin gene family, maps to chromosome 7q31.1 and encodes for **Cav-1** (21-24 kD), an integral membrane protein capable of forming caveolae, plasma membrane invaginations which regulate protein trafficking and signal transduction in cholesterol homeostasis and have been implicated in cell transformation (Williams and Lisanti, 2005). Cav-1 and 2 are expressed in most cell types, while the expression of Cav-3 is muscle-specific. The Cav-1 scaffolding domain shares homology with the SOCS pseudosubstrate domain, suggesting a similar negative regulatory function regarding Jak2-Stat5a/b signaling. Indeed, Cav-1 was demonstrated to inhibit Jak2 kinase activity and suppress Stat5a/b signaling (Jasmin, Mercier, Sotgia and Lisanti, 2006).

The Protein Inhibitors of Activated Stat, or **PIAS,** act as E3 ligases for the small ubiquitin-like modifier (SUMO) protein and negatively regulate Jak2-Stat5a/b signaling. PIAS1, PIAS3, PIASx, PIASy and several alternative splicing variants of PIASx inhibit Stat function directly (Chung, Liao, Liu *et al.*, 1997, Schmidt and Muller, 2003). Predictably, downregulation of PIAS may result in enhanced activation of Stat5a/b in prostate tumors. Intriguingly, the predominant form of Stat5a/b which binds DNA in human PCa cells was found to be N-terminally truncated (Dagvadorj *et al.,* 2010). This may provide an explanation as to why PIAS3, which physically interacts only with the N-terminal domain of Stat5a/b, can block Stat5a/b-regulated transcription in breast, but not prostate, cancer cells.

4. TARGET VALIDATION OF STAT5A/B FOR PROSTATE CANCER THERAPY

4.1. Active Stat5a/b Expression in Clinical Prostate Cancer

In the last decade, studies have emerged which support the involvement of Stat5a/b in the clinical progression of PCa. It has been reported that Stat5a/b is constitutively active in human PCa cells, but not in normal prostate epithelium (Ahonen, Xie, LeBaron *et al.*, 2003). A study involving 114 paraffin-embedded clinical PCa samples investigated active Stat5a/b distribution in tissues of varying histological grade and concluded that active Stat5a/b is strongly associated with high-grade PCa (Li, Ahonen, Alanen *et al.*, 2004). Tissue microarrays prepared from 357 PCa patients accompanied by 30-year clinical follow-up data further confirmed that expression of active Stat5a/b is correlated with poorly differentiated, high-grade PCa. Furthermore, active Stat5a/b status predicted early cancer recurrence following initial treatment in PCa patients. Even in PCa samples of intermediate Gleason grades, active Stat5a/b emerged as an independent prognostic marker of early disease recurrence (Li, Zhang, Glass *et al.*, 2005). Recently, high nuclear Stat5a/b expression was identified as a significant predictor of both early recurrence and PCa-specific death following radical prostatectomy and early PCa-specific death in patients treated by deferred palliative therapy (Mirtti *et al.,* 2012). The above findings strongly support the role and importance of active Stat5a/b in PCa progression and long-term clinical outcome, and further studies investigating (1) the distribution of specific Stat5 isoforms in PCa and (2) stratification of PCa patients by Stat5a/b status are warranted.

Recurrent PCa often behaves in a hormone-refractory manner, or more appropriately, is castrate-resistant. In CRPC, the AR and AR-regulated genes continue to be expressed, suggesting that AR signaling is somehow maintained despite minimization of circulating androgens and pharmacological blockade of AR (Isaacs and Isaacs, 2004). Importantly, it was demonstrated that active Stat5a/b increased transcriptional activity of AR in PCa cells, while ligand-bound AR, in turn, increased transcriptional activity of Stat5a/b (Tan *et al.,* 2008). Active Stat5a/b also promoted the nuclear translocation of AR under androgen deprivation conditions, while ligand-bound AR was capable of promoting Stat5a/b nuclear translocation in the absence of PRL stimulation. This biological and functional synergy extended to a physical interaction between Stat5a/b and AR, as detected by co-immunoprecipitation of the two proteins, both transfected and endogenous (Tan, Dagvadorj, Shen *et al.*, 2008). Given that both Stat5a/b and AR function as growth-promoting, pro-survival transcription factors in PCa, it is highly plausible that their cooperative action underlie castrate-resistant growth of

PCa. Further investigation is needed to clarify the mechanisms underlying Stat5a/b-AR synergy and extend these findings to PCa growth *in vivo.*

4.2. Stat5a/b as a Predictive Factor in Prostate Cancer

PCa prognosis includes probable outcomes, duration, recurrence, complications, death and survival rates. Since many PCas are low-grade and grow slowly, survival rates are excellent when the disease is detected in the early stages. The median duration of response of primary PCa to hormonal ablation is less than three years (Trachtenberg *et al.,* 1982). Patients progressing to CRPC typically receive additional hormonal manipulations and conventional chemotherapy. However, these interventions are of limited value, and advanced, metastatic CRPC is a lethal disease. Stat5a/b may serve as a useful prognostic and predictive marker for identifying those PCa patients most likely to progress to castrate-resistant disease who would benefit from targeted therapy.

Stat5a/b is attractive as a PCa biomarker for numerous reasons. As previously mentioned, Stat5a/b demonstrates persistent activation in PCa cells, but not in the normal adjacent prostate epithelium (Ahonen, Xie, LeBaron *et al.*, 2003). Active Stat5a/b was shown to be associated with high histological grade in PCa (Li, Ahonen, Alanen *et al.*, 2004) and predictive of early disease recurrence after initial treatment by radical prostatectomy or transurethral resection, even in intermediate stage PCas (Gleason scores 3 and 4) (Li, Zhang, Glass *et al.*, 2005). In primary PCa, Stat5a/b was more likely to be active in patients who had been treated with androgen ablation prior to radical prostatectomy, when compared with patients who did not receive adjuvant androgen deprivation therapy. Furthermore, Stat5a/b was found to be active in 95% of castrate-resistant human PCas (Tan, Dagvadorj, Shen *et al.*, 2008). Finally, analysis of nuclear Stat5a/b expression in two cohorts of clinical PCas treated by either (1) radical prostatectomy or (2) deferred palliative therapy revealed nuclear Stat5a/b as an independent predictive marker of PCa-specific death for both groups (Mirtti *et al.,* 2012). Additionally, in PCas of intermediate Gleason score (6-7), high levels of nuclear Stat5a/b predicted increased risk of surgical therapy failure and early disease recurrence (Mirtti *et al.,* 2012). Confirmation of these findings in future prospective studies would establish Stat5a/b as one of the few reliable biomarkers for recurrence of lethal PCa after initial therapy.

4.3. The Jak2/Stat5a/b Signaling Pathway in the Regulation of Prostate Cancer Cell Viability and Invasive Behavior

The Jak2/Stat5a/b signaling pathway is critical for the viability of human PCa cells *in vitro* and *in vivo*. Analysis of the phenotypes of Stat5a knockout mice (Nevalainen, Ahonen, Yamashita *et al.*, 2000) provided valuable information on the role of Stat5a/b in normal prostate tissues. Stat5a-/- mice exhibited a defective prostate epithelium characterized by abnormal architecture, acinar cyst formation, local disorganization of the gland and luminal shedding of epithelial cells. Broken prostate acini were filled with desquamated, granular epithelial cells embedded in a dense, coagulated secretory material. Notably, Stat5a-/- mice did not show any increase in the overall size of the prostate gland or morphological signs of epithelial hyperplasia. Stat5b was able to compensate for the lack of Stat5a in the mammary glands of Stat5a-/- mice after multiple pregnancies (Liu, Gallego, Smith, Robinson and Hennighausen, 1998, Nevalainen, Xie, Bubendorf, Wagner and Rui, 2002), while similarly compensating to some degree for Stat5a in the prostates of Stat5a-deficient mice.

Stat5a/b inhibition in human PCa cells using adenoviral expression of a dominant-negative Stat5a/b induced extensive apoptotic death of the cells, as detected by changes in cell morphology, decreased cell viability, DNA fragmentation and activation of caspases 3 and 9 (2003). Furthermore, Stat5a/b inhibition *via* antisense oligonucleotides, RNA interference or adenoviral dominant-negative Stat5a/b triggered extensive apoptosis of cultured PCa cells and inhibited xenograft tumor growth in nude mice. Cyclin-D1 and Bcl-X_L were identified as Stat5a/b target genes in PCa cells (Dagvadorj, Kirken, Leiby, Karras and Nevalainen, 2008). A recent study compared the two Stat5 isoforms and found a preferential role for Stat5b in promotion of PCa cell growth and viability (Gu *et al.,* 2010a). In cell lines derived from the TRAMP mouse model of PCa (Kazansky, Spencer and Greenberg, 2003), inhibition of Stat5a/b by inducible expression of a carboxy-terminal truncated Stat5b mutant decreased cell growth in soft agar and tumor formation in nude mice. A side-by-side comparison of Stat5a/b with Stat3 demonstrated that Stat5a/b inhibition resulted in massive apoptosis of PCa cells and reduced both subcutaneous and orthotopic prostate xenograft tumor growth, while the effects of Stat3 inhibition on PCa cell and tumor growth were marginal (Gu *et al.,* 2010a).

A recent paper provides the first evidence of Stat5a/b promotion of metastatic behavior of human PCa cells *in vitro* and *in vivo* (Gu *et al.,* 2010b). In an experimental lung metastasis model, introduction of active Stat5 (Stat5aS710F) into PCa cells prior to tail-vein injection into nude mice enhanced formation of lung metastases by 11-fold compared to unmodified cells. Moreover, Stat5a/b activity was associated with hallmarks of the epithelial-to-mesenchymal (EMT) transition that precedes metastasis, including increased cell migration, decreased cell surface E-cadherin expression and increased heterotypic adhesion of PCa cells to endothelial cells (Gu *et al.,* 2010b). These data suggest that Stat5a/b may be an especially robust therapeutic target protein for advanced, disseminated PCa.

5. TARGETING THE JAK2/STAT5A/B PATHWAY IN PROSTATE CANCER

5.1. Pharmacological Inhibitors of Jak2

Constitutive activation of Jak2 is conferred by an activating somatic mutation, V617F, which is common in numerous myeloproliferative disorders, including polycythemia vera (74-97%), essential thrombocythemia (33-57%) and idiopathic myelofibrosis (35-50%). Jak2 translocations also occur with some frequency in acute myeloid leukemia (AML). Consequently, Jak2 inhibitors were first developed in the context of these disorders. Although the V617F mutation was determined to be absent in both locally confined PCa and CRPC (Gu *et al.,* 2010c), Jak2 inhibition remains a promising strategy for disrupting Stat5 signaling in PCa.

Researchers at the University of Texas, M.D. Anderson Cancer Center (Houston, TX) generated WP1066, also known as (*E*)-3(6-bromopyridin-2-yl)-2-cyano-*N*-(S0-1-phenylethyl)acrylamide, a cell-permeable AG-490 tyrphostin analog which functions as a small-molecule Jak2 inhibitor. WP1066 inhibits phosphorylation of

Stat3, Stat5 and Akt by Jak2 (Ferrajoli *et al.,* 2007) and displays potent antitumor effects in malignant glioma, AML and other hematologic malignancies (Iwamarou *et al.,* 2007, Hussain *et al.,* 2007). The compound is orally bioavailable, efficiently crosses the blood-brain barrier and demonstrates a variety of *in vivo* activities, including anti-tumor immune activation, in a variety of preclinical models. Specifically, WP1066 treatment of the AML cell lines OCIM2 and K562 resulted in activation of caspase-3 and caspase-dependent apoptotic cell death. Additionally, WP1066 suppresses proliferation and induces apoptosis in human erythroid cells carrying the JAK2 V617F mutation.

Currently, a number of Jak2 inhibitors are under development by the pharmaceutical industry (Hedvat *et al.,* 2009). These include the combined Jak1/2 inhibitors ruxolitinib (*Incyte/Novartis*) and baricitinib (*Incyte/Eli Lilly*), which have demonstrated significant benefits for patients with psoriasis, myelofibrosis and rheumatoid arthritis in Phase IIb/III clinical trials (Harrison *et al.,* 2012, Verstovsek *et al.,* 2012).

5.2. Pharmacological Inhibitors of Stat5a/b

Therapeutic targeting of Stat5a/b has previously been achieved for the treatment of pathophysiological conditions. Nifuroxazide (*Merck*) is a cell-permeable and orally available nitrofuran-based antidiarrheal agent that effectively suppresses the activation of Stat1, 3 and 5a/b in human sarcoma U3A cells by specifically inhibiting tyrosine phosphorylation involving Jak2, Tyk2 or Stat3.

Phosphotyrosyl peptides or peptidomimetics inhibit Stat3 dimerization by binding the Stat3 SH2 domain (Turkson, Kim, Zhang *et al.*, 2004, Turkson, Ryan, Kim *et al.*, 2001); a similar application has not yet been reported for Stat5a/b. Peptide aptamers selected from combinatorial libraries were capable of blocking Stat5a/b dimerization and DNA binding (Nagel-Wolfrum, Buerger, Wittig *et al.*, 2004). Decoy oligonucleotides, which mimic Stat5a/b DNA-binding sites and sequester Stat5a/b from its target genes, successfully inhibited expression of the Stat5a/b target gene cyclin D1 in NRK-49F kidney cells (Guh, Huang, Chen *et al.*, 2001).

6. SUMMARY

PCa remains a leading cause of cancer-related mortality for men in the US, with a significant number of patients progressing to lethal, incurable CRPC despite aggressive therapy for local disease using a variety of therapeutic approaches. However, recent advances in treatment of both locally advanced as well as CRPC may substantially improve the therapeutic landscape. Therapeutic options now include a diverse array of pharmacological agents and biologic products, most notably the novel anti-androgen, enzalutamide (formerly MDV-3100); the androgen synthesis inhibitor, abiraterone; and the cell-based immunotherapy sipuleucel-T. However, further studies are required to optimally integrate these new therapies with existing treatment paradigms. Most importantly, the lack of curative treatment for CRPC, stemming from the poorly understood transition between hormone-responsive cancer and CRPC, underscores a major unmet medical need.

Identification of new therapeutic targets, such as the components of the Jak2-Stat5a/b signaling pathway, may provide a new critical strategy for treatment of advanced PCa. Transcription factor and signaling protein Stat5a/b, along with its upstream activating kinase Jak2, have been validated as therapeutic targets in PCa. A rationale for clinical use of Stat5a/b inhibitors is provided by the multiple detrimental effects regulated by Stat5a/b in PCa: (1) maintenance of PCa cell growth and viability; (2) enhancement of AR transcriptional activity in spite of androgen deprivation; and (3) promotion of invasive behavior associated with metastasis. Future work will be directed towards: (1) determining the molecular mechanisms which mediate the effects of Stat5a/b in PCa; and (2) developing novel pharmacological Stat5a/b inhibitors for direct therapeutic targeting of Stat5a/b in PCa. Importantly, active Stat5a/b expression identifies those patients at risk for disease recurrence, progression to CRPC and poor clinical outcome who would benefit most from targeted therapy. Active Stat5a/b in PCa may also provide a biomarker for patient selection for Stat5a/b-targeting therapies. Efforts are now underway in both academia and industry to translate laboratory proof-of-concept findings of Stat5a/b as a critical regulator of PCa cell viability into clinically efficacious Jak2-Stat5a/b targeted therapies for PCa.

ACKNOWLEDGEMENTS

P.V. and S.G. acknowledge their Fellowships at KCC, Thomas Jefferson University. We finally thank the personnel of Dr. Nevalainen's laboratory for helpful discussions.

CONFLICT OF INTEREST

The authors confirm that this chapter content has no conflict of interest.

REFERENCES

Aaronson, D. S. & Horvath, C. M. (2002) 'A road map for those who don't know JAK-STAT', *Science,* 296, 1653-5.

Ahonen, T. J., Harkonen, P. L., Laine, J., Rui, H., Martikainen, P. M. & Nevalainen, M. T. (1999) 'Prolactin is a survival factor for androgen-deprived rat dorsal and lateral prostate epithelium in organ culture', *Endocrinology,* 140, 5412-21.

Ahonen, T. J., Harkonen, P. L., Rui, H. & Nevalainen, M. T. (2002) 'PRL signal transduction in the epithelial compartment of rat prostate maintained as long-term organ cultures *in vitro*', *Endocrinology,* 143, 228-38.

Ahonen, T. J., Xie, J., LeBaron, M. J., Zhu, J., Nurmi, M., Alanen, K., Rui, H. & Nevalainen, M. T. (2003) 'Inhibition of transcription factor Stat5 induces cell death of human prostate cancer cells', *J Biol Chem,* 278, 27287-92.

Alexander, W. S. & Hilton, D. J. (2004) 'The role of suppressors of cytokine signaling (SOCS) proteins in regulation of the immune response', *Annu Rev Immunol,* 22, 503-29.

Alibhai, S. M., Breunis, H., Timilshina, N., Johnston, C., Tomlinson, G., Tannock, I., Krahn, M., Fleshner, N. E., Warde, P., Canning, S. D., Klotz, L. & Naglie, G. (2010) 'Impact of androgen-deprivation therapy on physical function and quality of life in men with nonmetastatic prostate cancer', *J Clin Oncol,* 28, 5038-45.

Ambrosio, R., Fimiani, G., Monfregola, J., Sanzari, E., De Felice, N., Salerno, M.C., Pignata, C., D'Urso, M. & Ursini, M.V. (2002) 'The structure of human STAT5A and STAT5B genes reveals two regions of nearly identical sequence and an alternative tissue specific STAT5B promoter', ***Gene,*** 285, 311-8.

American Cancer Society. (2012) 'Cancer Facts & Figures 2012', *Atlanta: American Cancer Society*, 1-64.

Aoki, N. & Matsuda, T. (2000) 'A cytosolic protein-tyrosine phosphatase PTP1B specifically dephosphorylates and deactivates prolactin-activated STAT5a and STAT5b', *J Biol Chem*, 275, 39718-26.

Azam, M., Lee, C., Strehlow, I. & Schindler, C. (1997) 'Functionally distinct isoforms of Stat5 are generated by protein processing', *Immunity*, 6, 691-701.

Barahmand-pour, F., Meinke, A., Eilers, A., Gouilleux, F., Groner, B. & Decker, T. (1995) 'Colony-stimulating factors and interferon-gamma activate a protein related to MGF-Stat 5 to cause formation of the differentiation-induced factor in myeloid cells', *FEBS Lett,* 360, 29-33.

Basaria, S., Lieb, J., 2nd, Tang, A. M., DeWeese, T., Carducci, M., Eisenberger, M. & Dobs, A. S. (2002) 'Long-term effects of androgen deprivation therapy in prostate cancer patients', *Clin Endocrinol (Oxf)*, 56, 779-86.

Becker, S., Groner, B. & Muller, C. W. (1998) 'Three-dimensional structure of the Stat3beta homodimer bound to DNA', *Nature,* 394, 145-51.

Begitt, A., Meyer, T., van Rossum, M. & Vinkemeier, U. (2000) 'Nucleocytoplasmic translocation of Stat1 is regulated by a leucine-rich export signal in the coiled-coil domain', Proc Natl Acad Sci U S A, 97, 10418-23.

Berthold, D. R., Pond, G. R., Soban, F., de Wit, R., Eisenberger, M. & Tannock, I. F. (2008) 'Docetaxel plus prednisone or mitoxantrone plus prednisone for advanced prostate cancer: updated survival in the TAX 327 study', *J Clin Oncol*, 26, 242-5.

Beuvink, I., Hess, D., Flotow, H., Hofsteenge, J., Groner, B. & Hynes, N. E. (2000) 'Stat5a serine phosphorylation. Serine 779 is constitutively phosphorylated in the mammary gland, and serine 725 phosphorylation influences prolactin-stimulated *in vitro* DNA binding activity', *J Biol Chem,* 275, 10247-55.

Blasko, J. C., Ragde, H. & Grimm, P. D. (1991) 'Transperineal ultrasound-guided implantation of the prostate: morbidity and complications', *Scand J Urol Nephrol Suppl,* 137, 113-8.

Bria, E., Cuppone, F., Giannarelli, D., Milella, M., Ruggeri, E. M., Sperduti, I., Pinnaro, P., Terzoli, E., Cognetti, F. & Carlini, P. (2009) 'Does hormone treatment added to radiotherapy improve outcome in locally advanced prostate cancer?: meta-analysis of randomized trials', *Cancer,* 115, 3446-56.

Candotti, F., Oakes, S. A., Johnston, J. A., Gilliani, S., Schumacher, R. F., Mella, P., Fiorini, M., Ugazio, A. G., Badolato, R., Bozzi, F., Macchi, P., Strina, D., Vezzoni, R., Blaese, R. M, O'Shea J. J. & Villa A. (1997) 'Structural and functional basis for JAK3-deficient severe combined immunodeficiency', *Blood*, 90, 3996-4003.

Catalona, W. J. & Bigg, S. W. (1990) 'Nerve-sparing radical prostatectomy: evaluation of results after 250 patients', *J Urol,* 143, 538-43; discussion 544.

Chatterjee-Kishore, M., Wright, K. L., Ting, J. P. & Stark, G. R. (2000) 'How Stat1 mediates constitutive gene expression: a complex of unphosphorylated Stat1 and IRF1 supports transcription of the LMP2 gene', *Embo J,* 19, 4111-22.

Chen, X., Vinkemeier, U., Zhao, Y., Jeruzalmi, D., Darnell, J. E., Jr. & Kuriyan, J. (1998) 'Crystal structure of a tyrosine phosphorylated STAT-1 dimer bound to DNA', *Cell,* 93, 827-39.

Chen, T., Wang, L. H. & Farrar, W. L. (2000) 'Interleukin 6 activates androgen receptor-mediated gene expression through a signal transducer and activator of transcription 3-dependent pathway in LNCaP prostate cancer cells', *Cancer Res*, 60, 2132-5.

Chopin, L. K., Veveris-Lowe, T. L., Philipps, A. F. & Herington, A. C. (2002) 'Co-expression of GH and GHR isoforms in prostate cancer cell lines', *Growth Horm IGF Res,* 12, 126-36.

Chung, C. D., Liao, J., Liu, B., Rao, X., Jay, P., Berta, P. & Shuai, K. (1997) 'Specific inhibition of Stat3 signal transduction by PIAS3', *Science,* 278, 1803-5.

Copeland, N. G., Gilbert, D. J., Schindler, C., Zhong, Z., Wen, Z., Darnell, J. E., Jr., Mui, A. L., Miyajima, A., Quelle, F. W., Ihle, J. N. & *et al.,* (1995) 'Distribution of the mammalian Stat gene family in mouse chromosomes', *Genomics,* 29, 225-8.

D'Amico, A. V., Manola, J., Loffredo, M., Renshaw, A. A., DellaCroce, A. & Kantoff, P. W. (2004) '6-month androgen suppression plus radiation therapy *vs.* radiation therapy alone for patients with clinically localized prostate cancer: a randomized controlled trial', *Jama,* 292, 821-7.

Dagvadorj, A., Collins, S., Jomain, J. B., Abdulghani, J., Karras, J., Zellweger, T., Li, H., Nurmi, M., Alanen, K., Mirtti, T., Visakorpi, T., Bubendorf, L., Goffin, V. & Nevalainen, M. T. (2007) 'Autocrine prolactin promotes prostate cancer cell growth *via* Janus kinase-2-signal transducer and activator of transcription-5a/b signaling pathway', *Endocrinology,* 148, 3089-101.

Dagvadorj, A., Kirken, R. A., Leiby, B., Karras, J. & Nevalainen, M. T. (2008) 'Transcription Factor Stat5 Promotes Growth of Human Prostate Cancer Cells *In Vivo*', *Clinical Cancer Research,* 14, 1317-24.

Dagvadorj, A., Tan, S. H., Liao, Z., Xie, J., Nurmi, M., Alanen, K., Rui, H., Mirtti, T. & Nevalainen M. T. (2010) 'N-terminal truncation of Stat5a/b circumvents PIAS3-mediated transcriptional inhibition of Stat5 in prostate cancer cells', *Int J Biochem Cell Biol*, 42, 2037-46.

Dall'Era, M. A., Cooperberg, M. R., Chan, J. M., Davies, B. J., Albertsen, P. C., Klotz, L. H., Warlick, C. A., Holmberg, L., Bailey, D. E. Jr., Wallace, M. E., Kantoff, P. W. & Carroll, P. R. (2008) 'Active surveillance for early-stage prostate cancer: review of the current literature', *Cancer*, 112, 1650-9.

Darnell, J. E., Jr. (1997) 'STATs and gene regulation', *Science,* 277, 1630-5.

Darnell, J. E., Jr., Kerr, I. M. & Stark, G. R. (1994) 'Jak-STAT pathways and transcriptional activation in response to IFNs and other extracellular signaling proteins', *Science,* 264, 1415-21.

de Bono, J. S., Logothetis, C. J., Molina, A., Fizazi, K., North, S., Chu, L., Chi, K. N., Jones, R. J., Goodman, O. B. Jr., Saad, F., Staffurth, J. N., Mainwaring, P., Harland, S., Flaig, T. W., Hutson, T. E., Cheng, T., Patterson, H., Hainsworth, J. D., Ryan, C. J., Sternberg, C. N., Ellard, S. L., Fléchon, A., Saleh, M., Scholz, M., Efstathiou, E., Zivi, A., Bianchini, D., Loriot, Y., Chieffo, N., Kheoh, T., Haqq, C. M., Scher, H. I. & COU-AA-301 Investigators (2011) 'Abiraterone and increased survival in metastatic prostate cancer', *N Engl J Med*, 364, 1995-2005.

de Bono, J. S., Oudard, S., Ozguroglu, M., Hansen, S., Machiels, J. P., Kocak, I., Gravis, G., Bodrogi, I., Mackenzie, M. J., Shen, L., Roessner, M., Gupta, S., Sartor, A. O.; TROPIC Investigators (2010) 'Prednisone plus cabazitaxel or mitoxantrone for metastatic castration-resistant prostate cancer progressing after docetaxel treatment: a randomised open-label trial', *Lancet*, 376, 1147-54.

de Groot, R. P., Raaijmakers, J. A., Lammers, J. W., Jove, R. & Koenderman, L. (1999) 'STAT5 activation by BCR-Abl contributes to transformation of K562 leukemia cells', *Blood,* 94, 1108-12.

Decker, T., Lew, D. J., Mirkovitch, J. & Darnell, J. E., Jr. (1991) 'Cytoplasmic activation of GAF, an IFN-gamma-regulated DNA-binding factor', *Embo J,* 10, 927-32.

Denham, J. W., Steigler, A., Lamb, D. S., Joseph, D., Mameghan, H., Turner, S., Matthews, J., Franklin, I., Atkinson, C., North, J., Poulsen, M., Christie, D., Spry, N. A., Tai, K. H., Wynne, C., Duchesne, G., Kovacev, O. & D'Este, C. (2005) 'Short-term androgen deprivation and radiotherapy for locally advanced prostate cancer: results from the Trans-Tasman Radiation Oncology Group 96.01 randomised controlled trial', *Lancet Oncol,* 6, 841-50.

Eggener, S. E., Scardino, P. T., Walsh, P. C., Han, M., Partin, A. W., Trock, B. J., Feng, Z., Wood, D. P., Eastham, J. A., Yossepowitch, O., Rabah, D. M., Kattan, M. W., Yu, C., Klein, E. A. & Stephenson, A. J. (2011) 'Predicting 15-year prostate cancer specific mortality after radical prostatectomy', *J Urol*, 185, 869-75.

Ehret, G. B., Reichenbach, P., Schindler, U., Horvath, C. M., Fritz, S., Nabholz, M. & Bucher, P. (2001) 'DNA binding specificity of different STAT proteins. Comparison of *in vitro* specificity with natural target sites', *J Biol Chem,* 276, 6675-88.

Feldman, B. J. & Feldman, D. (2001) 'The development of androgen-independent prostate cancer', *Nat Rev Cancer*, 1, 34-45.

Ferrajoli, A., Faderl, S., Van, Q., Koch, P., Harris, D., Liu, Z., Hazan-Halevy, I., Wang, Y., Kantarjian, H. M., Priebe, W. & Estrov, Z. (2007) 'WP1066 disrupts Janus kinase-2 and induces caspase-dependent apoptosis in acute myelogenous leukemia cells', *Cancer Res*, 67, 11291-9.

Fowler, F. J., Jr., Barry, M. J., Lu-Yao, G., Wasson, J. H. & Bin, L. (1996) 'Outcomes of external-beam radiation therapy for prostate cancer: a study of Medicare beneficiaries in three surveillance, epidemiology, and end results areas', *J Clin Oncol,* 14, 2258-65.

Foxwell, B. M., Beadling, C., Guschin, D., Kerr, I. & Cantrell, D. (1995) 'Interleukin-7 can induce the activation of Jak 1, Jak 3 and STAT 5 proteins in murine T cells', *Eur J Immunol,* 25, 3041-6.

Friesen, H. & Astwood, E. B. (1965) 'HORMONES OF THE ANTERIOR PITUITARY BODY', *N Engl J Med*, 272, 1328-35.

Gewinner, C., Hart, G., Zachara, N., Cole, R., Beisenherz-Huss, C. & Groner, B. (2004) 'The coactivator of transcription CREB-binding protein interacts preferentially with the glycosylated form of Stat5', *J Biol Chem,* 279, 3563-72.

Ghoreschi, K., Laurence, A. & O'Shea J. J. (2009) 'Janus kinases in immune cell signaling', *Immunol Rev*, 228, 273-87.

Ginzburg, S. & Albertsen, P. C. (2011) 'The timing and extent of androgen deprivation therapy for prostate cancer: weighing the clinical evidence', *Endocrinol Metab Clin North Am*, 40, 615-23, ix.

Gouilleux, F., Pallard, C., Dusanter-Fourt, I., Wakao, H., Haldosen, L. A., Norstedt, G., Levy, D. & Groner, B. (1995) 'Prolactin, growth hormone, erythropoietin and granulocyte-macrophage colony stimulating factor induce MGF-Stat5 DNA binding activity', *Embo J,* 14, 2005-13.

Gouilleux, F., Wakao, H., Mundt, M. & Groner, B. (1994) 'Prolactin induces phosphorylation of Tyr694 of Stat5 (MGF), a prerequisite for DNA binding and induction of transcription', *Embo J,* 13, 4361-9.

Goureau, A., Garrigues, A., Tosser-Klopp, G., Lahbib-Mansais, Y., Chardon, P. & Yerle, M. (2001) 'Conserved synteny and gene order difference between human chromosome 12 and pig chromosome 5', *Cytogenet Cell Genet,* 94, 49-54.

Gu, L., Dagvadorj, A., Lutz, J., Leiby, B., Bonuccelli, G., Lisanti, M. P., Addya, S., Fortina, P., Dasgupta, A., Hyslop, T., Bubendorf, L. & Nevalainen M. T. (2010a) 'Transcription factor Stat3 stimulates metastatic behavior of human prostate cancer cells *in vivo*, whereas Stat5b has a preferential role in the promotion of prostate cancer cell viability and tumor growth', *Am J Pathol*, 176, 1959-72.

Gu, L., Vogiatzi, P., Puhr, M., Dagvadorj, A., Lutz, J., Ryder, A., Addya, S., Fortina, P., Cooper, C., Leiby, B., Dasgupta, A., Hyslop, T., Bubendorf, L., Alanen, K., Mirtti, T. &

Nevalainen, M. T. (2010b) 'Stat5 promotes metastatic behavior of human prostate cancer cells *in vitro* and *in vivo*', *Endocr Relat Cancer*, 17, 481-93.

Gu, L., Zhu, X.H., Visakorpi, T., Alanen, K., Mirtti, T., Edmonston, T. B. & Nevalainen, M. T. (2010c) 'Activating mutation (V617F) in the tyrosine kinase JAK2 is absent in locally-confined or castration resistant prostate cancer', *Anal Cell Pathol (Amst)*, 33, 55-9.

Guh, J. Y., Huang, J. S., Chen, H. C., Hung, W. C., Lai, Y. H. & Chuang, L. Y. (2001) 'Advanced glycation end product-induced proliferation in NRK-49F cells is dependent on the JAK2/STAT5 pathway and cyclin D1', *Am J Kidney Dis,* 38, 1096-104.

Haddad, B., Pabon-Pena, C. R., Young, H. & Sun, W. H. (1998) 'Assignment1 of STAT1 to human chromosome 2q32 by FISH and radiation hybrids', *Cytogenet Cell Genet,* 83, 58-9.

Halmos, G., Schally, A. V., Czompoly, T., Krupa, M., Varga, J. L. & Rekasi, Z. (2002) 'Expression of growth hormone-releasing hormone and its receptor splice variants in human prostate cancer', *J Clin Endocrinol Metab,* 87, 4707-14.

Harrison, C., Kiladjian, J.-J., Al-Ali, H. K., Gisslinger, H., Waltzman, R., Stalbovskaya, V., McQuitty, M., Hunter, D. S., Levy, R., Knoops, L., Cervantes, F., Vannucchi, A. M., Barbui, T. & Barosi, G. (2012) 'JAK inhibition with ruxolitinib *versus* best available therapy for myelofibrosis', *New Engl J Med,* 366, 787-98.

Hedvat, M., Huszar, D., Herrmann, A., Gozgit. J. M., Schroeder, A., Sheehy, A., Buettner, R., Proia, D., Kowolik, C. M., Xin, H., Armstrong, B., Bebernitz, G., Weng, S., Wang, L., Ye, M., McEachern, K., Chen, H., Morosini, D., Bell, K., Alimzhanov, M., Ioannidis, S., McCoon, P., Cao, Z. A., Yu, H., Jove, R. & Zinda, M. (2009) 'The JAK2 inhibitor AZD1480 potently blocks Stat3 signaling and oncogenesis in solid tumors', *Cancer Cell,* 16, 487-97.

Horvath, C. M., Wen, Z. & Darnell, J. E., Jr. (1995) 'A STAT protein domain that determines DNA sequence recognition suggests a novel DNA-binding domain', *Genes Dev,* 9, 984-94.

Hou, J., Schindler, U., Henzel, W. J., Wong, S. C. & McKnight, S. L. (1995) 'Identification and purification of human Stat proteins activated in response to interleukin-2', *Immunity,* 2, 321-9.

Humphrey, P. A. (2012) 'Histological variants of prostatic carcinoma and their significance', *Histopathology*, 60, 59-74.

Hussain, S. F., Kong, L. Y., Jordan, J., Conrad, C., Madden, T., Fokt, I., Priebe, W. & Heimberger, A. B. (2007) 'A novel small molecule inhibitor of signal transducers and activators of transcription 3 reverses immune tolerance in malignant glioma patients' *Cancer Res*, 67, 9630-6.

Ihle, J. N. (2001) 'The Stat family in cytokine signaling', *Curr Opin Cell Biol,* 13, 211-7.

Isaacs, J. T. & Isaacs, W. B. (2004) 'Androgen receptor outwits prostate cancer drugs', *Nat Med,* 10, 26-7.

Iwamaru, A., Szymanski, S., Iwado, E., Aoki, H., Yokoyama, T., Fokt, I., Hess, K., Conrad, C., Madden, T., Sawaya, R., Kondo, S., Priebe, W. & Kondo, Y. (2007) 'A novel inhibitor of the STAT3 pathway induces apoptosis in malignant glioma cells both *in vitro* and *in vivo*', *Oncogene*, 26, 2435-44.

Jasmin, J. F., Mercier, I., Sotgia, F. & Lisanti, M. P. (2006) 'SOCS proteins and caveolin-1 as negative regulators of endocrine signaling', *Trends Endocrinol Metab,* 17, 150-8.

John, S., Vinkemeier, U., Soldaini, E., Darnell, J. E., Jr. & Leonard, W. J. (1999) 'The significance of tetramerization in promoter recruitment by Stat5', *Mol Cell Biol,* 19, 1910-8.

Kamizono, S., Hanada, T., Yasukawa, H., Minoguchi, S., Kato, R., Minoguchi, M., Hattori, K., Hatakeyama, S., Yada, M., Morita, S., Kitamura, T., Kato, H., Nakayama, K. & Yoshimura, A. (2001) 'The SOCS box of SOCS-1 accelerates ubiquitin-dependent proteolysis of TEL-JAK2', *J Biol Chem,* 276, 12530-8.

Kantoff, P. W., Higano, C. S., Shore, N. D., Berger, E. R., Small, E. J., Penson, D. F., Redfern, C. H., Ferrari, A. C., Dreicer, R., Sims, R. B., Xu, Y., Frohlich, M. W., Schellhammer, P. F. & IMPACT Study Investigators. (2010) 'Sipuleucel-T immunotherapy for castration-resistant prostate cancer', *N Engl J Med*, 363:411-22.

Kawashima, T., Bao, Y.C., Minoshima, Y., Nomura, Y., Hatori, T., Hori, T., Fukagawa, T., Fukada, T., Takahashi, N., Nosaka, T., Inoue, M., Sato, T., Kukimoto-Niino, M., Shirouzu, M., Yokoyama, S. & Kitamura, T. (2009) 'A Rac GTPase-activating protein, MgcRacGAP, is a nuclear localizing signal-containing nuclear chaperone in the activation of STAT transcription factors', *Mol Cell Biol*, 29, 1796-813.

Kazansky, A. V., Spencer, D. M. & Greenberg, N. M. (2003) 'Activation of signal transducer and activator of transcription 5 is required for progression of autochthonous prostate cancer: evidence from the transgenic adenocarcinoma of the mouse prostate system', *Cancer Res,* 63, 8757-62.

Kindblom, J., Dillner, K., Ling, C., Tornell, J. & Wennbo, H. (2002) 'Progressive prostate hyperplasia in adult prolactin transgenic mice is not dependent on elevated serum androgen levels', *Prostate,* 53, 24-33.

Kindblom, J., Dillner, K., Sahlin, L., Robertson, F., Ormandy, C., Tornell, J. & Wennbo, H. (2003) 'Prostate hyperplasia in a transgenic mouse with prostate-specific expression of prolactin', *Endocrinology,* 144, 2269-78.

Klotz, L., Boccon-Gibod, L., Shore, N. D., Andreou, C., Persson, B. E., Cantor, P., Jensen, J. K., Olesen, T. K. & Schroder, F. H. (2008) 'The efficacy and safety of degarelix: a 12-month, comparative, randomized, open-label, parallel-group phase III study in patients with prostate cancer', *BJU Int,* 102, 1531-8.

Lawton, C. A., Winter, K., Byhardt, R., Sause, W. T., Hanks, G. E., Russell, A. H., Rotman, M., Porter, A., McGowan, D. G., DelRowe, J. D. & Pilepich, M. V. (1997) 'Androgen suppression plus radiation *versus* radiation alone for patients with D1 (pN+) adenocarcinoma of the prostate (results based on a national prospective randomized trial, RTOG 85-31). Radiation Therapy Oncology Group', *Int J Radiat Oncol Biol Phys,* 38, 931-9.

Lawton, C. A., Winter, K., Grignon, D. & Pilepich, M. V. (2005) 'Androgen suppression plus radiation *versus* radiation alone for patients with stage D1/pathologic node-positive adenocarcinoma of the prostate: updated results based on national prospective randomized trial Radiation Therapy Oncology Group 85-31', *J Clin Oncol,* 23, 800-7.

Lawton, C. A., Winter, K., Murray, K., Machtay, M., Mesic, J. B., Hanks, G. E., Coughlin, C. T. & Pilepich, M. V. (2001) 'Updated results of the phase III Radiation Therapy Oncology Group (RTOG) trial 85-31 evaluating the potential benefit of androgen suppression following standard radiation therapy for unfavorable prognosis carcinoma of the prostate', *Int J Radiat Oncol Biol Phys,* 49, 937-46.

Leek, J. P., Hamlin, P. J., Bell, S. M. & Lench, N. J. (1997) 'Assignment of the STAT6 gene (STAT6) to human chromosome band 12q13 by *in situ* hybridization', *Cytogenet Cell Genet,* 79, 208-9.

Leonard, W. J. & O'Shea, J. J. (1998) 'Jaks and STATs: biological implications', *Annu Rev Immunol,* 16, 293-322.

Letsch, M., Schally, A. V., Busto, R., Bajo, A. M. & Varga, J. L. (2003) 'Growth hormone-releasing hormone (GHRH) antagonists inhibit the proliferation of androgen-dependent and -independent prostate cancers', *Proc Natl Acad Sci U S A,* 100, 1250-5.

Levy, D. E. & Darnell, J. E., Jr. (2002) 'Stats: transcriptional control and biological impact', *Nat Rev Mol Cell Biol,* 3, 651-62.

Li, H., Ahonen, T. J., Alanen, K., Xie, J., LeBaron, M. J., Pretlow, T. G., Ealley, E. L., Zhang, Y., Nurmi, M., Singh, B., Martikainen, P. M. & Nevalainen, M. T. (2004) 'Activation of signal transducer and activator of transcription 5 in human prostate cancer is associated with high histological grade', *Cancer Res,* 64, 4774-82.

Li, H., Zhang, Y., Glass, A., Zellweger, T., Gehan, E., Bubendorf, L., Gelmann, E. P. & Nevalainen, M. T. (2005) 'Activation of signal transducer and activator of transcription-5 in prostate cancer predicts early recurrence', *Clin Cancer Res,* 11, 5863-8.

Liao, Z., Gu, L., Shen, F., Dagvadorj, A., Gupta, S., Pattabiraman, N., Nevalainen, M., Trabulsi, E. J., Gomella, L. G. & McCue, P. (2011) Identification of a Small-molecule inhibitor of Stat5a/b through Structure-based Screen for Therapy Development for Prostate cancer. American Society of Clinical Oncology (ASCO) Genitourinary Cancers Symposium, Orlando, Fl, February 17-19, 2011.

Lim, A. J., Brandon, A. H., Fiedler, J., Brickman, A. L., Boyer, C. I., Raub, W. A., Jr. & Soloway, M. S. (1995) 'Quality of life: radical prostatectomy *versus* radiation therapy for prostate cancer', *J Urol,* 154, 1420-5.

Lin, J. X., Mietz, J., Modi, W. S., John, S. & Leonard, W. J. (1996) 'Cloning of human Stat5B. Reconstitution of interleukin-2-induced Stat5A and Stat5B DNA binding activity in COS-7 cells', *J Biol Chem,* 271, 10738-44.

Litterst, C. M., Kliem, S., Lodrini, M. & Pfitzner, E. (2005) 'Coactivators in gene regulation by STAT5', *Vitam Horm,* 70, 359-86.

Litterst, C. M., Kliem, S., Marilley, D. & Pfitzner, E. (2003) 'NCoA-1/SRC-1 is an essential coactivator of STAT5 that binds to the FDL motif in the alpha-helical region of the STAT5 transactivation domain', *J Biol Chem,* 278, 45340-51.

Liu, J. X., Mietz, J., Modi, W. S., John, S. & Leonard, W. J. (1996) 'Cloning of human Stat5B. Reconstitution of interleukin-2-induced Stat5A and Stat5B DNA binding activity in COS-7 cells', *J Biol Chem,* 271, 10738-44.

Liu, X., Gallego, M. I., Smith, G. H., Robinson, G. W. & Hennighausen, L. (1998) 'Functional release of Stat5a-null mammary tissue through the activation of compensating signals including Stat5b', *Cell Growth Differ,* 9, 795-803.

Liu, X., Robinson, G. W., Gouilleux, F., Groner, B. & Hennighausen, L. (1995) 'Cloning and expression of Stat5 and an additional homologue (Stat5b) involved in prolactin signal transduction in mouse mammary tissue', *Proc Natl Acad Sci U S A,* 92, 8831-5.

Llovera, M., Pichard, C., Bernichtein, S., Jeay, S., Touraine, P., Kelly, P. A. & Goffin, V. (2000) 'Human prolactin (hPRL) antagonists inhibit hPRL-activated signaling pathways involved in breast cancer cell proliferation [In Process Citation]', *Oncogene,* 19, 4695-705.

Loblaw, D. A., Mendelson, D. S., Talcott, J. A., Virgo, K. S., Somerfield, M. R., Ben-Josef, E., Middleton, R., Porterfield, H., Sharp, S. A., Smith, T. J., Taplin, M. E., Vogelzang, N. J., Wade, J. L. Jr., Bennett, C. L., Scher, H. I. & American Society of Clinical Oncology. (2004) 'American Society of Clinical Oncology recommendations for the initial hormonal management of androgen-sensitive metastatic, recurrent, or progressive prostate cancer', *J Clin Oncol*, 22, 2927-41.

Loblaw, D. A., Virgo, K. S., Nam, R., Somerfield, M. R., Ben-Josef, E., Mendelson, D. S., Middleton, R., Sharp, S. A., Smith, T. J., Talcott, J., Taplin, M., Vogelzang, N. J., Wade, J. L., 3rd, Bennett, C. L. & Scher, H. I. (2007) 'Initial hormonal management of androgen-sensitive metastatic, recurrent, or progressive prostate cancer: 2006 update of an American Society of Clinical Oncology practice guideline', *J Clin Oncol,* 25, 1596-605.

Lütticken, C., Wegenka, U. M., Yuan, J., Buschmann, J., Schindler, C., Ziemiecki, A., Harpur, A.G., Wilks, A. F., Yasukawa, K., Taga, T. & *et al.,* (1994) 'Association of transcription factor APRF and protein kinase Jak1 with the interleukin-6 signal transducer gp130', *Science*, 263, 89-92.

Magne, S., Caron, S., Charon, M., Rouyez, M. C. & Dusanter-Fourt, I. (2003) 'STAT5 and Oct-1 form a stable complex that modulates cyclin D1 expression', *Mol Cell Biol,* 23, 8934-45.

Marg, A., Shan, Y., Meyer, T., Meissner, T., Brandenburg, M. & Vinkemeier, U. (2004) 'Nucleocytoplasmic shuttling by nucleoporins Nup153 and Nup214 and CRM1-dependent nuclear export control the subcellular distribution of latent Stat1', *J Cell Biol,* 165, 823-33.

Maurer, A. B., Wichmann, C., Gross, A., Kunkel, H., Heinzel, T., Ruthardt, M., Groner, B. & Grez, M. (2002) 'The Stat5-RARalpha fusion protein represses transcription and differentiation through interaction with a corepressor complex', *Blood,* 99, 2647-52.

McBride, K. M., Banninger, G., McDonald, C. & Reich, N. C. (2002) 'Regulated nuclear import of the STAT1 transcription factor by direct binding of importin-alpha', *Embo J,* 21, 1754-63.

McBride, K. M., McDonald, C. & Reich, N. C. (2000) 'Nuclear export signal located within theDNA-binding domain of the STAT1 transcription factor', *Embo J,* 19, 6196-206.

Melen, K., Kinnunen, L. & Julkunen, I. (2001) 'Arginine/lysine-rich structural element is involved in interferon-induced nuclear import of STATs', *J Biol Chem,* 276, 16447-55.

Meyer, T., Gavenis, K. & Vinkemeier, U. (2002) 'Cell type-specific and tyrosine phosphorylation-independent nuclear presence of STAT1 and STAT3', *Exp Cell Res,* 272, 45-55.

Meyer, W. K., Reichenbach, P., Schindler, U., Soldaini, E. & Nabholz, M. (1997) 'Interaction of STAT5 dimers on two low affinity binding sites mediates interleukin 2 (IL-2) stimulation of IL-2 receptor alpha gene transcription', *J Biol Chem,* 272, 31821-8.

Mirtti, T., Leiby, B. E., Abdulghani, J., Aaltonen, E., Pavela, M., Mamtani, A., Alanen, K., Egevad, L., Granfors, T., Josefsson, A., Stattin, P., Bergh, A. & Nevalainen, M. T. (2012) 'Nuclear Stat5a/b predicts early recurrence and prostate cancer-specific death in patients treated by radical prostatectomy', *Hum Pathol,* [Epub ahead of print]. doi: 10.1016/j.humpath.2012.06.001.

Miyoshi, K., Cui, Y., Riedlinger, G., Robinson, P., Lehoczky, J., Zon, L., Oka, T., Dewar, K. & Hennighausen, L. (2001) 'Structure of the mouse Stat 3/5 locus: evolution from Drosophila to zebrafish to mouse', ***Genomics***, 71, 150-5.

Mui, A. L., Wakao, H., Harada, N., O'Farrell, A. M. & Miyajima, A. (1995a) 'Interleukin-3, granulocyte-macrophage colony-stimulating factor, and interleukin-5 transduce signals through two forms of STAT5', *J Leukoc Biol,* 57, 799-803.

Mui, A. L., Wakao, H., O'Farrell, A. M., Harada, N. & Miyajima, A. (1995b) 'Interleukin-3, granulocyte-macrophage colony stimulating factor and interleukin-5 transduce signals through two STAT5 homologs', *Embo J,* 14, 1166-75.

Nagel-Wolfrum, K., Buerger, C., Wittig, I., Butz, K., Hoppe-Seyler, F. & Groner, B. (2004) 'The interaction of specific peptide aptamers with the DNA binding domain and the dimerization domain of the transcription factor Stat3 inhibits transactivation and induces apoptosis in tumor cells', *Mol Cancer Res,* 2, 170-82.

Nakajima, H., Brindle, P. K., Handa, M. & Ihle, J. N. (2001) 'Functional interaction of STAT5 and nuclear receptor co-repressor SMRT: implications in negative regulation of STAT5-dependent transcription', *Embo J,* 20, 6836-44.

National Comprehensive Cancer Network (NCCN), http://www.nccn.org/index.asp.

Nevalainen, M. T., Ahonen, T. J., Yamashita, H., Chandrashekar, V., Bartke, A., Grimley, P. M., Robinson, G. W., Hennighausen, L. & Rui, H. (2000) 'Epithelial defect in prostates of Stat5a-null mice', *Lab Invest,* 80, 993-1006.

Nevalainen, M. T., Valve, E. M., Ahonen, T., Yagi, A., Paranko, J. & Harkonen, P. L. (1997a) 'Androgen-dependent expression of prolactin in rat prostate epithelium *in vivo* and in organ culture', *Faseb J,* 11, 1297-307.

Nevalainen, M. T., Valve, E. M., Ingleton, P. M. & Harkonen, P. L. (1996) 'Expression and hormone regulation of prolactin receptors in rat dorsal and lateral prostate', *Endocrinology,* 137, 3078-88.

Nevalainen, M. T., Valve, E. M., Ingleton, P. M., Nurmi, M., Martikainen, P. M. & Harkonen, P. L. (1997b) 'Prolactin and prolactin receptors are expressed and functioning in human prostate', *J Clin Invest,* 99, 618-27.

Nevalainen, M. T., Valve, E. M., Makela, S. I., Blauer, M., Tuohimaa, P. J. & Harkonen, P. L. (1991) 'Estrogen and prolactin regulation of rat dorsal and lateral prostate in organ culture', *Endocrinology,* 129, 612-22.

Nevalainen, M. T., Xie, J., Bubendorf, L., Wagner, K. U. & Rui, H. (2002) 'Basal activation of transcription factor signal transducer and activator of transcription (Stat5) in nonpregnant mouse and human breast epithelium', *Mol Endocrinol,* 16, 1108-24.

O'Donnell, A., Judson, I., Dowsett, M., Raynaud, F., Dearnaley, D., Mason, M., Harland, S., Robbins, A., Halbert, G., Nutley, B. & Jarman, M. (2004) 'Hormonal impact of the 17alpha-hydroxylase/C(17,20)-lyase inhibitor abiraterone acetate (CB7630) in patients with prostate cancer', *Br J Cancer*, 90, 2317-25.

Omlin, A. & de Bono, J. S. (2012) 'Therapeutic options for advanced prostate cancer: 2011 update', *Curr Urol Rep*, 13, 170-8.

Pallard, C., Gouilleux, F., Benit, L., Cocault, L., Souyri, M., Levy, D., Groner, B., Gisselbrecht, S. & Dusanter-Fourt, I. (1995a) 'Thrombopoietin activates a STAT5-like factor in hematopoietic cells', *Embo J,* 14, 2847-56.

Pallard, C., Gouilleux, F., Charon, M., Groner, B., Gisselbrecht, S. & Dusanter-Fourt, I. (1995b) 'Interleukin-3, erythropoietin, and prolactin activate a STAT5-like factor in lymphoid cells', *J Biol Chem,* 270, 15942-5.

Parker, C., Heinrich, D., O'Sullivan, J. M. & *et al.,* (2012) 'Overall survival benefit and safety profile of radium-223 chloride, a first-in-class alpha-pharmaceutical: Results from a phase III randomized trial (ALSYMPCA) in patients with castration-resistant prostate cancer (CRPC) with bone metastases', ASCO GU *J Clin Oncol*, 30 (suppl 5), Abstract 8.

Paukku, K., Yang, J. & Silvennoinen, O. (2003) 'Tudor and nuclease-like domains containing protein p100 function as coactivators for signal transducer and activator of transcription 5', *Mol Endocrinol,* 17, 1805-14.

Peng, B., Sutherland, K. D., Sum, E. Y., Olayioye, M., Wittlin, S., Tang, T. K., Lindeman, G. J. & Visvader, J. E. (2002) 'CPAP is a novel stat5-interacting cofactor that augments stat5-mediated transcriptional activity', *Mol Endocrinol,* 16, 2019-33.

Pilepich, M. V., Caplan, R., Byhardt, R. W., Lawton, C. A., Gallagher, M. J., Mesic, J. B., Hanks, G. E., Coughlin, C. T., Porter, A., Shipley, W. U. & Grignon, D. (1997) 'Phase III trial of androgen suppression using goserelin in unfavorable-prognosis carcinoma of the prostate treated with definitive radiotherapy: report of Radiation Therapy Oncology Group Protocol 85-31', *J Clin Oncol,* 15, 1013-21.

Pilepich, M. V., Winter, K., Lawton, C. A., Krisch, R. E., Wolkov, H. B., Movsas, B., Hug, E. B., Asbell, S. O. & Grignon, D. (2005) 'Androgen suppression adjuvant to definitive radiotherapy in prostate carcinoma--long-term results of phase III RTOG 85-31', *Int J Radiat Oncol Biol Phys,* 61, 1285-90.

Potosky, A. L., Davis, W. W., Hoffman, R. M., Stanford, J. L., Stephenson, R. A., Penson, D. F. & Harlan, L. C. (2004) 'Five-year outcomes after prostatectomy or radiotherapy for prostate cancer: the prostate cancer outcomes study', *J Natl Cancer Inst,* 96, 1358-67.

Ram, P. A. & Waxman, D. J. (1999) 'SOCS/CIS protein inhibition of growth hormone-stimulated STAT5 signaling by multiple mechanisms', *J Biol Chem,* 274, 35553-61.

Reich, N. C. & Liu, L. (2006) 'Tracking STAT nuclear traffic', *Nat Rev Immunol,* 6, 602-12.

Riddle, O., Bates, R.W. & Dykshorn, S.W. (1933) 'The preparation, identification and assay of prolactin-a hormone of the anterior pituitary', *Am J Physiol*, 105, 191-216.

Roach, M., 3rd, Bae, K., Speight, J., Wolkov, H. B., Rubin, P., Lee, R. J., Lawton, C., Valicenti, R., Grignon, D. & Pilepich, M. V. (2008) 'Short-term neoadjuvant androgen deprivation therapy and external-beam radiotherapy for locally advanced prostate cancer: long-term results of RTOG 8610', *J Clin Oncol,* 26, 585-91.

Rouet, V., Bogorad, R. L., Kayser, C., Kessal, K., Genestie, C., Bardier, A., Grattan, D. R., Kelder, B., Kopchick, J. J., Kelly, P. A. & Goffin, V. (2010) 'Local prolactin is a target to prevent expansion of basal/stem cells in prostate tumors', *Proc Natl Acad Sci U S A*, 107, 15199-15204.

Russell, S. M., Johnston, J. A., Noguchi, M., Kawamurra, M., Bacon, C. M., Friedmann, M., Berg, M., McVicar, D. W., Witthuhn, B. A., Silvennoinen, O., Goldmann, A. S., Schmalstieg, F. C., Ihle, J. N., O'Shea J. J. & Leonard, W. J. (1994) 'Interaction of IL-2Rb and gc C\chains with Jak1 and Jak3: Implication for XSCID and XCID', *Science*, 266, 1042-5.

Sanda, M. G., Dunn, R. L., Michalski, J., Sandler, H. M., Northouse, L., Hembroff, L., Lin, X., Greenfield, T. K., Litwin, M. S., Saigal, C. S., Mahadevan, A., Klein, E., Kibel, A., Pisters, L. L., Kuban, D., Kaplan, I., Wood, D., Ciezki, J., Shah, N. & Wei, J. T. (2008) 'Quality of life and satisfaction with outcome among prostate-cancer survivors', *N Engl J Med,* 358, 1250-61.

Scher, H. I., Fizazi, K., Saad, F., Taplin, M. E., Sternberg, C. N., Miller, M. D., de Wit, R., Mulders, P., Chi, K. N., Shore, N. D., Armstrong, A. J., Flaig, T. W., Fléchon, A., Mainwaring, P., Fleming, M., Hainsworth, J. D., Hirmand, M., Selby, B., Seely, L., de Bono, J. S. & the AFFIRM Investigators. (2012) 'Increased Survival with Enzalutamide in Prostate Cancer after Chemotherapy', *N Engl J Med*, [Epub ahead of print].

Schindler, C. & Darnell, J. E., Jr. (1995) 'Transcriptional responses to polypeptide ligands: the JAK-STAT pathway', *Annu Rev Biochem,* 64, 621-51.

Schindler, C. W. (2002) 'Series introduction. JAK-STAT signaling in human disease', *J Clin Invest,* 109, 1133-7.

Schmidt, D. & Muller, S. (2003) 'PIAS/SUMO: new partners in transcriptional regulation', *Cell Mol Life Sci,* 60, 2561-74.

Schmitt-Ney, M., Doppler, W., Ball, R. K. & Groner, B. (1991) 'Beta-casein gene promoter activity is regulated by the hormone-mediated relief of transcriptional repression and a mammary-gland-specific nuclear factor', *Mol Cell Biol,* 11, 3745-55.

Schmitt-Ney, M., Happ, B., Ball, R. K. & Groner, B. (1992a) 'Developmental and environmental regulation of a mammary gland-specific nuclear factor essential for transcription of the gene encoding beta-casein', *Proc Natl Acad Sci U S A,* 89, 3130-4.

Schmitt-Ney, M., Happ, B., Hofer, P., Hynes, N. E. & Groner, B. (1992b) 'Mammary gland-specific nuclear factor activity is positively regulated by lactogenic hormones and negatively by milk stasis', *Mol Endocrinol,* 6, 1988-97.

Schwaller, J., Parganas, E., Wang, D., Cain, D., Aster, J. C., Williams, I. R., Lee, C. K., Gerthner, R., Kitamura, T., Frantsve, J., Anastasiadou, E., Loh, M. L., Levy, D. E., Ihle, J. N. & Gilliland, D. G. (2000) 'Stat5 is essential for the myelo- and lymphoproliferative disease induced by TEL/JAK2', *Mol Cell,* 6, 693-704.

Schwartz, L. H., LaTrenta, L. R., Bonaccio, E., Kelly, W. K., Scher, H. I., Panicek, D. M. (1998) 'Small cell and anaplastic prostate cancer: correlation between CT findings and prostate-specific antigen level', Radiology. 208, 735-8.

Sekimoto, T., Imamoto, N., Nakajima, K., Hirano, T. & Yoneda, Y. (1997) 'Extracellular signal-dependent nuclear import of Stat1 is mediated by nuclear pore-targeting complex formation with NPI-1, but not Rch1', *Embo J,* 16, 7067-77.

Sekimoto, T., Nakajima, K., Tachibana, T., Hirano, T. & Yoneda, Y. (1996) 'Interferon-gamma-dependent nuclear import of Stat1 is mediated by the GTPase activity of Ran/TC4', *J Biol Chem,* 271, 31017-20.

Silva, C. M. (2004) 'Role of STATs as downstream signal transducers in Src family kinase-mediated tumorigenesis', *Oncogene,* 23, 8017-23.

Small, E. J. & Vogelzang, N. J. (1997) 'Second-line hormonal therapy for advanced prostate cancer: a shifting paradigm', *J Clin Oncol*, 15, 382-8.

Soldaini, E., John, S., Moro, S., Bollenbacher, J., Schindler, U. & Leonard, W. J. (2000) 'DNA binding site selection of dimeric and tetrameric Stat5 proteins reveals a large repertoire of divergent tetrameric Stat5a binding sites', *Mol Cell Biol,* 20, 389-401.

Stahl, N., Boulton, T. G., Farruggella, T., Ip, N.Y., Davis, S., Witthuhn, B. A., Quelle, F.W., Silvennoinen, O., Barbieri, G., Pellegrini, S. & *et al.,* (1994) 'Association and activation of Jak-Tyk kinases by CNTF-LIF-OSM-IL-6 beta receptor components', *Science*, 63, 92-5.

Stangelberger, A., Schally, A. V., Varga, J. L., Zarandi, M., Szepeshazi, K., Armatis, P. & Halmos, G. (2005) 'Inhibitory effect of antagonists of bombesin and growth hormone-releasing hormone on orthotopic and intraosseous growth and invasiveness of PC-3 human prostate cancer in nude mice', *Clin Cancer Res,* 11, 49-57.

Stocklin, E., Wissler, M., Gouilleux, F. & Groner, B. (1996) 'Functional interactions between Stat5 and the glucocorticoid receptor', *Nature,* 383, 726-8.

Stricker, P. & Grueter, R. (1928) 'Action du lobe anterieur de l'hypophyse sur la montee laiteuse', *Compt Rend Soc Biol,* 99, 1978–1980.

Tan, S. H., Dagvadorj, A., Shen, F., Gu, L., Liao, Z., Abdulghani, J., Zhang, Y., Gelmann, E. P., Zellweger, T., Culig, Z., Visakorpi, T., Bubendorf, L., Kirken, R. A., Karras, J. & Nevalainen, M. T. (2008) 'Transcription factor Stat5 synergizes with androgen receptor in prostate cancer cells', *Cancer Res,* 68, 236-48.

Tassone, P., Neri, P., Burger, R., Savino, R., Shammas, M., Catley, L., Podar, K., Chauhan, D., Masciari, S., Gozzini, A., Tagliaferri, P., Venuta, S., Munshi, N. C. & Anderson, K. C.

(2005) 'Combination therapy with interleukin-6 receptor superantagonist Sant7 and dexamethasone induces antitumor effects in a novel SCID-hu *In vivo* model of human multiple myeloma', *Clin Cancer Res*, 11, 4251-4258.

Thomis, D. C., Gurniak, C. B., Tivol, E., Sharpe, A. H. & Berg, L. J. (1995) 'Defects in B lymphocyte maturation and T lymphocyte activation in mice lacking Jak3', *Science*, 270:794-7.

Trachtenberg, J. & Walsh, P. C. (1982) 'Correlation of prostatic nuclear androgen receptor content with duration of response and survival following hormone therapy in advanced prostatic cancer', *J Urol*, 127, 466-71.

Trachtenberg, J., Halpern, N. & Pont, A. (1983) 'Ketoconazole: a novel and rapid treatment for advanced prostatic cancer', *J Urol*, 130, 152-3.

Tran, C., Ouk, S., Clegg, N. J., Chen, Y., Watson, P. A., Arora, V., Wongvipat, J., Smith-Jones, P. M., Yoo, D., Kwon, A., Wasielewska, T., Welsbie, D., Chen, C. D., Higano, C. S., Beer, T. M., Hung, D. T., Scher, H. I., Jung, M. E. & Sawyers, C. L. (2009) 'Development of a second-generation antiandrogen for treatment of advanced prostate cancer', *Science*, 324, 787-90.

Turkson, J., Kim, J. S., Zhang, S., Yuan, J., Huang, M., Glenn, M., Haura, E., Sebti, S., Hamilton, A. D. & Jove, R. (2004) 'Novel peptidomimetic inhibitors of signal transducer and activator of transcription 3 dimerization and biological activity', *Mol Cancer Ther,* 3, 261-9.

Turkson, J., Ryan, D., Kim, J. S., Zhang, Y., Chen, Z., Haura, E., Laudano, A., Sebti, S., Hamilton, A. D. & Jove, R. (2001) 'Phosphotyrosyl peptides block Stat3-mediated DNA binding activity, gene regulation, and cell transformation', *J Biol Chem,* 276, 45443-55.

Ungureanu, D., Saharinen, P., Junttila, I., Hilton, D. J. & Silvennoinen, O. (2002) 'Regulation of Jak2 through the ubiquitin-proteasome pathway involves phosphorylation of Jak2 on Y1007 and interaction with SOCS-1', *Mol Cell Biol,* 22, 3316-26.

Verstovsek, S., Mesa, R. A., Gotlib, J., Levy, R. S., Gupta, V., DiPersio, J. F., Catalano, J. V., Deininger, M., Miller, C., Silver, R. T., Talpaz, M., Winton, E. F., Harvey, J. H., Arcasoy, M. O., Hexner, E., Lyons, R. M., Paquette, R., Raza, A., Vaddi, K., Erickson-Viitanen, S., Koumenis, I. L., Sun, W., Sandor, V. & Kantarjian, H. M. (2012) 'A double-blind, placebo-controlled trial of ruxolitinib for myelofibrosis', *N Engl J Med,* 366, 799-807.

Vinkemeier, U. (2004) 'Getting the message across, STAT! Design principles of a molecular signaling circuit', *J Cell Biol,* 167, 197-201.

Vinkemeier, U., Moarefi, I., Darnell, J. E., Jr. & Kuriyan, J. (1998) 'Structure of the amino-terminal protein interaction domain of STAT-4', *Science,* 279, 1048-52.

Wakao, H., Gouilleux, F. & Groner, B. (1994) 'Mammary gland factor (MGF) is a novel member of the cytokine regulated transcription factor gene family and confers the prolactin response', *Embo J,* 13, 2182-91.

Wakao, H., Schmitt-Ney, M. & Groner, B. (1992) 'Mammary gland-specific nuclear factor is present in lactating rodent and bovine mammary tissue and composed of a single polypeptide of 89 kDa', *J Biol Chem,* 267, 16365-70.

Wallner, K., Roy, J. & Harrison, L. (1996) 'Tumor control and morbidity following transperineal iodine 125 implantation for stage T1/T2 prostatic carcinoma', *J Clin Oncol,* 14, 449-53.

Wang, Z., Prins, G. S., Coschigano, K. T., Kopchick, J. J., Green, J. E., Ray, V. H., Hedayat, S., Christov, K. T., Unterman, T. G. & Swanson, S. M. (2005) 'Disruption of Growth Hormone Signaling Retards Early Stages of Prostate Carcinogenesis in the C3(1)/Tag Mouse', *Endocrinology*, 146, 5188-96.

Wartmann, M., Cella, N., Hofer, P., Groner, B., Liu, X., Hennighausen, L. & Hynes, N. E. (1996) 'Lactogenic hormone activation of Stat5 and transcription of the beta- casein gene in mammary epithelial cells is independent of p42 ERK2 mitogen-activated protein kinase activity', *J Biol Chem,* 271, 31863-8.

Weiss-Messer, E., Merom, O., Adi, A., Karry, R., Bidosee, M., Ber, R., Kaploun, A., Stein, A. & Barkey, R. J. (2004) 'Growth hormone (GH) receptors in prostate cancer: gene expression in human tissues and cell lines and characterization, GH signaling and androgen receptor regulation in LNCaP cells', *Mol Cell Endocrinol,* 220, 109-23.

Welte, T., Garimorth, K., Philipp, S. & Doppler, W. (1994) 'Prolactin-dependent activation of a tyrosine phosphorylated DNA binding factor in mouse mammary epithelial cells', *Mol Endocrinol,* 8, 1091-102.

Wennbo, H., Kindblom, J., Isaksson, O. G. & Tornell, J. (1997) 'Transgenic mice overexpressing the prolactin gene develop dramatic enlargement of the prostate gland', *Endocrinology,* 138, 4410-5.

Williams, T. M. & Lisanti, M. P. (2005) 'Caveolin-1 in oncogenic transformation, cancer, and metastasis', *Am J Physiol Cell Physiol,* 288, C494-506.

Xu, W., Yu, F., Yan, M., Lu, L., Zou, W., Sun, L., Zheng, Z. & Liu, X. (2004) 'Geldanamycin, a heat shock protein 90-binding agent, disrupts Stat5 activation in IL-2-stimulated cells', *J Cell Physiol,* 198, 188-96.

Xu, X., Kreye, E., Kuo, C. B. & Walker, A. M. (2001) 'A molecular mimic of phosphorylated prolactin markedly reduced tumor incidence and size when du145 human prostate cancer cells were grown in nude mice', *Cancer Res,* 61, 6098-104.

Yamamoto, K., Kobayashi, H., Arai, A., Miura, O., Hirosawa, S. & Miyasaka, N. (1997) 'cDNA cloning, expression and chromosome mapping of the human STAT4 gene: both STAT4 and STAT1 genes are mapped to 2q32.2-->q32.3', *Cytogenet Cell Genet,* 77, 207-10.

Yang, E., Henriksen, M. A., Schaefer, O., Zakharova, N. & Darnell, J. E., Jr. (2002) 'Dissociation time from DNA determines transcriptional function in a STAT1 linker mutant', *J Biol Chem,* 277, 13455-62.

Yang, J., Chatterjee-Kishore, M., Staugaitis, S. M., Nguyen, H., Schlessinger, K., Levy, D. E. & Stark, G. R. (2005) 'Novel roles of unphosphorylated STAT3 in oncogenesis and transcriptional regulation', *Cancer Res,* 65, 939-47.

Yang, J., Liao, X., Agarwal, M. K., Barnes, L., Auron, P. E. & Stark, G. R. (2007) 'Unphosphorylated STAT3 accumulates in response to IL-6 and activates transcription by binding to NFkappaB', *Genes Dev,* 21, 1396-408.

Yu, H. & Jove, R. (2004) 'The STATs of cancer--new molecular targets come of age', *Nat Rev Cancer,* 4, 97-105.

Zeng, Z. Z., Yellaturu, C. R., Neeli, I. & Rao, G. N. (2002) '5(S)-hydroxyeicosatetraenoic acid stimulates DNA synthesis in human microvascular endothelial cells *via* activation of Jak/STAT and phosphatidylinositol 3-kinase/Akt signaling, leading to induction of expression of basic fibroblast growth factor 2', *J Biol Chem,* 277, 41213-9.

Zhang, J. G., Farley, A., Nicholson, S. E., Willson, T. A., Zugaro, L. M., Simpson, R. J., Moritz, R. L., Cary, D., Richardson, R., Hausmann, G., Kile, B. J., Kent, S. B., Alexander, W. S., Metcalf, D., Hilton, D. J., Nicola, N. A. & Baca, M. (1999) 'The conserved SOCS box motif in suppressors of cytokine signaling binds to elongins B and C and may couple bound proteins to proteasomal degradation', *Proc Natl Acad Sci U S A,* 96, 2071-6.

Zhao, W., Jaganathan, S. & Turkson, J. (2010) 'A cell-permeable Stat3 SH2 domain mimetic inhibits Stat3 activation and induces antitumor cell effects *in vitro*', *J Biol Chem*, 285, 35855-65.

Zhong, Z., Wen, Z. & Darnell, J. E. J. (1994) 'Stat3: a STAT family member activated by tyrosine phosphorylation in response to epidermal growth factor and interleukin-6', *Science,* 264, 95-98.

Zhu, M., John, S., Berg, M. & Leonard, W. J. (1999) 'Functional association of Nmi with Stat5 and Stat1 in IL-2- and IFNgamma-mediated signaling', *Cell,* 96, 121-30.

Cutting Edge Therapies for Cancer in the 21st Century, 2014, 219-252

CHAPTER 8

Targeting Interleukin-6 for the Treatment of Castration-Resistant Prostate Cancer

Sonia Godoy-Tundidor[1], Sucharitha Balasubramaniam[2], Ana Romero-Weaver[3] and Zoran Culig[1,*]

[1]Department of Urology, Innsbruck Medical University, Anichstrasse 35, A-6020, Innsbruck, Austria; [2]Department of Cancer Biology, Thomas Jefferson University, Philadelphia, PA 19107, USA and [3]Department of Radiation Oncology, University of Pennsylvania School of Medicine, Philadelphia, PA 19104, USA

Abstract: The existence of a crosstalk between the androgen receptor (AR) pathway and interleukin-6 (IL-6) signaling in prostate cancer (PCa) is broadly recognized. IL-6 activates the AR in a ligand-independent manner leading to the transcription of prostate-specific antigen (PSA), the most widely used marker for the detection and monitoring of PCa. IL-6 expression is increased in the malignant epithelium of prostate cancer patients and its levels are enhanced in the plasma of patients with late-stage disease. Interestingly, IL-6 is able to shift from being a paracrine growth inhibitor to an autocrine growth stimulator in PCa cells. Hence, IL-6 has been implicated in the progression towards castration-resistant prostate cancer (CRPC), in which elevated levels are indicative of poor prognosis and predict resistance to chemotherapy with taxanes. We will depict here the IL-6 signaling pathway and its contribution to PCa. For this purpose, we will portray the molecular events that prompted the origin of LNCaP-IL-6+ cells, a model of advanced PCa, upon chronic exposure to IL-6. We will also examine the similarities between LNCaP-IL-6+ cells and late-stage prostatic carcinoma. In addition, we will reveal the effect of CNTO 328, a chimeric monoclonal antibody targeting IL-6, in LNCaP-IL-6+ cells, as well as discuss the latest results from clinical trials with CNTO 328 in CRPC patients. Finally, we will speculate on the possibility, not yet investigated, of administering CNTO 328 to patients before the onset of CRPC.

Keywords: Interleukin-6 (IL-6), prostate cancer, castration-resistant prostate cancer, androgen deprivation therapy, androgen receptor, androgen, antiandrogen, JAK/STAT, MAP kinase, VEGF, retinoblastoma, clinical trials, prostate specific antigen (PSA).

***Address correspondence to Zoran Culig:** Department of Urology, Innsbruck Medical University, Anichstrasse 35, A-6020 Innsbruck, Austria; Tel: +43 512 504 24818; Fax: +43 512 504 24817; E-mail: zoran.culig@i-med.ac.at

Pier Paolo Claudio and Paraskevi Vogiatzi (Eds)

1. INTRODUCTION

Castration-resistant prostate cancer (CRPC) is a term coined to include those cases of advanced prostate cancer (PCa) in which hormone therapy has failed (Scher *et al.,* 2004). In the past, CRPC was more frequently referred to as androgen-independent prostate cancer (AIPC), or hormone-refractory prostate cancer (HRPC), based on the belief that such tumors were able to grow in the absence of androgen (Feldman & Feldman 2001). However, it has recently been shown that some so-called "androgen-independent" tumors can jump-start their own intracrine production of androgens under castrate levels of gonadal hormones (Locke *et al.,* 2008). Thus, the expression CRPC emphasizes the ability of tumors to thrive after hormonal therapy, independently of whether *de novo* synthesis of androgens is involved.

Let's take a look at the standard of care for patients with locally advanced or metastatic prostate cancer. The survival and proliferation of PCa cells are, in principle, highly dependent on androgens and a functional androgen receptor (AR) signaling pathway (Feldman & Feldman 2001). For this reason, conventional therapies for tumors that have spread beyond the boundaries of the prostate aim at hindering the AR pathway. This is regularly accomplished by: a) depriving tumor cells of androgens; b) blocking the AR to impede androgen binding; or c) a combination of both (combined androgen blockade, CAB) (Loblaw *et al.,* 2004). Androgen deprivation involves either surgical castration (orchiectomy) or chemical castration with luteinizing hormone-releasing hormone (LHRH) agonists. Androgen receptor blockade is accomplished with antiandrogens or AR antagonists like bicalutamide (Casodex®) (Loblaw *et al.,* 2004). Once the androgen/AR axis is shut down, PCa cells stop growing and, with their survival mechanisms compromised, undergo apoptosis (Feldman & Feldman 2001). This results in tumor shrinkage and a reduction in prostate-specific antigen (PSA), a marker of AR activity (Feldman & Feldman 2001). Unfortunately, PCa cells develop resistance to therapies targeting the AR in most patients in less than three years (Loblaw *et al.,* 2004). In some cases the AR becomes activated in the absence of gonadal androgens and tumor growth resumes; in others, tumor cells turn on mechanisms to bypass AR signaling and proliferate (Feldman & Feldman 2001). Moreover, some cancer cells manage to flourish after losing AR expression altogether (Kinoshita *et al.,* 2000; Shah, Mehra & Chinnaiyan 2004). In all these circumstances, PCa evolves into an incurable disease, castration-resistant prostate cancer, for which limited therapeutic options are available. Though a number of patients temporarily benefit from chemotherapy with docetaxel (Taxotere®) (Tannock *et al.,* 2004), they ultimately surrender to the devastating effects of CRPC. Fig. **1** summarizes the classical therapies used for the management of prostate cancer patients.

The difficulty in abolishing unrelenting AR signaling poses a challenge for the treatment of certain types of CRPC. However, shutting down AR expression may not be desirable either, since AR loss has been associated with more aggressive phenotypes (Kinoshita *et al.,* 2000; Shah, Mehra & Chinnaiyan 2004). In a traditional view of the AR pathway, two different states were recognized: a free and a ligand-bound AR. In the presence of androgen, the receptor adopted an active conformation and AR signaling was turned on leading to survival and proliferation of prostate cancer cells (Feldman & Feldman 2001). In a free, inactive state, the AR was presumably turned off and the lack of androgen resulted in cellular apoptosis (Feldman & Feldman 2001). Research conducted in Kennedy's disease, a degenerative disease of motor neurons in which the AR plays a crucial role, has revealed that the unliganded AR is not passive, as it was previously thought (Ellerby *et al.,* 1999). In fact, in the absence of ligand, the AR is cleaved by caspases (Ellerby *et al.,* 1999) and transmits a signal permitting cell death (Ellerby *et al.,* 1999; Bredesen, Mehlen & Rabizadeh 2005), while androgen binding inhibits its proapoptotic activity (Ellerby *et al.,* 1999; Bredesen, Mehlen & Rabizadeh 2005). Thus, the AR has been classified by some researchers as a "Dependence Receptor" or DR (Bredesen, Mehlen & Rabizadeh 2005; Goldschneider & Mehlen 2010). According to the DR theory, AR-harboring cells become addicted to androgen in order to bypass the proapoptotic command of a free receptor (Goldschneider & Mehlen 2010). Hence, vanishing of the AR in clusters of castration-resistant prostate tumors may indicate a failure of androgen ablation to induce widespread apoptosis.

As mentioned above, intracrine production of androgens may lead to castration-resistant disease (Locke *et al.,* 2008), but this is not the only way prostate cancer cells use to escape from therapy. Actually, there are several well-described mechanisms for the progression towards CRPC, which include both AR- and non-AR-mediated paths (Feldman & Feldman 2001) (Fig. **2**). These mechanisms may not be mutually exclusive so more than one type could operate in a particular tumor.

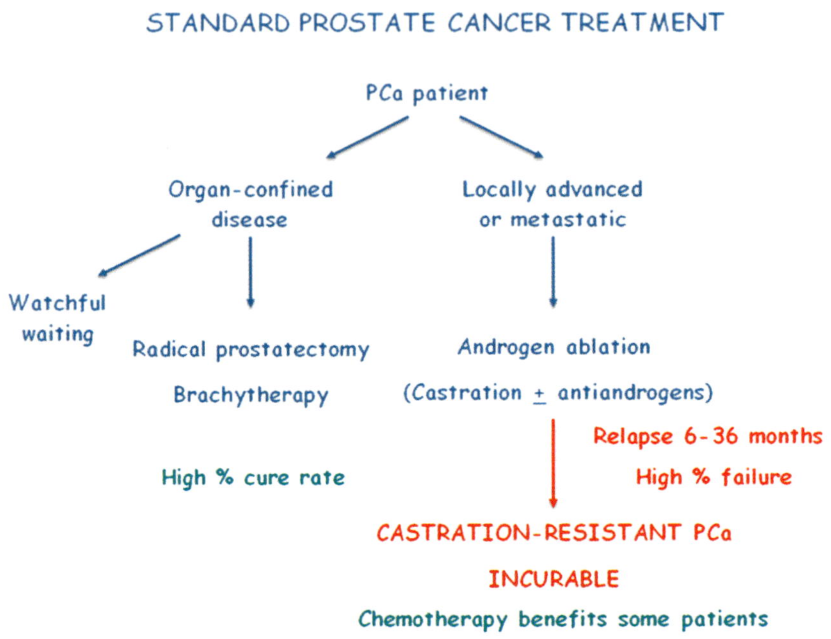

Figure 1: Standard therapies for the management of prostate cancer. Although clinically insignificant PCa may be monitored by watchful waiting, clinically significant organ-confined prostate cancer (PCa) is usually treated and cured by radical prostatectomy or brachytherapy. In the case of locally advanced PCa, androgen ablation *via* castration, administration of antiandrogens, or both, is the treatment of choice. However, PCa cells develop resistance to androgen receptor (AR)-targeted therapies in a short period of time, in which cancer cells develop a castration-resistant phenotype. Though chemotherapy may provide a survival benefit to patients with castration-resistant prostate cancer (CRPC), CRPC remains as an incurable and fatal disease. Thus, there is a great need for therapies directed towards CRPC.

Ligand-independent activation of the AR by interleukin-6 (IL-6) has been recognized as a paramount problem in patients with advanced PCa (Culig *et al.,* 2005). Thus, we will focus on the role of IL-6 in the development of CRPC, especially on the dramatic changes IL-6 imposes on PCa cells that allow them to circumvent the AR pathway. We will also reveal part of the reasoning behind IL-6-targeted therapies. In addition, we will discuss the results from clinical trials conducted with CNTO 328, a chimeric monoclonal anti-IL-6 antibody developed by Centocor, in patients with CRPC.

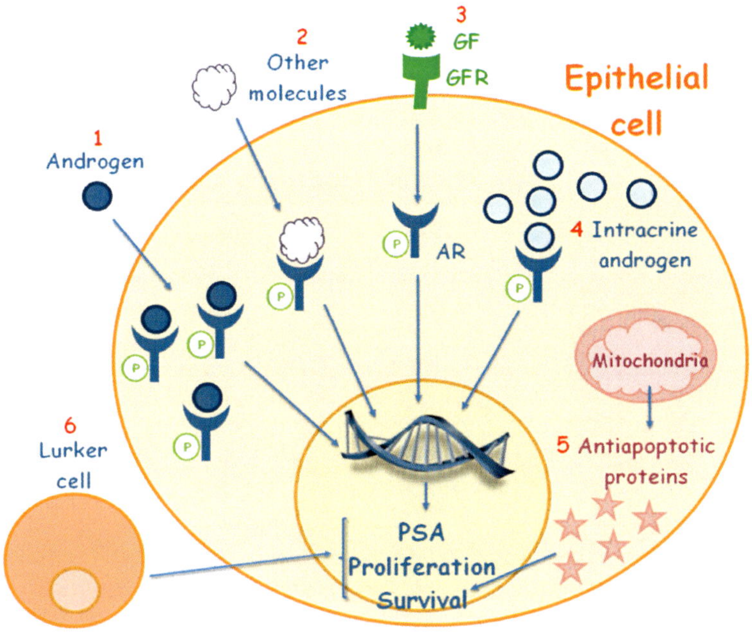

Figure 2: Mechanisms of development of castration-resistant prostate cancer (CRPC). 1. In some prostate cancer (PCa) cells, the androgen receptor (AR) becomes amplified in response to low levels of androgens, or the existing AR molecules become hypersensitive to androgens. AR coactivators are frequently overexpressed enhancing the sensitivity of the AR to residual androgens; 2. A "promiscuous" AR becomes activated by molecules other than androgens, such as antiandrogens, corticoids, *etc.*; 3. Activation of a receptor tyrosine kinase (RTK) by its corresponding ligand activates a phosphorylation cascade that results in phosphorylation and ligand-independent activation of the AR. Interleukin-6 (IL-6), insulin-like growth factor-1 (IGF-1), epidermal growth factor (EGF) and other growth factors and cytokines induce ligand-independent activation of the AR; 4. PCa cells may synthesize their own androgens *via* an intracrine mechanism; 5. The AR is bypassed through the increased production of antiapoptotic molecules such as Bcl-2 and Mcl-1; 6. Androgen-independent cells always present in the prostate (*i.e.*, "lurking" in the background) may be selected for after therapy getting amplified and repopulating the tumor.

2. THE INTERLEUKIN-6 SIGNALING PATHWAY

The human cytokine IL-6 is a 21-28 KDa glycoprotein consisting of 212 amino acids. It is encoded by the human *IL-6* gene, which is located at chromosome 7p21 (Akira, Taga & Kishimoto 1993). IL-6 behaves as a multifunctional hematopoietic cytokine tightly linked to inflammatory processes (Heinrich *et al.*, 2003). The IL-6 protein is normally synthesized and secreted by cells of the stroma/osteoblastic lineage, as well as by a wide range of unrelated cells and tissues (Bellido *et al.,* 1998; Kamimura & Hirano 2003). As a pleiotropic cytokine, IL-6 can activate target genes involved in apoptosis, survival, differentiation, and proliferation (Heinrich *et al.,* 2003). However, IL-6 functions, which are subject to strict regulatory mechanisms, are generally cell type- and context-specific. The versatility of IL-6 signaling can be understood by examining its canonical pathway, the JAK/STAT pathway, and its connections to other key signaling cascades such as the mitogen-activated protein kinase (MAPK) and the phosphatidylinositol 3-kinase (PI3K) pathways (Heinrich *et al.,* 2003). Fig. **3** illustrates the IL-6 pathway, particularly JAK/STAT and MAPK signaling, which are highly relevant to the topic covered in this chapter.

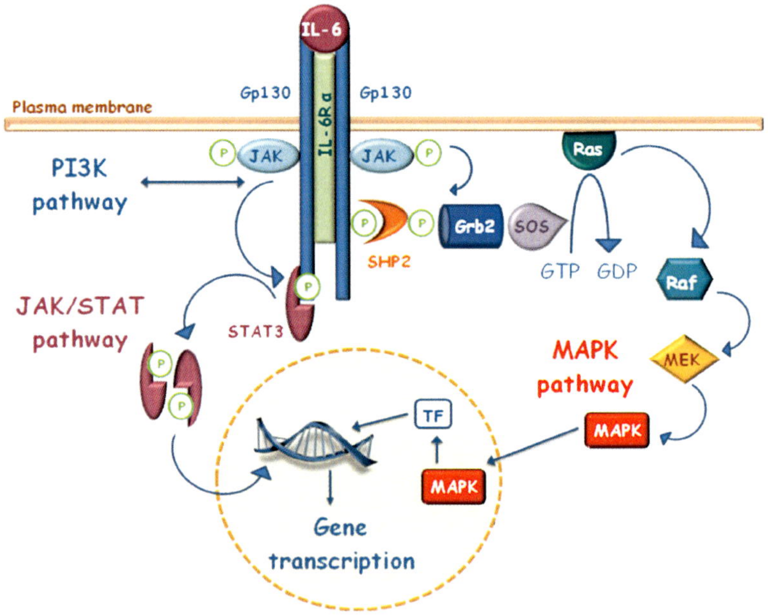

Figure 3: The interleukin-6 (IL-6) signaling pathway. IL-6 binds to the IL-6 receptor (IL-6R) complex activating the canonical JAK/STAT pathway (see text for full explanation). Alternatively, the gp130 subunit of the receptor provides connections to the MAPK and the PI3-K pathways.

IL-6 acts mainly *via* plasma membrane receptor complexes composed of the signal transducing subunit glycoprotein 130 (gp130) and a non-signaling α subunit (IL-6Rα) (Heinrich *et al.,* 2003). IL-6 binds to the IL-6Rα and then recruits two gp130 subunits, which form a homodimer. The gp130 homodimer in turn associates with, tyrosine phosphorylates, and activates janus kinases (JAK), especially JAK1 and JAK2. The activated JAKs phosphorylate and activate signal transducers and activators of transcription (STAT) family members STAT1, STAT5, and in particular, STAT3. STAT molecules can form homo or heterodimers and, in their active form, translocate to the nucleus, where they bind to the promoter of target genes activating their transcription (Heinrich *et al.,* 2003). In addition, gp130 provides a link to the MAPK and PI3K pathways (Grossmann, Huang & Tindall 2001; Heinrich *et al.,* 2003; Yang *et al.,* 2003). Often concealed in the shadows of the JAK/STAT pathway, the MAPK cascade plays a supreme role in the conquest of hormone resistance by IL-6 in prostate cancer. We will address this topic in greater detail throughout the chapter.

3. NEGATIVE REGULATION OF INTERLEUKIN-6 SIGNALING

Unrestrained cytokine signaling has the potential to disrupt cellular function. Thus, several compensatory mechanisms, most of them inherent to the IL-6 pathway, exist to modulate IL-6 signaling (Heinrich *et al.,* 2003). We briefly describe below, and portray on Fig. **4**, some of the mechanisms of negative regulation of the IL-6 pathway according to the molecules involved:

a. IL-6 cytokine: Modulation of IL-6 bioavailability can be accomplished by regulating the half-life of its mRNAs and by cytokine proteolysis (Heinrich *et al.,* 2003). p38 MAP kinase plays a key role in stabilizing short-lived IL-6 mRNAs by activating MAPK-activated protein kinase 2 (MK2 or MAPKAPK2) (Winzen *et al.,* 1999). The mature IL-6 protein is degraded *via* the proteasomal pathway.

b. IL-6 receptor: Upon cytokine binding, IL-6 receptors (IL-6Rs) internalize to prevent constitutive activation of the IL-6 pathway in target cells. In addition, the presence of soluble IL-6 receptors (sIL-6Rs) in the circulation may act like a buffer to equilibrate the response to IL-6 (Müller-Newen *et al.,* 1998).

c. SHPTP-2/SHP-2: An important event in IL-6 signaling is the phosphorylation of components of the signaling cascade. Thus, phosphatases must operate to prevent overstimulation and guarantee proper signal transmission (Heinrich *et al.,* 2003). SH2-domain-containing protein tyrosine phosphatase-2, or SHPTP-2/SHP-2, is a protein ubiquitously expressed in the cytoplasm that can work either as an adaptor or as a tyrosine phosphatase. As an adaptor, SHP-2 activates the MAPK cascade. However, as a phosphatase, SHP-2 negatively regulates the JAK/STAT pathway (Heinrich *et al.,* 2003). All tyrosine-phosphorylated components are potential substrates for the SHP-2 phosphatase (Heinrich *et al.,* 2003). *In vitro*, SHP-2 interacts with JAK1, JAK2 and TYK2, and is phosphorylated by JAK1 and JAK2 (Schaper *et al.,* 1998). STAT3 is a direct substrate of SHP-2 (Gunaje & Bhat 2001), while for STAT1, SHP-2 acts as a dual-specificity phosphatase (Wu *et al.,* 2002).

d. PIAS proteins: The protein inhibitors of activated STAT (PIAS) family encompasses five members in mammalians, which are important coregulators of the JAK/STAT pathway. PIAS3 specifically inhibits IL-6-induced STAT3-mediated gene expression (Chung *et al.,* 1997).

e. SOCS proteins: The suppressors of cytokine signaling (SOCS) family of classical feedback inhibitors consists of eight proteins. SOCS1 and SOCS3 are rapidly upregulated by IL-6 and inhibit cytokine signaling by acting on JAKs and abolishing the phosphorylation of gp130, STATs, and the JAKs themselves (Starr *et al.,* 1997). Although SOCS3 and SHP-2 are recruited to the same site within gp130, they downregulate the IL-6 pathway in a different manner (Lehmann *et al.,* 2003).

f. Half-life of other signaling components: Different components of the IL-6 pathway have distinctive half-lives. While SOCS1, SOCS2, and SOCS3 have very short lives, the half-life of JAK1, JAK2, TYK2, and gp130 is intermediate. However, STAT1, STAT3, and SHP2 have a slow turnover (Heinrich *et al.,* 2003).

g. Modulation through a cross-talk with other pathways: The canonical JAK/STAT pathway intersects with the MAPK and PI3K pathways. It is believed that the JAK/STAT and PI3K paths are mutually exclusive and, in some cases, an activated MAPK cascade inhibits JAK/STAT signaling (Sengupta *et al.,* 1998).

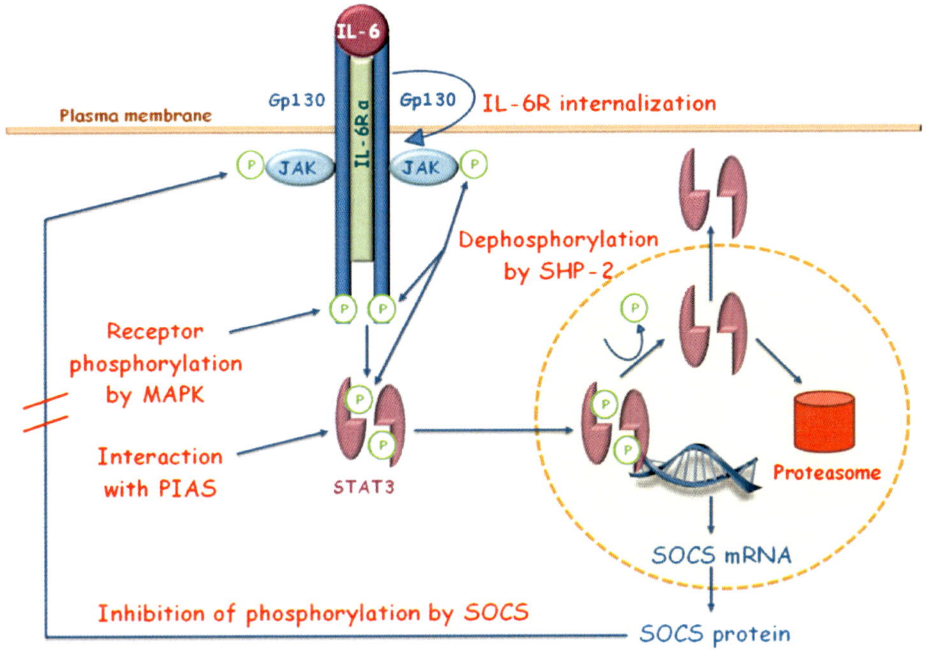

Figure 4: Negative regulation of the interleukin-6 (IL-6) signaling pathway. The IL-6 pathway can be modulated at several levels. For instance, the IL-6R is internalized upon cytokine binding to prevent overstimulation. SHP-2 dephosphorylates JAKs, gp130 and STAT3, while the MAP kinases phosphorylate the IL-6R. PIAS interact with activated STAT molecules and SOCS suppress cytokine signaling through the receptor by inhibiting its phosphorylation. Activated STAT molecules can also be dephosphorylated inside the nucleus and exported to the cytoplasm, or be degraded inside the proteasome. The different half-lives of mRNA and proteins of each element of the signaling pathway also play an important role in modulating the response to IL-6.

Though the IL-6 pathway could theoretically be interrupted at a few different levels, as described above, not every option may be feasible in the clinical practice. In this review, we will focus on an IL-6-targeting antibody that is currently in clinical trials, and part of the research findings backing its development, for the treatment of CRPC.

4. THE INTRICATE RELATIONSHIP BETWEEN INTERLEUKIN-6 AND THE PROSTATE

The first clue about a possible role for interleukin-6 in prostate cancer came from a study published twenty years ago (Siegall *et al.,* 1990). In their manuscript, Dr. Ira Pastan and coworkers described the presence of interleukin-6 receptor and the differential secretion of IL-6 in PCa cell lines. Four years later, they reported significant expression of IL-6R in all seventeen prostate carcinoma samples examined, suggesting that IL-6 might be involved in the growth of prostate tumors, and pointing to the IL-6R as a potential target for therapeutic intervention in PCa (Siegsmund, Yamazaki & Pastan 1994). A study of circulating IL-6 in seventy-three patients with CRPC prior to chemotherapy with suramin revealed that elevated IL-6 levels strongly correlate with PCa morbidity (Twillie *et al.,* 1995); based on their finding, the researchers proposed IL-6 as a candidate marker of PCa activity for prospective clinical testing (Twillie *et al.,* 1995).

The human prostate is a structured collection of glands organized into two well-differentiated compartments: the epithelium and the stroma. PCa takes place in the glandular epithelium. In earlier studies, the presence or absence of IL-6 and its receptors was reported in gross prostate specimens, without considering the specific cellular localization of these molecules. With the advent of modern techniques, it became possible to pinpoint the precise location of the cytokine and its receptors in both normal and diseased prostate. Thus, while in the normal prostate IL-6 expression was limited to basal epithelial cells (Hobisch *et al.,* 2000), the gp130 subunit from the IL-6R was confined to the stroma (Royuela *et al.,* 2004). However, expression of gp130 became widespread in both the epithelium and stroma of PCa tissue (Royuela *et al.,* 2004), and IL-6 in the epithelium (Hobisch *et al.,* 2000; Royuela *et al.,* 2004), confirming the development of autocrine and paracrine loops for IL-6 in carcinoma (Hobisch *et al.,* 2000). Hence, a clear distinction could be observed between healthy prostates and prostate cancer: whereas IL-6 signaling appeared to be missing in benign prostate epithelium, it really seemed to have spun out of control in prostatic carcinoma.

A great deal about the role of IL-6 in prostate cancer has been elucidated through a series of *in vitro* and *in vivo* experiments. Prostate tumors are highly heterogeneous and even research conducted with the same cellular model in separate laboratories sometimes yields conflicting results. This is probably due to differences in cell culture techniques, type of medium and additives used, passage number, and subtle variations in the genetic makeup of individual cell batches. Thus, for the purpose of clarity, we will not talk about all the literature available about IL-6 in PCa. Instead, we will try to explain how IL-6 may contribute to the progression towards CRPC based mainly on research conducted with a PCa model selected in the presence of IL-6. We would like to walk the readers through the story of LNCaP-IL-6+ cells, describing the alterations that make them closely resemble a group of castration-resistant prostate tumors. Groundwork on LNCaP-IL-6+ cells and xenograft models exposed some of the potential advantages and challenges of targeting IL-6 in CRPC. Again, the therapeutic potential of an anti-IL-6 antibody seems to be strongly determined by the specific makeup of target cells. Thus, we will compare the effects of an anti-IL-6 antibody, CNTO 328, in LNCaP-IL-6+ cells with those observed in other cellular/xenograft models. We would also like to discuss the results of clinical trials in which CNTO 328 was evaluated for the treatment of metastatic CRPC.

5. THE STORY OF LNCAP-IL-6+ CELLS: A MODEL OF ADVANCED CARCINOMA THAT MIRRORS LATE-STAGE PROSTATE CANCER IN PATIENTS

The LNCaP cell line, which was isolated from a lymph node metastasis in a prostate cancer patient (Horoszewicz *et al.,* 1980), represents a classical model for the study of prostatic carcinoma. LNCaP cells share similarities with early-stage PCa, such as a strong reliance on androgens to survive and proliferate (Horoszewicz *et al.,* 1983). Thus, they are androgen-dependent and express a functional, albeit mutated, AR (Tan *et al.,* 1997). LNCaP cells also express IL-6 receptors and respond to IL-6 in a paracrine manner, since they do not manufacture the cytokine themselves (Hobisch *et al.,* 1998). The first hint about the *modus operandi* of IL-6 in PCa came from studies performed over a decade ago at the University of Innsbruck, Austria. Dr. Hobisch and coworkers discovered that IL-6 was able to activate the AR and induce PSA expression, in a ligand-independent manner, in LNCaP cells (Hobisch *et al.,* 1998). Ligand-independent activation of the AR by IL-6 was abolished by the anti-androgen bicalutamide, confirming the involvement of the AR pathway. Hence, upon a short treatment with IL-6, both the AR and the IL-6 signaling pathways were activated through a pathway cross-talk (Hobisch *et al.,* 1998).

As stated before, IL-6 protein expression is elevated in prostate tumors (Hobisch *et al.,* 2000; Royuela *et al.,* 2004) and circulating IL-6 levels are higher in patients with metastatic carcinoma (Twillie *et al.,* 1995). Thus, enhanced serum IL-6 levels usually constitute a hallmark of advanced prostate cancer. A reason behind that rise may be that PCa occurs in elderly men and androgen levels decline with aging (Harman *et al.,* 2001); as androgens repress the expression of IL-6 (Keller, Chang & Ershler 1996), if androgen production diminishes IL-6 expression soars. Such hormone-cytokine interplay probably carries more weight in patients with advanced PCa treated with hormone ablation, which would lead to a greater rebound in IL-6 production.

In order to understand the behavior of prostate cancer cells in an IL-6-rich environment "around the clock", the LNCaP cell line was utilized once more. LNCaP cells with similar passage number were divided into two experimental conditions: while some cells were grown in regular growth medium, others were cultured in medium supplemented with 5 ng/ml exogenous IL-6 for several months (Hobisch *et al.,* 2001). After 20 passages, cells continuously grown in the presence of IL-6 had already acquired a different phenotype and constituted a distinct cell line. Interestingly, the longer they were nurtured with IL-6, the more pronounced and opposing their phenotype became from that of control cells growing in standard medium. Control cells, which were identical to parental LNCaP cells, were named LNCaP-IL-6- cells, whereas the ones constantly exposed to IL-6 were baptized as LNCaP-IL-6+ cells (Hobisch *et al.,* 2001).

LNCaP-IL-6+ cells acquired a significant growth advantage compared to control cells and, unlike them, secreted IL-6. Higher passages of LNCaP-IL-6+ cells produced larger amounts of the cytokine. Hence, prolonged exposure of LNCaP cells to IL-6 led to the development of an autocrine loop for IL-6 and the emergence of this new cell line (Hobisch *et al.,* 2001).

Since control cells did not express IL-6 and behaved so differently from IL-6-expressing LNCaP cells, it become important to assess their individual response to the cytokine. Thus, both cell lines were treated for a short period of time with IL-6. The discrepancy in cytokine response between the two cellular models was evident. Whereas exogenous IL-6 inhibited the growth of controls, it did not affect the proliferation of LNCaP-IL-6+ cells (Hobisch *et al.,* 2001). Dissecting the molecular mechanisms behind the different reactions also revealed striking dissimilarities. In control cells, IL-6 activated the IL-6R and downstream signaling *via* the classical JAK/STAT pathway, which resulted in phosphorylation and activation of STAT3 (Steiner *et al.,* 2003). Activated STAT3 has been reported to translocate to the nucleus, associate with the AR in an IL-6-dependent, but androgen-independent mode, and activate the transcription of AR target genes in LNCaP cells (Ueda, Bruchovsky & Sadar 2002). Ligand-independent activation of the AR by IL-6 in controls primarily led to increased PSA secretion and growth arrest, which could be reversed with the help of antiandrogens (Hobisch *et al.,* 2001). Furthermore, this activation was enhanced in the presence of androgen. In summary, short-term treatment of LNCaP-IL-6- cells with IL-6 halts cellular proliferation (Hobisch *et al.,* 2001) by preferentially stimulating the JAK/STAT pathway (Steiner *et al.,* 2003) and results in AR-induced gene transcription (Hobisch *et al.,* 2001). Hence, IL-6 acts as a paracrine growth inhibitor in LNCaP-IL-6- cells (Hobisch *et al.,* 2001).

On the other hand, LNCaP-IL-6+ cells shortly treated with exogenous IL-6 suffered from impaired binding of the cytokine to its receptor and, as a result, became partially resistant to IL-6 (Hobisch *et al.,* 2001). Thus, IL-6 was unable to phosphorylate and activate STAT3 in LNCaP-IL-6+ cells. This was in stark contrast with the strong activation of STAT3 achieved in control cells (Steiner *et al.* 2003). We must remember that, in LNCaP-IL-6+ cells, unrelenting exposure to IL-6 had resulted in endogenous secretion of IL-6 and the formation of an autocrine loop for the cytokine (Hobisch *et al.,* 2001). We hypothesized that the IL-6R must have been overwhelmed by the constant influx of IL-6 and become desensitized to further stimulation by the cytokine (Fisher *et al.,* 2004; Godoy-Tundidor 2004). Subsequent analysis of the IL-6 signaling pathway revealed that suppressor of cytokine signaling 3 (SOCS3), a negative feedback regulator of the

JAK/STAT pathway, was upregulated in LNCaP-IL-6+ cells but not in control cells (Puhr *et al.,* 2009). SOCS3 is expressed in prostate cancer and its expression is inversely correlated with that of phospho-STAT3 (Bellezza *et al.,* 2006). Taken together, the lack of phospho-STAT3 and the overexpression of SOCS3 clearly indicate inhibition of the JAK/STAT pathway both in LNCaP-IL-6+ cells and in PCa patients (Bellezza *et al.,* 2006).

Interestingly, ERK1/2 was constitutively expressed in LNCaP-IL-6+ cells and did not respond to additional challenge with IL-6 (Steiner *et al.,* 2003). ERK1/2 overexpression was associated with increased cellular proliferation in this cell model. The MAPK inhibitor PD98059 was able to reduce proliferation only in LNCaP-IL-6+ cells, leaving LNCaP-IL-6- cells unaffected (Steiner *et al.,* 2003). Of importance, MAPK activation has been linked to prostate cancer progression (Gioeli *et al.,* 1999). The levels of activated ERK1/2 increased with increasing tumor stage and Gleason score in PCa patients (Gioeli *et al.,* 1999). Moreover, MAPK activity was elevated in tumor samples from two patients after, but not before, androgen ablation therapy in recurrent tumors (Gioeli *et al.,* 1999).

In addition, LNCaP-IL-6+ cells secreted twenty times more vascular endothelial growth factor (VEGF) than control cells and upregulated expression of the VEGF receptor (VEGFR) Flk-1 (Steiner *et al.,* 2004). Thus, a powerful autocrine loop for VEGF also developed in LNCaP-IL-6+ cells. As VEGF signaling impinges on MAPK signaling, the autocrine loop for VEGF may have equally played a role in the upregulation of the MAPK pathway. It is believed that the conversion from paracrine to autocrine loops in growth factor production and signaling leads to persistent stimulation of the Ras pathway enabling transition to an androgen-independent state (Gioeli *et al.,* 1999). This hypothesis may explain the process taking place in LNCaP-IL-6+ cells, in which autocrine loops for IL-6 and VEGF develop. Enhanced expression of VEGF, a key molecule in the formation of new blood vessels, is also prevalent in advanced tumors (George *et al.,* 2001) and facilitates the metastatic process. Plasma VEGF levels inversely correlate with survival in metastatic CRPC and may be useful as a marker of tumor angiogenesis (George *et al.,* 2001).

Other major alterations occurring in LNCaP-IL-6+ cells included the loss of retinoblastoma (Rb) protein expression, which was abundantly expressed in control cells (Steiner *et al.,* 2003). Under normal circumstances, the Rb tumor suppressor can be found in two different configurations: hypo- or hyper-phosphorylated. In the hypophosphorylated form, Rb associates with the transcription factor E2F and works as a cellular brake, preventing entry into the cell cycle and eliciting growth arrest. However, when Rb is hyperphosphorylated, free E2F promotes cell cycle progression and proliferation. Thus, loss of Rb must have dramatically contributed to the uncontrolled proliferation, and progression towards androgen independence, of LNCaP-IL-6+ cells (Steiner *et al.,* 2003). Later research by other groups in Rb-depleted PCa cells demonstrated that Rb loss results in unchecked AR activity (Sharma *et al.,* 2010). Moreover, Rb loss in human PCa samples was mostly linked with progression to CRPC and the lack of Rb function was associated with poor clinical outcome (Sharma *et al.,* 2010).

One of the most interesting discoveries, though, was that late passages (80 and higher) of LNCaP-IL-6+ cells had reduced levels of AR mRNA and lacked AR protein expression (Debes *et al.,* 2005). In these "old" cells, IL-6 stimulated the expression of AR target genes, among them PSA, by enhancing the expression of the coactivator p300 (Debes *et al.,* 2005). The AR may eventually not be needed anymore to sustain tumor growth, since the proliferative machinery gets turned on by other molecules. Androgen receptor loss has also been reported in metastatic prostate cancer (Kinoshita *et al.,* 2000; Shah, Mehra & Chinnaiyan 2004). In a rapid autopsy study of androgen-independent prostate cancer metastases, AR expression was heterogeneous, as confirmed by the presence of AR-positive and AR-negative tumor populations, not only between patients but also within the same patient (Shah, Mehra & Chinnaiyan 2004). In that study, overall AR expression was downregulated in CRPC since 41.5% of tumor samples expressed less than 10% AR protein (Shah, Mehra & Chinnaiyan 2004). PSA expression, which was highly variable too, did not correlate with AR expression, suggesting that non-AR-mediated mechanisms might account for PSA expression in certain tumors (Shah, Mehra & Chinnaiyan 2004). Thus, the AR loss and AR-independent expression of PSA observed in LNCaP-IL-6+ cells is consistent with the behavior of AR-negative tumors in CRPC.

Moreover, in AR-negative LNCaP-IL-6+ cells, the antiapoptotic protein myeloid cell leukemia-1 (Mcl-1) was upregulated (Cavarretta *et al.,* 2007). This was in line with the overexpression of Mcl-1 observed in prostate cancer compared with benign prostate and, particularly, in advanced tumors (Krajewska *et al.,* 1996). Mcl-1 was expressed in almost 52 of 64 (81%) prostate tumor samples and nearly 9 of 24 (38%) PIN lesions (Krajewska *et al.,* 1996). Besides, the percentage of Mcl-1-positive cells was higher in metastases and tumors with high Gleason scores than in PIN and tumors with lower Gleasons (Krajewska *et al.,* 1996).

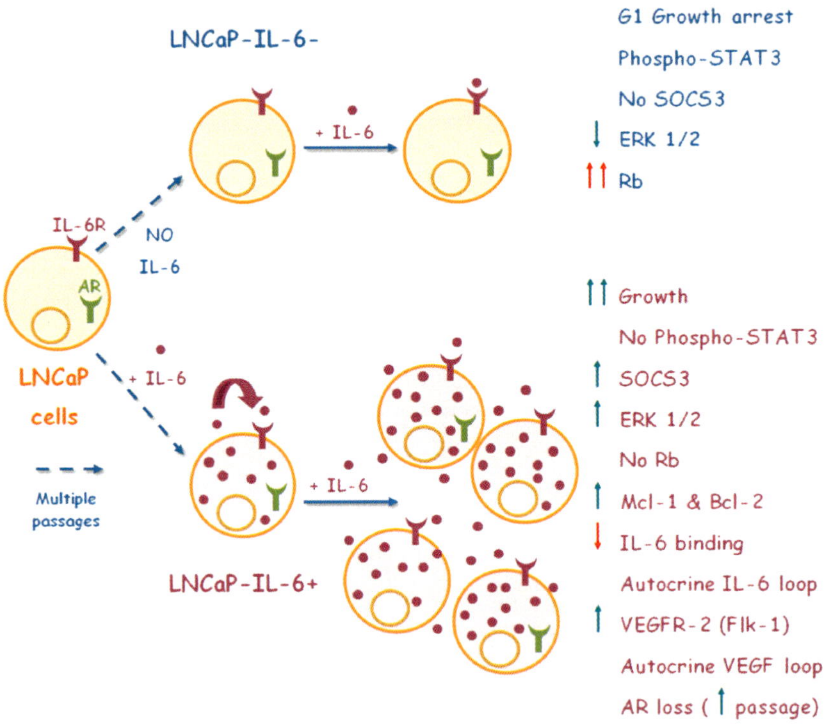

Figure 5: Interleukin-6 (IL-6) switches from paracrine growth inhibitor to autocrine growth stimulator in prostate cancer (PCa) cells. Chronic exposure to IL-6 in LNCaP cells leads to the generation of a new cell line, LNCaP-IL-6+ (lower panel), with multiple alterations consistent with those observed in castration-resistant prostate cancer (CRPC). The main differences between both cell lines are summarized in the figure.

In summary, the autocrine loop for IL-6 accelerated proliferation by abolishing Rb expression and enhancing MAPK expression (Steiner *et al.,* 2003), and circumvented apoptosis by upregulating Mcl-1 in LNCaP-IL-6+ cells (Cavarretta *et al.,* 2007). The development of a VEGF autocrine loop may have been critical in boosting the MAPK pathway in detriment of JAK/STAT signaling. Significantly, the growth arrest observed in LNCaP-IL6- cells, and the enhanced proliferation in LNCaP-IL-6+ cells, were further confirmed in their xenograft model counterparts; LNCaP-IL-6+ cells developed larger tumors than control cells when inoculated into nude mice, demonstrating a more aggressive phenotype (Steiner *et al.,* 2003). Thus, all these findings proved that IL-6 can switch from being a paracrine growth inhibitor acting *via* the JAK/STAT pathway in LNCaP-IL-6- cells, to an autocrine growth stimulator through upregulation of MAPK signaling in LNCaP-IL-6+ cells (Steiner *et al.,* 2003). The phenotypic changes fueled by IL-6 in prostate cancer are clearly implicated in the progression towards CRPC. Fig. **5** represents the alterations occurring in LNCaP cells under constant pressure from IL-6.

The major lesson we can learn from this PCa model is that there is a time and place for everything in cancer biology. Thus, when it comes to location, having an in-house factory for IL-6 in LNCaP-IL-6+ cells made all the difference between being in a quiescent state and achieving full-blown proliferation. However, without the correct timing, represented by continuous exposure to IL-6, the autocrine loop for IL-6 would have not occurred either. Time is essential also in that there might be a point of no return, after certain events have taken place, in a biological setting. In this case, the moment LNCaP-IL-6+ cells developed autocrine loops for IL-6 and VEGF, lost Rb expression, and upregulated MAPK and Mcl-1, might have pushed them through a boundary they may have been unable to cross back without therapeutic intervention. For this purpose, laboratory research continued in an effort to curtail IL-6's ability to sustain the survival and proliferation of LNCaP-IL-6+ cells.

6. TARGETING THE INTERLEUKIN-6 PATHWAY IN LNCAP-IL-6+ CELLS WITH CNTO 328

CNTO 328, also known as cCLB8 and siltuximab, is a human-mouse chimeric monoclonal antibody directed against human IL-6 (Zaki, Nemeth & Trikha 2004). It was engineered from a murine anti-human IL-6 antibody, CLB8 (Brakenhoff *et al.* 1990), to express a human Fc fragment at Centocor, Inc. (Zaki, Nemeth &

Trikha 2004). CNTO 328 binds to IL-6 with a Kd ~ 10^{-12} M and prevents IL-6 signaling through its receptors (Zaki, Nemeth & Trikha 2004). Besides prostate cancer, clinical trials are being conducted with siltuximab in a variety of cancer types and other illnesses such as Castleman's Disease (<http://clinicaltrials.gov/ct2/results?term=CNTO+328> 1 February 2011).

Within prostate cancer, the chimeric anti-IL-6 antibody exerts somewhat different responses depending on the specific cancer model. For instance, CNTO 328 inhibited cancer-associated cachexia in PC-3M PCa xenografts in nude mice, without impacting tumor growth (Zaki, Nemeth & Trikha 2004). On the other hand, CNTO 328 increased survival, abolished tumor growth, and reduced PSA levels in mice bearing the human androgen-dependent prostate cancer xenograft LuCaP 35 (Wallner *et al.,* 2006). CNTO 328, but not isotype control antibody, blocked the conversion of LuCaP 35 cells and tumor xenografts, upon androgen ablation and orchiectomy, respectively, from an androgen-dependent to an androgen-independent state (Wallner *et al.,* 2006). IL-6 inhibition stimulated apoptosis, inhibited cell growth, and halted expression of CBP and p300 coactivators in tumors from castrated animals (Wallner *et al.,* 2006). Similarly, the murine anti-human IL-6 antibody CLB8 (not the chimeric antibody CNTO 328) elicited apoptosis and a 60% reduction in tumor size in PC-3 xenografts (Smith & Keller 2001). Thus, since prostate tumors are highly heterogeneous, it is important to understand the mode of action of CNTO 328 across different experimental models. Such understanding will aid in the selection of target patient populations that may benefit from CNTO 328 therapy.

We have followed in this chapter the IL-6-triggered conversion of LNCaP cells from an androgen-dependent to a castration-resistant phenotype, which closely recapitulates the evolution of a cluster of tumors in patients with late-stage prostate cancer. The next step was to test whether disruption of IL-6 signaling by this anti-IL-6 antibody could revert the phenotype to a less aggressive one, or at least paralyze tumor growth. We will review here the key findings on the effect of CNTO 328 in LNCaP-IL-6+ cells and xenografts (Steiner *et al.,* 2006; Cavarretta *et al.,* 2007).

As reported earlier, IL-6 has the ability to induce apoptosis in control LNCaP-IL-6- cells, but not in LNCaP-IL-6+ cells (Cavarretta *et al.,* 2007). After a six-day treatment, 10 μg/ml CNTO 328 significantly reduced the viability of LNCaP-IL-6+ cells accompanied by a 30% decrease in the amount of the antiapoptotic protein Bcl-2, while having no effect on control cells (Steiner *et al.,* 2006). IL-6-overexpressing LNCaP cells usually express more Bcl-2 protein than controls but, in contrast, do not express the proapoptotic protein Bax. Such increased Bcl-2/Bax ratio strongly favors the survival of LNCaP-IL-6+ cells (Steiner *et al.,* 2006).

Neither endogenously secreted, nor exogenously added IL-6 could phosphorylate STAT3 in LNCaP-IL-6+ cells (Steiner *et al.,* 2003). Their deficient response to IL-6 was attributed to desensitization of IL-6 receptors unable to cope with overwhelming quantities of IL-6 (Fisher *et al.,* 2004; Godoy-Tundidor 2004), as well as to overexpression of SOCS3. Again, CNTO 328 was able to resensitize LNCaP-IL-6+ cells to the action of exogenous IL-6 (Steiner *et al.,* 2006). In particular, addition of 10 ng/ml IL-6 for 20 minutes in LNCaP-IL-6+ cells pre-treated with 5 μg/ml CNTO 328 increased STAT3 phosphorylation compared to cells pre-treated with control human immunoglobulin G (hIgG). Furthermore, pre-treatment with 10 μg/ml CNTO 328, but not with hIgG, decreased the ratio between phosphorylated and total (phosphorylated plus non-phosphorylated) ERK1/2 by 30% (Steiner *et al.,* 2006). Though IL-6R and SOCS3 expression were not assessed in response to CNTO 328, it seems that blocking superfluous IL-6 allowed the IL-6R to become resensitized to cytokine action. Thus, IL-6-overexpressing LNCaP cells responded to CNTO 328, which was able to reduce the activity of endogenous IL-6 (Steiner *et al.,* 2006).

In order to assess the response to CNTO 328 *in vivo,* experiments were conducted using LNCaP-IL-6+ xenografts (Steiner *et al.,* 2006). IL-6-overexpressing tumors were able to grow after castration, confirming their androgen-independent nature. Therapy with the anti-IL-6 antibody began after orchiectomy and experiments were performed until day 40. In two independent experiments, the mean weekly tumor volumes in mice treated with the antibody were lower than in control-treated animals. In parallel, tumors grew more in controls than in CNTO 328-treated mice. Although not statistically significant, there was a trend towards a reduction in tumor volume and a decrease in tumor growth in antibody-treated mice. Despite these results, the proliferative index, Ki67, was significantly lower in CNTO 328-treated animals. No difference between control and treated animals could be observed either in tumor VEGF or tumor-secreted VEGF serum levels (Steiner *et al.,* 2006).

Hence, CNTO 328 seemed to function mainly by resensitizing IL-6-overexpressing cells to IL-6 action *via* the JAK/STAT pathway, and improving their response to apoptosis (Steiner *et al.,* 2006). Small, non-significant changes were observed in tumor growth. Whether those changes could be amplified by modifying the experimental setup, for example using other concentrations of CNTO 328 or administering it at different time points, is an open question.

Some prostate carcinomas lose androgen receptor expression (Kinoshita *et al.,* 2000; Shah, Mehra & Chinnaiyan 2004). We have previously stated that late passages of LNCaP-IL-6+ cells lack AR protein (Debes *et al.,* 2005). Since AR loss is more frequent in late-stage, aggressive tumors (Kinoshita *et al.,* 2000; Shah, Mehra & Chinnaiyan 2004), AR deficiency could have a great impact in response to therapy. In an attempt to explore the mechanism of action of CNTO 328 in AR-negative tumors, "old" LNCaP-IL-6+ cells missing the AR were chosen for further studies (Cavarretta *et al.,* 2007). AR-negative LNCaP-IL-6+ cells showed enhanced resistance to IL-6-induced apoptosis, as well as to other proapoptotic stimuli, compared to LNCaP-IL-6- cells (Cavarretta *et al.,* 2007).

The next step was to determine if neutralization of endogenous IL-6 could reverse the resistance of AR-null LNCaP-IL-6+ cells to apoptosis (Cavarretta *et al.,* 2007). Thus, both IL-6-producing and control cells were treated with 10 μg/ml CNTO 328, in androgen-deprived conditions, for four days. Essentially, IL-6-overexpressing cells underwent apoptosis while control cells were not affected by the anti-IL-6 antibody. The amount of caspase-cleaved cytokeratin 18 (CK18) released from LNCaP-IL-6+ cells was 30% higher than that from hIgG-treated cells, demonstrating that CNTO 328 was able to sensitize AR-void LNCaP-IL-6+ cells to programmed cell death (Cavarretta *et al.,* 2007).

As cited earlier, the autocrine loop for IL-6 resulted in increased levels of the antiapoptotic protein Mcl-1 (Cavarretta *et al.,* 2007). AR-negative LNCaP-IL-6+ cells expressed twice as much Mcl-1 as controls, which could be downregulated by an Mcl-1-specific siRNA increasing apoptosis by 60% only in LNCaP-IL-6+ cells. Moreover, 10 μg/ml CNTO 328 reduced Mcl-1 expression by 40%, in IL-6-manufacturing cells, after six days. However, in Mcl-1-negative cells, CNTO 328 could not further enhance apoptosis, implying that endogenous IL-6 sustains cell survival and confers apoptotic resilience *via* Mcl-1 upregulation (Cavarretta *et al.,* 2007).

Constitutive activation of the classical MAP kinases, ERK1/ERK2, could also be downregulated by CNTO 328 in AR-deficient IL-6+ cells (Cavarretta *et al.,* 2007). In order to study a possible relationship between the MAPK pathway and Mcl-1 expression, the MAPK inhibitor PD 98059 was used. PD 98059 was able to diminish phospho-ERK1/2 expression in both control and AR-negative IL-6-expressing cells, but Mcl-1 was decreased only in AR-negative LNCaP-IL-6+ cells. Thus, the MAPK cascade was involved in upregulation of Mcl-1 by endogenous IL-6 (Cavarretta *et al.,* 2007). This conclusion was further supported by the fact that Mcl-1 levels increased in control cells after IL-6-induced activation of ERK1/2 (Cavarretta *et al.,* 2007).

In summary, the anti-IL-6 antibody CNTO 328 modulates the IL-6 pathway at several levels in IL-6-overexpressing cells *in vitro* (Steiner *et al.,* 2006; Cavarretta *et al.,* 2007). CNTO 328 binds to excess IL-6 allowing resensitization of the IL-6R to the cytokine, rerouting of available IL-6 through the JAK/STAT pathway, reduction in MAPK signaling, downregulation of the antiapoptotic proteins Mcl-1 and Bcl-2, and increased apoptosis (Steiner *et al.,* 2004; Cavarretta *et al.,* 2007). Still, CNTO 328 was not able to reduce tumor volume in mice bearing LNCaP-IL-6+ xenografts, though cell proliferation was significantly downregulated. Interestingly, the ineffectiveness of CNTO 328 on tumor growth had also been observed in PC-3M xenografts (Zaki, Nemeth & Trikha 2004). PC-3M cells were isolated from liver metastases (Kozlowski *et al.,* 1984) of PC-3 cells injected into the spleen of nude mice, and may have been more aggressive than parental PC-3. This was in contrast with the evident reduction in tumor growth achieved by CNTO 328 in LuCaP 35 cells (Wallner *et al.,* 2006). However, while LuCaP cells were still androgen-dependent, LNCaP-IL-6+ cells represented a model of androgen-independent, therapy-resistant cancer with multiple alterations. Since multiple mechanisms may be involved in the progression to CRPC, therapy with an anti-IL-6 antibody may not suffice to halt tumor growth in LNCaP-IL-6+ cells. Here we have described how IL-6 impinges upon, at least, two of such mechanisms: ligand-independent activation of the AR and enhanced expression of antiapoptotic proteins. Yet, the results from these different PCa models (Zaki, Nemeth & Trikha 2004; Wallner *et al.,* 2006; Steiner *et al.,* 2006; Cavarretta *et al.,* 2007) were encouraging enough to conduct clinical trials with CNTO 328 in patients with CRPC. In the next section, we will review the latest results from trials with the anti-IL-6 antibody in prostate cancer.

7. RESULTS FROM CLINICAL TRIALS WITH CNTO 328 IN PATIENTS WITH METASTATIC CASTRATION-RESISTANT PROSTATE CANCER

Until January 2011, three interventional clinical trials for CNTO 328 in patients with metastatic hormone-refractory prostate cancer had been registered at the ClinicalTrials.gov site of the NIH (<http://www.clinicaltrials.gov/ct2/results?term=CNTO+328+and+prostate+cancer> 1 February 2011), including a Phase I and two Phase II studies. One of the Phase II trials comparing CNTO 328 in combination with mitoxantrone *vs.* mitoxantrone alone, with ID NCT00385827, was terminated during the enrollment period, when an interim analysis showed more fatalities in the combined treatment (<http://clinicaltrials.gov/ct2/show/NCT00385827?term=CNTO+328+and+prostate+cancer&rank=2> 1 February 2011). Failure of that trial was attributed to biases in the study design and execution during its presentation at the 2010 Genitourinary Cancers Symposium (GUC) of the American Society for Clinical Oncology (ASCO) (<http://www.asco.org/ASCOv2/Meetings/Abstracts?&vmview=abst_detail_view&confID=73&abstractID=30763> 1 February 2011).

Results have also been presented, to a certain extent, about the other two trials. The first trial, *A Phase I Study of a Chimeric Antibody Against Interleukin-6 (CNTO 328) Combined With Docetaxel in Subjects With Metastatic Hormone-Refractory Prostate Cancer*, with ID NCT00401765, was designed to assess the safety and tolerability of multiple dosing regimens of CNTO 328 administered in combination with docetaxel, the efficacy and pharmacodynamics (PD) of the antibody plus docetaxel, and the pharmacokinetics (PK) of docetaxel and CNTO 328 (<http://www.clinicaltrials.gov/ct2/show/NCT00401765?term=CNTO+328+and+prostate+cancer&rank=1> 1 February 2011). Results for this trial were presented at the 2009 GUC Symposium (<http://www.asco.org/ASCOv2/Meetings/Abstracts?&vmview=abst_detail_view&confID=64&abstractID=20244> 1 February 2011). Briefly, chemotherapy-naïve patients with metastatic CRPC were given a run-in cycle of docetaxel followed by CNTO 328 in three dose-escalation groups (6 mg/kg q2w -each 2 weeks -, and 9 and 12 mg/kg q3w) in combination with 75 mg/m^2 q3w docetaxel. Thirty-three patients were treated with docetaxel and twenty-nine with CNTO 328 plus docetaxel. In each group, one case of dose limiting toxicity (DLT) was observed, and the maximum tolerated dose (MTD) for the combined therapy was not reached. There were no deaths related to treatment, and the combination regimen was in general well tolerated with the most frequent ≥ grade 3 adverse events being hematological (neutropenia, 69%; leukopenia, 62%; and lymphopenia, 31%). Twenty-one (72%) of the twenty-nine patients treated with the anti-IL-6 antibody had a decline in PSA ≥ 30% within three months. Sixteen (55%) patients had confirmed PSA responses ≥ 50%, and twenty-one subjects had unconfirmed reductions in PSA between ≥ 75% and ≥ 90%. In twenty-eight patients with detectable C-reactive protein (CRP) levels, this marker for IL-6 activity could not be detected after therapy. The study concluded that the combination therapy was safe, with proven biological and anti-tumor effects in CRPC patients, and merited further study (<http://www.asco.org/ASCOv2/Meetings/Abstracts?&vmview=abst_detail_view&confID=64&abstractID=20244> 1 February 2011).

In the second trial, *A Phase II Study of CNTO 328, A Monoclonal Antibody Against Interleukin-6 (IL-6), in Patients With Hormone Refractory Prostate Cancer*, with ID NCT00433446, patients received only the biologic therapy consisting of the chimeric anti-IL-6 antibody (<http://clinicaltrials.gov/ct2/show/NCT00433446?term=CNTO+328+and+prostate+cancer&rank=3>1February 2011). The primary goal of this Phase II study was to confirm the PSA response rate (50% reduction) in taxane-refractory CRPC patients treated with CNTO 328. The secondary goals were to assess overall survival (OS), progression-free survival (PFS), and objective response rate (confirmed and unconfirmed; complete response, CR; and partial response, PR) in treated patients with measurable disease, as well as to assess the quantitative and qualitative toxicities of the regimen (<http://clinicaltrials.gov/ct2/show/NCT00433446?term=CNTO+328+and+prostate+cancer&rank=3> 1 February 2011). Fifty-three patients who had been previously treated with taxanes were eligible for the study (Dorff *et al.,* 2010). Fifty-two of them received a median of four cycles and only one patient completed twelve rounds of treatment. There were two cases of grade 4 toxicity (one instance of cerebral ischemia and another of disseminated intravascular coagulation) and ten cases of grade 3 toxicity (Dorff *et al.,* 2010). Two patients had an overall PSA response rate of 3.8% (95% CI, 0.5-13%). Among thirty-one patients with measurable disease, none had a RECIST (Response Evaluation Criteria in Solid Tumors) response, but seven had stable disease. The median PFS was 1.6 months (95% CI, 1.6-1.7) and median OS 11.6 months (95% CI, 7.5-19.0) after a median follow-up of 14.8 months (Dorff *et al.,* 2010).

Several surrogate markers were correlatively measured at baseline and after treatment with CNTO 328 (Dorff *et al.,* 2010). The list of markers included, among others, molecules related to the IL-6 pathway (IL-6, sgp130, and CRP) and the neuroendocrine markers neuron-specific enolase (NSE) and Chromogranin A (ChrA). Soluble gp130 levels slightly rose after treatment and enhanced OS significantly correlated with baseline sgp130 levels above the median (Dorff *et al.,* 2010). High levels of sgp130 are desirable because sgp130 binds to IL-6 and prevents IL-6 signaling (Müller-Newen *et al.,* 1998). C-reactive protein, whose gene is a target of IL-6, was reduced after CNTO 328 treatment. In particular, CRP plasma levels declined in thirty-two of thirty-eight patients at six weeks, indicating biological activity of the anti-IL-6 antibody (Dorff *et al.,* 2010).

Yet, the most impressive change was that detected in IL-6. Though it is unclear why, IL-6 blood levels sky-rocketed over 400-fold after treatment, from a median baseline of 12.5 pg/mL (range: 1.6-33.0) to 4,831 pg/mL (range: 3,450-8,637) (Dorff *et al.,* 2010). Patients with baseline IL-6 levels above 12.5 pg/mL had a significantly shorter OS than those with baseline values below 12.5 pg/mL (53% *vs.* 94%, respectively; $p = 0.02$) (Dorff *et al.,* 2010). It is important to remember that these patients had already failed therapy with taxanes. In an earlier study, serum IL-6 levels higher than 16 mg/mL predicted resistance to docetaxel in

CRPC patients and pretreatment IL-6 levels correlated with PSA response (Domingo-Domenech *et al.,* 2006). Similarly, IL-6 levels predicted chemotherapy resistance in androgen-independent prostate cancer patients with bone metastases; while overall IL-6 levels decreased by 35% in PSA responders, IL-6 increased by 76% in non-responders (p = 0.03) (Ignatoski *et al.,* 2009). Thus, it may be crucial to determine serum IL-6 levels in patients with advanced PCa early in the equation treatment, and attempt to reduce such levels soon enough to prevent the appearance of chemotherapy resistance.

Dexamethasone has been shown to decrease IL-6 levels (Ray, LaForge & Sehgal 1990). In the Phase I trial comparing docetaxel alone with CNTO 328 plus docetaxel in chemotherapy-naïve patients, all patients received an infusion of 75 mg/m^2 docetaxel on week 1 of every cycle. Dexamethasone was also administered 12 hours, 3 hours, and 1 hour before the beginning of every docetaxel infusion through cycle 3, allowing doctors to decide how dexamethasone should be taken afterwards. The data from this trial showed that CNTO 328 plus docetaxel was superior to taxane alone in this group of patients. IL-6 levels were not mentioned in the study, but IL-6 activity was clearly reduced since the levels of the IL-6-induced protein CRP became undetectable in twenty-eight patients after treatment. Perhaps the addition of dexamethasone and the inclusion of the anti-IL-6 antibody improved the sensitivity of cancer cells to docetaxel by decreasing IL-6 levels and hindering IL-6 signaling, respectively. We cannot predict yet if the combined regimen will be effective in a Phase II trial, since the Phase II study we have mentioned evaluated only siltuximab as a second-line therapy in taxane-refractory patients. Overall the latter trial was dealing with a population more difficult to treat and following a different treatment plan. Thus, taxane-resistant CRPC patients did not receive premedication, as opposed to patients enrolled in the Phase I trial. In addition, they were treated with only one dose of antibody, 6 mg/kg, for a maximum of 12 cycles instead of 17. Hence, these patients seemed to receive less antibody than the ones in the Phase I study, even though they were already resistant to chemotherapy. We would anticipate that this "lighter" regimen with CNTO 328 may not be sufficient to elicit a strong response in chemotherapy-resistant patients with more aggressive tumors, as compared to CRPC patients not previously exposed to chemotherapy. This has already been observed in animal models bearing "belligerent" tumors, in which CNTO 328 had some effect but failed to halt tumor growth (Zaki, Nemeth & Trikha 2004; Steiner *et al.,* 2006). Still, CNTO 328 was well tolerated and exerted biological activity, albeit not a clinical response, in taxane-refractory CRPC patients (Dorff *et al.,* 2010).

Taken together, CNTO 328 has proven to be safe in both chemotherapy-naïve (<http://www.asco.org/ASCOv2/Meetings/Abstracts?&vmview=abst_detail_view &confID=64&abstractID=20244> 1 February 2011) and chemotherapy-resistant (Dorff *et al.,* 2010) patients with metastatic castration-resistant prostate cancer. CNTO 328 was able to diminish IL-6 signaling in both groups of patients, although it only showed clinical efficacy in chemotherapy-naïve patients treated also with docetaxel. The results from the Phase I trial really encourage further studies with the combined treatment in a similar cohort of patients. As for CNTO 328 as sole therapy, we do not have data to assess whether it would be a good option for chemotherapy-naïve patients, but it seems that it may not be sufficient to stop taxane-refractory tumors at least unless different doses/administration schedules are used. However, we cannot exclude the possibility that siltuximab could benefit taxane-resistant patients, in combination with other agents. In the meanwhile, and provided that elevated levels of IL-6 increase the risk of developing resistance to chemotherapy (Domingo-Domenech *et al.,* 2006; Ignatoski *et al.,* 2009), it may be a good idea to investigate whether siltuximab could be used in patients before the development of castration-resistant prostate cancer.

8. FINAL DISCUSSION

Due to its extraordinary heterogeneity, metastatic CRPC has been defined as a group of diseases even within the same patient, in which metastases from different sites often have distinct phenotypes and genotypes (Shah, Mehra & Chinnaiyan 2004). For example, median PSA expression ranged from 3.03% in the prostate to 60.61% in the bone of one patient with CRPC. Besides, PSA expression was highly variable within the bone, ranging from 14.67% to 77.86% (Shah, Mehra & Chinnaiyan 2004). Such variability complicates the search for effective therapies targeting CRPC, for which few alternatives exist nowadays. Current treatments aim at improving the quality of life of patients, prolonging survival, and palliating cancer-associated pain but, so far, none of them are able to cure CRPC.

One of the therapies used to fight CRPC consists in the administration of docetaxel accompanied by the corticosteroids prednisone and dexamethasone. In a Phase III study, the TAX 327 trial, treatment with docetaxel and prednisone every three weeks achieved superior survival and better response rates regarding serum PSA levels, pain, and quality of life than mitoxantrone and prednisone (Tannock *et al.,* 2004). Though statistically significant, the median survival benefit of docetaxel reached less than three months (Tannock *et al.,* 2004). Mitoxantrone plus prednisone can be used in CRPC patients who do not tolerate docetaxel; however, this combination affords no survival benefit compared to prednisone alone (Tannock *et al.,* 1996). In addition, a number of CRPC patients develops resistance to docetaxel, further narrowing their therapeutic options. Although the origin of resistance to docetaxel is not well understood, IL-6 seems to be tightly linked to it. IL-6, which is considerably elevated in PCa patients (Twillie *et al.,* 1995), predicts resistance to docetaxel and is associated with decreased survival in CRPC patients (Domingo-Domenech *et al.,* 2006; Ignatoski *et al.,* 2009; George *et al.* 2005). Docetaxel induced NF-κB activation and IL-6 production, which could be inhibited by the IKK-2 inhibitor PS-1145, in androgen-independent PCa cell lines (Domingo-Domenech *et al.,* 2006). Moreover, combined treatment with docetaxel and PS-1145 prevented docetaxel-stimulated activation of NF-κB, decreased IL-6 expression, and increased sensitivity to docetaxel (Domingo-Domenech *et al.,* 2006).

Thus, reducing IL-6 levels may be essential for docetaxel treatment to tackle CRPC efficiently. The question is: when should therapy aimed at shrinking IL-6 levels be administered to patients? We have already discussed, based on results from a Phase II trial (Dorff *et al.,* 2010), that the anti-IL-6 antibody CNTO 328 alone may be of little benefit in taxane-refractory patients. On the other hand, concomitant administration of CNTO 328 with docetaxel in chemotherapy-naïve CRPC patients demonstrated promising results in a Phase I trial. As we mentioned earlier, chronic exposure to IL-6 imparts dramatic changes on PCa cells (Hobisch *et al.,* 2001; Steiner *et al.,* 2003; Debes *et al.,* 2005; Cavarretta *et al.,* 2007; Puhr *et al.* 2009) and high quantities of IL-6 are already present in the epithelium of carcinomas with low Gleason grades (Hobisch *et al.,* 2000; Royuela *et al.,* 2004). This suggests that the autocrine loop for IL-6, accompanied by a myriad of molecular alterations, may develop early in the natural history of PCa. Hence, those changes may precede the onset of advanced prostate cancer, which is usually treated with androgen ablation.

Paradoxically, overexpression of IL-6 in advanced tumors provides several routes of escape from androgen deprivation therapies. For instance, IL-6 can activate the AR in a ligand-independent fashion in AR-bearing tumors, while assisting other tumor cells in losing AR expression. Additionally, IL-6-producing tumors lose Rb protein expression (Steiner *et al.,* 2003) and Rb deficiency has been shown to facilitate bypass of first-line hormone therapy (Sharma *et al.,* 2007). Together with shifts towards preferential activation of pathways involved in proliferation (MAPK), survival (Mcl-1 and Bcl-2), and angiogenesis (VEGF), IL-6 confers resistance to androgen deprivation techniques. Approximately 85% of patients respond initially to hormone therapy, but PCa progresses to CRPC in practically all patients in a median time of 24 months (Parmar *et al.,* 2008). As we know that it is just a matter of time until androgen ablation fails, why not utilize CNTO 328 in combination with hormone therapy prior to the development of CRPC? Furthermore, would it be possible to combine androgen ablation, not only with CNTO 328, but also with docetaxel?

Although this triple-target therapeutic approach may seem unrealistic, a new methodology for the design of clinical trials allowing the simultaneous evaluation of different agents and their combinations (Parmar *et al.,* 2008; James *et al.,* 2009) may yield new insights into advanced PCa treatment. This new tactic is currently being assessed in three clinical studies (Parmar *et al.,* 2008). One of them, the STAMPEDE (systemic therapy for advancing or metastatic prostate cancer) trial, is being conducted in the UK with the purpose of accelerating the development of therapies for CRPC patients (James *et al.,* 2009). They differ from conventional trials in that they have multiple arms and stages and rely on intermediate outcomes to proceed from one stage to the next one (Parmar *et al.,* 2008). They are more efficient than standard trial designs, allow for the simultaneous evaluation of several treatments *vs.* one sole control group, permit a faster evaluation of such treatments, and require fewer patients (Parmar *et al.,* 2008). For instance, in the STAMPEDE trial there are six arms: a control arm, consisting of hormone therapy (HT); and five experimental arms: HT + zoledronic acid, HT + celecoxib, HT + docetaxel, HT + zoledronic acid + celecoxib, and HT + zoledronic acid + docetaxel (Parmar *et al.,* 2008; James *et al.,* 2009). There are also five stages: a pilot stage with safety as main outcome; three intermediate activity stages assessing failure-free survival; and a final efficacy stage measuring overall survival (Parmar *et al.,* 2008; James *et al.,* 2009). At the end of stage I, each experimental arm is compared against the control based on the designated outcome for that stage (*e.g.* safety for stage I) (Parmar *et al.,* 2008). If the results are satisfactory for a specific arm of stage I, accrual continues for stage II, and so on, until performing the final primary analysis. However, for those experimental conditions that do not pass the test at certain stage (for example, if failure-free survival were lower in the HT + celecoxib group than in control), accrual is discontinued but a secondary analysis of the data will be performed at the end (Parmar *et al.,* 2008).

Hence, a multi-arm, multi-stage trial could be designed to evaluate three new combination therapies at once, comparing them to standard hormone therapy, in therapy-naïve advanced PCa patients: HT + CNTO 328, HT + docetaxel, and HT + CNTO 328 + docetaxel. The objective of such trial would be to elucidate whether the onset of CRPC could be delayed during the androgen-dependent stage of PCa, by introducing therapies that seem to provide benefits in castration-resistant disease such as CNTO 328 and docetaxel.

ACKNOWLEDGEMENT

Research performed in Dr. Culig´s laboratory was supported by the Austrian Science Fund (FWF) and Centocor, Inc.

CONFLICT OF INTEREST

The author(s) confirm that this chapter content has no conflict of interest.

REFERENCES

Akira, S, Taga, T & Kishimoto, T (1993), 'Interleukin-6 in biology and medicine', *Advances in Immunology,* no. 54, pp. 1-78.

Bellezza, I, Neuwirt, H, Nemes, C, *et al.*, (2006), 'Suppressor of cytokine signaling-3 antagonizes cAMP effects on proliferation and apoptosis and is expressed in human prostate cancer', *The American Journal of Pathology,* no. 169, pp. 2199-208.

Bellido, T, O'Brien, CA, Roberson, PK & Manolagas, SC (1998), 'Transcriptional activation of the p21^{WAF1,CIP1,SDI1} gene by interleukin-6 type cytokines. A prerequisite for their pro-differentiating and anti-apoptotic effects on human osteoblastic cells', *The Journal of Biological Chemistry,* no. 273, pp. 21137-44.

Brakenhoff, JP, Hart, M, De Groot, ER, Di Padova, F & Aarden, LA (1990), 'Structure-function analysis of human IL-6. Epitope mapping of neutralizing monoclonal antibodies with amino- and carboxyl-terminal deletion mutants', *Journal of Immunology,* no. 145, pp. 561-8.

Bredesen, DE, Mehlen, P & Rabizadeh, S (2005), 'Receptors that mediate cellular dependence', *Cell Death & Differentiation,* no. 12, pp. 1031-43.

Cavarretta, IT, Neuwirt, H, Untergasser, G, *et al.,* (2007), 'The antiapoptotic effect of IL-6 autocrine loop in a cellular model of advanced prostate cancer is mediated by Mcl-1', *Oncogene,* no. 26, pp. 2822-32.

Chung, CD, Liao, J, Liu, B, *et al.,* (1997), 'Specific inhibition of Stat3 signal transduction by PIAS3', Science no. 278, pp. 1803-5.

Culig, Z, Steiner, H, Bartsch, G & Hobisch, A (2005), 'Mechanisms of endocrine therapy-responsive and -unresponsive prostate tumours', *Endocrine-Related Cancer,* no. 12, 229-44.

Debes, JD, Comuzzi, B, Schmidt, LJ, Dehm, SM, Culig, Z & Tindall, DJ (2005), 'p300 regulates androgen receptor-independent expression of prostate-specific antigen in prostate cancer cells treated chronically with interleukin-6', *Cancer Research,* no. 65, pp. 5965-73.

Domingo-Domenech, J, Oliva, C, Rovira, A, *et al.*, (2006), 'Interleukin-6, a nuclear factor-kappaB target, predicts resistance to docetaxel in hormone-independent prostate cancer and nuclear factor-kappaB inhibition by PS-1145 enhances docetaxel antitumor activity', *Clinical Cancer Research,* no. 15, pp. 5578-86.

Dorff, TB, Goldman, B, Pinski, JK, *et al.,* (2010), 'Clinical and correlative results of SWOG S0354: A Phase II trial of CNTO328 (siltuximab), a monoclonal antibody against interleukin-6, in chemotherapy-pretreated patients with castration-resistant prostate cancer', *Clinical Cancer Research,* no. 16, pp. 3028-34.

Ellerby, LM, Hackam, AS, Propp, SS, *et al.,* (1999), 'Kennedy's disease: caspase cleavage of the androgen receptor is a crucial event in cytotoxicity', *Journal of Neurochemistry,* no. 72, pp. 185-95.

Feldman, BJ & Feldman, D (2001), 'The development of androgen-independent prostate cancer', *Nature Reviews Cancer,* no. 1, pp. 34-45.

Fisher, P, Lehmann, U, Sobota, RM, *et al.,* (2004), 'The role of the inhibitors of interleukin-6 signal transduction SHP2 and SOCS3 for desensitization of Interleukin-6 signalling', *The Biochemical Journal,* no. 378, pp. 449-60.

George, DJ, Halabi, S, Shepard, TF *et al.,* (2005), 'The prognostic significance of plasma interleukin-6 levels in patients with metastatic hormone-refractory prostate cancer: results from cancer and leukemia group B 9480', *Clinical Cancer Research,* no. 11, pp. 1815-20.

George, DJ, Halabi, S, Shepard, TF, *et al.,* (2001), 'Prognostic significance of plasma vascular endothelial growth factor levels in patients with hormone-refractory prostate cancer treated on Cancer and Leukemia Group B 9480', *Clinical Cancer Research,* no. 7, pp. 1932-6.

Gioeli, D, Mandell, JW, Petroni, GR, Frierson Jr., HF & Weber, MJ (1999), 'Activation of mitogen-activated protein kinase associated with prostate cancer progression', *Cancer Research,* no. 59, pp. 279-94.

Godoy-Tundidor, S (2004), 'Interleukin-6 and related cytokines in the regulation of androgen receptor activity and prostate cancer cell growth, PhD thesis, University of Innsbruck.

Goldschneider, D & Mehlen, P (2010), 'Dependence receptors: a new paradigm in cell signaling and cancer therapy', *Oncogene,* no 29, pp. 1865-82.

Grossmann, ME, Huang, H & Tindall, DJ (2001), 'Androgen receptor signaling in androgen-refractory prostate cancer', *Journal of the National Cancer Institute,* no. 93, pp. 1687-97.

Gunaje, JJ & Bhat, GJ (2001), 'Involvement of tyrosine phosphatase PTP1D in the inhibition of interleukin-6 induced Stat3 signaling by α-thrombin', *Biochemical and Biophysical Research Communications,* no. 288, pp. 252-7.

Harman, SM, Metter, EJ, Tobin, JD, Pearson, J & Blackman, MR (2001), 'Longitudinal effects of aging on serum total and free testosterone levels in healthy men', *The Journal of Clinical Endocrinology and Metabolism,* no. 86, pp. 724-731.

Heinrich, PC, Behrmann, I, Haan, S, Hermanns, HM, Müller-Newen, G & Schaper, F (2003), 'Principles of interleukin (IL)-6-type cytokine signalling and its regulation', *The Biochemical Journal,* no. 374, pp. 1-20.

Hobisch, A, Eder, IE, Putz, T, *et al.,* (1998), 'Interleukin-6 regulates prostate-specific protein expression in prostate carcinoma cells by activation of the androgen receptor', *Cancer Research,* no. 58, pp. 4640-5.

Hobisch, A, Ramoner, R, Fuchs, D, *et al.,* (2001), 'Prostate cancer cells (LNCaP) generated after long-term interleukin 6 (IL-6) treatment express IL-6 and acquire an IL-6 partially resistant phenotype', *Clinical Cancer Research,* no. 7, pp. 2941-8.

Hobisch, A, Rogatsch, H, Hittmair, A, *et al.,* (2000), 'Immunohistochemical localization of interleukin-6 and its receptor in benign, premalignant and malignant prostate tissue', *The Journal of Pathology,* no. 191, pp. 239-44.

Horoszewicz, JS, Leong, SS, Chu, TM, *et al.,* (1980), 'The LNCaP cell line - a new model for studies on human prostatic carcinoma', *Progress in Clinical and Biological Research,* no. 37, pp. 115-32.

Horoszewicz, JS, Leong, SS, Kawinski, E, *et al.,* (1983), 'LNCaP model of human prostatic carcinoma', Cancer Research, no. 43, pp. 1809-18.

Ignatoski, KM, Friedman, J, Escara-Wilke, J, *et al.,* (2009), 'Change in markers of bone metabolism with chemotherapy for advanced prostate cancer: Interleukin-6 response is a potential early indicator of response to therapy', *Journal of Interferon and Cytokine Research,* no. 29, pp. 105-12.

James, ND, Sydes, MR, Clarke, NW, *et al.,* (2009), 'Systemic therapy for advancing or metastatic prostate cancer (STAMPEDE): a multi-arm, multistage randomized controlled trial', *BJU International,* no. 103, pp. 464-9.

Kamimura, D & Hirano, T (2003), 'Interleukin-6', In: HL Henry & AW Norman (Eds.), *Encyclopedia of Hormones,* Academic Press, Oxford.

Keller, ET, Chang, C & Ershler, WB (1996), 'Inhibition of NFκB activity through maintenance of IκBα levels contributes to dihydrotestosterone-mediated repression of the interleukin-6 promoter', *The Journal of Biological Chemistry,* no. 271, pp. 26267-75.

Kinoshita, H, Shi, Y, Sandefur, C, *et al.,* (2000), 'Methylation of the androgen receptor minimal promoter silences transcription in human prostate cancer', *Cancer Research,* no. 60, pp. 3623-30.

Kozlowski, JM, Fidler, IJ, Campbell, D, Xu, ZL, Kaighn, ME & Hart, IR (1984), 'Metastatic behavior of human tumor cell lines grown in the nude mouse', *Cancer Research,* no. 44, pp. 3522-9.

Krajewska, M, Krajewski, S, Epstein, JI, *et al.,* (1996), 'Immunohistochemical analysis of bcl-2, bax, bcl-X, and mcl-1 expression in prostate cancers', *The American Journal of Pathology,* no. 148, pp. 1567-76.

Lehmann, U, Schmitz, J, Weissenbach, M, *et al.,* (2003), 'SHP2 and SOCS3 contribute to Tyr-759-dependent attenuation of interleukin-6 signaling through gp130', *The Journal of Biological Chemistry,* no. 278, pp. 661-71.

Loblaw, DA, Mendelson, DS, Talcott, JA, *et al.,* (2004), 'American Society of Clinical Oncology recommendations for the initial hormonal management of androgen-sensitive metastatic, recurrent, or progressive prostate cancer', *Journal of Clinical Oncology,* no. 22, pp. 2927-41.

Locke, JA, Guns, ES, Lubik, AA, *et al.,* (2008), 'Androgen levels increase by intratumoral *de novo* steroidogenesis during progression of castration-resistant prostate cancer', *Cancer Research,* no. 68, pp. 6407-15.

Müller-Newen, G, Küster, A, Hemmann, U, *et al.,* (1998), 'Soluble interleukin-6 receptor potentiates the antagonistic activity of soluble gp130 on interleukin-6 responses', *Journal of Immunology,* no. 161, pp. 6347-55.

Parmar, MKB, Barthel, FM-S, Sydes, M, *et al.,* (2008), 'Speeding up the evaluation of new agents in cancer', *Journal of the National Cancer Institute,* no. 100, pp. 1204-14.

Puhr, M, Santer, FR, Neuwirt, H, *et al.,* (2009), 'Down-regulation of suppressor of cytokine signaling-3 causes prostate cancer cell death through activation of the extrinsic and intrinsic apoptosis pathways', *Cancer Research,* no. 69, pp. 7375-84.

Ray, A, LaForge, K & Sehgal, P (1990), 'On the mechanism for efficient repression of the interleukin-6 promoter by glucocorticoids: enhancer, TATA box, and RNA start site (Inr motif) occlusion', *Molecular and Cellular Biology,* no. 10, pp. 5736-46.

Royuela, M, Ricote, M, Parsons, MS, García-Tuñón, I, Paniagua, R & De Miguel, MP (2004), 'Immunohistochemichal analysis of the IL-6 family of cytokines and their receptors in benign, hyperplastic, and malignant human prostate', *The Journal of Pathology,* no. 202, pp. 41-9.

Schaper, F, Gendo, C, Eck, M, *et al.,* (1998), 'Activation of the protein tyrosine phosphatase SHP2 *via* the interleukin-6 signal transducing receptor protein gp130 requires tyrosine Jak1 and limits acute-phase protein expression', *The Biochemical Journal,* no. 335, pp. 557-65.

Scher, HI, Buchanan, G, Gerald, W, Butler, LM & Tilley, WD (2004), 'Targeting the androgen receptor: improving outcomes for castration-resistant prostate cancer', *Endocrine-Related Cancer,* no. 11, pp. 459-76.

Sengupta, TK, Talbot, ES, Scherle, PA & Ivashkiv, LB (1998), 'Rapid inhibition of interleukin-6 signaling and Stat3 activation mediated by mitogen-activated protein kinases', *Proceedings of the National Academy of Sciences of the United States of America,* no. 95, pp. 11107-12.

Shah, RB, Mehra, R, Chinnaiyan, AM, *et al.,* (2004), 'Androgen-independent prostate cancer is a heterogeneous group of diseases: lessons from a rapid autopsy program', *Cancer Research,* no. 64, pp. 9209-16.

Sharma, A, Comstock, CES, Knudsen EK, *et al.,* (2007), 'Retinoblastoma tumor suppressor status is a critical determinant of therapeutic response in prostate cancer cells', *Cancer Research,* no. 67, pp. 6192-203.

Sharma, A, Yeow, W-S, Ertel, A, *et al.*, (2010), 'The retinoblastoma tumor suppressor controls androgen signaling and human prostate cancer progression', *The Journal of Clinical Investigation,* no. 120, pp. 4478-92.

Siegall, CB, Schwab, G, Nordan, RP, FitzGerald, DJ & Pastan, I (1990), 'Expression of the interleukin 6 receptor and interleukin 6 in prostate carcinoma cells', *Cancer Research,* no. 50, pp. 7786-8.

Siegsmund, MJ, Yamazaki, H & Pastan, I (1994), 'Interleukin 6 receptor mRNA in prostate carcinomas and benign prostate hyperplasia', *The Journal of Urology,* no. 151, pp. 1396-9.

Smith, PC & Keller, ET (2001), 'Anti-interleukin-6 monoclonal antibody induces regression of human prostate cancer xenografts in nude mice', *The Prostate,* no. 48, pp. 47-53.

Starr, R, Wilson, TA, Viney, EM, *et al.*, (1997), 'A family of cytokine-inducible inhibitors of signalling', *Nature,* no. 387, pp. 917-21.

Steiner, H, Berger, AP, Godoy-Tundidor, S, *et al.*, (2004), 'An autocrine loop for vascular endothelial growth factor is established in prostate cancer cells generated after prolonged treatment with interleukin-6', *European Journal of Cancer,* no. 40, pp. 1066-72.

Steiner, H, Cavarretta, IT, Moser, PL, *et al.*, (2006), 'Regulation of growth of prostate cancer cells selected in the presence of interleukin-6 by the anti-interleukin-6 antibody CNTO 328', *The Prostate,* no. 66, pp. 1744-52.

Steiner, H, Godoy-Tundidor, S, Rogatsch, H, *et al.*, (2003), 'Accelerated *in vivo* growth of prostate tumors that up-regulate interleukin-6 is associated with reduced retinoblastoma protein expression and activation of the mitogen-activated protein kinase pathway', *The American Journal of Pathology,* no. 162, pp. 655-63.

Tan, J, Sharief, Y, Hamil, KG, *et al.*, (1997), 'Dehydroepiandrosterone activates mutant androgen receptors expressed in the androgen-dependent human prostate cancer xenograft CWR22 and LNCaP cells', *Molecular Endocrinology,* no. 11, pp. 450-9.

Tannock, IF, de Wit, R, Berry, WR, *et al.*, (2004), 'Docetaxel plus prednisone or mitoxantrone plus prednisone for advanced prostate cancer', *New England Journal of Medicine,* no. 351, pp. 1502-1512.

Tannock, IF, Osoba, D, Stockler, MR, *et al.*, (1996), 'Chemotherapy with mitoxantrone plus prednisone or prednisone alone for symptomatic hormone-resistant prostate cancer: a Canadian randomized trial with palliative end points', *Journal of Clinical Oncology,* no. 14, pp. 1756-64.

Twillie, DA, Eisenberger, MA, Carducci, MA, Hseih, WS, Kim, WY & Simons, JW (1995), 'Interleukin-6: a candidate mediator of human prostate cancer morbidity', *Urology,* no. 45, pp. 542-9.

Ueda, T, Bruchovsky, N & Sadar, MD (2002), 'Activation of the androgen receptor N-terminal domain by interleukin-6 *via* MAPK and STAT3 signal transduction pathways', *The Journal of Biological Chemistry,* no. 277, pp. 7076-85.

Wallner, L, Dai, J, Escara-Wilke, J, *et al.*, (2006), 'Inhibition of interleukin-6 with CNTO328, and anti-interleukin-6 monoclonal antibody, inhibits conversion of androgen-dependent prostate cancer to an androgen-independent phenotype in orchiectomized mice', *Cancer Research,* no. 66, pp. 3087-95.

Winzen, R, Kracht, M, Ritter, B, *et al.*, (1999), 'The p38 MAP kinase pathway signals for cytokine-induced mRNA stabilization *via* MAP kinase-activated protein kinase 2 and a AU-rich region-targeted mechanism', *The EMBO Journal,* no. 18, pp. 4969-80.

Wu, TR, Hong, YK, Wang, XD, *et al.,* (2002), 'SHP-2 is a dual-specificity phosphatase involved in Stat1 dephosphorylation at both tyrosine and serine residues in nuclei', *The Journal of Biological Chemistry,* no. 277, pp. 47572-80.

Yang, L, Wang, L, Lin, H-K, *et al.,* (2003), 'Interleukin-6 differentially regulates androgen receptor transactivation *via* PI3K-Akt, STAT3, and MAPK, three distinct signal pathways in prostate cancer cells', *Biochemical and Biophysical Research Communications,* no. 305, pp. 462-9.

Zaki, MH, Nemeth, JA & Trikha, M (2004), 'CNTO 328, a monoclonal antibody to IL-6, inhibits human tumor-induced cachexia in nude mice', *International Journal of Cancer,* no. 111, pp. 592-5.

Cutting Edge Therapies for Cancer in the 21st Century, 2014, 253-270

CHAPTER 9

Role of Gastrokine 1 in Gastric Cancer: A Potential Diagnostic Marker and Antitumor Drug

Maria Irene Scarano[1,2,#], Emili Rippa[1,#,*], Filomena Altieri[1], Chiara Stella Di Stadio[1], Giuseppina Miselli[1] and Paolo Arcari[1]

[1]Department of Molecular Medicine and Medical Biotechnologies, University of Naples Federico and CEINGE, Advanced Biotechnologies, Naples, Italy and [2]Department of Biochemistry and Microbiology, Joan C. Edwards School of Medicine, Marshall University, Huntington, WV, USA

Abstract: Gastric cancer is still one of the prevalent leading causes of cancer-related deaths worldwide. The high mortality rate is mainly due to late-stage diagnosis, which has a very poor prognosis (five-year survival rates are as little as 3-10%). By contrast, early stage gastric cancer is highly curable with five-year survival rates exceeding 90%. Early detection is therefore the single most important factor influencing the outcome for gastric cancer patients. However, there are currently no biomarkers of acceptable sensitivity and specificity to detect early stage gastric cancer. Gastric infection with *Helicobacter pylori* (*H. pylori*) seems to be a risk factor for gastric cancer. Epidemiological studies have shown that patients that test serum positive to *H. pylori* infection are associated with a three- to six-fold increase in the risk of gastric cancer, findings that are compatible with pathological links between *H. pylori*-associated gastritis, pre-cancerous lesions, and subsequent cancer of the stomach. In a previous study, moving from genomic to proteomic investigation, we have identified a protein, gastrokine 1 (GKN1), a stomach-secreted protein previously named AMP-18 (18kDa Antrum Mucosa Protein) that was highly expressed in normal tissues and significantly down-regulated in *H. pylori* positive patients with respect to *H. pylori* negative subjects. In addition, we have also found that GKN1 is normally expressed in gastric mucosa but not in primary tumours, both at the transcriptional and translational levels. On the basis of these findings, we propose that GKN1 can be used as a new molecular marker that could be useful to predict early cell transformation and might be a potential novel target for gastric cancer therapeutics. Moreover, we have also found that recombinant GKN1 affect cancer cell growth and that the transient expression of GKN1 in human gastric cancer also inhibits cell growth and induces apoptosis, thus suggesting the importance of GKN1 in preventing cancer development in gastric tissues. Finally, we hypothesize that GKN1 might act as a tumor suppressor and thus foresee its importance as an antitumor drug.

***Address correspondence to Maria Irene Scarano:** Department of Biochemistry and Microbiology, Marshall University, Joan C. Edwards School of Medicine, Translational Genomics Research Institute, 1600 Medical Drive, Huntington WV, 25705, USA; Tel: (267) 886 8528; E-mail: scarano@ceinge.unina.it
[#]MIS and ER contributed equally to this book chapter.

Keywords: Gastrokine-1, non-atrophic gastritis, chronic atrophic gastritis, intestinal metaplasia, dysplasia, Gastric Cancer, prognostic biomarker, cDNA microarrays, gene expression, mRNA, *Helicobacter pylori*, Fas, Fas ligand, Caspase-3, Apoptosis.

1. INTRODUCTION

The molecular mechanisms of neoplastic transformation include genetic alterations (point mutations, deletions and gene rearrangements) that lead to the production of altered proteins with respect to their wild-type counterpart (Rosenberg, 2001). These proteins might be specific tumour markers and, as such, they can be considered useful targets for the development of therapeutic and molecular diagnostic strategies. In the past years, a great effort has been devoted to the possibility of performing a detailed genetic analysis of tumour tissues by means of DNA microarray. These techniques include differential display, cDNA membrane arrays (Clontech), cDNA microarrays and serial analysis of gene expression (Oien, *et al.*, 2003; Hippo, *et al.*, 2002; Mori, *et al.*, 2002; El-Rifai, *et al.*, 2001; Yoshikawa, *et al.*, 2000). However, RNA-based expression strategies are limited by the poor correlation between RNA and protein expression. Moreover, measurements made at the mRNA level will fail to detect posttranslational modifications of proteins and protein isoforms (Orrù, *et al.*, 2003; Griffin, *et al.*, 2002; Gygi, *et al.*, 1999). Gene expression at the mRNA level is not necessarily correlated to the expression of the protein that particular gene codes for. Therefore, we cannot always predict whether it is directly responsible for the phenotypic behavior of the neoplasia. For example, in eukaryotic cells, a different transcriptional and translational activity of a given gene may exist; the expression of this gene can be also post-translationally regulated by its degradation. More recently, the method of global analysis of cellular proteins, known as proteomics, has shown great promise in identifying novel diagnostic and prognostic biomarkers for human cancers (Li, *et al.*, 2008; Vlahou and Fountoulakis, 2005; Michener, *et al.*, 2002; Petricoin, *et al.*, 2002).

Tumour markers are often characterized by the presence of mutations in the amino acid sequence and/or by post-translational modifications (phosphorylation, acetylation) that modify some molecular properties of the protein such as the isoelectric point and the molecular mass, thus allowing their separation by bidimensional electrophoresis on polyacrylamide gel, followed by their identification by mass spectrometry (2D-MS) (Baek, *et al.*, 2004; Orrù, *et al.*, 2003). Moreover, tumour associated proteins or peptides can be released in the blood and thus used as serum markers of the neoplasia (Anderson and Anderson, 2003), or they can induce specific serum antibody titers (Mintz, *et al.*, 2003).

Gastric cancer, despite its declining incidence rate, remains as the fourth most common cancer and the second cause of cancer-related death worldwide (Ferlay *et al.*, 2010) Gastric cancers are often characterized by two distinct histological types of adenocarcinomas, each having different epidemiological and pathophysiological features (Lauren, 1965). The intestinal-type generally evolves through a relatively well-defined sequence of histological lesions, namely non-atrophic gastritis, chronic atrophic gastritis, intestinal metaplasia, and dysplasia (Correa, 1995; Correa, 1992). On the contrary, the diffuse subtype is also preceded by years of chronic *H. pylori*-associated gastritis, although the molecular pathways and histologic changes involved in progression to cancer are less characterized. A multistage process in which several alteration of genetic and epigenetic nature accumulates characterizes the progress of gastric carcinogenesis. The chronic active gastritis is the primary condition related to *H. pylori* colonization, causing an elevated risk of gastric adenocarcinoma, both intestinal type and diffuses type. (Bornschein and Malfertheiner, 2011). Anyhow, the propensity to develop disease is an aspect that remains unclear but may depend on host characteristic, particular bacterial factors such as the virulence of the infecting strains or to the specific interactions between host and microbe, besides the environmental factors (Kabir, 2009).

2. GASTROKINES AND GASTRIC CANCER

The importance of *H. pylori* infection in promoting gastric cancer is already well known. Exposure of gastric epithelial cells to the bacterium determines a complex inflammatory and immune reactions associated to production of neutrophils, release of cytokines and reactive oxygen species (ROS) and induction of nitric oxide synthase (NO) that in turn may cause genetic alterations leading to cancer in a subset of subjects. *H. pylori* infection, a necessary but not sufficient cause, is associated with a 5.9-fold increased risk of non-cardia gastric cancer in a combined analysis of nested case control studies (Helicobacter and Cancer Collaborative Group, 2001). A prospective cohort study in Japan highlighted that gastric cancer developed in 2.9 % of 1,246 *H. pylori*-infected persons over 7.8 years. In contrast, none of the 280 *H. pylori*-uninfected persons developed gastric cancer (Wu, *et al.,* 2000). It is noteworthy that the prevalence of *H. pylori* infection and incidence of gastric cancer vary among different countries. This highlights the importance of host genetic factors and other factors beyond *H. pylori* infection in the carcinogenesis of gastric cancer (Leung, *et al.,* 2008).

In order to search for possible informative biomarkers for gastric cancer, the protein profile of malignant and non-malignant gastric tissues was extensively analysed. From these analyses, a secreted protein, specifically expressed in gastric mucosa, gastrokine 1 (GKN1), formerly foveolin or AMP18 kDa (AMP18) was identified. The expression of this protein was found to be markedly reduced or completely absent in stomach carcinomas. Gastrokine1 belongs to a family of genes encoding stomach-specific proteins formed by 3 known members: GKN1 (Martin, *et al.*, 2003), GKN2 (Du, *et al.*, 2003) and GKN3 (Menheniott, *et al.*, 2010). Gastrokine expression is coordinately down-regulated in *H. pylori* infection and frequently is lost in gastric carcinoma (Moss, *et al.*, 2008; Nardone, *et al.*, 2007). Collectively, these studies argue that gastrokines participate at the *H. pylori* host susceptibility and function as gastric tumor-suppressor genes. In recent studies, TFF1, a small protein synthesized and secreted by the gastric epithelial cells, was demonstrated, in most gastric adenocarcinomas, to be down-regulated or absent (Kjellev *et al.*, 2009; Machado *et al.*, 1996). Moreover, a previous study showed that the TFF1-deficient mice developed antropyloric adenoma (Lefebvre *et al.*, 1996) therefore TFF1 appears to be involved in gastric carcinogenesis. The recent demonstration of a GKN2/trefoil factor (TFF1) heterodimer in gastric mucus suggests that gastrokines may have an important role in the regulation of TFFs function (Westley, *et al.*, 2005).

The human GKN1 gene has been localized in a region of chromosome 2p13 of about 6 kb and contains 6 exons (Yoshikawa, *et al.*, 2000). The protein is made of 185 amino acid residues and contains a N-terminal signal peptide. GKN1 is expressed only in normal human stomach, in all areas (cardia, body and antrum), but is absent in gastric adenocarcinomas, gastro-oesophageal adenocarcinoma cell lines, and other normal and tumour gastro-intestinal tissues including placenta and ovary (Oien, *et al.*, 2004). The protein is characterized by the presence of a central domain known as BRICHOS (Martin, *et al.*, 2003; Shiozaki, *et al.*, 2001). BRICHOS domain is made of 100 amino acid residues and contains several motifs of likely functional significance. It is present also in other proteins such as BRI2 (Sanchez-Pulido, *et al.*, 2002), related to familial British dementia; chondromodulin-I (ChM-I), associated with chondrosarcoma; and lung surfactant protein C (SP-C), linked with Respiratory Distress Syndrome.

3. CHARACTERIZATION OF GKN1 EXPRESSION IN NORMAL AND GASTRIC TUMOR TISSUES

3.1. Expression of GKN1 in Normal Gastric Tissues and in Pre-Malignant and Malignant Gastric Tissues

Employing immunohistochemistry (IHC), western blot (WB), immunofluorescence (IF) and flow cytometry assay, we investigated on the expression level, biological activity and regulation mechanism of GKN1. The expression of GKN1 was examined in normal gastric tissue, pre-malignant (non-atrophic gastritis, chronic atrophic gastritis, intestinal metaplasia and gastric dysplasia) and different malignant histopathological types of gastric cancer (intestinal and diffuse). The goal of these experiments was to ascertain whether there is any relation between the different histopathological states and the levels of GKN1 expression.

Methodology: A large population of patients who underwent upper gastrointestinal endoscopy in our university hospitals were enrolled. Tissues of gastric tumors and their corresponding distant non-tumor tissues were collected from 28 subjects with gastric cancer (intestinal and diffuse types) who underwent surgery. Interview has been performed focusing on diet and lifestyle habits, family history and other toxic environmental factors. A positive gastric cancer family history was also carefully verified. All tissue specimens were diagnosed by pathologist and confirmed by an experienced pathologist. Specimens were also collected for culture test, histological and immunohistochemical tests and for molecular approach (RT-PCR, Western Blot).

The clinical and histological characteristics of the 65 dyspeptic patients (36 *H. pylori* negative and 29 *H. pylori* positive) are reported in Table **1A**. Only 5 of the *H. pyl*ori negative cases had minimal infiltration of lymphomonocytes in the lamina propria. *H. pylori* infection was present in 29/65 patients suffering from active gastritis (25 mild-moderate and 4 severe); moreover 10 patients showed mild or moderate atrophy that was associated in 4 cases with focal antral complete IM. Among the 29 subjects with infection 21 (72%) were positive for CagA strain. The characteristics of the 28 patients with Gastric Cancer (GC) (20 intestinal and 8 diffuse) are outlined in Table **1B**.

Table 1: Clinical and histopathological characteristics of the dyspeptic (A) and gastric cancer (B) patients

A	***H. pylori* - Negative n. 36**	***H. pylori* - Positive n. 29**
Age (yrs) Mean ± SD	44 ± 15	39 ± 20
Sex M/F	20/16	18/11
LMN (lymphocytes and monocytes)		
Absent	31 (86%)	0 (0%)
Mild	5 (14%)	8 (28%)
Moderate	0 (0%)	17 (58%)
Severe	0 (0%)	4 (14%)
PMN (polymorphonuclear cells)		
Absent	36 (100%)	0 (0%)
Mild	0 (0%)	10 (32%)
Moderate	0 (0%)	12 (41%)
Severe	0 (0%)	7 (27%)
Atrophy		
Absent	36 (100%)	19 (66%)
Mild	0 (0%)	6 (21%)
Moderate	0 (0%)	4 (14%)
Severe	0 (0%)	0 (0%)
IM (intestinal metaplasia)		
Absent	36 (100%)	25 (86%)
Present	0 (0%)	4 (14%)
Anti-*H. pylori* IgG	0 (0%)	29 (100%)
Anti-CagA IgG	0 (0%)	21 (72%)

B	**Intestinal Type n. 20**	**Diffuse Type n. 8**
Age (yrs) Mean ± SD	63 ± 11	54 ± 14
Sex M/F	12/8	4/4
Grade of Differentiation		
Well	4 (20%)	0 (0%)
Moderate	8 (40%)	0 (0%)
Poor	8 (40%)	8 (100%)
Stage		
Early	4 (25%)	0 (0%)
Advanced	16 (75%)	8 (100%)
Anti-*H. pylori* IgG	16 (80%)	6 (75%)
Anti-CagA IgG	14 (70%)	3 (38%)

The intestinal type was well differentiated in 4, moderately differentiated in 8 and poorly differentiated in the remaining 8 cases, while four were in the early stage and the remaining 16 in the advanced stage. Diffuse type of GC was poorly differentiated and advanced in all cases. The non-tumoural areas of intestinal type of GC showed a variable degree of atrophic gastritis with diffuse IM, instead, the peritumoural areas of diffuse type of GC showed a variable degree of non-dysplastic inflammation. *H. pylori* infection was not revealed in the tumoural areas in all cases. It is interesting to point out, however, that *H. pylori* infection was detected, in the peritumoral areas, in 6 cases (4 early and 2 advanced). Anti-*H. pylori* IgG antibodies were detected in 16/20 patients with intestinal histotype GC and in 6 out of 8 with diffuse type GC. Anti-CagA antibodies were detectable in 17/28 cases (14 intestinal and 3 diffuse histotype). Tissue distribution of GKN1 expression was evaluated by immunohistochemistry and by Western blot analysis on tissues and cell extracts obtained from normal and pathological human samples. For immunohistochemical studies, 7-micron sections of frozen unfixed gastric tissues were used. The percentages of immunoreactive cells were scored as follows: 0-5% = negative; 5-25% = low staining; 25-50% = moderate staining; >50% = intense staining. The study was carried out using a commercial anti-

GKN1 monoclonal antibody from Abnova (Taiwan). As reported in Fig. **1**, the immunohistochemical evaluation of the surgical specimens generally evinced a lack of GKN1 in cancer specimens.

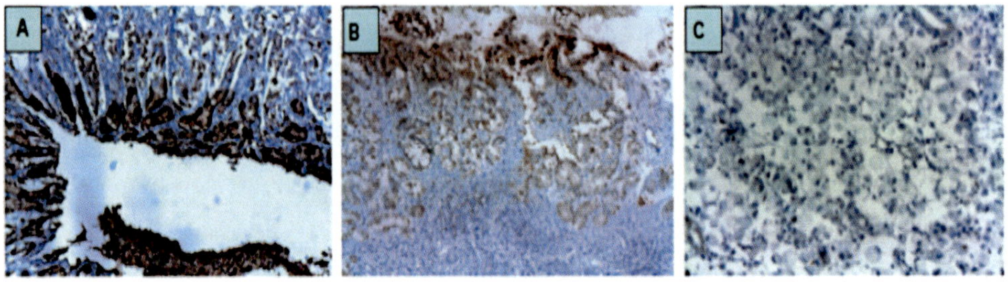

Figure 1: Immunohistochemical detection of GKN1 protein in surgical specimens from: **A**) Normal Gastric Mucosa; **B**) Intestinal metaplasia; **C**) Intestinal type gastric cancer; (Rippa *et al.,* 2011).

GKN1 expression was also evaluated by Western blot (WB) analysis (Fig. **2**). GKN1 protein expression was detected in all *H. pylori*-negative subjects whereas GKN1 was dramatically down-regulated in *H. pylori*-positive gastritis. Densitometric evaluation of the bands showed a significantly lower level in *H. pylori*-positive patients compared to the *H. pylori*-negative subjects (0.19 ±0.02 *vs.* 0.44 ± 0.07, $p < 0.005$). In contrast, GKN1 protein expression was not detectable in any of the tumoral areas but was expressed in non-tumoral areas. The hystopathological aspect of the tumor specimens correlated the GKN1 expression with tumor subtype and was a strong indication that GKN1 could be employed as a useful prognostic biomarker.

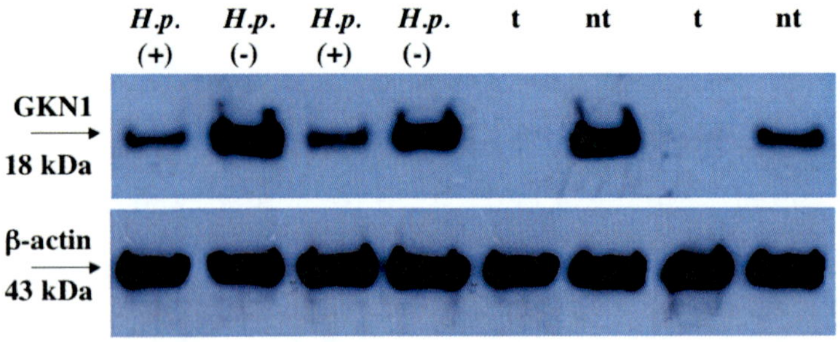

Figure 2: Expression of GKN1 in human specimens. *H.p.* (+), *H. pylori*-positive cases; *H.p.* (-), *H. pylori*-negative cases; t, tumoral area; nt, non-tumoral area.

This hypothesis could be enforced by the analysis of the expression of other new possible markers of gastric adenocarcinoma like the intestinal trefoil factor (ITF), the enhancer of zeste homolog 2 (EZH2) or transgelin in order to correlate their expression with clinico-pathological factors (Huang, *et al.*, 2008; Moss, *et al.*, 2008; Mattioli, *et al.*, 2007; Dhar, *et al.*, 2005; Yamachika, *et al.*, 2002).

4. CHARACTERIZATION OF THE MOLECULAR AND FUNCTIONAL ROLE OF GKN1

4.1. Effect of GKN1 Over-Expression in Gastric Cancer Cell Lines

Although a detailed function remains to be identified, GKN1 appears to be important in maintaining mucosal integrity and could play a role in cell proliferation and differentiation. GKN1 protects the intestinal mucosal barrier by acting on specific tight junction proteins and stabilizing peri-junctional action by increasing accumulation of specific tight and adherens junction proteins and also promotes healing by facilitating restitution and proliferation following injuries (Walsh-Reitz *et al.*, 2005; Toback, *et al.*, 2003. The protective function of GKN1 might be ascribed to the presence of the BRICHOS domain. In fact, it has been found that the BRICHOS domain of another gastric protein, GKN2, originally named GDDR, related to GKN1, is also down-regulated in gastric cancer. This protein was described as TFZ1 due to its binding to tumor suppressor proteins such as the trefoil protein 1 (TFF1). Taken together, this remarks suggested that this interaction seems to be important in the regulation of the integrity of the mucosa (Baus-Loncar *et al.*, 2007; Otto *et al.*, 2006; Bruce *et al.*, 2005). The down-regulation of GKN1 observed in *H. pylori*-infected gastric mucosal epithelial cells (Nardone, *et al.*, 2007), the loss of its expression in gastric cancer in precancerous lesion (Moss *et al.*, 2008; Nardone *et al.*, 2008) and its absence in human gastric cancer cell lines (AGS and MKN28) (Oien *et al.*, 2004; Segal *et al.*, 1996; Motoyama, *et al.*, 1986) indicated that GKN1 participates in the host response to *H. pylori* and might exert a gastric tumor suppressor function (Du *et al.*, 2003). It is plausible that GKN1 acts as a tumor suppressor though the regulation of epigenetic modifications, cell cycle or loss of heterozygosis, as it was observed for other tumor suppressor genes such as TFF1. (Carvalho, *et al.*, 2002). Moreover, conflicting results have been reported: Martin *et al.*, (2003) have proposed that GKN1 protein exerts mitogenic effects on IEC-6 cells when compared with EGF, whereas Shiozaki *et al*., (2001) have found that this protein can inhibit growth in MKN28 cells after transfection. Therefore, if GKN1 shows the ability to stimulate or inhibit the proliferation of gastric cells, it is important to define its role in inflammatory bowel disease (IBD) or in gastric carcinogenesis. To this aim, we initiated a systematic study to define the molecular mechanism of the protein in the processes of proliferation and signaling transduction. Thus, besides the analysis of GKN1 expression in tissues specimens at normal, premalignant and malignant gastric mucosa level, we investigated on the effects of GKN1 on gastric cancer cells either by treating the cell with exogenous recombinant GKN1 (rGKN1) or by its cDNA-mediated overexpression.

Methodology: Recombinant GKN1 (rGKN1) was expressed in *P. pastoris* and purified according to the procedure reported by Pavone *et al*., 2012. Cell proliferation was assessed using a MTT [3-(4,5-dimethylthiazol-2-yl)-2,5-diphenyltetrazolium bromide] assay (Sigma). Cell proliferation was expressed as the percentage of formazan formation in the treated samples, compared to the negative control treated only with solvent (Pavone *et al*., 2012). For transient expression of GKN1 in gastric cancer cells, the coding sequence of full-length human GKN1 cDNA was cloned into the eukaryotic expression vectors pcDNA 3.1 (Invitrogen USA). As experimental systems, human gastric carcinoma epithelial cell lines AGS and MKN28 (Motoyama, *et al*., 1986) were used. Cells were cultured in DMEM F12 (Dulbecco's modified Eagle'smedium) in a humidified incubator with 5% CO_2 at 37° C and transfected in 60 mm-diameter dishes with expression plasmids (construct and void vector; 4μ (Rippa *et al*., 2011).

The ability of rGKN1 to affect cell proliferation *in vitro* using different cell cultures was evaluated. The results reported in Fig. **3** showed that rGKN1 possessed an anti-proliferative activity after 24 h of treatment of the AGS cell line at a concentration of μM. It was also observed that the anti-proliferative action was dose dependent. In fact, the inhibition of cell growth increased at increasing rGKN1 concentration. This activity resulted instead less marked using a non-gastric cancer cell line (H1355) or a normal cell line (HEK 293), although for the latter higher concentrations of rGKN1 were required. These results strongly indicated that rGKN1 was able to exert its function specifically on gastric cancer cells.

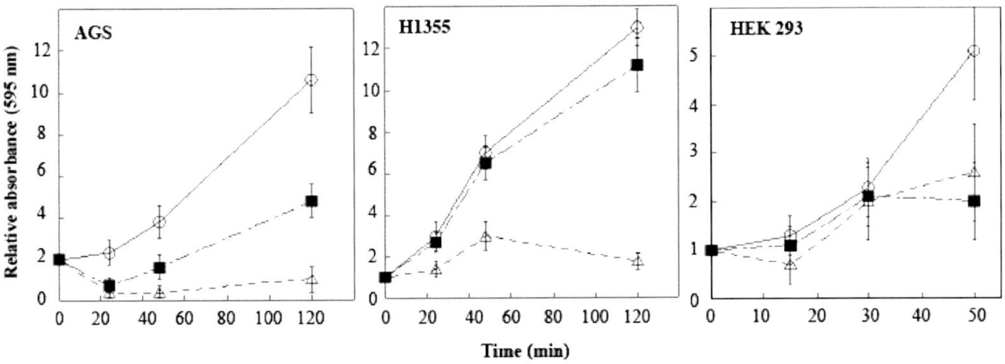

Figure 3: Effect of recombinant GKN1 on cell growth. The effect of GKN1 on cell growth was evaluated by the MTT assay after incubation of the cells with GKN1 at different times and concentrations. AGS cell growth in the absence (○) or in the presence of 0.5 μM (■) or 3 μM (△) GKN1. H1355 cells growth in the absence (○) or in the presence of 0.5 μM (■) or 3 μM (△) GKN1. HEK 293 cells growth in the absence (○) or in the presence of 5.5 μM (■) or 18 μM (△) GKN1, respectively.

The effects of the transient expression of GKN1 on cell growth and apoptosis were evaluated by cytofluorimetry (Fig. **4**). It was found that the expression of GKN1 in MKN28 cells, compared to control, reduced cell growth (Rippa, *et al.*, 2011). In agreement with our results, Shiozaky *et al.*, 2001 reported that transfection with CA11 gene reduced colony formation of MKN-28 gastric cancer cells. Also a novel mammal gastrokine, GKN3, reduced the growth of GKN3-overexpressing MKN28 cells (Menheniott, *et al.*, 2010). Because tissue repair is linked to many signals coming from the local environment it is important to understand why gastric cells are addressed to undergo apoptosis, proliferation or survive, following the inflammatory process. Therefore, gastric epithelial cell apoptosis could be influenced by GKN1 during inflammation. The Fas-ligand (FasL) system has been recognized as the major pathway for the induction of apoptosis in a variety of human normal and neoplastic cells (Nagata, 1996; Itoh and Nagata, 1993; Suda, *et al.*, 1993). The CD95 receptor (APO-1/Fas) belongs to TNFR superfamily and is a type I transmembrane protein (Itoh, *et al.*, 1991). Therefore, restoration of GKN1 could increase the level of expression of Fas, normally extremely low, in MKN28 cells (Osaki, *et al.*, 2001). We observed that restoration of GKN1 expression in negative GC cells (MKN28) induces a significant increase of Fas expression and this appears to be specific as also demonstrated by the enhancement of the Fas mRNA transcription. CD95 receptor and ligand system was also described in infection by *H. pylori*, however in this case other apoptotic factors are involved as well (Rudi *et al.*, 1998). These include TRIAL and its receptor subtypes (Martin, *et al.*, 2004; Yang, *et al.*, 2003). Because *H. pylori*-associated chronic gastritis involves apoptosis of gastric epithelial cells by activation of the CD95 receptor and ligand system, cells overexpressing GKN1 showed an increase in apoptosis that is mainly due to the exposure of the MKN28 cells to FasL compared to that observed in the control cells. In addition, when FasL binds to Fas, intracellular death caspases are activated, resulting in apoptotic demise of the cell (Chen, *et al.*, 1999). Also, a time-dependent increase in apoptotic cells was observed in GKN1 transfected cells and, as expected, cleaved forms of caspase-3, normally present as a 32 kDa inactive precursor (Zou, *et al.*, 1997), were found. This finding, evaluated by Western blot and fluorimetric assay suggest that GKN1-transfected cells were signalled to die (Schlegel, *et al.*, 1996; Wang, *et al.*, 1996; Nicholson, *et al.*, 1995). However, GKN1- induced apoptosis is suppressed when caspase-3 and caspase-8 are inhibited (Yoon, *et al.*, 2011).

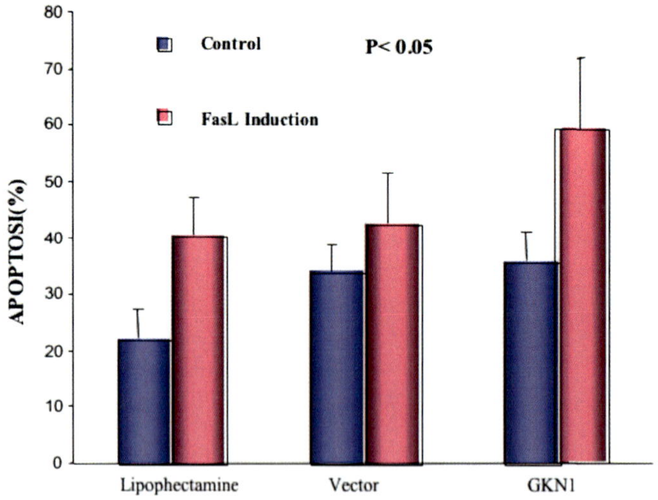

Figure 4: Effects of transfected GKN1 on cell death. Cell death was measured after transfection by TUNEL assay. Representative flow cytometry of cells treated with lipophectamine, cells transfected with empty pcDNA 3.1, cells transfected with GKN1 before and after incubation with antibody anti-FasL. Value from five independent experiments with similar results.

CONCLUSIONS

In the present study we have investigated expression of GKN1, mRNA and protein, in tissues specimen from normal and *H. pylori* infected gastric mucosa, atrophic gastritis, intestinal metaplasia, dysplasia, gastric cancer cell line and gastric cancer. We found that GKN1 is down-regulated and lost progressively in *H. pylori*-infected gastric mucosa and GC tissues but is abundant present in the adjacent non-cancer tissues as well as in normal gastric mucosa in agreement with other previous studies. The immunohistochemical analysis of human specimens showed a progressive decrease of GKN1 expression thus suggesting that the decrease of GKN1 is an early event in gastric precancer or cancer, and the presence of GKN1 may protect gastric mucosa from neoplasia. Thus GKN1 may be a potential biomarker candidate for early detection of gastric cancer. Moreover, the effects of GKN1 on gastric cancer cells were investigated; our data indicated that restoration of protein in cancer cells induced Fas-pathway mediated apoptosis and suggest that GKN1 may play an important role as a tumor suppressor gene. In conclusion, GKN1 appears as a modulator of apoptosis during the early stages of acute gastric injury and may influence tissue repair and be instrumental in determining the individual host response.

ACKNOWLEDGEMENTS

MIS and PA were partly funded by University of Naples 'Federico II', Italy: "International Exchange Program between foreign University and Research Institute for mobility of researchers".

CONFLICT OF INTEREST

The authors confirm that this chapter content has no conflict of interest.

REFERENCES

Anderson, N.L. and Anderson, N.G. 2002. The human plasma proteome: history, character, and diagnostic prospects. *Molecular and Cellular Proteomics*, 1, pp. 845-67. Erratum in: *Molecular and Cellular Proteomics*; 2003, 2, pp.50.

Baek, H.Y., Lim, J.W., Kim, H., Kim, J.M., Kim, J.S., Jung, H.C. and Kim, K.H. 2004. Oxidative stressrelated proteome changes in *Hilicobacter pylori*-infected human gastric mucosa. *Biochemical Journal*, 15, pp. 291-9.

Baus-Loncar, M., Lubka, M., Pusch, C.M., Otto, W.R., Poulsom, R. and Blin, N. 2007. Cytokine Regulation of the Trefoil Factor Family Binding Protein GKN2 (GDDR/TFIZ1/blottin) in Human Gastrointestinal Epithelial Cells. *Cellular Physiology and Biochemistry*, 20, pp. 193-20.

Bornschein, J. and Malfertheiner, P. 2011. Gastric carcinogenesis. *Langenbecks Arch Surg*, 396, pp. 729-42.

Bruce, R., Westley, S., Griffin, M. and May, F.E.B. 2005. Interaction between TFF1, a Gastric Tumor Suppressor Trefoil Protein, and TFIZ1, a Brichos Domain Containing Protein with Homology to SP-C. *Biochemistry*, 44, pp. 7967-75.

Carvalho, R., Kayademir, T., Soares, P., Canedo, P., Sousa, S., Oliveira, C., Leistenschneider, P., Seruca, R., Gött, P., Blin, N., Carneiro, F. and Machado, J.C. 2002. Loss of heterozygosity and promoter methylation, but not mutation, may underlie loss of TFF1 in gastric carcinoma. *Laboratory Investigation*, 82, pp. 1319-26.

Chen, M.K., Strande, L.F., Beierle, E.A., Kain, M.S., Geldziler, B.D. and Doolin, E.J. 1999. Fas-Mediated Induction of Hepatocyte Apoptosis in a Neuroblastoma and Hepatocyte Coculture Model. *Journal of Surgical Research*, 84, pp. 82-7.

Correa, P. and Piazuelo, M,B. 2008. Natural history of *Helicobacter pylori* infection. *Digestive and Liver Disease*, 40, pp. 490-6.

Correa, P. 1992. Human gastric carcinogenesis: a multistep and multifactorial process--First American Cancer Society Award Lecture on Cancer Epidemiology and Prevention. *Cancer Research*, 52, pp. 6735-40.

Correa, P. 1995. *Helicobacter pylori* and gastric carcinogenesis. *American Journal of Surgical Pathology*, 19 pp. S37-43.

Dhar, D.K., Wang, T.C., Tabara, H., Tonamoto, Y., Maruyama, R., Tachibana, M., Kubota, H. and Nagasue, N. 2005. Expression of Trefoil Factor family members correlates with patients prognosis and neoangiogenesis. *Human Cancer Biology*, 11, pp. 6472-78.

Du, J.J., Dou, K.F., Peng, S.Y., Wang, W.Z., Wang, Z.H., Xiao, H.S., Guan, W.X., Liu, Y.B. and Gao, Z,Q. 2003. Down-regulated full-length novel gene GDDR and its effect on gastric cancer. *Zhonghua Yi Xue Za Zhi*, 83, pp. 1166-68.

El-Omar, E.M., Rabkin, C.S., Gammon, M.D., Vaughan, T.L., Risch, H.A., Schoenberg, J.B., Stanford, J.L., Mayne, S.T., Goedert, J., Blot, W.J., Fraumeni, J.F. Jr and Chow, W.H. 2003. Increased risk of noncardia gastric cancer associated with proinflammatory cytokine gene polymorphisms. *Gastroenterology*, 124, pp. 1193-201.

El-Rifai, W., Frierson, H.F., Harper, J.C., Powell, S.M. and Knuutila, S. 2001. Expression profiling of gastric adenocarcinoma using cDNA array. *International Journal of Cancer*, 92, pp. 832–38.

Ferlay, J., Parkin, D.M. and Steliarova-Foucher, E. 2010. Estimates of cancer incidence and mortality in Europe in 2008. *Eur J Cancer*, 46, pp. 765-81.

Forman, D., Newell, D.G. and Fullerton, F. 1991. Association between infection with *Helicobacter pylori* and risk of gastric cancer: evidence from prospective investigation. *BMJ*, 302, pp. 1302-05.

Goldstone, A.R., Quirke, P. and Dixon, M,F. 1996. *Helicobacter pylori* infection and gastric cancer. Journal of Pathology, 179, pp. 129-37.

Griffin, T.J., Gygi, S.P., Ideker, T., Rist, B., Eng, J., Hood, L. and Aebersold, R. 2002. Complementary profiling of gene expression at the transcriptome and proteome levels in *Saccharomyces cerevisiae*. *Molecular and Cellular Proteomics*, 1, pp. 323-33.

Gygi, S.P., Rochon, Y., Franza, B.R. and Aebersold, R. 1999. Correlation between protein and mRNA abundance in yeast. Molecular and Cellular Biology, 19, pp. 1720-30.

Helicobacter and Cancer Collaborative Group. 2001. Gastric cancer and Helicobacter pylori: a combined analysis of 12 case control studies nested within prospective cohorts. *Gut*, 49, pp. 347-53.

Hippo, Y., Taniguchi, H., Tsutsumi, S., Machida, N., Chong, J.M., Fukayama, M., Kodama, T. and Aburatani, H. 2002. Global gene expression analysis of gastric cancer by oligonucleotide microarrays. *Cancer Research*, 62, pp. 233-40.

Holcombe, C. 1992. *Helicobacter pylori*: the African enigma. *Gut*, 33, pp. 429-431.

Huang, Q., Huang, Q., Chenn, W., Wang, L., Lin, W., Lin, J. and Lin, X. 2008. Identification of transgelin as a potential novel biomarker for gastric adenocarcinoma based on proteomics technology. *Journal of Cancer Research and Clinical Oncology*, 134, pp. 1219-27.

Itoh, N. and Nagata, S. 1993. A novel protein domain required for apoptosis. Mutational analysis of human Fas antigen. *Journal of Biological Chemistry*, 268, pp. 10932-7.

Itoh, N., Yonehara, S., Ishii, A., Yonehara, M., Mizushima, S., Sameshima, M., Hase, A., Seto, Y. and Nagata, S. 1991. The polypeptide encoded by the cDNA for human cell surface antigen Fas can mediate apoptosis. *Cell*, 66, pp. 233-43.

Kabir, S. 2009. Effect of Helicobacter pylori eradication on incidence of gastric cancer in human and animal models: underlying biochemical and molecular events. *Helicobacter*, 14, pp. 159-171.

Kjellev, S. 2009. The trefoil factor family – small peptides with multiple functionalities. *Cell Mol Life Sc*, 66, pp. 1350-1369.

Lauren, P. 1965. The Two Histological Main Types of Gastric Carcinoma: Diffuse and So-Called Intestinal-Type Carcinoma. An Attempt at a Histo-Clinical Classification. *Acta Pathologica et Microbiologica Scandinavica*, 64, pp. 31-49.

Lefebvre, O., Chenard, M.P., Masson, R. Linares J, Dierich A, LeMeur M, Wendling C, Tomasetto C, Chambon P. and Rio MC. 1996. Gastric mucosa abnormalities and tumorigenesis in mice lacking the pS2 trefoil protein. *Science*, 274, pp. 259-262.

Leung, W.K., Wu, M.S., Kakugawa, Y., Kim, J.J., Yeoh, K.G., Goh, K.L., Wu, K.C., Wu, D.C., Sollano, J., Kachintorn, U., Gotoda, T., Lin, J.T., You, W.C., Ng, E.K., Sung, J.J. and Asia Pacific Working Group on Gastric Cancer. 2008. Screening for gastric cancer in Asia: current evidence and practice. *Lancet Oncol*, 9, pp. 279-87.

Li, W., Li, J.F., Qu, Y., Chen, X.H., Qin, J.M., Gu, Q.L., Yan, M., Zhu, Z.G. and Liu, B.Y. 2008. Comparative proteomic analysis of human gastric cancer. *World Journal of Gastroenterology*, 14, pp. 5657-64.

Machado, J.C., Carneiro, F., Blin, N. and Sobrinho-Simoes M. 1996 Pattern of pS2 protein expression in premalignant and malignant lesion of gastric mucosa. *Eur J Cancer Prev*, 5, pp. 169-79.

Martin, J.H., Potthoff, A., Ledig, S., Cornberg, M., Jandl, O., Manns, M.P., Kubicka, S., Flemming, P., Athmann, C., Beil, W. and Wagner, S. 2004. Effect of *H. pylori* on the Expression of TRAIL, FasL and their Receptor Subtypes in Human Gastric Epithelial Cells and their Role in Apoptosis. *Helicobacter*, 9, pp. 371-86.

Martin, T.E., Powell, C.T., Wang, Z., Bhattacharyya, S., Walsh-Reitz, M.M., Agarwal, K. and Toback, F.G. 2003. A novel mitogenic protein that is highly expressed in cells of the gastric antrum mucosa. *American Journal of Physiology Gastrointestinal and Liver Physiology*, 285, pp. G332-43.

Mattioli, E., Vogiatzi, P., Sun, A., Abbaddessa, G., Angeloni, G., D'Ugo, D., Trani, D., Gaughan, J.P., Vecchio, F.M., Cevenini, G., Persiani, R., Giordano, A. and Claudio, P.P. 2007. Immunohistochemical analysis of pRb2/p130, VEGF, EZH2, p53, p16(INK4A), p27(KIP1), p21(WAF1), Ki-67 expression patterns in gastric cancer. *Journal of Cellular Physiology*, 210, pp. 183-191.

Menheniott, T.R., Peterson, A.J., O'connor, L., Lee, K.S., Kalantzis, A., Kondova, I., Bontrop, R.E., Bell, K.M. and Giraud, AS. 2010. A Novel Gastrokine in Mammals Marks Gastric Atrophy and shows evidence of adaptive gene loss in human. *Gastroenterology*, 138, pp. 1823-35.

Michener, C.M., Ardekani, A.M,. Petricoin, E.F., Liotta, L.A. and Kohn, E.C. 2002. Genomics and proteomics: application of novel technology to early detection and prevention of cancer. *Cancer Detection and Prevention*, 26, pp. 249-55.

Mintz, J.P., Kim, H., Kim-Anh, D., Wang, W., Zinner, R.G., Cristofanilli, M., Arap, M.A., Hong, W.K., Troncoso, P., Logothetis, C.H., Pasqualini, R., and Arap, W. 2003. Fingerprinting the circulating repertoire of antibodies from cancer patients. *Nature Biotechnology*, 21, pp. 57-63.

Mori, M., Mimori, K., Yoshikawa, Y., Shibuta, K., Utsunomiya, T., Sadanaga, N., Tanaka, F., Matsuyama, A., Inoue, H. and Sugimachi, K. 2002. Analysis of the gene-expression profile regarding the progression of human gastric carcinoma. *Surgery*, 131, pp. S39-47.

Moss, S.F., Lee, J.W., Sabo, E., Rubin, A.K., Rommel, J., Westley, B.R., May, F.E., Gao, J., Meitner, P.A., Tavares, R. and Resnick, M.B. 2008. Decreased expression of gastrokine 1 and trefoil Factor Interacting Protein TFIZ1/GKN2 in gastric cancer: influence of tumor histology and relationship to prognosis. *Clinical Cancer Research*, 14, pp. 4161-7.

Motoyama, T., Hojo, H., and Watanabe, H. 1986. Comparison of seven cell lines derived from human gastric carcinomas. *Acta Pathologica Japonica*, 36, pp. 65-83.

Nabewera, H.M. and Logan, R.P. 1999. Epidemiology of *Helicobacter pylori* infection: transmission, translocation and extragastric reservoirs. *Journal of Physiology and Pharmacology*, 50, pp. 711-22.

Nagata, S. 1996. Apoptosis by death factor. *Cell*, 88, pp. 355-65.

Nardone, G, Martin, G., Rocco, A., Rippa, E., La Monica, G., Caruso, F. and Arcari, P. 2008. Molecular expression of Gastrokine 1 in normal mucosa and in *Helicobacter pylori*-related preneoplastic and neoplastic gastric lesions. *Cancer Biology and Therapy*, 7, pp. 1890-95

Nardone, G., Rippa, E., Martin, G., Rocco, A, Siciliano, R.A., Fiengo, A. Cacace, G., Malorni, A., Budillon, G. and Arcari, P. 2007. Gastrokine 1 expression in patients with and without *Helicobacter pylori* infection. *Digestive and Liver Disease*, 39, pp. 122-29.

Nicholson, W.D., Ali, A., Thornberry, N.A., Vailancourt, J.P., Ding, C.K., Gallant, M., Gareau, Y., Griffin, P.R., Labelle, M., Lazebnik, Y.A., Munday, N.A., Raji, S.M., Smulson, M.E., Yamin, T.T., Yu, V.L. and Miller, D.K. 1995. Identification and inhibition of the ICE/CED-3 protease necessary for mammalian apoptosis. *Nature*, 376, pp. 37-43.

Oien, K.A., McGregor, F., Butler, S., Ferrier, R.K., Downie, I., Bryce, S., Burns, S. and Keith, W.N. 2004. Gastrokine 1 is abundantly and specifically expressed in superficial gastric epithelium, down-regulated in gastric carcinoma, and shows high evolutionary conservation. *Journal of Pathology*, 203, pp. 789-97.

Oien, K.A., Vass, J.K., Downie, I., Fullarton, G. and Keith, W.N. 2003. Profiling, comparison and validation of gene expression in gastric carcinoma and normal stomach. *Oncogene*, 22, pp. 4287-300.

Orrù, S., Caputo, I., D'Amato, A., Ruoppolo, M. and Esposito, C. 2003. Proteomics Identification of Acylacceptor and Acyl-donor Substrates for Transglutaminase in a Human Intestinal Epithelial Cell Line: implications for celiac disease. *Journal of Biological Chemistry*, 278, pp. 31766-73.

Osaki, M., Kase, S., Kodani, I., Watanabe, M., Adachi, H. and Ito, H. 2001. Expression of Fas and Fas ligand in human gastric adenomas and intestinal-type carcinomas: correlation with proliferation and apoptosis. *Gastric Cancer*, 4, pp. 198-205.

Otto, W.R., Patel, K., McKinnell, I., Evans, M.D., Lee, C.Y., Frith, D., Hanrahan, S., Blight, K., Blin, N., Kayademir, T., Poulsom, R., Jeffery, R., Hunt, T., Wright, N.A., McGregor, F. and Oien, K.A. 2006. Identification of blottin: A novel gastric trefoil factor family-2 binding protein. *Proteomics*, 6, pp. 4235-45.

Parsonnet, J., Friedman, G.D., Oremtreich, N. and Vogelman, H. 1997. Risk for gastric cancer in people with CagA positive or CagA negative *Helicobacter pylori* infection. *Gut*, 40, pp. 297-301.

Pavone, L.M., Del Vecchio, P., Mallardo, P., Altieri, F., De Pasquale, V., Rea, S., Martucci, N.M., Di Stadio, C.S., Pucci, P., Flagiello, A., Masullo, M., Arcari, P. and Rippa, E. 2013. Structural characterization and biological properties of human gastrokine 1. *Mol Biosyst*, 9, pp. 412-21.

Petricoin, E.F., Ardekani, A.M., Hitt, B.A., Levine, P.J., Fusaro, V.A., Steinberg, S.M., Mills, G.B., Krieg, R.C., Paweletz, C.P., Liotta, L.A. and Petricoin, E.F. 2002. Clinical proteomics for cancer biomarker discovery and therapeutic targeting. *Technology in Cancer Research and Treatment*, 4, pp. 263-72.

Pisani, P., Parkin, D.M., Bray, F. and Ferlay, J. 1999. Estimates of the worldwide mortality from 25 cancers in 1990. *International Journal of Cancer*, 83. pp. 18-29.

Rippa, E., La Monica, G., Allocca, R., Romano, M.F., De Palma, M. and Arcari, P. 2011. Overexpression of gastrokine 1 in gastric cancer cells induces Fas-mediated apoptosis. *Journal of Cellular Physiology*, 226, pp. 2571-8.

Rosenberg, S.A. 2001. Progress in human tumour immunology and immunotherapy. *Nature*, 411, pp. 380-4.

Rudi, J., Kuck, D., Strand, S., von Herbay, A., Mariani, S.M. Krammer, P.H., Galle, P.R. and Stremmel, W. 1998. Involvement of the CD95 (APO-1/Fas) receptor and ligand system in *Helicobacter pylori*-induced gastric epithelial apoptosis. *J Clin Invest*, 102, pp. 1506–1514.

Sanchez-Pulido, L., Devos, D. and Valencia, A. 2002. BRICHOS: a conserved domain in proteins associated with dementia, respiratory distress and cancer. *Trends in Biochemical Science*, 27, pp. 329-32.

Schlegel, J., Peters, I., Orrenius, S., Miller, D.K., Thornberry, N.A., Yamin, T.T. and Nicholson, D.W. 1996. CPP32/apopain is a key interleukin 1 beta converting enzyme-like protease involved in Fasmediated apoptosis. *Journal of Clinical Investigation*, 271, pp. 1841-4.

Segal, E.D., Falkow, S. and Tompkinset, L.S. 1996. *Helicobacter pylori* attachment to gastric cells induces cytoskeletal rearrangements and tyrosine phosphorylation of host cell proteins. *Proceedings of the National Academy of Sciences USA*, 93, pp. 1259-64.

Shiozaki, K., Nakamori, S., Tsujie, M., Okami, J., Yamamoto, H., Nagano, H., Dono, K., Umeshita, K., Sakon, M., Furukawa, H., Hiratsuka, M., Kasugai, T., Ishiguro, S. and Monden, M. 2001. Human stomach-specific gene, CA11, is down-regulated in gastric cancer. *International Journal of Oncology*, 19, pp. 701-7.

Suda, T., Takahashi, T., Golstein, P. and Nagata, S. 1993. Molecular cloning and expression of the Fas ligand, a novel member of the tumor necrosis factor family. *Cell*, 75, pp. 1169-78.

Toback, F.G., Walsh-Reitz, M.M., Musch, M.W., Chang, E.B., Del Valle, J., Ren, H., Huang, E. and Martin, T.E. 2003. Peptide fragments of AMP-18, a novel secreted gastric antrum mucosal protein, are mitogenic and motogenic. *American Journal of Physiology Gastrointestinal and Liver Physiology*, 285, pp. G344-53.

Vlahou, A. and Fountoulakis, M. 2005. Proteomic approaches in the search for disease biomarkers. *Journal of Chromatogr B Analytical Technologies in the Biomedical Life Sciences*, 814, pp. 11-9.

Walsh-Reitz, M.M., Huang, E.F., Musch. M.W., Chang, E.B., Martin, T.E., Kartha, S. and Toback, F.G. 2005. AMP18 protects barrier function of colonic epithelial cells: role of tight junction proteins. *American Journal of Physiology Gastrointestinal and Liver Physiology*, 289, pp. G163-71.

Wang, X., Zelenski, N.G., Yang, J., Sakai, J., Brown, M.S. and Goldstein, J.L. 1996. Cleavage of sterol regulatory element binding proteins (SREBPs) by cpp32 during apoptosis. *EMBO Journal*, 15, pp. 1012–20.

Watanabe, T., Tada, M. and Nagai, H. 1998. *Helicobacter pylori* infection induces gastric cancer in Mongolian gerbils. *Gastroenterology*, 115, pp. 642-48.

Westley, B.R., Griffin, S.M. and May, F.E. 2005. Interaction between TFF1, a gastric tumor suppressor trefoil protein, and TFIZ1, a brichos domain-containing protein with homology to SP-C. *Biochemistry*, 44, pp. 7967-75.

Whary, M.T., Sundina, N., Bravo, L.E., Correa, P., Quinones, F., Caro, F. and Fox, J.G. 2005. Intestinal helminthiasis in Colombian children promotes a Th2 response to Helicobacter pylori: possible implications for gastric carcinogenesis. *Cancer Epidemiology, Biomarkers and Prevention*, 14, pp. 1464-9.

Wu, C.Y., Tseng, J.J., Chou, M.M., Lin, S.K., Poon, S.K. and Chen, G.H. 2000. Correlation between Helicobacter pylori infection and gastrointestinal symptoms in pregnancy. *Adv Ther*, 17, pp. 152-8.

Yamachika, T., Werther, J.L., Bodian, C., Babyatsky, M., Tatematsu, M., Yamamura, Y., Chen, A. and Itzkowitz, S. 2002. Intestina Trefoil Factor: a marker of poor prognosisi in gastric carcinoma. *Clinical Cancer Research*, 8, pp. 1092-99.

Yang, Y., Deng, C.S., Peng, J.Z., Wong, B.C.Y., Lam, S.K. and Xia, H.H.X. 2003. Effect of *Helicobacter pylori* on apoptosis and apoptosis related genes in gastric cancer cells. *Molecular Pathology*, 56, pp. 19-24.

Yoon, J.H., Song, J.H., Zhang, C., Jin, M., Kang, Y.H., Nam, S.W., Lee, J.Y. and Park, W.S. 2011. Inactivation of Gastrokine 1 gene in gastric adenomas and carcinomas. *Journal of Pathology*, published on line in Wiley Online Library.

Yoshikawa, Y., Mukai, H., Hino, F., Asada, K. and Kato, I. 2000. Isolation of two novel genes, own-regulated in gastric cancer. *Japanese Journal of Cancer Research*, 91, pp. 459-63.

Zou, H., Henzel, W.J., Liu, X., Lutschg, A. and Wang, X. 1997. Apaf-1, a Human Protein Homologous to C. elegans CED-4, Participates in Cytochrome c–Dependent Activation of Caspase-3. *Cell*, 90, pp. 405-13.

Send Orders for Reprints to reprints@benthamscience.net
Cutting Edge Therapies for Cancer in the 21st Century, 2014, 271-351 271

CHAPTER 10

Nuclear Medicine Spectrum in Neuroendocrine Tumour Management: Molecular-Based Apogee Effectuating Improved Outcomes

Pipitsa Valsamaki*

Nuclear Medicine Department, "Alexandra" University General Hospital, Athens, Greece

Abstract: Nuclear medicine imaging and treatment play a particularly prominent role in the management of Neuroendocrine Tumours (NET), consistently pertaining to the molecular level on the ground of specific properties of neuroendocrine neoplastic cells. NET may be sporadic or appear as part of an inherited syndrome, originate from the diffuse neuroendocrine system and consist of Amine Precursor Uptake and Decarboxylation (APUD) cells; these cells produce and store hormones which account for a broad spectrum of subsequent clinical manifestations. NET cells also characteristically overexpress specific cell membrane peptide receptors like somatostatin receptors (sstr). Clinically non-functional NET contribute further to their relatively common delayed diagnosis.

Histologic assessment with relative immunohistochemical indices, remains the gold standard for NET diagnosis. Measurement of serum or urinary, specific or non-specific, hormonal markers, aids in the diagnostic NET investigation, with high sensitivity, in addition to follow-up and possibly prognostic value. Involved localization modalities include endoscopic ultrasound (EUS), computerized tomography (CT), magnetic resonance imaging (MRI) and radionuclide methods.

Nuclear imaging exploits radiopharmaceuticals similar in molecular structure to the tumour-synthesized substances or incorporated into various tumour cellular metabolic processes, to selectively visualize NET. Established scintigraphic studies on primary and metastatic NET imaging, apply radiolabelled synthetic somatostatin (sst) analogues [like indium-111-diethylene triamine pentaacetic acid-octreotide (^{111}In-DTPA-octreotide)] to bind on sstr, iodine-131/123 meta-iodo-benzylguanidine ($^{131/123}$I-MIBG) to be actively transported and stored within neurosecretory granules of APUD cells as a chemical nor-epinephrine analogue, and pentavalent technetium-99m dimercaptosuccinic acid [^{99m}Tc(V)-DMSA] to be taken up by cells exhibiting accelerated proliferation. Positron emission tomography (PET) or PET/CT studies are

***Address correspondence to Pipita Valsamaki:** Nuclear Medicine Department "Alexandra" University General Hospital Athens, Greece; Tel/Fax: 0030 210 3381736; E-mail: pivals@gmail.com

also helpful for NET evaluation, by employing ^{68}Ga-labelled sst analogues such as [^{68}Ga-DOTA^{0},Tyr^{3}]octreotide (^{68}Ga-DOTATOC), [^{68}Ga-DOTA^{0},Tyr^{3}]octreotate (^{68}Ga-DOTATATE) and ^{68}Ga-DOTANOC for sstr binding, ^{18}F-DOPA, ^{11}C-5-HTP and ^{11}C-hydroxyephedrine (^{11}C-HED) for APUD mechanism exploitation, and ^{18}F-FDG-PET for NET of low-differentiation and high proliferative activity. The traditional whole-body bone scan with ^{99m}Tc-methylene diphosphonate (^{99m}Tc-MDP) adds to staging and prognostic data through the identification of skeletal metastases. Altogether, in patients bearing NET, radionuclide imaging provides non-invasive diagnosis, staging, restaging, treatment planning, prediction of therapy response, selection of patients for targeted (radio- or non-radiolabelled) therapy, and follow-up for detection of relapse or disease progression.

Keywords: Neuroendocrine tumours, pheochromocytoma, neuroblastoma, ^{111}In-DTPA-octreotide, ^{131}I-MIBG, ^{99m}Tc(V)-DMSA, ^{68}Ga-DOTATOC, PRRT, ^{90}Y-DOTATOC, ^{177}Lu-DOTATATE, multiple endocrine neoplasia syndromes, APUD cells, carcinoids, MRI, PET, scintigraphy, isotope.

1. INTRODUCTION

Neuroendocrine Tumours (NET) comprise a genetically heterogeneous group of neoplasms derived from diffuse neuroendocrine system. Most NET are sporadic in nature, but they may also appear as part of an inherited syndrome, like Multiple Endocrine Neoplasia syndromes (MEN I and MEN II), Von Hippel-Lindau disease and neurofibromatosis. In general, NET are rare and affect both genders with equal frequency, usually at 40-50 years of age, except for neuroblastoma which involves children. According to Surveillance, Epidemiology, and End Results (SEER) database, increased prevalence of NET has been recorded during the last years, with the annual incidence rising worldwide 3 to 5/100.000 population (Yao *et al.*, 2008).

The neuroendocrine system originates from the embryonal neural crest tissue found in the hypothalamus, pituitary gland, thyroid gland, adrenal medulla and the gastrointestinal tract and consists of Amine Precursor Uptake and Decarboxylation (APUD) cells. NET may arise from any of these sites. Gastroenteropancreatic (GEP)-NET in particular arise from the neuroendocrine cells found in the pancreas, the gut and its derivatives like the bronchial tree (Khanna *et al.*, 2008, Nisa *et al.*, 2011). The most common GEP-NET, arising from enterochromaffin cells of the gastrointestinal tract are carcinoids. They are clinically less aggressive than the more common intestinal adenocarcinoma and typically occur as well-circumscribed round submucosal lesions (Fass, 2008). The APUD cells characteristically possess the ability to take up and incorporate amine precursors in their cytoplasm, which are utilized for the production, storage and secretion of peptides and amines. They contain granules in which they store two kinds of substances: a) amines, *i.e.* dopamine, catecholamines (adrenaline and nor-adrenaline) and serotonin, and b) peptides, like somatostatin, substance P, insulin, glucagon *etc.* These substances are secreted by APUD cells and act as neurotransmitters, neuromodulators and/or hormones. The produced peptides/ hormones/neurotransmitters are bound at their action site by specific cell membrane receptors and lead to specific symptom expression. Thus NET disease entities usually provoke a wide spectrum of clinical manifestations, which may disorientate and prevent prompt diagnosis and treatment; both prerequisites for complete cure. The patients often present at the general practitioner, when already bearing metastatic disease and/or being seriously ill and thus having limited treatment options.

The classification of NET contributes to the evaluation of their biologic behaviour and thus their correct management and according to relevant guidelines (ENET, AJC, WHO), includes: a) their anatomic site of origin, with broad generalizations, such as: i) the pancreatic and bronchial NET comprise distinct entities and may be related to hormone hypersecretion syndromes, ii) the NET originating from the small intestine and the proximal large intestine are relatively homogeneous tumours closely related to the typical carcinoid syndrome and iii) the NET derived from the distal large intestine and the rectum are usually non-functional. b) the grade, which expresses the tumour proliferating ability and thus its aggressivity: low, G1- typically develop slowly; intermediate, G2- bear a less predictable, medium aggressive course; and high grade, G3- are extensively aggressive. The most important factors in determining the grade are the number of mitoses (mitotic count per HPF) and the immunohistochemical proliferation index Ki-67 (MIB-1). c) the histopathological parameters: the discrimination between well- from poorly-differentiated NET, is one of the most significant distinctions of these neoplasms, since the biologic behaviour of the well-differentiated group is commonly rather indolent, while the poorly-differentiated neuroendocrine carcinomas are particularly aggressive, hence directly influencing the treatment decision. d) the TNM stage which determines the disease extent: local, regional, distant metastatic, and e) the functionality: the tumours may secrete hormones or amines (functioning) and may provoke plenty of symptoms, like the carcinoid syndrome which appears in 8%-35% of the patients; on the other hand, non-functioning tumours produce peptides without adding to distinct clinical manifestation, but may cause symptoms due to increased mass effect (*e.g.* pain, obstruction, hemorrhage) (Nisa *et al.*, 2011).

The diagnostic approach of NET encompasses specific (gastrin, insulin, catecholamines, vanillylmandelic acid- VMA *etc.*) or non-specific (chromogranin-A (CgA), synaptophysin, neuron specific enolase (NSE)) serum or urinary hormonal indices with high sensitivity and possibly prognostic value, as well as specifically indicated imaging methods, including endoscopic ultrasound (EUS), computerized tomography (CT), magnetic resonance imaging (MRI) and radionuclide imaging methods. Nuclear imaging utilizes a variety of underlying pathophysiological and biochemical associated alterations and based on radiopharmaceuticals either similar in molecular structure to the tumour-synthesized hormones or incorporated into various tumour cellular metabolic processes (Fass, 2008), selectively visualizes NET and accordingly offers therapeutic options. Specifically nuclear NET imaging uses radiolabelled synthetic somatostatin (sst) analogues [like indium-111-diethylene triamine pentaacetic acid-octreotide (^{111}In-DTPA-octreotide)], iodine-131/123 meta-iodo-benzylguanidine ($^{131/123}$I-MIBG), pentavalent technetium-99m dimercaptosuccinic acid [^{99m}Tc(V)-DMSA] and various positron-emitting radionuclides in positron emission tomography (PET). In addition, the traditional whole-body study with technetium-99m-methylene diphosphonate (^{99m}Tc-MDP) provides staging and prognostic data by identifying skeletal metastases with high sensitivity and low cost.

2. RADIONUCLIDE IMAGING OF NEUROENDOCRINE TUMOURS

Nuclear medicine imaging and treatment have an established and constantly expanding role into the core of cancer management, including NET. Nuclear medicine imaging encompasses non-invasive diagnosis, staging, restaging, treatment planning, prediction of therapy response, and evaluation of response to treatment in patients suffering from NET, in concordance with associated laboratory data. Low radiation absorbed doses and minimum adverse effects allow for the radionuclide studies to be repeated. Radionuclide imaging consists of planar gamma (γ-) cameras, 3D depiction by single photon emission computed tomography (SPECT) as well as PET. SPECT or PET co-registration with CT or MRI increases the sensitivity of both studies even more (Koopmans *et al.*, 2008). In order to overcome the difficulty of fusion of non-rigid moving anatomy, such as the thorax, hybrid imaging systems have been created (Zaidi *et al.*, 2007). Combined PET/MR was the first conception, but SPECT/CT and PET/CT were the first to become commercially available. The advantages of a combined system have been proved in oncological imaging by PET/CT especially regarding staging and radiotherapy planning. The continuing technological improvements in association with the ongoing elucidation and exploitation of the underlying NET cellular processes and related mechanisms of radiopharmaceuticals uptake, have induced alternative imaging and treatment options with promising results and perspectives.

I. Scintigraphy With ^{123}I- or ^{131}I-labelled MIBG

Radioiodinated ^{131}I-MIBG was developed and employed in 1980 at the University of Michigan Medical Centre, Ann Arbor, Michigan, U.S.A., as the first localization procedure in all patients with either clinical or biochemical indications of pheochromocytoma (PCC) (Cheung *et al.*, 1988). MIBG is a combination of the benzyl group of bretylium and the guanidine group of guanethidine, structurally resembling norepinephrine and guanethidine (a neurosecretory granule depleting agent). MIBG is taken up mostly by the Na^+-dependent type-I amine active transport mechanism and stored within vesicles or neurosecretory granules of catecholamine-producing cells possibly by displacing norepinephrine. The uptake–re-uptake system preserves norepinephrine in sympathetic neurons (Fass, 2008).

MIBG labelled with either ^{123}I or ^{131}I is used for the scintigraphic study of the adrenergic nervous system, the adrenal medulla as well as paragangliomas and other neuroendocrine tissues. Apart from localizing neural crest tumors of the

APUD system (APUDomas), ^{131}I-MIBG constitutes a valuable treatment option (Troncone *et al.*, 2004). Thus, specifically, scintigraphy with $^{123/131}$I-MIBG is indicated for functional diagnosis, anatomical localization, staging, and follow-up of NET in terms of determination of prognosis or exclusion of a subclinical relapse, as well as planning of ^{131}I-MIBG therapy and evaluation of treatment response. Regarding therapy planning, the tumour uptake and residence time are evaluated on imaging. Yet, individualized dosimetric evaluation is needed, since the ICRP Tables supply only an indicative value limited to diagnostic procedures (ICRP, 1987, 1998, Stabin *et al.*, 1998). For the evaluation of tumour response to therapy, the intensity of MIBG uptake and the number of focal MIBG uptake sites are measured upon imaging (Boubaker *et al.*, 2003, Perel *et al.*, 1999).

The intravenously injected tracer undergoes rapid blood clearance and accumulates in adrenergic presynaptic nerve endings and cells of the adrenal medulla either by transport within catecholamine-storage granules *via* an ATPase-dependent and reserpine-sensitive mechanism like in PCC, or by binding to extra-granular cytoplasmic structures like in neuroblastoma. The tracer remains as monoamineoxidase and catechol-0-methyltransferase and is not further metabolized; thus it shows minor binding to postsynaptic receptors and induces minor or no pharmacological response (Sisson *et al.*, 1986). Forty to seventy-five percent of the administered dose is excreted unchanged in the urine within 24 hours and 70% to more than 95% within 96 hours, while the rest is excreted through the gut, saliva, sweat and respiration. The use of ^{123}I-MIBG is advantageous over ^{131}I-MIBG, having a 10 fold greater imaging ability due to its higher specific radioactivity, the feasibility of SPECT, the lower radiation burden to the patient and the faster scintigraphic procedure. Nevertheless, the readily available ^{131}I-MIBG is extensively used in clinical routine principally in adults due to its longer half-life and the associated option of delayed images as well as its lower cost (Table **1**) (Swanson *et al.*, 1981).

Table 1: Physical properties and availability features of ^{131}I- and ^{123}I-MIBG

	^{131}I	**^{123}I**
Half-life t1/2 (h)	193	13
Production	Nuclear reactor Te-130	Cyclotron

		^{131}I	^{123}I
			Xe-124
Radiation emission	mean β- maximum β- MeV	0.192 0.61 (89.9%)	
	γ keV	364 (81.2%)	159 (83.4%)
Tissue penetration (particle range)	mean	0.6mm	-
	maximum	2mm	-
Daughter isotope		Xe-131	Te-123
Whole-body radiation dose (cGy/37 MBq)	adult	0.89	0.053
	1 year old	4.4	0.22

Radiopharmaceutical uptake and/or storage has been reported to be inhibited by a variety of drugs which may be received by the patient, including antihypertensives (like labetalol, guanethidine, reserpine, iv phenoxybenzamine, calcium channel blockers), sympathomimetics, nasal decongestants, tricyclic and related antidepressants, antipsychotics, sedating antihistamines, opioid analgesics and CNS stimulants. Such interfering agents should be discontinued, each for a specific time period prior to scintigraphy in order to ensure tumour uptake and visualization (Khagaghi *et al.*, 1989, Bombardieri *et al.*, 2010). In case of clinical factors prohibiting such drug interruption, the study may be postponed or be performed under unchanged medication in consultation with the referring physician (Bombardieri *et al.*, 2010). The possibility of impaired diagnostic accuracy should be considered and reported (Solanki *et al.*, 1992, Lassmann *et al.*, 2007). Breastfeeding should be discontinued for 48 hours when using ^{123}I-MIBG, and terminated for ^{131}I-MIBG imaging. In pregnancy possible harm *versus* benefit assessment directs the clinical decision in order for the method to be applied. Furthermore, radiation protection of the thyroid gland is pursued through justified blockade by stable iodine per os. This is especially important in children, the thyroid being more radiosensitive than in adults and doses should be adjusted according to EANM Paediatric Committee guidelines (Olivier *et al.*, 2002 Bombardieri *et al.*, 2010).

Each radioiodinated MIBG dose is slowly administered intravenously over at least 2-5 minutes. When the tracer is rapidly administered, rare potential adverse effects include blood pressure increase, vomiting, tachycardia, pallor, abdominal pain, allergic reactions, flush and asthmatic spasms. Increased fluid intake by the patients is advised so that excretion of unbound radiopharmaceutical is enhanced. The appropriate administered activities and imaging procedures for ^{131}I- and ^{123}I-MIBG, are described in Table **2**. Normal $^{123/131}$I-MIBG radioactivity distribution visualizes the heart (intensely or faintly) and lungs early, the liver, spleen (sometimes absent in children), salivary glands and bladder throughout the entire examination, and in about 20% of patients the colon in the delayed images. Normally the adrenal medulla is only faintly visualized in less than 20% of cases at 48 hours (the percentage recently increasing, possibly due to increased ^{131}I-MIBG specific activity), a finding more frequently observed with ^{123}I-MIBG, which may also image the kidneys, nasal mucosa and lacrimal glands (Nakajo *et al.*, 1983, Bombardieri *et al.*, 2010). Diagnostic or mostly post-therapeutic imaging may demonstrate focal uptake in cerebellum, basal nuclei and thalamic regions (Dwamena *et al.*, 1998). Muscle activity may be recognized but bones are always photopenic (Nakajo *et al.*, 1983, Troncone *et al.*, 2004).

Table 2: Protocol for $^{123/131}$I-MIBG scintigraphy

	^{123}I-MIBG Scintigraphy	**^{131}I-MIBG Scintigraphy**
Preparation	- Withdrawal of interfering drugs (1-2 weeks prior to scintigraphy) and patient stabilization on alternative medication, if clinically feasible - Thyroid blockade: Stable iodine per os, starting 24 h before tracer injection and continued for 24-48 h pi, for ^{123}I-MIBG or 48-72 h pi, for ^{131}I-MIBG Adults: Lugol solution 1% at 1 drop/kg/day with a maximum of 40 (20 drops twice daily) Children: 32 mg/day of potassium iodide for children 1 month to 3 years old, 65 mg for 3 to 13 years old, and 130 mg for older than 13 years; the recommended dose for newborns is 16 mg only on the day before tracer injection Alternatively potassium perchlorate may be used for rapid blockade on the day of injection in emergencies, or in patients with allergy to iodine	
Administration route and activity	iv 400 MBq (10.8 mCi) children: 20-400 MBq	iv 40-80 MBq (1.2-2.2 mCi) children: 35-80 MBq
	The pediatric doses are calculated based on reference adult doses scaled to	

	^{123}I-MIBG Scintigraphy	**^{131}I-MIBG Scintigraphy**
	body weight according to the schedule proposed by the EANM Paediatric Task Group	
Post-injection (pi) preparation	hydration	
Imaging	early at 2-3 h and delayed at 24 and 48 h pi	early at 24 h and potentially delayed at 48, 72 and 96 h pi
	whole-body anterior and posterior spot images according to clinical setting	
Collimator	low or medium-energy parallel-hole	high-energy parallel-hole
Energy window	20% at 159 keV	20% at 360 keV

In adrenal medullary hyperplasia, which is associated with MEN IIA and MEN IIB syndromes, MIBG scintigraphy shows increased bilateral adrenal uptake both on early and delayed imaging, while CT and MRI become positive only at advanced stage. There have been reports indicating a restricted role of ^{123}I-MIBG scintigraphy in precocious detection of nodular (diameter of tumor nodules < 1 cm) medullary hyperplasia, which in hypertensive patients could potentially represent a phase in the natural history of PCC. Nevertheless MIBG has a decisive place in the imaging diagnostic armamentarium of adrenal medullary hyperplasia (Valk *et al.*, 1981, Van der Harst *et al.*, 2001).

Scintigraphy with MIBG is the method of choice for PCC confirmation and is a valuable screening test, based on its high sensitivity, *i.e.* 86% for benign and 92.4% for malignant lesions, with only 1-5% of false positive results; the corresponding unilateral focal tumour uptake in the posterior view of the abdomen constitutes the characteristic appearance (Shapiro *et al.*, 1985, Troncone *et al.*, 1990, Mozley *et al.*, 1994). PCC may be benign or malignant, uni- or bilateral, solitary or multiple and may originate from chromaffin cells of the adrenal medulla (intra-adrenal PCC), the sympathetic chain ganglia in the paraspinal region or the parasympathetic nervous system of the head, neck and middle mediastinum (extra-adrenal PCC or paragangliomas, except for tumours arising from the branchiomeric region and comprising carotid body paragangliomas or chemodectomas) (Pacak *et al.*, 2001). The typically chromaffin-positive sympathoadrenal NET often produce catecholamines resulting in the corresponding clinical manifestations. On the contrary, the typically chromaffin-negative parasympathetic NET are usually clinically silent. While the incidence of PCC in hypertensive patients is approximately 0.1%-0.5%, around 60% of patients with PCC/paraganglioma develop protracted hypertension and the rest show increased blood pressure during an attack. Patients may also be asymptomatic, with the PCC/paraganglioma prevalence being 4% in patients with adrenal incidentaloma (Sisson *et al.*, 1981, Troncone *et al.*, 2004). In patients with bilateral or multiple PCC, bearing a prevalence of 0.001%-0.01% in adults, there is usually an association with a neuroendocrine syndrome such as MEN IIA (Fig. **1**), MEN IIB, von Recklinghausen's neurofibromatosis and von Hippel Lindau disease; they might additionally be combined with inherited PCC transmitted as an autosomal dominant trait. MIBG imaging can localize all types of paragangliomas (Kalff *et al.*, 1982, Nakajo *et al.*, 1983, McEwan *et al.*, 1985). Large PCC/paragangliomas exceeding a diameter of 1.5 cm are readily depicted by CT, while MIBG scintigraphy detects both large and small lesions; the invaluable inherent advantage of MIBG is the feasibility for whole-body investigation and thus the recognition of unifocal lesion in close relationship to other structures or recurrent, multifocal, or metastatic disease (Sisson *et al.*, 1981, Mozley *et al.*, 1994, Troncone *et al.*, 2004).

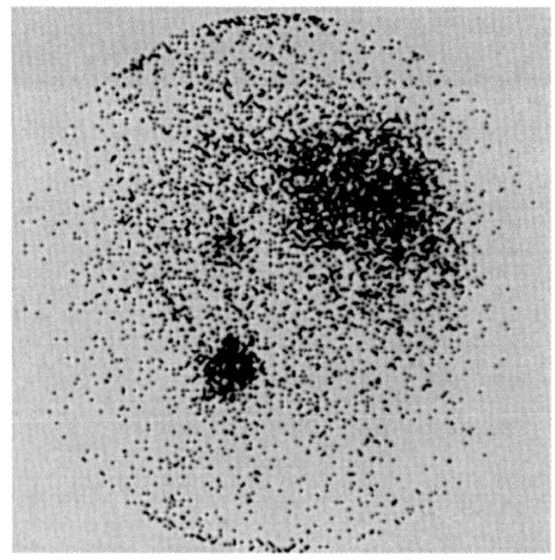

Figure 1: ^{131}I-MIBG scintigraphy in a 47 years old man with MEN IIA syndrome, who had thyroidectomy due to MTC and bilateral semi-adrenalectomy due to PCC 16 years before. He was referred to our department due to elevated adrenaline and metanephrine levels in 24-h urine collection. The posterior abdominal view at 24 h pi shows relatively increased radiopharmaceutical uptake at the anatomical position of the adrenals, with broadened limits particularly on the left, indicating bilateral PCC relapse. The depicted large (max dia: 3.5 cm) lesion with intense tracer uptake located towards the midline and below the level of the lower pole of the left kidney was as of neuroendocrine origin, possibly paraganglioma. All findings were matched on CT imaging.

(All figures are herein published with the courtesy of Dr. Vassilios Papantoniou, Head of the Nuclear Medicine Department of University General Hospital "Alexandra" in Athens, Greece).

Radiopharmaceutical intensity of uptake corresponds to the quantity of neuroendocrine granules of the imaged tumour. Therefore the presence necrotic foci and dispersed neuroendocrine elements within a large malignant PCC may prevent significant radiotracer uptake. Decreased MIBG uptake by the heart and salivary glands may be expected in the background of hypercatecholaminemia of PCC/paraganglioma; restoration of uptake should follow postoperatively along with normal catecholamine levels (Welchick *et al.*, 1989, Suga *et al.*, 2000). Overall radiolabelled MIBG has been proved to be superior to US and radiographs and equivalent to CT and MRI (Shulkin *et al.*, 1998, Troncone *et al.*, 2004). Venous sampling of catecholamines may indicate the level of a given lesion, but it cannot survey the entire body. On the other hand, the few false-positive results still clarify the nature of the lesion since they are mainly attributed to adrenal hyperplasia post contralateral adrenalectomy, or to other NET.

Neuroblastoma is highly malignant and the second most common solid tumour in childhood, often presenting at an advanced stage. It usually originates from the adrenal medulla in neonates and children below 5 years of age. The clinical symptoms are related to the locally increased mass effect, the distant metastases and the secretion of norepinephrine, L-DOPA and dopamine. Scintigraphy with MIBG detects neuroblastomas in 90% of the cases (Troncone *et al.*, 2004). Apart from detection, MIBG scintigraphy is also crucial for staging, monitoring response to therapy and distinguishing residual/recurrent tumour from scar. Accurate localization of the full extent of the disease, including the frequent metastases in the limbs and skull, before initiating therapy is important, because the prognosis in neuroblastoma is highly dependent on staging. Traditional staging investigations include CT and MRI, bone scan, and bone marrow aspiration biopsy. The specificity of MIBG scintigraphy approaches 100%, whereas sensitivity for staging has been reported to be 90%-95% in various studies (Shulkin *et al.*, 1992, Lebtahi *et al.*, 1995, Perel *et al.*, 1999, Shapiro, 1995, Troncone *et al.*, 2004). The highest sensitivity, at the order of 91-97%, involves potential revealing more bone deposits than bone scan with ^{99m}Tc-MDP but in approximately 10% of the cases, ^{99m}Tc-MDP may also reveal false-negative-MIBG lesions; hence both methods are influential in detecting skeletal neuroblastoma (Shulkin *et al.*, 1992, Lebtahi *et al.*, 1995, Shapiro, 1995, Perel *et al.*, 1999, Troncone *et al.*, 2004). In neuroblastoma, the radiotracer remains within the cytoplasm and its retention is pertinent to the rapid reuptake of the tracer percentage that escaped from the cell (Lebtahi *et al.*, 1995). The preferred tracer is ^{123}I-MIBG due to the better image quality and the lower radiation burden to the patient. The lesion uptake is a useful guide for the application of therapeutic ^{131}I-MIBG.

Detection of other NET by $^{123/131}$I-MIBG is limited but appears complementary to other imaging modalities. Medullary thyroid carcinoma (MTC) originates from the neural crest-derived parafollicular C cells of the thyroid. Despite the high specificity of MIBG in MTC detection (95%), the method sensitivity is quite low 34% (Kaltsas *et al.*, 2001, Modlin *et al.*, 2006). About 70% of carcinoids are able to concentrate radiolabelled MIBG (De Herder *et al.*, 2003, Troncone *et al.*, 2004). Only few of other NET tumours show faint MIBG uptake, commonly with wide inhomogeneity among the different tumour sites. More than half of gangioloneuromas, few cases of schwannoma, retinoblastoma, Merkel cell tumours, and APUDomas of unknown origin are visualized on ^{131}I-MIBG scintigraphy.

II. Scintigraphy with Radiolabelled Synthetic Somatostatin Analogues

Neuroendocrine tumours share another common characteristic, namely the overexpression of one or more of the five known different somatostatin receptor ($sstr_{1\text{-}5}$) subtypes, usually $sstr_2$, which consists of $sstr_{2a}$ and $sstr_{2b}$. Sstr are integral membrane glycoproteins which belong to the superfamily of G-protein-coupled receptors (GPCRs) and 7 regions of their molecule traverse the cell membrane (transmembrane domains). The common feature of sstr overexpression by NET, enables their *in vivo* imaging and targeted therapy with appropriate radiolabelled synthetic somatostatin analogues.

Somatostatin (sst) is a regulatory neuropeptide, produced by neurons and endocrine cells in the pituitary, the hypothalamus, the brainstem, the gastrointestinal system and the pancreas, in two biologically active forms: as 14-peptide, sst-14 and as 28-peptide, sst-28. Its actions, accomplished through its binding to sstr, comprise: a) the inhibition of normal and cancer cell proliferation, b) the inhibition of neurotransmitter and hormone synthesis and secretion by neuroendocrine cells, c) the regulation of the immune response, through the expression in lymphocytes and macrophages and d) the inhibition of hormone secretion, like growth hormone (GH), calcitonin, serotonin, insulin, glucagon, gastrin, vasoactive intestinal peptide (VIP), GH releasing hormone, cholecystokinin A/B, substance P, secretin, neurotensin, glucocorticoids, thyroxine and oestradiol. Endogenous sst presents short biological half-life *in vivo* (2-4 min) and cannot be used for medical purposes. Therefore, synthetic sst analogues have been produced; they have comparatively slower blood clearance and hence longer half-life (~90 min), accompanied by particularly high selectivity and specificity for the different sstr subtypes, thereby retaining the capacity to exert most of the biological actions of the native peptide (De Herder *et al.*, 2003). Somatostatin receptors are distributed in different tissues and are overexpressed by NETs (APUD system) as well as by certain other tumours (Table **3**).

Table 3: Tumour somatostatin receptor mapping

NET	Other Tumours
• Pheochromocytoma	Meningioma
• Neuroblastoma	CNS glioma
• Carcinoid	Hodgkin's disease
• Paraganglioma	Non-Hodgkin lymphoma
• Parasympathetic paraganglioma (chemodectoma – glomus tumor)	Melanoma
	Hypernephroma
• Anterior pituitary adenoma	Hepatocellular cancer
– Thyrotropinoma	Breast cancer
– Prolactinoma	Uterine cervical cancer
– GH-secreting tumour	Prostate cancer
– Non-functional tumours	Thyroid cancer
• Pancreatic islet cell tumours (GEP tumors)	Sarcomas
– Gastrinoma (Zollinger-Ellison syndrome)	
– Insulinoma	
– Glucagonoma	
– VIP-oma	
– Non-classified APUDoma	
• Medullary thyroid cancer	

NET	Other Tumours
• Neuroendocrine cancer of the neck • Tumours related to MEN I and MEN II syndromes • Tumours related to type I neurofibromatosis • Tumours related to Carney syndrome • Small cell lung cancer • Merkel cell skin tumour	

The specificity of sstr radiotracers is based on their selective binding to certain sstr subtypes. In general, scintigraphy with radiolabelled oligopeptides (like octreotide, bombesin, substance P) refers to imaging at the cellular level *via* specific molecules (Molecular Nuclear Medicine), such as the receptors. Each molecule of radiolabelled sst analogue is bound on the cellular sstr, which in turn is internalized by cell membrane invagination. Then the complex radiotracer-sstr is split into its initial components by acidification within intracellular storage granules. The radiotracer, which is prevented from exiting through the cell membrane due to its polarity, enters and remains in the lysosomes and the sstr is externalized on the cell membrane, in order to continue its function.

Table 4: Protocols for somatostatin receptor scintigraphy

	^{111}In-DTPA-Octreotide	**^{99m}Tc-Depreotide**	**^{99m}Tc-Tektrotyd**
Preparation	- withdrawal of long-acting nonradiolabelled sst analogues for 4-6 weeks, with switch to short-acting subcutaneous formulations up to 12-24 h prior to scintigraphy, if clinically feasible - previous surgical operations, chemotherapy or radiotherapy should be completed by 1 mo prior to scintigraphy		
Administration Route and Activity	iv 222 MBq	iv 550-740 MBq	iv 400 MBq
Post-Injection Preparation	hydration		
	laxatives may be given between 24 and 48 h imaging to diminish radioactive bowel content, if high		
Imaging	4 h pi: high background radioactivity but negligible bowel content 24 h pi 48, 72 and 96 h pi: especially useful for differentiating lesion from radioactive bowel content at 24-h scintigraphy	2-4 h pi	

	^{111}In-DTPA-Octreotide	**^{99m}Tc-Depreotide**	**^{99m}Tc-Tektrotyd**
	whole-body scan planar and SPECT images		
	two sets of planar and SPECT images according to clinical setting, at 4 and 24 h or 24 and 48 h pi, with at least one SPECT acquisition, since the tracer concentration in the sites of diseases may become significant later		
Collimator	medium-energy, parallel hole	low-energy, parallel hole	
Energy Window	20% at 172 keV and at 245 keV	20% at 140 keV	
SPECT	360 ° rotation 120 projections; 45 sec/projection 64×64 word acquisition matrix	360 ° rotation 120 projections; 30 sec/projection 128×128 word acquisition matrix	

The main radiolabelled sst analogues that have been worldwide used for diagnostic purposes are: ^{111}In-DTPA-octreotide (^{111}In-DTPA-D-Phe-octreotide or ^{111}In-pentetreotide, OctreoScan®; Covidien, Mallinckrodt, Inc., Petten, The Netherlands), ^{111}In-DOTATOC, ^{111}In-DOTA-lanreotide, ^{99m}Tc-depreotide (NeoTect® [Diatide Inc.]; NeoSpect® [Nycomed]) and ^{99m}Tc-hydrazinonicotinyl-Tyr3-octreotide (^{99m}Tc-EDDA-HYNIC-TOC or ^{99m}Tc-Tektrotyd) (Blum *et al.*, 1999, Kwekkeboom *et al.*, 1999, Virgolini *et al.*, 2002, Gabriel *et al.*, 2003, 2004, Bushnell *et al.*, 2004, Kahn *et al.*, 2004, Valsamaki *et al.*, 2004, 2006, Graham *et al.*, 2011). Each of these radiolabelled synthetic sst analogues presents unique affinity profile for specific sstr subtypes. Specifically, ^{111}In-DTPA-octreotide preferentially binds to sstr$_2$, moderately to sstr$_5$ and less to sstr$_3$, ^{111}In-DOTATOC to sstr$_2$ and less to sstr$_3$ and sstr$_5$, ^{111}In-DOTA-lanreotide to sstr$_2$, sstr$_3$, sstr$_4$ and sstr$_5$ while less to sstr$_1$, ^{99m}Tc-depreotide to sstr$_2$, sstr$_3$ and sstr$_5$, and ^{99m}Tc-EDDA-HYNIC-TOC to sstr$_2$, while less to sstr$_3$ and sstr$_5$ (De Jong *et al.*, 1998, Virgolini *et al.*, 2002, Gnanasegaran *et al.*, 2005, IJNM). The performance of ^{99m}Tc-depreotide was under investigation with variable results for the detection of malignant pulmonary nodules or masses, mediastinal nodal metastasis, lymphomas, TC, PCC and neuroblastoma, but was never carefully studied for general NET imaging (Blum *et al.*, 1999, Bushnell *et al.*, 2004, Kahn *et al.*, 2004, Valsamaki *et al.*, 2004, 2006, Graham *et al.*, 2011). In 2010, the European Commission issued a decision to withdraw the marketing authorization for ^{99m}Tc-depreotide, apparently in accordance with the manufacturer's request based on commercial reasons (Graham *et al.*, 2011). Scintigraphy with ^{99m}Tc-EDDA-HYNIC-TOC has been found to visualize sstr-expressing tumours, such as primary or secondary TC lesions, pulmonary nodules, carcinoid, pancreatic NET, and pituitary tumour (De Jong *et al.*, 1998, Decristoforo *et al.*, 2000, Gabriel *et al.*, 2003, 2004, Gnanasegaran *et al.*, 2005 IJNM, Gambini *et al.*, 2008, 2009, Chen *et al.*, 2009, Jing *et al.*, 2011). Also, ^{99m}Tc-EDDA-HYNIC-TOC scintigraphy has been reported to be more sensitive than ^{131}I-MIBG imaging in the detection of extraadrenal PCC (Chen *et al.*, 2009). Despite the advantageous physical characteristics, associated improved image quality, easier availability, and lower cost and radiation burden of the ^{99m}Tc-labelled sst analogues, none has hitherto gained widespread acceptance and use, probably in part owing to differential intensity of sstr-binding affinity. Protocols for sstr-scintigraphy are described in Table **4**. ^{111}In-DTPA-octreotide has been successfully used since 1994 and remains the most widely applied for scintigraphic purposes; the eight-amino-acid sst analogue octreotide labelled with ^{111}In is chelated with DTPA (De Jong *et al.*, 2003). The chelate DTPA contributes to the rapid renal clearance, with 85% of the administered activity found in urine within 24 hours, while a small percentage (2%) is excreted *via* the hepatobiliary tract. Its plasma half-life is around 2 h. To date, sstr scintigraphy with ^{111}In-DTPA-octreotide is considered among the well-established procedures in patients with NET (Fig. **2** and Table **5**). Amendment in further treatment in patients with NET is guided by sstr-scintigraphy results and appears particularly valuable in patients with GEP-NET, occurring at an estimated level of 30%. Particularly in the detection of PCC and neuroblastoma, the method of choice is $^{131/123}$I-MIBG scintigraphy; however, ^{111}In-DTPA-octreotide is indicated as complementary method, in order to increase the sensitivity with or without the use of SPECT or SPECT/CT.

Table 5: Indications for radionuclide imaging with ^{111}In-DTPA-octreotide and $^{123/131}$I-MIBG in NET

- Determination of the neuroendocrine nature of a mass, complementary to the rest imaging methods.
- Detection and localization of primary (even small occult) tumours.
- Staging/detection of metastatic lesions.
- Restaging/evaluation of the therapeutic outcome.
- Selection of patients for targeted radionuclide therapy.
- As prognostic parameter of the clinical response to therapy.
- Follow-up for detection of relapse or progression of disease.

Herein it is worth noting that the absence of lesion visualization upon scintigraphy with radiolabelled synthetic sst analogues, does not necessarily imply complete absence of neuroendocrine elements or receptors, bearing in mind the variety of receptor subtypes and their quantities (density). Overall the sensitivity of ^{111}In-DTPA-octreotide regarding NET detection has been reported to range from 80% to almost 100% in carcinoids and 60-90% in pancreatic NET, mostly depending on tumour type and lesion size, and the method specificity is only relatively lower due to uptake in many other sstr-expressing tumours, granulomas, autoimmune diseases as well as inflammatory processes (Krenning *et al.*, 1993, Kwekkeboom *et al.*1993, Westlin *et al.*, 1993, De Kerviler *et al.*, 1994, Kalkner *et al.*, 1995, Gibril *et al.*, 1995, 1996, Zimmer *et al.*, 1996, Lebtahi *et al.*, 1997, Virgolini *et al.*, 2005, Teunissen *et al.*, 2011).

Normal scintigraphic pattern with ^{111}In-DTPA-octreotide encompasses depiction of tissues due to receptor binding, namely the spleen and in a proportion of patients the thyroid, adrenals and/or pituitary gland, as well as due to tracer excretion. Tracer reabsorption in the renal tubular cells after glomerular filtration results in intense kidney visualization. The urinary bladder and the bowel are commonly visualized to an unpredictable extent (Krenning *et al.*, 1992, Jacobsson *et al.*, 2003). Light diet or the use of laxatives and scanning at 48 h may sometimes be required to differentiate between non-specific bowel uptake and sstr-positive abdominal lesions. Prior to imaging patients are also adviced to temporarily discontinue the therapeutic use of «cold» sst analogues according to their duration of action, based on the concept of possible competition between «cold» and radiolabelled octreotide at the receptor site with resultant false negative scans.

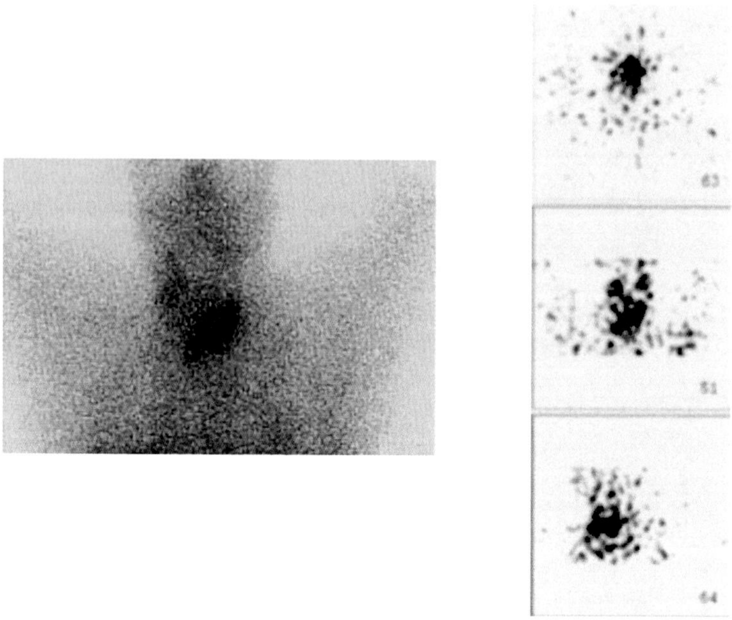

Figure 2: Planar ^{111}In-DTPA-octreotide anterior cervicothoracic (left) and SPECT cervical images (right) in a 44 years old male bearing MTC with extensive perithyroid and lymphatic invasion, about 1.5 month post-thyroidectomy. Abnormally increased density of $sstr_{2,3 \text{ and } 5}$ is seen at the lower cervical area, particularly on the left, extending into the anterior upper mediastinum. Increased tracer uptake is also evident at the right lateral cervix. The findings indicate residual disease.

The reported notion of generally higher sensitivity for NET detection with ^{111}In-DTPA-octreotide than with ^{131}I-MIBG, has been compensated by the small numbers of different patients of these studies (Taal *et al.*, 1996) and by the demonstration of ^{123}I-MIBG-avid lesions which are not visualized by sstr scintigraphy, *i.e.* there can be quantitative and qualitative differences in uptake pattern (Ramage *et al.*, 1996, Taal *et al.*, 1996, Kaltsas *et al.*, 2001). Hence a complementary role in NET imaging may be expected for both methods (Krenning *et al.*, 1993, Ramage *et al.*, 1996). Nevertheless most pancreatic islet cell tumours are depicted by ^{111}In-DTPA-octreotide which may also identify previously unsuspected orbital lesions and appears more likely to visualise primary tumours, like MTC, as well as metastatic foci (Krenning *et al.*, 1993, Kwekkeboom *et al.*, 1993, Höfnagel, 1994). However, ^{123}I-MIBG scintigraphy remains the method of choice for detecting adrenomedullary tumours; occasional non-^{123}I-MIBG-avid lesions may be revealed by ^{111}In-DTPA-octreotide that is indicated as an adjunctive diagnostic tool for staging malignant PCC (Krenning *et al.*, 1993). The necessity of both scans is also associated with the selection of patients who would benefit from corresponding or combined therapies.

III. Scintigraphy With ^{99m}Tc(V)-DMSA

During the last decades the tumour-seeking properties of the radiotracer ^{99m}Tc(V)-DMSA have been investigated and established regarding NET and soft tissue tumors, such as MTC and lung, breast, brain, and metastatic bone lesions (Ohta *et al.*, 1984, Hirano *et al.*, 1995, Papantoniou *et al.*, 2005). No special patient preparation is required, except for adequate hydration. Whole-body scan (at 8 cm/min) is performed 2-3 h pi of 370 MBq tracer activity. Static images of 500 kounts may also be acquired at corresponding areas under investigation. Foci of increased tracer uptake in the thyroid bed that correspond to ^{99m}Tc-pertechnetate-photopenic findings, confirm TC diagnosis. Post-operative metastatic lesions, exhibit mild to intense tracer uptake, especially in soft tissues (Fig. **3**). Absence of non-specific hepatic uptake enables lucid identification of hepatic metastases. In case of scintimammography, lateral and anterior prone early (at 10-20 min) and late planar images (at 60-70 minutes) are acquired after iv administration of 925 to 1,100 MBq tracer activity. Acquisitions are obtained using a special positioning pad. Any focally increased accumulation is regarded as associated with invasive pathology, whereas any other pattern of a more widespread diffuse uptake indicates pre-invasive lesions, such as ductal carcinoma *in situ* (DCIS) and epithelial hyperplasia (Papantoniou *et al.*, 2005, 2006). Based on *in vivo* scintigraphic and *in vitro* studies, the cellular uptake mechanism of the tracer is closely related to cellular proliferation, focal adhesion kinase (FAK) activation, neo-angiogenesis and overexpression of several growth factors such as calcitonin-gene related peptide (CGRP), VEGF and platelet-derived growth factor (PDGF) (Denoyer *et al.*, 2004, 2005, Papantoniou *et al.*, 2011, 2012). Vascular endothelial GF and PDGF have been long identified among the positive regulators of angiogenesis which is a very well recognized powerful control point in tumour development (Tonini *et al.*, 2003). The neo-angiogenic neuropeptide CGRP has been attributed with an additional proliferative role, possibly exerted through the PDGF/PDGFreceptorsystem (Papantoniou *et al.*, 2012). Interestingly, the tracer reflects phosphate ion (Pi) transport and metabolism; it enters cancer cells specifically *via* the type III Na/Pi co-transporter, this uptake being motivated by the cellular levels of phosphorylated (*i.e.* activated) FAK, a keystone of accelerated proliferation (Papantoniou *et al.*, 2012). Favourably adding to this knowledge, ^{99m}Tc(V)-DMSA quantitatively predicts rhenium-188(V)-DMSA [^{188}Re(V)-DMSA] distribution (Blower *et al.*, 2000). In advanced breast cancer stages, ^{99m}Tc(V)-DMSA uptake in metastatic lesions may guide therapeutic ^{188}Re(V)-DMSA administration, as propounded by Papantoniou and colleagues in Greece. Currently this protocol is under process in collaboration with Djokic and colleagues (Vince Institute of Nuclear Sciences, Belgrade, Serbia) (Papantoniou *et al.*, 2012). Hence new horizonts may also appear regarding therapeutic options of all NET.

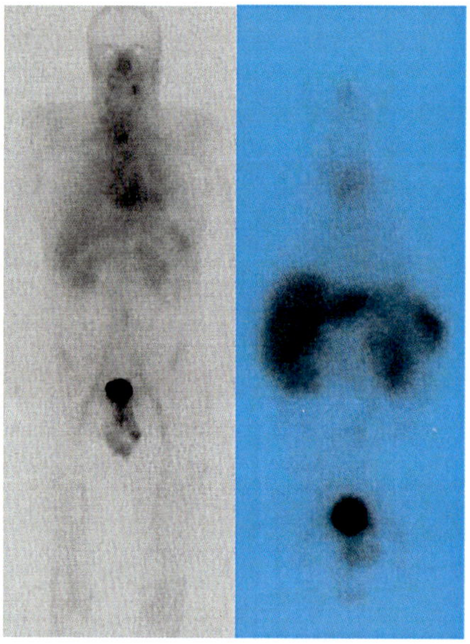

Figure 3: ^{99m}Tc(V)-DMSA (left) and ^{111}In-DTPA-octreotide (right) whole-body scintigraphy in the same patient with MTC (**2**) demonstrate compatible findings; relatively more clearly visible on ^{99m}Tc(V)-DMSA.

IV. Imaging with PET

Simultaneously significant positron-emitting radiotracers have been developed for NET imaging with PET, mainly gallium-68-(^{68}Ga-)DOTA-peptides (-TOC, -NOC, -BOC, -TATE), carbon-11-5-hydroxy-tryptophan (^{11}C-5-HTP), ^{18}F-dihydroxy-phenyl-alanine (^{18}F-DOPA) and ^{11}C-L-dihydroxy-phenyl-alanine (^{11}C-L-DOPA).

The positron-emitting radioisotopes are created in a cyclotron, like fluorine-18 (^{18}F) and ^{11}C or in a generator like ^{68}Ga. The most widely used isotope is ^{18}F due to the practicality of transport with a half-life of 109.8 min. From a practical point of view, the only two FDA-(Food and Drug Administration, American Health Authority)-approved tracers for oncologic imaging are ^{18}F-fluoro-D-deoxyglucose (^{18}F-FDG) a substrate for hexokinase in glucose metabolism and [^{18}F]fluoride ions such as ^{18}F-NaF that are incorporated in the hydroxyapatite crystals in bone for bone imaging. The radiolabelled glucose analogue ^{18}F-FDG is transported across the plasma membrane into cells down a concentration gradient through facilitated transport by the glucose transport proteins such as glut 1 and glut 3. Glut 1 and glut 3 are overexpressed in tumour cell membranes. Hexokinase in the cell phosphorylates the ^{18}F-FDG into 6-Phospho-^{18}F-FDG, which is not transported by the glut transporters and cannot be further metabolized, thus remaining and accumulating in the cell as opposed to normal glucose. The rate-limiting step for FDG uptake and retention in most tissues is phosphorylation rather than transport. The rate of glycolysis is far greater in neoplastic tissues than in the normal tissues and correlates with ^{18}F-FDG PET uptake (Larson *et al.*, 1999). The tumour activity per dose injected per body mass constitutes the standardized uptake value (SUV), the common measurement used by PET and is proportional to the glucose metabolic rate within the normal range of serum glucose concentration (Huang *et al.*, 2000). The percentage change of post-therapy SUV from the pre-therapy SUV defines the metabolic response. In some cancers, the maximum SUV has been demonstrated to predict prognosis (Koopmans *et al.*, 2008).

Unfortunately, the most powerful and commonly applied PET radiotracer in oncology, namely ^{18}F-FDG, does not usually depict NET, unless they are dedifferentiated and retain high proliferative activity, the so-called "flip-flop phenomenon" (Adams *et al.*, 1998). In fact a recent publication has determined a negative correlation between ^{18}F-FDG uptake and disease prognosis as well as increased overall sensitivity of 86% by combining ^{111}In-DTPA-octreotide and ^{18}F-FDG-PET as compared with ^{111}In-DTPA-octreotide alone yielding 89% sensitivity (Binderup *et al.*, 2010). Hence ^{18}F-FDG-PET may provide complementary diagnostic and staging information particularly in GEP-NET patients with negative ^{111}In-DTPA-octreotide or a high proliferation index Ki-67 of 15%, since these tumours show often more aggressive behaviour and faster growth (Belhocine *et al.*, 2002). Finally, the reported superior specificity of FDG-PET compared to the ^{99m}Tc-MDP bone scan, especially for bone marrow metastases, favors the ongoing debate about the relative merits of each technique (Fogelman *et al.*, 2005).

In accordance with traditional γ-camera sstr scintigraphy, various ^{68}Ga-labelled sst analogues have been explored by the use of ^{68}Ga, with half-life 68.1 min, that can be chelated with DOTA to form stable complexes with sst analogues. Promising results by studies in patients with the first clinically applicable ^{68}Ga-labelled sst analogue [^{68}Ga-DOTA0,Tyr3]octreotide (^{68}Ga-DOTATOC, with $ssstr_2$ binding) urged for the development of other ^{68}Ga-labelled sst analogues in order to increase their sensitivity or broaden their affinity profile, such as ^{68}Ga-DOTANOC (binding to $sstr_2$, $sstr_3$ and $sstr_5$) and [^{68}Ga-DOTA0,Tyr3]octreotate (^{68}Ga-DOTATATE, $sstr_2$-binding) (Hofmann *et al.*, 2001, Maecke *et al.*, 2005, Wild *et al.*, 2005, Gabriel *et al.*, 2007, Ambrosini *et al.*, 2008, Fanti *et al.*, 2008, Kayani *et al.*, 2008, Krausz *et al.*, 2011). The clinical introduction of these positron-emitting radionuclide-labelled sst analogues is advantageous over the γ-emitting analogues, in terms of superb image quality with better spatial resolution, easy accessibility and availability of the ^{68}Ga-generator, favourable acquisition protocol, with relative short scanning time, and low radiation exposure to the patient (Krausz *et al.*, 2011). It has been suggested that imaging of malignant PCC by ^{68}Ga-DOTATATE may be indicated for therapy with ^{90}Y-DOTATATE, coupled with optimal therapy planning based on separation of blood background activity from sstr binding by pharmacokinetic data analysis; however, up till now there exist no accurate results comparing findings by ^{68}Ga-labelled sst analogues *versus* ^{111}In-DTPA-octreotide scintigraphy (Hofmann *et al.*, 2001, Buchmann *et al.*, 2007, Ambrosini *et al.*, 2008, Fanti *et al.*, 2008, Krausz *et al.*, 2011).

Gastroenteropancreatic NET imaging with PET, apart from labelled sst analogues, also includes ^{18}F-DOPA or ^{11}C-L-DOPA and ^{11}C-5-HTP, due to neuroendocrine cell uptake of the catecholamine precursor DOPA and the direct precursor for the serotonin pathway 5-HTP, respectively (Eriksson *et al.*, 2002, Becherer *et al.*, 2004, Orlefors *et al.*, 2005, Koukouraki *et al.*, 2006, Win *et al.*, 2007). Recent studies have proposed staging in patients with carcinoid by ^{11}C-5-HTP and in patients with endocrine pancreatic NET by ^{18}F-DOPA. Carcinoid tumours produce serotonin which increases the dilation of blood vessels and platelet (PLT) aggregation. Serotonin is synthesized from the amino acid tryptophan by hormone-producing enterochromaffin cells in the gut and bronchi. Serotonin is metabolized in the liver to 5-hydroxyindole acetic acid (5-HIAA) and eventually excreted in the urine. Better tumour visualization, even for small, occult lesions has been reported by ^{11}C-5-HTP-PET than CT and sstr scintigraphy (Koopmans *et al.*, 2008). In addition, ^{11}C-5-HTP-PET may be indicated for treatment monitoring based on the strong correlation during treatment between changes in the transport rate constant at repeated PET and those of urinary HIAA. Per os administration of carbidopa [(2S)-3-(3,4-dihydroxyphenyl)-2-hydrazinyl-2-methyl-propanoic acid] to the patients before PET blocks the aromatic amino acid decarboxylase enzyme, thereby decreasing the decarboxylation rate of ^{11}C-5-HTP and resulting in a 300% higher tumour uptake, 600% less urinary radioactivity concentration and a reduction of streak artefacts.

Additional PET tracers have been used in NET imaging such as radiolabelled catecholamine analogues ^{11}C-hydroxyephedrine (^{11}C-HED) and ^{11}C-epinephrine (^{11}C-EPI). Specifically, ^{11}C-EPI has depicted PCC and ^{11}C-HED has localized both PCC and neuroblastomas with high sensitivity, specificity and accuracy (Ilias *et al.*, 2003, Shulkin *et al.*, 1995, Trampal *et al.*, 2004). Another sympathoneuronal imaging agent, 6-^{18}F-dopamine (^{18}F-DA) has been developed considering that dopamine is a better substrate for the norepinephrine transporter than most other amines, including norepinephrine. ^{18}F-DA is highly specific for the localization of both adrenal and extra-adrenal PCC, including metastatic lesions (Ilias *et al.*, 2003). However, when ^{123}-MIBG or ^{18}F-DA fails to localize lesions seen on conventional imaging studies, ^{18}F-FDG may be recommended as an ancillary test for the diagnosis and localization of metastatic PCC, particularly aggressive PCC (Mamede *et al.*, 2006). Also, it has recently been postulated that when ^{18}F-DOPA provides better visualization of PCC lesions than ^{18}F-DA, the reason may adhere to differences in expression of the vesicular monoamine transporters 1 and 2 (VMAT1 and VMAT2) (Martiniova *et al.*, 2012).

Finally, several adrenocortical tracers have been applied in order to enable the differential diagnosis of adrenocortical carcinomas *versus* other adrenal tumours such as PCC. Inhibition of an important enzyme in the biosynthesis of cortisol and aldosterone in the adrenal cortex, namely 11b-hydroxylase, has been accomplished by various PET-radiopharmaceuticals like ^{11}C-metomidate (^{11}C-MTO), ^{11}C-etomidate (^{11}C-ETO), ^{18}F-metomidate (^{18}F-FMTO) and ^{18}F-etomidate (^{18}F-FETO) (Hennings *et al.*, 2006, Wadsak *et al.*, 2006). Researchers have stated that due to the binding of MTO to the 11b-hydroxylase activity, ^{11}C-MTO is useful even in the presence of extended necrosis.

In conclusion, although conventional imaging techniques such as EUS, multi-detector CT and new MRI sequences are used to image NET with considerable improvement, nuclear medicine sstr imaging with the gold standard ^{111}In-DTPA-octreotide scintigraphy remains to provide crucial data on primary and metastatic NET foci during the initial diagnostic work-up (Kaltsas *et al.*, 2004, Teunissen *et al.*, 2011). Scintigraphy with ^{123}I-MIBG may be useful in patients with MIBG-avid but ^{111}In-DTPA-octreotide non-avid lesions (Kaltsas *et al.*, 2001). In addition, possibility of differential uptake of ^{123}I-MIBG and ^{111}In-DTPA-octreotide in different metastases within the same patient, should be considered in view of further clinical management (Quigley *et al.*, 2005). Interestingly, ^{99m}Tc(V)-DMSA imaging has been proved valuable for metastatic MTC as well as breast lesions but has not been extensively utilized in NET imaging. Among the available alternative γ-emitting or PET radionuclide imaging modalities for NET detection, none of them is approved by the European Medicines Evaluation Agency (EMEA, European Health Authority) and/or FDA (Daly *et al.*, 2006). PET metabolic imaging of GEP-NET with ^{18}F-DOPA and ^{11}C-HTP shows promise. In the future, PET/CT with ^{68}Ga-labelled sst analogues, if available, will become the modality of choice for sstr imaging. Moreover in GEP-NET patients, the reported increased overall sensitivity of 92% when combining ^{68}Ga-DOTATATE PET/CT and ^{18}F-FDG-PET/CT, especially in intermediate- and high-grade NET, might incorporate ^{18}F-FDG-PET in the NET diagnostic work-up (Kayani *et al.*, 2008). Finally, regarding current NET visualization, sstr scintigraphy remains the imaging method of choice, with interchangeable complementary role of $^{123/131}$I-MIBG scintigraphy, having the inherent advantage of patient selection for potential corresponding peptide receptor radionuclide therapy (PRRT) or ^{131}I-MIBG therapy.

3. TARGETED RADIONUCLIDE THERAPY OF NEUROENDOCRINE TUMOURS

On the whole, malignant NET have poor prognosis and aggressive multimodality treatment is required for primary and metastatic tumours that continue to grow and cause symptoms (Öberg, 2004, Kaltsas *et al.*, 2005, Nisa *et al.*, 2011). The main treatment goal is diminishing hormone overproduction by NET, because associated mortality is often related to the consequences of peptide hypersecretion rather than tumour progression (Öberg, 1998). The available therapeutic options are applicable in specific clinical settings, present variable response rates and include: a) surgical removal of the primary tumour mass; surgery may provide definite cure when successful and is often the initial approach. Reported effectiveness in <5% of all patients may possibly be connected with the presence of metastases in 90% of the patients at the time of appearance (Higgins *et al.*, 1979, Prinz *et al.*, 1981, Raut *et al.*, 2006). b) cytoreductive therapies with Radio Frequency Ablation (RFA) or with chemo-embolization, as in case of subtotal resection or co-existence of hepatic metastases. In case of relapse, the indicated drug treatment may consist of: ci) sst analogues with or without interferon (IFN); «cold» sst as monotherapy (which is mainly indicated in patients with functional tumours) or in combination with IFN seldom induces tumour shrinkage based on CT/MRI assessment. Reported results do not appear encouraging for IFN. cii) new targeted agents that have shown improvement of Progression-Free Survival (PFS): ciia) monoclonal antibodies against the vascular endothelial growth factor (anti-VEGF, bevacizumab). ciib) kinase inhibitors; monotherapy with the mTOR inhibitor everolimus or the multiple (including VEGF and PDGF pathway) tyrosine kinase inhibitor sunitinib, mainly aims at pancreatic NET. ciii) chemotherapy; response rates range from 15 to 30%, quickly subside in general and are inferior in functional tumours. Therapy postponement due to side-effects is frequent; lower toxicity is reported with temozolomide-based chemotherapy compared to the streptozotocin-based regime. civ) internal radiotherapy with the administration of targeted ^{131}I-MIBG or PRRT. Applied molecular biology constitutes the basis of the therapeutic approach targeting at the cellular level, in particular targeted radionuclide therapy. Long-term experience shows effective use of ^{131}I-MIBG therapy, especially in PCC and neuroblastoma. Also, encouraging results have been published during the last years by specialized centres worldwide, which highlight PRRT benefits and pertain mainly to the treatment of progressive GEP-NET that do not respond to conventional therapeutic regimes. Prerequisites for targeted radionuclide therapy include high selective uptake of the diagnostic (thus also the corresponding therapeutic) agent by the primary NET and the metastatic foci and sufficient particulate radiation for tissue destruction. The use of ^{99m}Tc(V)-DMSA and respective therapeutic agents has not been till now clinically established worldwide, with the exception of certain breast and MTC applications, and will not be herein further discussed.

I. Targeted ^{131}I-MIBG Therapy of Pheochromocytoma and Neuroblastoma

Through the identification of PCC, neuroblastomas, MTC, carcinoid and other APUDomas by ^{131}I-MIBG emerged the prospect of corresponding radionuclide therapy (Sisson *et al.*, 1984, McEwan *et al.*, 1985) due to the favourable physical characteristics of ^{131}I. Treatment with ^{131}I-MIBG is indicated in inoperable, metastatic or recurrent PCC, neuroblastoma, carcinoid and MTC (Table **6**).

The unique advantage of all targeted internal radiotherapies like ^{131}I-MIBG therapy is the selective targeting of all sites of disease, including distant metastases. Disease depiction on $^{123/131}$I-MIBG scintigraphy is *sine qua non* for the initiation of treatment; thus patient selection for targeted metabolic ^{131}I-MIBG therapy is based on high $^{131/123}$I-MIBG uptake upon imaging, in order for at least 20 cGy/mCi to be delivered to the tumour foci by the therapeutic infusion. Ideally, drugs implemented in the radiopharmaceutical uptake and/or retention should be discontinued for the proper time interval prior to ^{131}I-MIBG administration for therapeutic or diagnostic purposes, as herewith previously analyzed (Bombardieri *et al.*, 2010, Giammarile *et al.*, 2008, Solanki *et al.*, 1992). However, patients with metabolically active catecholamine-secreting tumours (*i.e.* PCC and paraganglioma) often receive alpha and beta blockers for symptom control before ^{131}I-MIBG and are thus recommended not to change their medication due to the risk of developing symptoms after drug withdrawal. Thyroid blockade is also required for therapy with ^{131}I-MIBG in order to prevent post-radiation fibrosis of the thyroid parenchyma from glandular uptake of free iodine. Thyroid protection is accomplished by oral stable iodine, combined with potassium perchlorate to facilitate the wash-out of the radio-iodine from the thyroid (Giammarile *et al.*, 2008).

According to EANM 2008 guidelines (Giammarile *et al.*, 2008), therapy with ^{131}I-MIBG is absolutely contraindicated in case of pregnancy, breastfeeding, survival expectancy less than 3 months, unless in case of intractable bone pain, and end-stage renal failure. Relative contraindications include unacceptable medical risk for patient isolation, unmanageable urinary incontinence, rapidly deteriorating renal function (GFR<30ml/min), myelosuppression, *i.e.* haemoglobin (Hb<9g/dl, white blood cells (WBC)<$4x10^9$/l, and PLT<$100x10^9$/l. In case of massive bone marrow invasion or significantly decreased renal function, the therapeutic dose should be reduced and the patient should be closely followed-up.

Treatment protocols vary between different centres. The usual administered activities range between 3.7 and 11.2 GBq, commonly repeated at 1-6 months intervals (not less than 1 month in children and 1.5 in adults) driven by PLT levels. Repeated high ^{131}I-MIBG doses of 7.4 GBq are usually required every 3-5 weeks in children with neuroblastoma due to its aggressivity; thus accordingly relatively serious myelotoxicity may ultimately not be avoided. The therapeutic dose of ^{131}I-MIBG is diluted in 50-100 ml saline or glucose solution, in compliance with the manufacturer's instructions, and administered by slow intravenous infusion usually over 90 min (45 min-4 h). The infused ^{131}I-MIBG solution contains high specific activity of up to 1.48 GBq/mg, in order to minimize the MIBG content to less than 5 mg and thus prevent side-effects. During the infusion, the patient should be continuously monitored by ECG and determination of vital signs, since unstable blood pressure is expected. Ondansetron is the anti-emetic of choice advised prophylactically, commencing on the day of treatment and continued for 3 days.

Ordinarily, ^{131}I-MIBG treatment is well-tolerated with short-term side effects limited to nausea or vomiting within 24-72 h pi. In patients with PCC and neuroblastoma hypertensive crises due to carecholamine release may be expected, while flushing predominates in carcinoid tumours due to serotonin release. Mild hepatic dysfunction with spontaneous recovery, and temporary myelosuppression may appear 4–6 weeks posttherapy. Only incidentally patients may develop significant side effects in terms of severe myelosuppression, especially in the presence of extensive bone marrow metastatic spread, or hepatic failure in patients with widespread liver metastases (Bongers *et al.*, 1997). Rarely, deterioration of renal function is observed, mainly in patients whose kidneys have been compromised, *e.g.* by intensive pretreatment with cisplatin and ifosfamide. Delayed side effects may comprise hypothyroidism by inadequate or lacking thyroid blockade and persistent haematologic abnormalities. Induction of leukaemia or other solid tumours has not been reported but cannot be excluded. The frequency and severity of most haematologic side effects are significantly less than the chemotherapy-associated and are evidently related to the cumulative administered activity (Bomanji *et al.*, 2003, Safford *et al.*, 2004).

Table 6: Synopsis of ^{131}I-MIBG therapy criteria, indications, preparation, procedure and adverse effects

Prerequisite	**$^{123/131}$I-MIBG-Positive Tumours**
Indications	Inoperable/ malignant PCC Inoperable/ malignant paraganglioma Inoperable/ malignant carcinoid tumour Stage III / IV neuroblastoma Inoperable/ malignant MTC
Basic haematology and biochemistry criteria	Hb >10 g/dl WBC >3x10^9/l PLT >100x10^9/l GFR >40ml/min
Preparation	- Withdrawal of interfering drugs (1-2 weeks prior to therapy) and patient stabilization on alternative medication, if clinically feasible - Thyroid blockade: starting 24-48 h before infusion and continued for 10-15 days posttherapy: Adults: Lugol solution 1% at 1 drop/kg/day with a maximum of 40 (20 drops twice daily) and potassium perchlorate capsules of 400mg/day Children: capsules of KI of 16-65 mg/day and of $KClO_4$ of 100-300 mg/day (dose adjusted per kg of body weight)
Procedure	- Slow iv infusion *via* an indwelling cannula or central venous line using a lead-shielded infusion system, usually over 90 min (45 min-4 h) of activities ranging between 3.7 and 11.2 GBq ^{131}I-MIBG diluted in 50-100 ml saline or glucose solution (manufacturer's instructions) with continuous ECG and vital signs monitoring

Prerequisite	$^{123/131}$I-MIBG-Positive Tumours
	- Ondansetron per os for 3 days - Enhanced hydration before, during and after infusion - Infusion of the ^{131}I-MIBG should be reduced or stopped, at least temporarily, if hypertension occurs; short acting alpha or beta blockers should be available for emergency use in case of catecholamine surge during or after infusion
Possible adverse effects	Acute: nausea or vomiting In PCC and neuroblastoma: hypertensive crises In carcinoid: flushing Long-term: - myelosuppression: usually mild and transient - hepatic dysfunction: usually mild and transient - renal function deterioration: rare - hypothyroidism: by inadequate thyroid blockade

Clinical reports show ^{131}I-MIBG-therapy efficacy in patients bearing NET with avid accumulation of $^{123/131}$I-MIBG (Drazin *et al.*, 1985, Shulkin *et al.*, 1990, Höfnagel *et al.*, 1991, Shapiro *et al.*, 1991, De Kraker *et al.*, 1995, Taal *et al.*, 1996, Pathirana *et al.*, 2001, Yanik *et al.*, 2002, Safford *et al.*, 2004, DuBois *et al.*, 2004, Sywak *et al.*, 2004, Pashankar *et al.*, 2005). Patients with malignant PCC, treated with various large doses of ^{131}I-MIBG, have shown partial response in 18 to 88%, in terms of more than 50% decline in catecholamine and metabolite levels and greater decrease in tumour volume (Shapiro *et al.*, 1991). Improvement has also been recorded pertinent to retroperitoneal metastases, bone pain, and blood pressure.

Neuroblastoma is the most common extracranial tumour in childhood and presents the greatest clinical variability as compared to all solid childhood tumours. Metastatic neuroblastoma at the age above 1 year, retains the worse prognosis over all childhood tumours. More than 50% of children initially appearing at the general practitioner already suffer from stage IV disease. If the primary focus or the surgical remnant is eligible to surgical operation followed by chemotherapy, neuroblastoma may be cured. If the disease persists, intensive chemotherapy is the treatment of choice. Initial response therapy is usually followed by drug resistance, unresponsiveness and relapse. The prolonged and intense uptake of the diagnostic dose of $^{123/131}$I-MIBG by most neuroblastomas has facilitated treatment of inoperable/metastatic disease with large doses of ^{131}I-MIBG (Shulkin *et al.*, 1990).

In patients with neuroblastoma, ^{131}I-MIBG therapy is justified for slowly progressive disease, tumour refractory to chemotherapy, clinical manifestations due to tumour-related biochemical activity or painful bone metastases. The toxicity by therapeutic doses of ^{131}I-MIBG is lower than the corresponding chemotherapy-induced. Results from preoperative ^{131}I-MIBG therapy in 33 children with inoperable/advanced neuroblastoma, demonstrated adequate tumour volume reduction in order for surgery to be performed in 63.6% (De Kraker *et al.*, 1995, Pashankar *et al.*, 2005). Single-agent ^{131}I-MIBG therapy at a fixed dose (3.7-7.4 GBq) administered to 53 adults and children with metastatic or recurrent neuroblastoma due to failure of conventional treatment, resulted in 56% objective response accompanied by impressive palliative effect (Höfnagel *et al.*, 1991). Notably haematologic toxicity was observed in 53 patients receiving ^{131}I-MIBG at a dose of 0.666MBq/kg; 70% with neutropenia, 91% requiring red cell transfusions and 96% PLT transfusion. The need for autologous stem cell reconstitution in 19 patients induced stem cell availability as a prerequisite before treatment initiation (DuBois *et al.*, 2004). According to another study, combined ^{131}I-MIBG therapy followed by multiagent chemotherapy (melphalan, carboplatin, etoposide) and autologous bone marrow tranasplantation (ABMT), was administered in order to improve survival in twelve patients with 4 refractory/8 metastatic neuroblastoma; 3 out of 8 patients with metastatic disease achieved complete remission (CR) and 2/8 partial remission (PR) with acceptable toxicity (Yanik *et al.*, 2002).

In patients with metastatic carcinoid, reported tumour responses after ^{131}I-MIBG therapy range from 13 to 35% (Shapiro *et al.*, 1991, Höfnagel, 1994, Safford *et al.*, 2004). Greatest objective tumour shrinkage assessed by CT or MRI based on WHO criteria, has reached 15% in a study of 52 patients. Biochemical response, as indicated by more than 50% reduction in the tumour marker levels such as CgA or 5-HIAA was demonstrated in 37-46%, and symptom relief in 49-87% (Shapiro *et al.*, 1991, Taal *et al.*, 1996, Pathirana *et al.*, 2001, Safford *et al.*, 2004). Among the few survival reports in ^{131}I-MIBG-treated patients with NET, two studies reported survival benefit when patients with carcinoid tumour were treated with at least 15 GBq ^{131}I-MIBG during 6 months (Shapiro *et al.*, 1991, Sywak *et al.*, 2004).

Overall, therapy with ^{131}I-MIBG induces satisfactory responses, by means of neoadjuvant intervention enabling surgical approach upon previously inoperable tumours, improvement of symptomatology, and remission of metastatic foci. In patients with GEP-NET who do not qualify for PRRT based on sstr-negative scintigraphy, and present MIBG-avid lesions, ^{131}I-MIBG therapy should be considered as an alternative treatment option with substantial potential for tumour size reduction, effective palliation and survival benefit (Teunissen *et al.*, 2011).

II. Targeted Somatostatin Receptor Radionuclide Therapy of Neuroendocrine Tumours

Somatostatin and its synthetic analogues bind to sstr 1 through 5 that are overexpressed in NET. Somatostatin receptors belong to the superfamily of G-coupled protein receptors, allowing for agonist (ligand) binding with subsequent sstr desensitization, cyclic AMP production, and internalization (Drazin *et al.*, 1985). This internalization following the ligand-sstr binding, offers a useful route for targeted transport of cytotoxic radiolabelled sst analogues to the neoplastic cell nucleus. ^{111}In-DTPA-octreotide, the herein above-described $sstr_2$ preferring sst analogue with γ and Auger electron decay characteristics, which constitutes the standard means for the scintigraphic evaluation of NET patients, has also been applied in high activities for NET targeted radiotherapy. Thus the overexpression of sstr subtypes by differentiated NET defines the principle allowing for sstr imaging by radiolabelled-sst analogues, and «cold» or radiolabelled sst analogue therapy. High energy therapeutic radionuclides are administered in the setting of high density of cancer cell sstr expression in order to selectively eliminate cancer cells, while sparing healthy tissues (Reubi, 2003, Rinke *et al.*, 2009, Cancer, 2010). Regarding the induced biologic effects, PRRT principally targets DNA by producing several different lesions either directly through DNA ionization or indirectly through free radical interaction with DNA (Kassis *et al.*, 2005). Precondition for sst-analogue-based PRRT, is the abnormally increased uptake (at least as high as normal liver uptake on planar images) on the relevant imaging by ^{111}In-DTPA-octreotide in the NET tissues; possibly also by other sstr-imaging agents, although missing available direct correlations (Krenning *et al.*, 1989). During the past decades the radiolabelled sst analogues applied for therapeutic purposes consist of a sstr-subtype(s)-targeted peptide compound, labelled with high doses of Auger- or β^--particle-emitting radionuclides, namely ^{111}In or yttrium-90 (^{90}Y)/ lutetium-177 (^{177}Lu)/ rhenium-186/188 ($^{186/188}$Re), respectively (Table **7**).

Table 7: Physical characteristics of ^{111}In, ^{90}Y, ^{177}Lu, ^{188}Re and ^{186}Re

Radionuclides		**^{111}In**	**^{90}Y**	**^{177}Lu**	**^{188}Re**	**^{186}Re**
Half-life (h)		67.2	64.1	161	16.95	89.28
Production		Cd-122	Sr-90	Lu-176	W-186	Re-185
Radiation emission	mean β^- maximum β^- (MeV)		0,93 2,279	0, 14 0,497	0.213	0.107
	γ (keV)	171 245	-	113 (6.2%) 208.4 (10.4%)	155	137
	AE (keV)	0.5-25				
	CE (keV)	218-245				
Tissue penetration (particle range)	mean-max	0.02-10μm (Auger electrons)	4-12mm	0.5-2mm	11mm	5mm
	Maximum	200-550μm (CE)		2mm		
Daughter isotope		Cd-111	Zr-90	Hf-177	Os-188	Os-186

AE: Auger electrons, CE: conversion electrons.

Currently, besides tumour uptake on the ^{111}In-DTPA-octreotide, sst-analogue-based PRRT is administered to patients with NET according to additional ENETS consensus guidelines. Permission to perform PRRT should be individually obtained based on national legislation. Ethical committee approval should be acquired and eligible patients suffer from inoperable, histologically-proven NET, have a life-expectancy of at least 3-6 months, have a >50% Karnofski Performance Score or >4 Performance Score (ECOG) and should sign an informed consent form. Laboratory examinations should be focused on the exclusion of relative and absolute contraindications, including impaired renal (*i.e.* creatinine clearance <40-50ml/min), haematologic (*i.e.* Hb <8g/dl), PLT <$75x10^9$/l, WBC <$2x10^9$/l,) hepatic (*i.e.* total bilirubin >3xupper normal limit or albumin <30g/l and increased prothrombin time) and cardiac function, as well as pregnancy and lactation (Kwekkeboom *et al.*, 2009, Graham *et al.*, 2011). Main indications and criteria for sst-based PRRT, as well as commonly used dose schemes for ^{90}Y- and ^{177}Lu-labelled sst analogues, are herewith supplied (Fig. **4**, Table **8**). Multidisciplinary discussion is ideal for determining suitability and clinical decision making.

Table 8: Synopsis of sst-based PRRT criteria and indications; common practice and adverse effects with ^{90}Y- and ^{177}Lu-labelled sst-analogues

Prerequisite	**^{111}In-DTPA-Octreotide-Positive Tumours**
Indications	Inoperable sympathoadrenal system tumours (PCC, neuroblastoma and paraganglioma) Inoperable functioning GEP-NET Inoperable MTC NET of unknown origin
Basic haematology and biochemistry criteria	Hb >10 g/dl WBC >$3x10^9$/l PLT >$100x10^9$/l GFR >40ml/min
Preparation	- Withdrawal of «cold» sst analogues for a period 2fold the dosing interval or long-acting analogues 6 weeks before PRRT, and switch to short-acting subcutaneous formulations up to 12-24 h before PRRT, if clinically feasible - Previous surgical operations or radiotherapy should be performed until at least 2 mo before PRRT initiation - Previous chemotherapy should be completed by 1 mo prior to PRRT
Procedure	- Ondansetron 8mg iv ~ 30 min before PRRT administration - Individualized dose adjustment by risk factors: age, co-existing hypertension or diabetes mellitus, prior chemotherapy or PRRT-related toxicity and exceptionally high kidney uptake on ^{111}In-DTPA-octreotide scintigraphy - Possibly ACE inhibitors and Ag-II antagonists
	^{90}Y-DOTATOC: - Amino acids iv infused, *e.g.* 500 ml of Hartman (Hepa 8% amino acid; 500ml/h). After 30 min, slow iv administration of 4.4 GBq ^{90}Y-DOTATOC in 100 ml physiological saline over 20-30 min. Continuing with additional 1500 ml of amino acids infused over

Prerequisite	**^{111}In-DTPA-Octreotide-Positive Tumours**
	~ 3-3.5 h , - Time interval between treatments: 8 weeks (7-10 possible) - Total treatment cycles: 3 (*i.e.* total dose: 13.32 GBq) **^{90}Y-LANREOTIDE: -** Slow iv administration of 1.2 GBq over about 30 min - Time interval between treatments: 4-6 weeks - Total treatment cycles: 6 Can give second set of treatment with a 6 month break maximum is 6 treatments. **^{90}Y-DOTATATE:**. - Amino acids iv infused (*e.g.* 1 litre Viamin 18) at a rate of 1litre per 4 hours or slower; if vomiting occurs, 8 mg per os odansetron supplied. After 30 min, slow iv administration of 3-4 GBq ^{90}Y-DOTATATE over 20-30 min. Continuing the amino acids until finished - Time interval between treatments can be 6-8 weeks - Total treatment cycles: 3 **^{177}Lu-DOTATATE: -** Amino acids iv infused, *e.g.* an infusion of lysine 2.5%, arginine 2.5% in 1 l 0.9% NaCl; 250ml/h. After 30 min, slow iv co-administration of 7.4 GBq ^{177}Lu-DOTATATE in 100 ml physiological saline *via* a second pump system over 20-30 min. Continuing with amino acids infused over ~ 3.5 h - Time interval between treatments: 8 weeks (6-10 possible) - Total treatment cycles: 4 (*i.e.* total dose: 29.6 GBq)
	Post-therapeutic imaging ^{90}Y-labelled analogues: a Brehmsstrahlungs scintigraphy at 24 h pi ^{177}Lu-labelled analogues: the γ-emission at photopeaks of 113 and 208 keV enables scintigraphy at 24h pi
	- Enhanced hydration before, during and after infusion - Patients on long-acting sst formulations should receive also short-acting analogues in the first 7-10 days after their long- acting formulation has been restarted
Most common adverse effects	Acute: nausea, vomiting (mostly associated with amino acid coinfusion), abdominal discomfort and localized NET- related pain; usually mild and tolerable Long-term:- myelosuppression; usually mild and transient but dose- limiting - renal function deterioration; usually mild and transient but for ^{90}Y-and ^{177}Lu-labelled sst analogues, dose- limiting - hepatic dysfunction; usually mild and transient

PRRT with ^{111}In-DTPA-Octreotide

Somatostatin-based PRRT has been introduced into clinical practice since the 1990's through a multicentre trial by the administration of high doses of ^{111}In-DTPA-octreotide in GEP-NET patients, with overall encouraging reported results pertaining to symptom relief and biochemical response (Anthony *et al.*, 2002, Valkema *et al.*, 2002, Buscombe *et al.*, 2003, Delpassand *et al.*, 2008). At least 92% of the patients had documented progressive disease (PD) at study entry; hence stable disease (SD) and minor response (MR) could imply a therapeutic benefit, even though there were only few partial remissions (Teunissen *et al.*, 2011). Upon evaluation of 26 GEP-NET patients, mostly bearing carcinoid neoplasms with carcinoid syndrome and a few pancreatic islet cells neoplasms, who were treated with at least two-monthly doses (of 6.6 GBq) of ^{111}In-DTPA-octreotide, clinical benefit was noted in 62%, SD in 81% and PR in 8% of patients. The treatment was proved safe and well-tolerated, with median survival of 18 months, thereby overall increased expected survival (Anthony *et al.*, 2002). Another review study of 16 patients suffering from disseminated NET (10 with carcinoid, 2 MTC, and 1 each with a gastrinoma, glucagonoma, fibrolamellar cancer and malignant histiocytoma) who had received ^{111}In-DTPA-octreotide at total cumulative activities from 3.1 to as high as 36.6 GBq, divided in 1- to 3-month intervals over a 2.5-year period, reported a mean PFS of 12.25 months (median, 9 months) and no significant toxicity. Seventy percent of patients had some benefit for at least 6 months after the end of treatment, including 2 CR and 3 PR, but only 31% of patients had sustained benefit at 18 months from this treatment (Buscombe *et al.*, 2003). Other researchers have recorded the therapeutic and adverse effects of ^{111}In-DTPA-octreotide administration at total cumulative activities of 20 to 160 GBq, in 40 patients with NET. Stabilization of previously progressive neoplasms was observed in 14 patients, MR in 6 patients and PR in 1 patient. The side effects involved mostly mild bone marrow toxicity and indices related to impaired spermatogenesis. The administration of 100 GBq was considered as the maximal tolerable dose, due to the development of myelodysplastic syndrome (MDS) or leukemia in 3/6 patients who received larger doses with estimated bone marrow radiation dose of more than 3 Gy (Valkema *et al.*, 2002). Yet in one of these three patients, ^{111}In-DTPA-octreotide therapy followed chemotherapy, which could have contributed to or caused this severe complication. In a more recently completed study enrolling 29 patients with progressive GEP-NET, high-activity PRRT was administered in 18/29 (62%) patients with total cumulative activities up to 37.3 GBq, given in two cycles, while 4/29 were decreased and 7/29 decided not to participate (Delpassand *et al.*, 2008). Three months after the second cycle, PR had been accomplished in 2/18 (11%) and SD in 16/18 (89%) patients. Moreover, in eight patients (44%), CgA or at least one hormone levels were reduced by 50% compared to pretreatment levels.

Among the ^{111}In-DTPA-octreotide therapy-related adverse effects, transient bone marrow suppression was the most frequent encountered toxicity, with dose-limited tolerability (Valkema *et al.*, 2002, Teunissen *et al.*, 2011). The radiopharmaceutical undergoes predominantly urinary excretion as pre-mentioned and the radiation of the short-range (maximal 10 μm) Auger electrons originating from the cells of the proximal tubules has not been not been proved harmful for the renal function (Valkema *et al.*, 2002). Renal insufficiency has been reported in one of 26 patients and was probably related to pre-existing retroperitoneal fibrosis and not therapy-related (Anthony *et al.*, 2002). Transient grade-4 hepatic toxicity developed in 3 patients with widespread hepatic metastases and with treatment-associated necrosis on CT.

The clinical studies with ^{111}In-DTPA-octreotide, show that the favourable effects on symptom control are unfortunately not accompanied by tumour regression, thus rendering this radiolabelled peptide not ideal for PRRT, at least in GEP-NET with large metastatic foci, possibly owing to the small particle range and resultant short tissue penetration (Buscombe *et al.*, 2003, Delpassand *et al.*, 2008, Kwekkeboom *et al.*, 2009). Based on experimental observations in rats, clinical studies might prove that ^{111}In-DTPA-octreotide efficiently treats micro-metastases or prevents metastatic spread during initial surgery (Slooter *et al.*, 1999). In the meantime, intensive research has led to the construction of newer analogues with higher affinity profiles that can be linked to β^-- or alpha- (α-) emitting radionuclides for better targeting and destruction of sstr-expressing tumours.

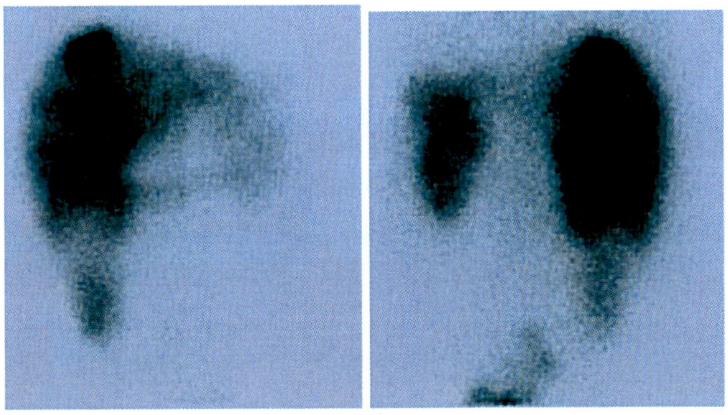

Figure 4: Planar anterior (left) and posterior (right) abominal views with ^{111}In-DTPA-octreotide in a 65 years old female patient with primary NET of the rectum accompanied by hepatic metastases, show both the primary and the metastatic foci. The patient was diagnosed with recurrent disease and was treated with 3 cycles of ^{90}Y-DOTATOC at 4.4 GBq/cycle, with 8-weeks intercycle intervals at University General Hospital "Alexandra" in Athens, Greece. No significant adverse effect has been observed. Vomiting associated with the amino acid infusions, was the only consistent symptom encountered by the patient. Imaging re-evaluation is pending.

Newer Somatostatin-Based PRRT Radiopharmaceutical

The current newer radiopharmaceuticals exploit the chelate 1,4,7,10-tetraazacyclododecane-1,4,7,10-tetraacetic acid (DOTA) which links the octreopeptide to a b-emitting therapeutic radionuclide such as ^{90}Y or ^{177}Lu in a stable complex: [^{90}Y-DOTA^{0}TYR^{3}]-octreotide (^{90}Y-DOTATOC, SMT-487 or generically known as ^{90}Y-edotreotide; Onalta® [Molecular Insight Pharmaceuticals]), [^{90}Y-DOTA]-lanreotide, [^{90}Y-DOTA^{0},TYP^{3}]-octreotate and [^{177}Lu-DOTA^{0},TYR^{3}]-octreotate (^{177}Lu-DOTATATE) (De Jong *et al.*, 1997, Van Essen *et al.*, 2007, Khanna *et al.*, 2008). The first promising DOTA-chelated somatostatin analogue was conjugated in 1996 (Behe *et al.*, 1996). Based on *in vitro* studies, each radiopharmaceutical retains high affinity towards specific sstr subtypes; in particular, ^{90}Y-DOTATOC mainly for sstr$_2$ and sstr$_5$ and moderate for sstr$_3$, ^{90}Y-lanreotide for sstr$_2$, sstr$_3$, sstr$_4$ and sstr$_5$ while lower for sstr$_1$, and ^{177}Lu-DOTATATE ninefold higher affinity for sstr$_2$ (De Jong *et al.*, 1997, Gnanasegaran *et al.*, 2005 IJNM). Consequently, as the radiopharmaceutical binds to sstr on NET cells, the emitted β^- radiation by ^{90}Y or ^{177}Lu is tumouricidal. The β^- ray emitters such as ^{131}I, ^{90}Y, ^{186}Re and ^{188}Re have a tissue range of several millimeters, which can generate a ''crossfire'' effect so that receptor-negative cells in a tumour can also be treated. Accordingly, the emitted β^- particles by ^{90}Y have a maximum tissue penetration of 12mm and thus maximum action spectrum up to ~500 cells (cell diameter: ~20μm), enabling ^{90}Y to deliver high radiation doses to NET cells which overexpress sstr but also to adjacent areas with potentially low sstr levels, *i.e.* with poor differentiation or perfusion as well as heterogeneous tumors. Therefore β^- ray therapy with ^{90}Y-sst analogues is preferred for large tumours. The emitted β^- particles by ^{177}Lu have a maximum tissue penetration of ~2mm, which is effective in NET cell destruction, yet with limited influence on adjacent cells, a fact of particular importance for small NET burden. An outline of reported PRRT results derived from worldwide experience is provided in Table **9**, regarding the most commonly agents used, *i.e.* ^{90}Y-DOTATOC and ^{177}Lu-DOTATATE.

Optimal treatment protocols for ^{90}Y- and ^{177}Lu-labelled sst analogues have not yet been established due to lack of randomized clinical trials. Available treatment schemes regarding the cycle dose, intercycle interval and cumulative dose of each radiopharmaceutical may be individualized, *i.e.* adjusted according to factors like the occurrence of side effects, and must therefore depend on local expertise and clinical judgment. Patients are hospitalized for 2-3 days for the procedure, in accordance with radiation protection regulations.

Furthermore, before each therapy cycle, certain laboratory evaluations are required and include liver function (SGOT, SGPT, albumin, bilirubin), kidney function (creatinine, BUN; creatinine clearance on indication), haematology (Hb, WBC plus differential, PLT number), Cg-A and/or other serum tumour markers if elevated at baseline (Kwekkeboom *et al.*, 2009). The patients should receive written instructions regarding travel and contact with others after each treatment, according to national and international legislation. Also, after each therapy cycle, blood cell counts are preferably performed at 4 and 6 weeks, and repeated every 2 weeks in case of WHO toxicity grade 3 or 4.

During each therapy cycle, the measured activity of ^{90}Y-DOTATOC/^{177}Lu-DOTATATE is administered slowly by iv route over 20-30 min in 100 ml physiological saline. Concommitant iv infusion of amino acid solutions which contain lysine and arginine is essential to reduce kidney radiation-absorbed dose when performing PRRT. Starting 30 min before the administration of the radiopharmaceutical, 2.5% lysine, 2.5% arginine in 1 liter normal saline can be infused in 4 h. Alternatively, a recently applied protocol used 25 g of lysine diluted in 1 liter of normal saline infused over 4 h, starting 30-60 min before radiolabelled sst analogue injection, followed by an additional 12.5 g of lysine diluted in 500 ml of normal saline, over 3 h, twice daily on day 2 and day 3 post-therapy (Bodei *et al.*, 2011). Other commercially available amino acid solutions may be used, such as Aminosteril N-Hepa 8% at an infusion rate of 500 ml/h (Fresenius AG, Bad Homburg, Germany), or Baxter Synthamin (at 500 ml/h) (Kwekkeboom *et al.*, 2009).

Therapy discontinuation may be advocated in case of patient clinical deterioration or imaging-based disease progression during the treatment period. Also prolonged (*i.e.* more than 2-3 months) WHO grade 3 or 4 haematologic, renal, or hepatic toxicity may constitute a reason to discontinue treatment, or to modify the cycle dose/intercycle interval, according to the local protocol. On the contrary, an increase in serum tumour markers may not be used as a relevant guide, since it may be temporary and attributed to tumour lysis (Kwekkeboom *et al.*, 2009).

Clinical and biochemical response should always be accompanied by imaging response assessment. Follow-up laboratory and imaging monitoring should ideally be performed after 3 and 6 months, and thereafter every 6 months. Considering that factors besides changes in tumour burden may also influence serum tumour marker levels, such as medication (*e.g.* sst analogues), there are no accepted criteria for biochemical responses, but recommendations define tumour marker response as a decrease in serum levels of $\geq$50% of baseline. Symptomatic responses should preferentially be reported according to the WHO toxicity criteria. Imaging response is validated by accepted standards, *i.e.* WHO, RECIST (Response Evaluation Criteria In Solid Tumors), or SWOG (South West Oncology Group) criteria. The follow-up imaging modality (CT or MRI) and technique should be identical to baseline, keeping in mind that CT and MRI may underestimate responses in case of cystic or necrotic tumours. The use of the validated EORTC QLC-30 questionnaires is recommended for assessment of the quality of life, if possible with additional NET-specific questions that are currently in the process of validation. Follow-up should be ideally continued lifelong.

The value of radionuclide therapy largely relies on the predictability of the patterns of biodistribution of the radiopharmaceutical. Imaging ^{90}Y and ^{177}Lu could apply for the assessment/monitoring of the therapeutic plan and outcome. The β^- particles emitted from ^{90}Y interact with the tissue to produce Brehmsstrahlung radiation, which cannot be easily imaged due to its continuous energy spectrum (Shen *et al.*, 1994). For PRRT with ^{90}Y-labelled analogues, quality control with a small activity test dose and a Brehmsstrahlungs scintigraphy 1 h after infusion is not recommended. However, a Brehmsstrahlungs whole-body scan at 24 h pi (Fig. **5**) may prove helpful when using medium- or high-energy collimators, at an energy window of 55-285 keV or at 75 keV photopeak and 50% windows, respectively (Shen *et al.*, 1994, Gnanasegaran *et al.*, 2005). Despite the limited resolution of Brehmsstrahlungs imaging and thus inability to distinguish all tumour sites and calculate total tumour uptake, localization of the ^{90}Y-labelled sst analogues at the tumour sites has been documented (Gopinath *et al.*, 2004, Gnanasegaran *et al.*, 2005). For PRRT with ^{177}Lu-labelled analogues, the γ-emission at photopeaks of 113 and 208 keV enables both post-therapeutic imaging and dosimetric determinations and, if feasible, blood and urine collections, may be performed. Naturally, simplified methods are required in order to enable individual dosimetry in routine clinical practice (Kwekkeboom *et al.*, 2009).

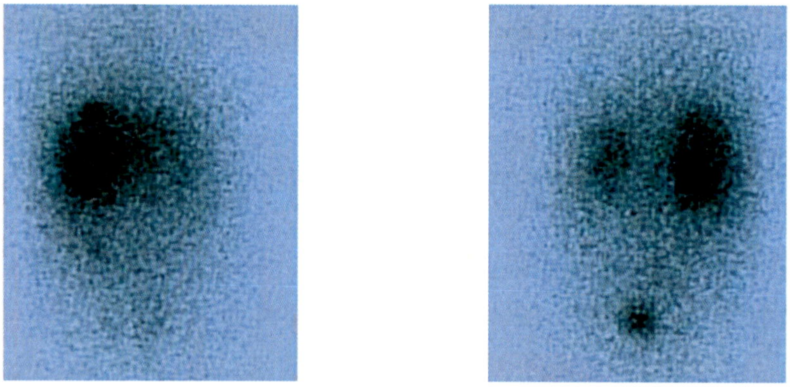

Figure 5: Anterior (left) and posterior (right) Brehmsstrahlungs whole-body scan 24 h post administration of the third ^{90}Y-DOTATOC dose of 4.4 GBq to the same patient with metastatic NET depicted in Fig. **4**.

PRRT-Associated Acute and Long-Term Adverse Effects

PRRT is considered a safe treatment; reported frequency of serious side-effects is low (Imhof *et al.*, 2011, Pfeifer *et al.*, 2011). Acute adverse effects are mild and temporary such as nausea, vomiting and localized NET-related pain within 24 hours after the administration of ^{90}Y-DOTATOC or ^{177}Lu-DOTATATE. The latter has also been reported to cause mild alopecia. Notably, nausea and vomiting are mostly considered to be associated with the coinfusion of renal protective amino acid solutions rather than the PRRT itself (Rolleman *et al.*, 2003). Long-term adverse effects are generally few and mild; they are attributed to absorbed dose and mainly involve the kidneys, bone marrow, and to a lesser extent, the liver. Myelotoxicity has been reported in relatively low rates. Serious but reversible grade II myelotoxicity has been recorded in up to 15%. A literature-based minimum percentage of development of MDS might be associated with preceding first-line cytotoxic treatments. Maximum tolerated absorbed dose for the highly radiosensitive bone marrow cells has been defined at levels below 2 Gy. Hepatotoxicity has been recorded in even lower rates, with mild- usually grade II- and reversible character. PRRT-related nephrotoxicity is attributed to the tubular reabsorption of the radiolabelled peptides, thereby increasing the dose delivered to the kidneys. The megalin/cubulin system in the proximal tubule cells seems to play an important synergistic role in the reabsorption process of the radiolabelled peptides, thus increasing renal parenchyma irradiation (Rolleman *et al.*, 2010). Thus efforts have been focused on methods that interfere with this reabsorption pathway in order to achieve kidney protection. Such methods include coinfusion of basic amino acids, the bovine gelatin-containing solution Gelofusine or albumin fragments. Cotreatment with amifostine (Ethylol), a radiation protector, or with blockers of the renin-angiotensin-aldosterone system are still under research. Amino acids such as arginine and lysine are already typically used in the clinical setting during PRRT and may effectively ensure renal protection. However, despite the efforts to develop the absolute protective recipe, serious PRRT-related nephrotoxicity was still reported in low rates. Studies of long-term follow-up of patients treated with PRRT, have suggested a PRRT-triggered process at the level of the glomerulus that continues long after the radiation exposure; yet no clinically notable impairment of tubular function occurred, in agreement with histopathologic findings of radiation nephropathy. Renal biopsies of patients treated with ^{90}Y-DOTATOC who encountered nephrotoxicity revealed typical signs of thrombotic microangiopathy involving glomeruli, arterioles and small arteries accompanied by tubular atrophy and interstitial fibrosis (Valkema *et al.*, 2005). Thus, the spectrum of PRRT-related nephropathy and external-beam radiation nephropathy fits within the multifactorial pathophysiology of chronic kidney disease, finally leading to end-stage renal disease (Valkema *et al.*, 2005). Obviously, the used radionuclide plays an important role in the potential nephrotoxicity. The low-energy Auger electrons of ^{111}In do not penetrate tissue far enough (only 10 μm) to leave the tubular cell, hence justifying the low nephrotoxicity encountered in relevant studies. On the other hand, the β^- particles from ^{90}Y and ^{177}Lu travel long enough (up to 12 mm and 2 mm, respectively), thus may potentially reach the glomeruli and induce lesions. The maximum ^{90}Y-DOTATOC and ^{177}Lu-DOTATATE per-cycle and cumulative treatment dose have been under intensive investigation. For ^{90}Y-DOTATOC, a protocol with fixed cumulative activity of 13.3 GBq, divided into 3 equal cycles of 4.4 GBq, is well-tolerated and avoids the risk factor of a high dose per cycle. Additional consistent recommendations comprise concomitant amino acid infusion, and individualized dose-adjustment; the latter should be guided by assessing other possible risk factors, including age, co-existing hypertension or diabetes mellitus, prior chemotherapy and exceptionally high kidney uptake on ^{111}In-DTPA-octreotide scintigraphy. Moreover, based on the central role of the renin-angiotensin system in the process of renal microvascular injury, the efficacy of angiotensin-converting enzyme (ACE) inhibitors and angiotensin II (Ag-II) blockade in diminishing the incidence of renal failure has been demonstrated (Moulde *et al.*, 1998, Cohen *et al.*, 2003).

On the whole, taking into account that both kidneys and bone marrow absorbed radiation doses vary widely between patients, individualized tailored dosimetry for each patient is the ideal method for treating patients with PRRT (Forrer *et al.*, 2009). The highest possible radiation dose to the tumour should be combined with a maximally well-tolerated dose to the dose-limiting organs. Therefore, fixed dose regimens with relatively few side effects, may actually be implicated in undertreatment of a proportion of patients (Teunissen *et al.*, 2011).

^{90}Y-Labelled Somatostatin Analogues for PRRT

^{90}Y-DOTATOC

Somatostatin-based PRRT with ^{90}Y-DOTATOC was developed and introduced into clinical practice by Otte and colleagues in 1997 in Basel, Switzerland, who treated a patient with sstr-positive abdominal metastases of a neuroendocrine carcinoma of unknown origin and reported good response with symptom relief (Otte *et al.*, 1997, Nisa *et al.*, 2011). Initial reports on a small patient group with sstr-positive metastatic NET, showed that ^{90}Y-DOTATOC was efficient in inducing PR in 2/10 patients and SD in 6/10 (Otte *et al.*, 1998). The introduction of tyrosine into the third position of the octreotide sequence increases the hydrophilicity and receptor affinity of the peptide, and conjugation with a high energy β^- emitter such as ^{90}Y at elevated specific activities of up to 55.5-62.9 GBq/μmol, allows for selective irradiation of the sstr-positive tumour (Chinol *et al.*, 2002). Chelation with DOTA inhibits the release of ^{90}Y that would otherwise build up in bone. DOTA-d-Phe(1)-Tyr(3)-octreotide (DOTATOC) retains both its receptor-binding properties and its physiological function when labelled with ^{90}Y. Yttrium-90 is a high-energy β^- emitter with a mean tissue penetration of approximately 5 mm (max 12 mm) and a decay half-life of 64.1 hours, rendering it particularly effective for tumour treatment. ^{90}Y-DOTATOC is administered iv, binds to sstr on the target cells, with an increased affinity for $sstr_2$, expressed by most NET, and exerts cytotoxic effects *via* irradiation.

Since 1997 several clinical results have been published focusing on NET patients treated with ^{90}Y-DOTATOC. According to a recent comprehensive review of the several clinical phase I and phase II trials with ^{90}Y-DOTATOC therapy carried out in centres mainly in Europe and in cooperation with USA, clinical experience gained for over a decade proves that it is still a powerful agent for targeting large infiltrative NET in selected patients (Nisa *et al.*, 2011). The accomplishment of an objective response in nearly a quarter of the patients as well as symptomatic improvement and stability of the disease in more than half of the patients treated with ^{90}Y-DOTATOC justifies its use even in end stage disease. However, it is highlighted that a multidisciplinary approach is advocated aiming at precocious diagnosis of NET and prompt application of the appropriate therapy for a more satisfactory outcome.

In the above-mentioned analysis from 13 centres, a total number of 774 patients (mean age 41.25 years) bearing different types of NET (526 GEP-NET and 248 others such as carcinoids, MTC, breast cancer, paragangliomas, meningiomas, small cell lung cancer and NET of unknown primary origin), ^{90}Y-DOTATOC was administered after failure and/or unsuitability of conventional treatment means. Various dose regimes were applied, from 1.74-27 MBq/m^2, divided in 2-16 cycles, either in equal doses or single dose escalation, at time intervals mostly ranging from 4-9 weeks (Otte *et al.*, 1999, Paganelli *et al.*, 1999, 2001, 2002, Waldherr *et al.*, 2001, 2002, Valkema *et al.*, 2001, 2006, Chinol *et al.*, 2002, Bodei *et al.*, 2003, 2004, Forrer *et al.*, 2006, Frilling *et al.*, 2006, Nisa *et al.*, 2011). Patients suffering from symptomatic SD or progressive NET were selected for PRRT, based on sufficiently high uptake of the tracer in NET tissues on sstr scintigraphy, due to its direct correlation with tumour regression after therapy. Renal protection was pursued in most trials by employing amino acids such as lysine ± arginine infusion immediately before, during and/or right after therapy at different concentrations and combinations. Renal dosimetric measurements were utilized in some centres for planning treatment so as not to exceed 27 Gy to the kidneys. Response to therapy was evaluated by standard WHO and/or SWOG criteria in most centres and side effects were reported based on the WHO toxicity grade criteria. The overall objective response rate for all treated tumours was 24% (Nisa *et al.*, 2011). Disease stabilization was achieved in 54% patients, while PD was observed in 18%.

The group from Basel published the results of their phase I clinical study applying PRRT with ^{90}Y-DOTATOC in 29 patients with 16 GEP-NET, 4 of unknown origin and 9 other NET. The administration of a mean cumulative dose of 6.12 GBq/m^2 divided over in 4 cycles, was effective in terms of SD in 69% of the patients and partial and minor responses in 21%, while the disease progressed in 10% of the patients. Forty-one patients bearing NET, encompassing 22 GEP-NET, were treated as part of the phase II trial by the same group with a cumulative dose of 6 GBq/m^2 ^{90}Y-DOTATOC administered over 4 cycles at 6-week intervals (Waldherr *et al.*, 2001). Complete remission was documented in 2% of the patients, PR in 22%, SD in 61% and PD in 15%. The overall response rate for GEP-NET was higher, specifically 36%. Waldherr and colleagues further treated 39 patients with progressive GEP and bronchial NET using a total radiopharmaceutical dose of 7.4 GBq/m^2 in conjunction with rigorous renal protection (Waldherr *et al.*, 2002). The outcome was remarkable in terms of both clinical improvement (63%) and objective response, showing CR in 5% and PR in 18%, while SD was noted in 69% and PD in 8% of the patients. The response rate was higher, *i.e.* 38%, in 13 patients with endocrine pancreatic tumours.

In a multicentre phase I trial designed to define the maximal tolerated single and 4-cycle dose of ^{90}Y-DOTATOC, 42 patients bearing progressive as well as stable NET including 21 with carcinoid, 10 with islet cell cancer and 11 with other types of NET, were treated with escalating doses divided in 4 cycles at 6- to 9-week intervals. The cumulative dose ranged from 1.7 to 27 GBq without reaching the maximum tolerable dose and was administered with concomitant amino acid infusion. Of 32 evaluable patients, 53% had SD, 13% had minor and mixed response, 9% had PR, and 25% had PD. Notably in 2/2 patients suffering from insulinoma and 1/1 from gastrinoma, complete symptomatic cure was accomplished. Overall, half of the patients experienced symptomatic improvement (Valkema *et al.*, 2001).

In the meantime, Paganelli and colleagues published the outcome of ^{90}Y-DOTATOC therapy in 20 patients suffering from carcinoid (17), breast cancer (1), MTC (1) and grade III meningioma (1). Fifty-five percent of the patients achieved MR/SD and 20% CR or PR. Progressive disease was observed in 25% of the patients. The treatment protocol comprised 3 treatment cycles, with dose escalation from 1.1 GBq/cycle in the first group of five individuals, up to 2.2 GBq/cycle in the last group of five patients (Paganelli *et al.*, 1999). The same researchers, reported their results on 30 patients, most of whom with carcinoid, three with MTC and one each with meningioma, grade III astrocytoma and SCLC. The treatment regime comprised 3 cycles of up to 2.59 GBq of the radiopharmaceutical per cycle (total 7.77 GBq) without renal protection (Paganelli *et al.*, 2001). The majority (64%) of patients achieved SD and 23% CR or PR with median duration of response being 18 months, while 13% had PD. In their next protocol, the group from Milan treated 87 patients, among them 57 with GEP-NET, 14 with MTC and 16 with other or of unknown origin NET, with ^{90}Y-DOTATOC at doses from 7.4 to 20.2 GBq/m^2 with no major adverse effects in doses up to 5.55 GBq/cycle (Paganelli *et al.*, 2002). Disease stability was mainly observed (49%), besides 23% PR and 5% CR. Twenty percent of the patients had PD and 3% could not be evaluated. Overall, in clinical studies derived from Milan, most of the patients bearing scintigraphically sstr-positive tumours, who obtained a favourable PRRT outcome, had GEP-NET.

Further results with ^{90}Y-DOTATOC therapy were published by the group from the European Institute of Oncology who proceeded with 256 patients, among whom 111 (mostly with GEP-NET) received cumulative activities of 7.4 GBq to 21.3 GBq divided in two or more cycles. During a 15-month mean follow-up in these patients, the objective response rate was 27% (5% CR and 22% PR), while disease stabilization was noted in 49%. Progressive disease endured in 20% and response assessment was not feasible for 4% of the patients (Chinol *et al.*, 2002).

The researchers from Basel and Milan attempted to establish the maximum tolerated dose of ^{90}Y-DOTATOC per cycle in conjunction with amino acid infusion in a collaborative phase I study (Bodei *et al.*, 2003). Forty patients with sstr-positive tumours, specifically 21 with GEP-NET, 11 with thyroid, 5 brain and 3 other NET, received 2 cycles of the radiopharmaceutical at an escalating activity ranging from 5.9 to 11.1 GBq. On the whole, the median duration of response was 9 months. One patient with MTC had CR and 17.5% of the patients had PR, 45% had SD, 32.5% had PD, while in one patient the response evaluation was not feasible. The objective response was 28.5% in patients with GEP-NET.

Bodei and colleagues collected and analyzed in a review the results of 141 patients treated with ^{90}Y-DOTATOC for different types of NET (Bodei *et al.*, 2004). The cumulative administered activities ranged from 7.4 to 26.4 GBq divided into 2-16 cycles at 4- to 6-week intervals. The overall objective response (PR and CR) was 26% and clinical benefit was observed in 76% patients who had PD and in 32% patients who had SD at the time of treatment. The majority of the patients who responded (69.7%) had GEP-NET.

In 2006, Valkema and colleagues published long-term follow-up and survival data on 58 patients treated with ^{90}Y-DOTATOC in combination with amino acid (lysine 2.5%/arginine 2.5%) infusion, for advanced GEP-NET in a multi-centre

(Rotterdam, The Netherlands; Brussels, Belgium; Tampa, USA) dose escalation phase I study (Valkema *et al.*, 2006). At baseline, 47 of the 58 patients had PD. Sixteen out of 52 patients with liver metastasis and 2/6 patients without liver metastasis were in the 'end stage'. Total activities up to 14.8 GBq/m^2 in 4 cycles or up to 9.3 GBq/m^2 in a single cycle were administered guided by a maximum estimated dose of 27 Gy to the kidneys and did not reach the maximum tolerated single dose. Of 36 symptomatic patients at baseline, 58% experienced symptom relief or improved Karnofsky score. The overall outcome in evaluable patients, encompassed PR in 8%, MR (25-50% tumour volume reduction) in 13%, SD in 50% and PD in 29%. Overall 33 (57%) patients experienced some improvement in their disease status; including conversion from PD into SD or improvement from SD to MR (by SWOG criteria). The median overall survival was 36.7 months and the median time to progression in the 41 patients who had either SD, MR, or PR was 30 months.

Moreover, treatment with a cumulative dose of 7.4 GBq/m^2 ^{90}Y-DOTATOC divided into two or more sessions at 8-10 weeks interval, was used as cutting edge therapy in 20 patients bearing progressive metastatic NET (18 GEP-NET, 1 paraganglioma and 1 unknown NET) not suitable for primary resection. Later on, therapy with ^{177}Lu-DOTATOC was advocated in six patients due to tumour relapse and/or due to small size and multilocularity of the neoplastic lesions. During a median follow-up period of 19.9 months, among 14 patients who received solely ^{90}Y-DOTATOC therapy, 21.4% had PR, 57.14% had SD and 21.4% had PD. Remarkably the therapy allowed the surgical resection of large metastatic deposits in two patients (Frilling *et al.*, 2006). In another study of patients with inoperable and advanced NET, PRRT was proposed to be advanced to first or second line therapy. Sixty-eight patients received ^{90}Y-DOTATOC mostly and/or ^{177}Lu-DOTATATE, and presented CR in 7.4%, PR in 16.2% and SD in 61.8%, based on RECIST criteria, while the PFS was 29 months (Pfeifer *et al.*, 2011).

Upon studying the efficacy and safety of treatment with 5.9-7.4 GBq/m^2 ^{90}Y-DOTATOC in 116 patients with metastatic NET, mostly (79) GEP-NET, Forrer and colleagues (Forrer *et al.*, 2006) from Basel reported that on the whole, CR was achieved in 4% of the patients, PR in 23% and SD including MR in 62%, while 11% patients had PD. In addition, the assessment of 57 patients for symptomatic response according to the National Cancer Institute-Common Toxicity Criteria (NCI-CTC) scoring system, revealed a substantial diminution of tumour-associated pain with subsequent cease of pain medication or switch to milder analgesics; also, carcinoid symptoms were significantly alleviated in 83% patients with diarrhea, 46% patients with flushes, 63% patients with wheezing and in 75% patients with pellagra.

From 2006 onwards, further studies adding to sst-based PRRT effectiveness in patients with NET have been published. Forrer and colleagues observed a remarkable mean duration of response of 18 months in 28 patients treated with ^{90}Y- and ^{177}Lu-DOTATOC due to inoperable paragangliomas and PCC (Forrer *et al.*, 2008). Twenty five patients received a total activity of 7.4 GBq/m^2 ^{90}Y-DOTATOC alone and three patients having mainly small metastatic lesions (<2 cm) were treated with one cycle of 3.7 GBq/m^2 ^{90}Y-DOTATOC, followed by 7.4 GBq/m^2 ^{177}Lu-DOTATOC. Disease progression during therapy in 2/28 patients resulted in treatment cessation. Out of the 26 patients who completed the treatment, 2 had PR, 5 had MR, 13 had conversion of PD to SD, 2 showed a mixed response (some lesions were bigger and some smaller) and 4 patients remained at PD.

Therapy with ^{90}Y-DOTATOC has unfortunately not produced objective response in patients with sstr-positive SCLC (Pless *et al.*, 2004). On the contrary, in a phase II trial on metastatic MTC, response to this therapy was found to be associated with long-term survival benefit (Iten *et al.*, 2007). Similar outcome has also been described for a patient with MTC cardiac metastasis (Bertagna *et al.*, 2009).

According to results published by Bushnell and colleagues in 2010, PRRT with three cycles of 4.4 GBq ^{90}Y-DOTATOC each, at 6-week intervals, remarkably produced objective tumour response (4) or SD (63) in 74.4% of 90 patients with metastatic carcinoid refractory to octreotide, with no treatment alternatives. In this multicentre phase II trial, the maximum cumulative administered activity of 13.3 GBq accompanied by renal protective amino acid infusion, was well-tolerated with an acceptable expected adverse event profile. The median progression-free survival was 16.3 months and was significantly greater for the 38 patients who had durable diarrhea improvement (18.2 months) than the 18 patients who did not

(7.9 months). The median overall survival was 26.9 months (Bushnell *et al.*, 2010). Earlier, the clinical effectiveness of PRRT had also been evaluated in 21 treated patients at the University of Iowa and VAMC Iowa City. A favourable clinical response was shown in 67% of these patients, with a significant decrease in the daily nonradioactive octreotide requirement; clinical response scoring system included evaluations of weight change, the Karnofsky score, a patient-reported health state score and tumour-related symptoms such as fatigue, abdominal pain, diarrhea, nausea or vomiting, and flushing (Graham *et al.*, 2011, Bushnell *et al.*, 2003). The outcome of this trial is comparable with the results of the second multicentre PRRT phase I study with this radiopharmaceutical (Valkema *et al.*, 2006, Teunissen *et al.*, 2011).

Noteworthy results regarding 17 children and young adults on ^{90}Y-DOTATOC phase I trial, due to refractory, sstr-expressing tumours were reported from Menda and colleagues at the University of Iowa. The scheme included 3 cycles of the therapeutic agent, administered over dose escalation from 1.11 GBq/m^2 to 1.85 GBq/m^2 per cycle, at a 6-week interval. The outcome comprised 12% PR, 29% MR and 35% SD, without any dose-limiting toxicity (Menda *et al.*, 2010).

Consistently favourable long-term outcome has been identified over a clinical phase II single-centre open-label trial, comprising 1,109 patients with neuroendocrine cancers (74% GEP-NET) who were treated with repeated cycles (1-10 cycles per patient; median, two) of 3.7 GBq/m^2 ^{90}Y-DOTATOC (Imhof *et al.*, 2011). Overall, 378 patients (34.1%) experienced morphologic response, 172 biochemical response (15.5%) and 329 clinical response (29.7%). Response to therapy was associated with longer survival, based on a median follow-up of 23 months. Multivariable regression revealed that tumoural uptake on the initial sstr-imaging was predictive for overall survival.

In a newer study coming from Basel, analysis was focused on long-term outcome in 359 patients with metastasized NET, after clinical introduction and dose escalation of PRRT with ^{90}Y-DOTATOC. Overall 60 patients were treated with low dose (cumulative up to 34.6 GBq; range 0.9-7.8 GBq/cycle), 77 patients with intermediate dose (up to 58.5 GBq; 2.0-7.4 GBq/cycle) and 222 patients with high dose (up to 62.2 GBq; 3.7-8.1 GBq/cycle) of the radiopharmaceutical. The median survival was 39 months (range: 1-158) in the low-dose group, 34 months (range: 1-118) in the intermediate-dose group and 29 months (range: 1-113) in the high-dose group (Marincek *et al.*, 2013).

Reported adverse effects attributed to PRRT with ^{90}Y-DOTATOC are generally mild and reversible, if adequate kidney protective measures are engaged and dose-limits are respected. In particular, acute side effects occuring after treatment administration are mainly described as mild and tolerable. Most patients experienced nausea, vomiting and flushing (grades 1-3), as well as abdominal pain that were typically associated with concommitant amino acid infusion and either subsided after infusion cessation or required significant additional therapy (Nisa *et al.*, 2011, Bushnell *et al.*, 2010). Warm sensation, paraesthesia and gastric heaviness have also been reported, while patients with carcinoid syndrome (grades 1-4) encountered symptoms of imprecise location in the form of flushing, diarrhea, vomiting, wheezing/dyspnea and pellagra, sometimes despite octreotide medication (Waldherr *et al.*, 2001, Waldherr *et al.*, 2002, Bodei *et al.*, 2003). One patient with pancreatic insulinoma required co-infusion of 5% glucose solution (Bodei *et al.*, 2003). Some patients with bone and/or liver metastasis experienced tumour-associated pain and weakness, occasionally requiring morphine administration (Waldherr *et al.*, 2001). No clinical manifestation of acute toxicity, like allergic reaction or fever was ever observed in any of the trials. Yet, some patients often experienced irradiation-related asthenia within the first week after therapy (Bodei *et al.*, 2004).

Moreover, mild and temporary bone marrow suppression was the most frequently encountered long-term adverse effect in patients treated with ^{90}Y-labelled sst analogues. Lymphocytopenia and anemia have been observed to be reversible within 3-4 weeks (Waldherr *et al.*, 2001). Acute grades 3 and 4 haematologic toxicity was collectively observed in 3-12% of the patients regarding PLT, 1-7% for Hb and 2-7% for WBC (Otte *et al.*, 1999, Waldherr *et al.*, 2002, Bodei *et al.*, 2003, Valkema *et al.*, 2006). Toxicity regarding the lymphocytic subpopulation reached grades 3 and 4 and was reported to mainly affect the B-cell subpopulation (Bushnell *et al.*, 2010, Sierra *et al.*, 2009). In line with these observations, 142/1,109 patients (12.8%) developed severe transient grade 3 to 4 haematologic toxicities (leucopenia, 67 patients; anemia, 11; thrombocytopenia, 64). Also, post-therapy two patients developed myeloproliferative diseases; one developed MDS after two treatment cycles and one, acute myeloid leukemia after four cycles (Imhof *et al.*, 2011). Liver toxicity is overall reported to be low; grade 3 hepatotoxicity was noticed in a minority of patients (De Jong *et al.*, 2002, Valkema *et al.*, 2006).

In addition, all trials were compatible in terms of determining that kidneys also belong to the dose-limiting organs with repeated administration of ^{90}Y-DOTATOC owing to potential interstitial irradiation that can occur from tubular peptide reabsorption. The co-infusion of positively charged amino acids such as L-lysine and L-arginine, has been introduced due to demonstrating a potential decline in renal dose through competitive inhibition on the proximal tubular reabsorption of the radiopeptide (Bodei *et al.*, 2004). Even so, the kidneys are often found to be dose-limiting. Renal toxicity has been reported in a relatively limited number of patients treated with ^{90}Y-labelled sst analogues with and without kidney protection (Teunissen *et al.*, 2011) and has been associated with several risk factors.

On initial studies without amino acid coinfusion, no major acute undesirable reactions were observed after ^{90}Y-DOTATOC injection up to 2.59 GBq per cycle, grade-2 nephrotoxicity was observed 6 months post-therapy in one patient after total dose of 3.33 GBq and renal toxicity (including grade-4) was noted in 4/5 patients who received more than 7.4 GBq/m^2 (Otte *et al.*, 1999, Paganelli *et al.*, 2001). In the latter report, biopsy confirmed radiation-induced thrombotic microangiopathy. In studies under renal protection, either no renal toxicity or delayed (5 months post-therapy) serum creatinine elevation (in one patient) was observed, among patients who received a maximum of 7.4 GBq/m^2 administered cumulative activity (Otte *et al.*, 1999, Waldherr *et al.*, 2001, 2002). Thus a cumulative administered activity of 7.5 GBq/m^2 was proposed as dose-limiting for the kidneys in PRRT with this agent. Nonetheless, the development of end-stage renal disease was reported in a patient treated with 5.6 GBq/m^2 of the radiopharmaceutical, suggesting that the limit of 7.5 GBq/m^2 may not be completely reliable to exclude nephrotoxicity (Cybulla *et al.*, 2001).

Adaptation of individualized dose scheme is frequently recommended on account of the kidney volume effect on the corresponding absorbed organ dose (Konijnenberg, 2003). In the background of a multicentre phase I trial, PET scan with ^{86}Y-DOTATOC was conducted in all patients before treatment, to predict the renal exposure expected with ^{90}Y-DOTATOC. The upper limit of cumulative radiation dose to the kidneys was 27 Gy. All patients received amino acids co-infusion and renal toxicity was mild (Valkema *et al.*, 2001). Since the ideal surrogate of ^{90}Y for dosimetry studies ^{86}Y-DOTATOC is not widely available, pre-therapeutic dosimetry can be performed on planar scintigraphic images using the readily available ^{111}In-DOTATOC (Forrer *et al.*, 2005). A thorough dosimetric study was performed by the European Institute of Oncology after iv injection of ^{111}In-DOTATOC in order to estimate the absorbed doses during ^{90}Y-DOTATOC treatment in 30 patients who were treated without kidney protection with 3 cycles (at 8 wks interval) of escalating doses from 1.11 to 2.59 GBq per cycle and 40 patients who received under renal protection 2 cycles of the agent starting from 2.96 GBq up to 5.55 GBq activities per cycle. Only mild reversible grade-1 renal toxicity was observed within the short period of follow-up. They determined that infusion of lysine with or without arginine before and after therapy offered approximately 30% protection, thereby setting the maximum cumulative activity of the radiopharmaceutical in the range of 12-18 GBq. Yet in these patients the dose limiting factor was bone marrow toxicity and the maximum tolerated dose was defined at 5.18 GBq (Chinol *et al.*, 2002, Paganelli *et al.*, 2002). The biodistribution study showed reduction of kidney uptake of ^{111}In-DOTATOC. In another study applying individualized renal dosimetry and synchronous infusion of protective amino acids, the renal toxicity was mild, once renal radiation dose did not exceed 27 Gy (De Jong *et al.*, 2002). According to Bodei and colleagues, setting the cumulative dose at the limited of ~27 Gy and using different combinations of amino acids infusion in 40 patients, prevented completely potential permanent renal toxicity over a 3-30 months follow-up period and resulted in only transient serum BUN and creatinine elevation in two patients (Bodei *et al.*, 2003).

Still, interestingly conventional dosimetry and nephrotoxicity do not always correlate in patients treated with ^{90}Y-DOTATOC (Barone *et al.*, 2005). The observed biological effective dose (BED) threshold for nephrotoxicity has been found 28 Gy in patients with risk factors including hypertension and diabetes, whereas 40 Gy in patients without risk factors (Bodei *et al.*, 2008). Also, Forrer and colleagues found grade-4 nephrotoxicity requiring hemodialysis in one out of 116 patients (Forrer *et al.*, 2006). When renal function became the focus of a study in 28 patients who had a cumulative radiation dose to the kidneys up to 38.7 Gy and a median follow-up 2.9 years, a median decline of creatinine clearance of 7.3%/year was observed (Valkema *et al.*, 2005). Pre-existing hypertension and/or diabetes in 5/9 patients whose creatinine clearance decline was reported to exceed 15%. Hence, cumulative and per-cycle renal radiation dose, age, hypertension and diabetes may be connected with nephrotoxicity (Valkema *et al.*, 2005, Bodei *et al.*, 2008). Valkema and colleagues restricted cumulative radiation dose to kidneys to 27 Gy and applied concomitant kidney protective amino acid infusions to all 58 patients; they observed dose-limiting toxicity in two patients (Valkema *et al.*, 2006). More recently, among 90 patients who received therapy-accompanying amino acid infusion, three (3.3%) encountered grade-3 to grade-4 renal or urinary toxicity, which lasted 6 days in two cases and 42 days in one (Bushnell *et al.*, 2010). Moreover, in a cohort of 1,109 patients, 102 patients (9.2%) experienced severe permanent renal toxicity (grade-4, 67 patients; grade-5, 35) and two patients experienced tumor lyses syndrome directly after ^{90}Y-DOTATOC with acute reversible kidney failure. There was no difference in the survival of patients with and without post-therapeutic kidney toxicity. Relevant statistical analyses identified that older age, low baseline glomerular filtration rate, and high kidney sstr-scintigraphic uptake were associated with the occurrence of severe nephrotoxicity (Imhof *et al.*, 2011). Finally, results of the long-term outcome in 359 patients enrolled in dose escalating treatment, suggest that fractionated ^{90}Y-DOTATOC treatment might allow to reduce nephrotoxicity and to improve overall survival. In the low-, intermediate- and high-dose group, the respective incidences of hematotoxicities grade 1-4 were 65.0%, 64.9% and 74.8%; the incidences of grade-4/5 nephrotoxicities were 8.4%, 6.5% and 14.0% (Marincek *et al.*, 2013).

Table 9: Reported responses in patients with NET treated with PRRT

Centre/ Publication Year	**Patient Number**	**CR**	**PR**	**SD**	**PD**
^{90}Y-DOTATOC					
Basel/2001	41	2%	22%	49%	15%
Milan/2001	30	23%	NA	13%	23
Basel/2001-2002	74	4%	20%	65%	11%
Milan/2002	87	5%	23%	48%	
Basel/2002	39	5%	18%	69%	8%
European institute of oncology/2002	256	5%	22%	49%	20%
Milan/2003	21	0	29%	52%	19%
Basel/2006	116	4%	23%	62%	11%
Rotterdam, Brussels and Tampa/2006	58	0	9%	53%	25%
Basel, Ontario, Los Angeles/2011	1,109	34.1%		5.2%	
^{177}Lu-DOTATATE					
Rotterdam/2008	310	2%	28%	35%	20%
Lund/2010	12	0	17%	50%	17%
Milan/2011	51	2	27	2	18%

Even with the wide variability regarding the features of the patients and their NET as well as their treatment schemes, ^{90}Y-DOTATOC consistently produced a favourable outcome with clinical and objective responses ranging up to a respective order of 100% and 34.1%, in treating a variety of sstr-positive tumours. Notably, PRRT with this radiopharmaceutical has been proved most effective in GEP-NET compared to other NET. The response rate of GEP-NET has been consistently better (28–38%) than the corresponding for other $sstr_2$-positive tumors that were treated (Nisa *et al.*, 2011). The median overall survival in a group of 58, 90 and 60 patients was 36.7, 26.9 and 39 months, respectively (Valkema *et al.*, 2006, Bushnell *et al.*, 2010, Marincek *et al.*, 2013). Furthermore, in the large patient cohort of 1,109 patients bearing a variety of NET, response according to RECIST was associated with a median survival of 53.8 months (Imhoff *et al.*, 2011). Hence, according to clinical experience for over a decade, treatment with ^{90}Y-DOTATOC along with rigorous renal protection is a powerful therapeutic tool with a profound palliative effect and long-term survival benefit for patients suffering from large infiltrative $sstr_2$-expressing NET.

^{90}Y-DOTA-Lanreotide and ^{90}Y-DOTATATE

Another radiolabelled sst analogue, namely lanreotide has been reported to present higher affinity for $sstr_3$ and $sstr_4$ compared to ^{111}In-DTPA-octreotide, without unambiguous support (Reubi, 2003). Treatment of 39 patients bearing GEP-NET with [^{90}Y-DOTA^0] lanreotide (^{90}Y-DOTA-Lanreotide) was reported to achieve 21% disease regression (defined as a >25% reduction in tumour size), 44% SD, while 36% of the patients had PD (Teunissen *et al.*, 2011). A plausible explanation would consider the predominant expression of $sstr_2$ by GEP-NET; radiolabeled DOTA-TOC/TATE presents higher affinity for sstr2 than radiolabelled lanreotide.

The ^{90}Y-labelled somatostatin analogue [DOTA^0,Tyr^3]octreotate (^{90}Y-octreotate or ^{90}Y-DOTATATE). DOTATATE is formed by replacing the C-terminal threoninol in DOTATOC with threonine and presents improved binding to sstr-positive tissues in animals (De Jong *et al.*, 1998, Baum *et al.*, 2004). The development of DOTATATE was considered advantageous over DOTATOC due to ninefold higher affinity for $sstr_2$, which became sevenfold when comparing the corresponding ^{90}Y-labelled sst analogues (Reubi, 2003). According to the first presentation of results following treatment of 75 NET patients with ^{90}Y-DOTATATE, PR was accomplished in 37% of the patients and disease stabilization in 52% (Baum *et al.*, 2004).

Clinical experience with ^{90}Y-DOTATATE is still limited; yet interestingly there exists a relevant case report from Bad Berka, suggesting PRRT application as first-line treatment (Kaemmerer *et al.*, 2009). Characteristically, a 33-year-old woman, who was diagnosed with an initially inoperable highly differentiated neuroendocrine pancreatic carcinoma, stage IV, received neoadjuvant PRRT comprising two cycles of this radiopharmaceutical, specifically at an initial activity of 6 GBq followed by 4.5 GBq approximately 4 months later, each with concomitant amino acid infusion (Jamar *et al.*, 2003, Kaemmerer *et al.*, 2009). The resultant significant downstaging of the tumour as identified on PET/CT using ^{68}Ga-DOTANOC and ^{18}F-FDG, allowed its subsequent surgical removal. Complete remission was revealed during follow-up for eighteen months. There was no significant hematotoxicity or nephrotoxicity. Nevertheless further clinical studies are warranted in order for the effectiveness of ^{90}Y-DOTATATE to be established.

^{177}Lu-Labelled Radiopharmaceuticals for PRRT

^{177}Lu-DOTATATE

Lutetium-177 emits medium energy β^- radiation (E_{max}=0.5 MeV) with maximum tissue penetration of 2 mm and two γ-photopeaks, at 113 and 208 KeV, enabling post-therapy scintigraphy and dosimetry. In a clinical comparison, the percent uptake of the injected dose of [^{177}Lu-DOTA^0,Tyr^3]octreotate (^{177}Lu-DOTATATE, Lutathera®), was 3- to 4-fold higher in 4 out of 5 tumours than with the corresponding with ^{111}In-DTPA-octreotide, while remaining comparable for kidneys, spleen and liver (Kwekkeboom *et al.*, 2001).

Initial evaluable results in 34 GEP-NET patients, who received 3.7, 5.6 or 7.4 GBq of ^{177}Lu-DOTATOC up to a final cumulative dose of 22.2-29.6 GBq at 6-9 week intervals, showed CR in 3% of the patients, PR in 35% and SD in 41%, whilst PD in 21%; also, few and mostly transient side effects were observed, the most common being mild bone marrow suppression (Kwekkeboom *et al.*, 2003). Later on, a published comparison of dosimetry in a therapeutic setting using 3.7 GBq ^{177}Lu-DOTATATE and 3.7 GBq ^{177}Lu-DOTATOC in the same patients, indicated that ^{177}Lu-DOTATATE represents an important improvement in view of the higher achievable tumour-absorbed doses with about equal doses to potentially dose-limiting organs and of the lower tissue penetration range of ^{177}Lu, if compared to ^{90}Y, which may be especially important for small tumours (Esser *et al.*, 2006).

According to a study of 504 GEP-NET patients, who received ^{177}Lu-DOTATATE therapy up to a cumulative dose of 27.8-29.6 GBq, mostly in four treatment cycles, at 6-10 week intervals, the favourable tumour response rates and PFS are accompanied by only a few adverse effects (Kwekkeboom *et al.*, 2008). Complete tumour remissions, PR, MR (decrease in size > 25% and < 50%) and SD occurred in 2%, 28%, 16% and 35% of 310 GEP-NET patients, respectively. Median time to disease progression was 40 months. Median overall survival from start of treatment was 46 months and from diagnosis, 128 months. In a small number of patients who had inoperable pancreatic NET without metastases, tumor shrinkage 6-12 months after this radiopharmaceutical, rendered these patients candidates for surgery (Kwekkeboom *et al.*, 2008). This neoadjuvant use of PRRT, although applicable in select cases only, is of great interest, as it may cure such patients. The eventual maximal shrinkage of the tumor may take months after completing the therapy. This is most likely due to the slow growing nature of these tumors; radiation biology axioms state that radiation damage to the DNA usually results in cell death only after their reproductive integrity is tested by one or more attempts at mitotic division (Whithers, 1992). Therefore, if such attempts at cell division are few, tumor size reduction will be slow.

In 2011, Bodei and colleagues published the results of a prospective phase I-II study of 51 patients with unresectable/metastatic sst_2-positive tumours, who received escalating activities of 3.7-5.18 GBq/cycle and of 5.18–7.4 GBq/cycle of ^{177}Lu-DOTATATE. Patients were affected by mainly GEP-NET. Cumulative activities in 21 patients ranged from 3.7 to 29.2 GBq (median 26.4 GBq in median 6 cycles,) and in 30 patients from 5.55 to 28.9 GBq (median 25.2 GBq in 4 cycles), based on dosimetry. Thirty-nine patients were progressive at enrolment. Fifteen of 46 evaluable patients (32.6%) achieved CR or PR. The median time to progression was 36 months and the overall survival was 68% at 36 months (Bodei *et al.*, 2011).

According to a recent review, analysis in NET patients treated with ^{177}Lu-DOTATATE indicated that the results are very encouraging in terms of both tumour regression and the patients' self-assessed quality of life, with median PFS more than 40 months (Kam *et al.*, 2012). Higher remission rates have been positively correlated with high uptake during pre-therapy ^{111}In-DTPA-octreotide, a limited number of liver metastases and a Karnofsky Performance Score higher than 70 (Kwekkeboom *et al.*, 2005, 2008). Furthermore, in patients with tumour regression during follow-up, a reduced tumour uptake after the third or fourth treatment in comparison with the scan after the first treatment was frequently observed. Compatible observations have been published regarding reduced sstr-mediated uptake after PRRT by the use of ^{68}Ga-DOTATATE in tumours after the first cycle of PRRT, which predicted the time to progression after completion of PRRT (one, two or three cycles) and was correlated with improvement in clinical symptoms. Possible reasons accounting for this decreased uptake may be the obviously decreased amount of viable sstr-expressing tumour cells as a reflection of the PRRT-induced cytotoxic therapeutic effect and/or NET cell dedifferentiation (Miederer *et al.*, 2009, Haug *et al.*, 2010). Yet, dedifferentiation may be excluded, considering the observed favourable effect on tumour response, time to progression and clinical symptoms in tumours with reduced uptake after PRRT. Also, the effect of PRRT on receptor expression and density on a single tumour cell still remains to be clarified.

In addition, PRRT with ^{177}Lu-DOTATATE has been applied to patients with progressive NET who had previously developed an objective tumour response in terms of remission or SD when treated with PRRT. Specifically in one study two additional cycles of 7.4 GBq were administered to patients previously successfully treated with ^{177}Lu-DOTATATE and resulted in 24% tumour remission, 31% SD and 45% disease progression out of 33 radiologically evaluated patients at three months after the last therapy. Notably the additional treatments were well tolerated with acceptable haematologic toxicity and without any serious delayed toxicity (Van Essen *et al.*, 2010). In another study, an additional cycle of 7.4 GBq ^{177}Lu-DOTATATE was administered in 27 patients with NET previously successfully treated with ^{90}Y-DOTATOC, resulting in remission in 26% of the patients and disease stabilization in 44% at 8-12 weeks after therapy (Forrer *et al.*, 2005).

In a study mainly addressing dosimetric issues relevant to PRRT, out of 12 evaluable patients treated with ^{177}Lu-DOTATATE (three or four cycles of 7.4 GBq), PR was reported in 17%, MR in 25% and SD in 42% (Garkavij *et al.*, 2010). Also, according to Gains and colleagues, 5 of 6 children who were treated with ^{177}Lu-DOTATATE due to refractory or relapsing high-risk neuroblastoma, achieved SD (Gains *et al.*, 2011).

The major side effects upon treatment with ^{177}Lu-DOTATATE are described in the study of the largest patient group in the relevant current literature

(Kwekkeboom *et al.*, 2008). Specifically any grade-3 or grade-4 haematologic toxicity occurred 4-8 weeks after 3.6% of administrations and serious adverse events (approximately 1%) that were likely attributable to the treatment, included MDS in 3/504 patients, and temporary, nonfatal, hepatotoxicity in 2/504 patients. Two patients had a decrease in renal function, which was most probably unrelated to the treatment. It is also noteworthy that side effects within the first 24 h were nausea in 25% of administrations, vomiting in 10%, and abdominal discomfort or pain in 10%. Six patients with very hormonally active NET, encountered a related clinical crisis within 2 days after administration, which rendered (re)hospitalization mandatory; complete recovery was accomplished following adequate medical care, including fluid infusion, high-dose iv administered somatostatin analogue, corticosteroids and correction of electrolyte disturbances (De Keizer *et al.*, 2008). Reversible mild alopecia was reported by 62% of the patients.

The kidneys belong to the dose-limiting organs for PRRT with ^{177}Lu-DOTATATE. According to a relevant study, the impact of PRRT on renal function has been reported to produce a median decline of 3.8%/year in creatinine clearance, suggesting that high administered cumulative activities may be feasible (Valkema *et al.*, 2005). The same researchers observed that a creatinine clearance decrease of more than 25% per year is required for end-stage renal disease to develop within 5 years; such a decrease in kidney function was found in only 1 of 37 patients treated with this radiopharmaceutical. In another more recent report, a median decrease of creatinine clearance of 21.7% 6 months after PRRT, 23.9% after 1 year and 27.6% after 2 years was observed, with cumulative renal absorbed doses of 8–37 Gy. Higher losses (>20%) occurred in patients with risk factors for renal toxicity, particularly hypertension and diabetes. In this study, cumulative bone marrow doses were <1.5 Gy and no major acute or delayed renal or haematologic toxicity occurred (one grade 3 leukopenia and thrombocytopenia), but blood elements showed a progressive mild drop during cycles, with recovery during follow-up (median 30 months). Thus, ^{177}Lu-DOTATATE was well tolerated up to 29 GBq cumulative activity (up to 7.4 GBq/cycle) and the maximum tolerated dose/cycle was not reached. However, it was concluded that the individual bone marrow function and the co-existence of risk factors for kidney toxicity after PRRT, may justify dividing cumulative activities into lower activity cycles (Bodei *et al.*, 2011).

Finally, ^{177}Lu-DOTATATE-induced hormone disturbances have been reported, in particular transient inhibitory effect on inhibin, suggesting an impact on spermatogenesis and mild reduction of gonadotropin hormones in postmenopausal women (Teunissen *et al.*, 2009).

Despite the considerable discrepancy in patient selection and applied protocols among the various studies, not only improvement in the quality of life, but also prolongation of survival in patients with advanced NET have been constantly reported after therapy with ^{177}Lu-DOTATATE (Teunissen *et al.*, 2004, Kwekkeboom *et al.*, 2005). The symptom scores for fatigue, insomnia and pain have been shown to decrease significantly, thereby improving the role, emotional and social function scales (Aaronson *et al.*, 1993). Additionally, the comparison between the outcome of PRRT with this agent and that of historical studies with single or combination chemotherapy regimens, revealed consistent differences suggesting a survival benefit of 40-72 months (Kwekkeboom *et al.*, 2005). Thus, treatment with ^{177}Lu-DOTATATE accompanied by kidney protective amino acid solutions, has evolved into an effective option, which may become the therapy of first choice in the clinical setting of advanced NET (Kam *et al.*, 2012).

^{177}Lu-DOTANOC

Preclinical data have introduced the sst analogue DOTANOC which presents a broader affinity profile than DOTATATE, as it binds with high affinity to $sstr_3$ and $sstr_5$ besides $sstr_2$ and suggest its potential imaging and therapeutic effectiveness when labelled with ^{111}In for patients with corresponding sstr-expressing tumours (Wild *et al.*, 2003). In a study focusing on dosimetric aspects, PRRT was performed using ^{177}Lu-DOTANOC and/or ^{177}Lu-DOTATATE in patients bearing NET with high sstr expression documented on ^{68}Ga-DOTANOC PET/CT (Wehrmann *et al.*, 2007). The observed high interpatient variability and the increased whole-body dose due to higher ^{177}Lu-DOTANOC uptake in normal tissue, indicated the need for individual patient dosimetry upon deciding whether to treat a patient with ^{177}Lu-DOTATATE or ^{177}Lu-DOTANOC. Preliminary results originate from Rotterdam, and include patients with TC, who were treated with 6.7–32.5 GBq ^{177}Lu-DOTANOC; one patient with follicular TC experienced PR and one with Hürthle cell TC showed clinical improvement; yet PD was noted in two patients- one with Huerthle cell and one with MTC (Valkema *et al.*, 2007). Unfortunately, published reports on NET responses in patients treated with this agent remain limited.

^{188}Re-Labelled Somatostatin Analogues for PRRT

Another radiolabelled peptide, namely ^{188}Re-P2045 (an analogue of ^{99m}Tc-depreotide) has been reported in a phase I trial in the United States, involving patients with metastatic or recurrent inoperable lung tumours. Based on positive sstr imaging with ^{99m}Tc-P2045, the patients were treated with escalating doses of ^{188}Re-P2045 (Edelman *et al.*, 2009, Graham *et al.*, 2011). Five out of 8 patients with PD at baseline who were treated with ^{188}Re-P2045 at 1.11-3.33 GBq/m^2, remained stable at 8 wk after therapy. There were no other grade-3 or 4 therapy-related toxicities, apart from one case of grade-3 lymphocytopenia (Edelman *et al.*, 2009).

Considering nuclear medicine therapeutic options, clinical decision making should be individualized based on: a) sstr-imaging by traditional γ-camera, or PET, with subsequent PRRT, b) $^{123/131}$I-MIBG imaging and associated ^{131}I-MIBG therapy and c) ^{99m}Tc(V)-DMSA imaging with respective $^{186/188}$Re(V)-DMSA treatment. Based on worldwide recorded experience, patients with NET, who either do not respond, or present contraindications to the conventional treatment options, are referred to specialized centres, in order to be treated with PRRT as palliative therapy. Symptom relief control can be achieved with all ^{111}In-, ^{90}Y- and ^{177}Lu-labelled sst analogue-based PRRT. The drawbacks hindering the direct comparison of PRRT results and the deduction of definite conclusions reside in the inhomogeneity of the relevant studies, with regard to the characteristics of the patients (*e.g.* total NET burden and differentiation, disease duration, extent of hepatic invasion, radiotracer uptake intensity, previous treatment regimes, co-existing disorders), the used sst analogue (different affinity profiles) and radionuclide (different physical properties), PRRT dose regimes and response criteria. Overall, acknowledging the inherent problems of interstudy comparisons, treatment with radiolabelled sst analogues is a potent means in the management of patients with inoperable or metastasized NET. The results obtained with the most extensively used ^{90}Y-DOTATOC and ^{177}Lu-DOTATATE are very encouraging in terms of clinical benefit, tumour shrinkage, and a duration of response exceeding 2 years. Thus, PRRT substantially contributes to the patients' quality of life improvement and survival prolongation (Teunissen *et al.*, 2011). In patients who benefit from PRRT, a repeated course remains a therapeutic option in case of relapse (Norton *et al.*, 2003). Randomized trials should establish the optimal radiolabelled sst analogue or combination of analogues and treatment schemes. Both ^{90}Y-DOTATOC and ^{177}Lu-DOTATATE have organ drug status in Europe and USA and are in progress of entering phase III protocols to FDA and EMEA. Reports suggesting the application of PRRT as first or second line treatment continue to emerge, since the oncology concept was changed from palliative to curative intent re-considering operability. PRRT appears increasingly useful for downstaging and downsizing well-differentiated NET, thereby achieving a higher operability rate (Pfeifer *et al.*, 2011, Kaemmerer *et al.*, 2009, Kwekkeboom *et al.*, 2008, O'Grady *et al.*, 2008, Nomura *et al.*, 2009). In addition, staging of the patient after every cycle is recommended in order to evaluate the response and the operability.

Novel PRRT-Related Therapeutic Approaches

To date, the β^- emitting ^{90}Y- and ^{177}Lu-labelled sst analogues have been the gold standard for PRRT. The α-emitting radionuclides, like the 10-day half-life Actinum-225 (^{225}Ac), are characterized by extremely high cytotoxic activity, and may be delivered to the target tumour cells, sparing normal tissues (Miederer *et al.*, 2008, Basuroy *et al.*, 2012). Miederer and colleagues have recently introduced the α-emitting generator nuclide ^{225}Ac labelling DOTATOC for PRRT in NET in comparison with ^{177}Lu-DOTATOC. The administration of 12-20 kBq reduced the growth rate of tumours, with improved therapeutic efficacy over ^{177}Lu-DOTATOC, and no significant toxicity in rodents (Miederer *et al.*, 2008). Initial results from ongoing clinical studies using an α-emitter for DOTATOC labelling, reside in 2012 (Morgenstern *et al.,* 2012). Specifically, treatment with of i.a. administered ^{213}Bi-DOTATOC in 17 patients with GEP-NET refractory to previous treatment with ^{90}Y- or ^{177}Lu-DOTATOC, resulted in short-term shrinkage of primary tumours as well as liver and bone metastases, while long-term outcome is pending. The maximum tolerable dose of 6 GBq of a single administration was not related with any significant toxicity. Another recently employed concept is the use of sstr-targeting antagonist instead of agonist ligands, for diagnostic and therapeutic applications (Wadas *et al.*, 2008, Cescato *et al.*, 2008, Nanda *et al.*, 2010). Clinical trials are currently underway (Reubi *et al.*, 2002). Other therapeutic approaches under research include locoregional administration of radiolabelled sst analogues and PRRT combinations with chemosensitisation agents such as 5-fluorouracil (5-FU) or its prodrug capecitabine. An appealing and pioneering means to deliver a higher concentration of the radiolabelled sst analogue activity to the target tumour, while reducing systemic toxicity would be by radiopeptide brachytherapy. Since NET show a particular predisposition for hepatic invasion, mostly perfused by the hepatic artery, hepatic intraarterial infusion of radiolabelled sst analogues was introduced. The technique involves a femoral artery puncture in the angiographic catheter lab, followed by identification and selective catheterization of the relevant hepatic artery, into which the radiolabelled sst analogue is infused (Gnanasegaran *et al.*, 2005, McStay *et al.*, 2005). On this basis, selective hepatic intra-arterial administered 1.2 GBq ^{90}Y-DOTA-lanreotide proved to be safe and effective in 19 patients bearing NET, resulting in 16% PR and 63% SD, with 61% clinical improvement and reduction in biologic marker levels. The 1-year reported survival rate was 63% and the median survival time was 15 months (McStay *et al.*, 2005). Further noteworthy results were reported by Limouris and colleagues. After multiple cycles (6.3±2.3 GBq/cycle; maximum of 15 per patient) of intra-arterially administered ^{111}In-DTPA-octreotide in 17 patients with NET liver metastases, CR was achieved in 6% of patients, PR in 47% and SD in 25%, according to RECIST (Limouris *et al.*, 2008). Recently recurrent high grade gliomas were successfully treated by local administration of 1.66-2.22 GBq of ^{90}Y-DOTATOC with only minor side-effects; 98 Gy/GBq was delivered to residual tumour tissue with kidneys irradiation of only 2.8 Gy/GBq (Heute *et al.*, 2010). Preliminary results from combination of PRRT by ^{177}Lu-DOTATATE with relatively low doses (1650 mg/m^2 per day for 2 weeks) of capecitabine in patients with GEP-NET, have been found feasible and safe concerning acute and subacute side effects (Van Essen *et al.*, 2008).

III. Selective Internal Radiation Therapy (SIRT) of Neuroendocrine Tumours

In patients with disseminated and inoperable liver disease, radioembolisation of liver metastases with intraarterial ^{90}Y-resin microspheres may offer a favourable long-term outcome, with PR or CR in 63% and median survival in the range of 36 to 70 months (King *et al.*, 2008, Murthy *et al.*, 2008, Kennedy *et al.*, 2008, Cao *et al.*, 2010, Basuroy *et al.*, 2012). The most beneficial treatment results are observed in patients with hepatic tumour burden of 20-50% by volume, well-differentiated tumour, female gender, and no extrahepatic disease (Saxena *et al.*, 2010). Contraindications to SIRT include vascular involvement, *e.g.* portal vein thrombosis, severe hepatic dysfunction, and large tumour burden. Encouraging effects with SIRT in patients suffering from NET hepatic invasion continue to emerge. Randomized clinical trials in this setting are required in order for the value of SIRT to be established among all locoregional therapies.

Apparently, multidisciplinary approach is warranted in the management of patients with NET, allowing for innovative concepts and progressively superior outcome.

ACKNOWLEDGEMENT

The author would like to take this opportunity to express her gratitude for the invaluable support, vision and foresight of Dr. Vassilios Papantoniou, Head of the Nuclear Medicine Department of University General Hospital "Alexandra" in Athens, Greece.

CONFLICT OF INTEREST

The authors confirm that this chapter content has no conflict of interest.

REFERENCES

Aaronson, N. K., Ahmedzai, S., Bergman, B., Bullinger, M., Cull, A., Duez, N. J., Filiberti, A., Flechtner, H., Fleishman, S. B., de Haes, J. C., Kaasa, S., Klee, M. C., Osoba, D., Razavi, D., Rofe, P. B., Schraub, S., Sneeuw, K. C. A., Sullivan, M. & Takeda, F. 1993. The European Organization for Research and Treatment of Cancer QLQ-C30: a quality-of-life instrument for use in international clinical trials in oncology. *J. Natl. Cancer Inst.*, 85, 365-376.

Adams, S., Baum, R., Rink, T., Schumm-Drager, P. M., Usadel, K. H. & Hor, G. 1998. Limited value of fluorine-18 fluorodeoxyglucose positron emission tomography for the imaging of neuroendocrine tumours. *Eur. J. Nucl. Med.*, 25, 79-83.

Ambrosini, V., Rubello, D., Nanni, C., Al-Nahhas, A. & Fanti S. 2008. ^{68}Ga-DOTA-peptides *versus* ^{18}F-DOPA PET for the assessment of NET patients. *Nucl. Med. Commun.*, 29, 415-417.

Anthony, L. B., Woltering, E. A., Espenan, G. D., Cronin, M. D., Maloney, T. J. & McCarthy, K. E. 2002. Indium-111-pentetreotide prolongs survival in gastroenteropancreatic malignancies. *Semin. Nucl. Med.*, 32, 123-132.

Barone, R., Borson-Chazot, F., Valkema, R., Walrand, S., Chauvin, F., Gogou, L., Kvols, L. K., Krenning, E. P., Jamar, F. & Pauwels, S. 2005. Patient-specific dosimetry in predicting renal toxicity with (90)Y-DOTATOC: relevance of kidney volume and dose rate in finding a dose-effect relationship. *J. Nucl. Med.*, 46, 99S-106S.

Basuroy, R., Srirajaskanthan, R. & Ramage, J. K. 2012. A multimodal approach to the management of neuroendocrine tumour liver metastases. *Int. J. Hepatol.*, 13.

Baum, R. P., Soldner, J., Schmucking, M. & Niesen A. 2004. Peptidrezeptorvermittelte Radiotherapie (PRRT) neuroendokriner Tumoren Klinischen Indikationen und Erfahrung mit ^{90}Yttrium-markierten Somatostatinanaloga. *Der Onkologe*, 10, 1098-1110.

Baum, R. P., Soldner, J., Schmucking, M. & Niesen, A. 2004. Intravenous and intra-arterial peptide receptor radionuclide therapy (PRRT) using Y-90-DOTA-Tyr3-octreotate (Y-90-DOTA-TATE) in patients with metastatic neuroendocrine tumors. *Eur. J. Nucl. Med.*, 31(suppl.2), S238 [abstract].

Becherer, A., Szabo, M., Karanikas, G., Wunderbaldinger, P., Angelberger, P., Raderer, M., Kurtaran, A., Dudczak, R. & Kletter, K. 2004. Imaging of advanced neuroendocrine tumors with ^{18}F-FDOPA PET. *J. Nucl. Med.*, 45, 1161-1167.

Behe, M., Heppeler, A. & Maecke, H. R. 1996. New somatostatin analogs for SPET and PET. *Eur. J. Nucl. Med.* 23, 1144 (abstract).

Belhocine, T., Foidart, J., Rigo, P., Najjar F, Thiry, A., Quatresooz, P. & Hustinx, R. 2002. Fluorodeoxyglucose positron emission tomography and somatostatin receptor scintigraphy for diagnosing and staging carcinoid tumours: correlations with the pathological indexes p53 and Ki-67. *Nucl. Med. Commun.* 23, 727-734.

Bertagna, F., Giubbini, R., Savelli, G., Pizzocaro, C., Rodella, C., Biasiotto, G., Lucchini, S., Maroldi, R., Rosenbaum, J. & Alavi A. 2009. A patient with medullary thyroid carcinoma and right ventricular cardiac metastasis treated by ^{90}Y-Dotatoc. Hell. J. *Nucl. Med.*, 12, 161-164.

Binderup, T., Knigge, U., Loft, A., Federspiel, B. & Kjaer, A. 2010. ^{18}F-fluorodeoxyglucose positron emission tomography predicts survival of patients with neuroendocrine tumors. *Clin Cancer Res,* 16, 978-985.

Binderup, T., Knigge, U., Loft, A., Mortensen, J., Pfeifer, A., Federspiel, B., Hansen, C. P., Hojgaard, L. & Kjaer, A. 2010. Functional imaging of neuroendocrine tumors: a head-to-head comparison of somatostatin receptor scintigraphy, ^{123}I-MIBG scintigraphy, and ^{18}F-FDG PET. *J. Nucl. Med.,* 51, 704-712.

Blower, P. J., Kettle, A. G., O'Doherty, M. J. & Knapp, F. F. 2000. ^{99m}Tc(V)DMSA quantitatively predicts Re-188(V) DMSA distribution. *Nucl. Med. Commun.*, 21, 370.

Blum, J. E., Handmaker, H. & Rinne, N. A. 1999. The utility of a somatostatin-type receptor binding peptide radiopharmaceutical (P829) in the evaluation of solitary pulmonary nodules. *Chest*, 115, 224-232.

Bodei, L., Cremonesi, M., Ferrari, M., Pacifici, M., Grana, C. M., Bartolomei, M., Baio, S. M., Sansovini, M. & Paganelli, G. 2008. Long-term evaluation of renal toxicity after peptide receptor radionuclide therapy with ^{90}Y-DOTATOC and ^{177}Lu-DOTATATE: the role of associated risk factors. *Eur. J. Nucl. Med. Mol. Imaging*, 35, 1847-1856 (epub 22 Apr 2008; erratum in Eur. J. Nucl. Med. Mol. Imaging 2008; 35:1928).

Bodei, L., Cremonesi, M., Zoboli, S., Grana, C., Bartolomei, M., Rocca, P., Caracciolo, M., Mäcke, H. R., Chinol, M. & Paganelli, G. 2003. Receptor-mediated radionuclide therapy with ^{90}Y-DOTATOC in association with amino acid infusion: a phase I study. *Eur. J. Nucl. Med. Mol. Imaging*, 30, 207-216.

Bodei, L., Cremonesi, M., Grana, C., Rocca, P., Bartolomei, M., Chinol, M. & Paganelli, G. 2004. Receptor radionuclide therapy with ^{90}Y-[DOTA]0-Tyr3-Octreotide (^{90}Y-DOTATOC] in neuroendocrine tumors. *Eur. J. Nucl. Med. Mol. Imaging*, 31, 1038-1046.

Bodei, L., Cremonesi, M., Grana, C. M., Fazio, N., Iodice, S., Baio, S. M., Bartolomei, M., Lombardo, D., Ferrari, M. E., Sansovini, M., Chinol, M. & Paganelli, G. 2011. Peptide receptor radionuclide therapy with ^{177}Lu-DOTATATE: the IEO phase I-II study. *Eur. J. Nucl. Med. Mol. Imaging*, 38, 2125-2135.

Bomanji, J. B., Wong, W., Gaze, M. N., Cassoni, A., Waddington, W., Solano, J. & Ell PJ. 2003. Treatment of neuroendocrine tumours in adults with ^{131}I-MIBG therapy. *Clin. Oncol.*, 15, 193-198.

Bombardieri, E., Giammarile, F., Aktolun, C., Richard P. Baum, Bischof Delaloye, A., Maffioli, L., Moncayo, R., Mortelmans, L.,

Pepe, G., Reske, S. N., Castellani, M. R. & Chiti, A. 2010. ^{131}I/^{123}I-Metaiodobenzylguanidine (mIBG) scintigraphy: procedures guidelines for tumour imaging. *Eur. J. Nucl. Med. Mol. Imaging*, 37, 2436–2446.

Bongers, V., de Klerk, J. M. H., Zonnenberg, B. A., de Kort, G., Lips, C. J. M. & van Rijk, P. P. 1997. Acute liver necrosis induced by iodine-131-MIBG in the treatment of metastatic carcinoid tumors. *J. Nucl. Med.*, 38, 1024-1026.

Boubaker, A. & Bischof Delaloye, A. 2003. Nuclear medicine procedures and neuroblastoma in childhood. Their value in the diagnosis, staging and assessment of response to therapy. *Q. J. Nucl. Med.*, 47, 31-40.

Brouwers, A. H., Jager, P. L. & de Vries, E. G. 2008. Improved staging of patients with carcinoid and islet cell tumors with ^{18}F-dihydroxy-phenyl-alanine and ^{11}C-5-hydroxy-tryptophan positron emission tomography. *J. Clin. Oncol.*, 26, 1489-1495.

Buchmann, I., Henze, M., Engelbrecht, S., Eisenhut, M., Runz, A., Schafer, M., Schilling, T., Haufe, S., Herrmann, T. & Haberkorn U. 2007. Comparison of ^{68}Ga-DOTATOC PET and ^{111}In-DTPAOC (DTPA-octreotide) SPECT in patients with neuroendocrine tumours. *Eur. J. Nucl. Med. Mol. Imaging*, 34, 1617-1626.

Buscombe, J. R., Caplin, M. E. & Hilson, A. J. 2003. Long-term efficacy of high-activity ^{111}In-pentetreotide therapy in patients with disseminated neuroendocrine tumors. *J. Nucl. Med.*, 44, 1-6.

Bushnell, D., O'Dorisio, T., Menda, Y., Carlisle, T., Zehr, P., Connolly, M., Karwal, M., Miller, S., Parker, S. & Bouterfa, H. 2003. Evaluating the clinical effectiveness of ^{90}Y-SMT 487 in patients with neuroendocrine tumors. J. *Nucl. Med.*, 44, 1556-1560.

Bushnell, D. L., Menda, Y., Madsen, M. T., Link, B. K., Kahn, D., Truhlar, S. M., Juweid, M., Shannon, M. & Murguia, J. S. 2004. ^{99m}Tc-depreotide tumour uptake in patients with non-Hodgkin's lymphoma. *Nucl. Med. Commun.*, 25, 839-843.

Bushnell., Jr. D. L., O'Dorisio, T. M., O'Dorisio, M. S., Menda, Y., Hicks, R. J., Van Cutsem, E., Baulieu, J-L., Borson-Chazot, F., Anthony, L., Benson, A. B., Oberg, K., Grossman, A. B., Connolly, M., Bouterfa, H., Li, Y., Kacena, K. A., LaFrance, N. & Pauwels, S. A. 2010. ^{90}Y-Edotreotide for metastatic carcinoid refractory to octreotide. *J. Clin. Oncol.*, 28, 1652-1659.

Cancer K. 2010. Antitumor effects of octreotide LAR, a somatostatin analog. *Nat. Rev. Endocrinol.*, 6, 188-189.

Cao, C. Q., Yan, T. D., Bester, L., Liauw, W. & Morris, D. L. 2010. Radioembolization with yttrium microspheres for neuroendocrine tumour liver metastases. *Br. J. Surg.*, 97, 537-543.

Chen, L., Li, F., Zhuang, H., Jing, H., Du, Y. & Zeng, Z. 2009. ^{99m}Tc-HYNIC-TOC scintigraphy is superior to ^{131}I-MIBG imaging in the evaluation of extraadrenal pheochromocytoma. *J. Nucl. Med.,* 50, 397-400.

Cescato, R., Erchegyi, J., Waser, B., Piccand, V., Mäcke, H. R., Rivier, J. E. & Reubi, J. C. 2008. Design and *in vitro* characterization of highly sst$_2$-selective somatostatin antagonists suitable for radiotargeting. *J. Med. Chem.*, 51, 4030-4037.

Cheung, P. S. Y., Thompson, N. W., Dmuchowski, C. F. & Sisson, J. C. 1988. Spectrum of pheochromocytoma in the ^{131}I-MIBG era. *World J Surg*, 12, 546-551.

Chinol, M., Bodei, L., Cremonesi, M. & Paganelli, G. 2002. Receptor-mediated radiotherapy with ^{90}Y-DOTA-Dphe1-Tyr3- octreotide: the experience of the European Institute of Oncology Group. *Semin. Nucl. Med.,* 32, 141-147.

Cohen, E. P., Hussain, S. & Moulder, J. E. 2003. Successful treatment of radiation nephropathy with angiotensin II blockade. *Int. J. Radiat. Oncol. Biol. Phys.,* 55, 190-193.

Cybulla, M., Weiner, S. M. & Otte, A. 2001. End-stage renal disease after treatment with ^{90}Y-DOTATOC. *Eur. J. Nucl. Med.*, 28, 1552-1554.

Daly, A. F., Jaffrain-Rea, M. L., Ciccarelli, A., Valdes-Socin, H., Rohmer, V., Tamburrano, G., Borson-Chazot, C., Estour, B,. Ciccarelli, E., Brue, T., Ferolla, P., Emy, P., Colao, A., De Menis, E., Lecomte, P., Penfornis, F., Delemer, B., Bertherat, J., Wémeau, J. L., De Herder, W., Archambeaud, F., Stevenaert, A., Calender, A., Murat, A., Cavagnini, F. & Beckers, A. 2006. Clinical characterization of familial isolated pituitary adenomas. *J. Clin. Endocrinol. Metab.*, 91, 3316-3323.

Decristoforo, C., Mather, S. J., Cholewinski, W., Donnemiller, E., Riccabona, G. & Moncayo, R. 2000. ^{99m}Tc-EDDA-HYNIC-TOC: a new ^{99m}Tc-labelled radiopharmaceutical for imaging somatostatin receptor-positive tumours; first clinical results and intra-patient comparison with ^{111}In-labelled octreotide derivatives. *Eur. J. Nucl. Med.,* 27, 1318-1325.

De Herder, W. W., Hofland. L. J., Van Der Lely, A. J. & Lambert, S. W. 2003. Somatostatin receptors in gastroentero-pancreatic neuroendocrine tumors. *Endocr Relat Cancer*, 10, 451-458.

De Jong, M., Bakker, W. H., Krenning, E. P., Breeman, W. A., van der Pluijm, M. E., Bernard, B. F., Visser, T. J., Jermann, E., Béhé, M., Powell, P. & Mäcke, H. R. 1997. Ytrium-90 and Indium-111 labelling, receptor binding and biodistribution of [DOTAO.D-Phe'/Tyr3] octreotide, a promising somatostatin analogue for radionuclide therapy. *Eur. J. Nucl. Med.*, 24, 368-371.

De Jong, M., Bakker, W. H., Breeman, W. A., Bernard, B. F., Hofland, L. J., Visser, T. J., Srinivasan, A., Schmidt, M., Behe, M., Mäcke, H. R. & Krenning, E. P. 1998. Pre-clinical comparison of [DTPA0] octreotide, [DTPA0,Tyr3] octreotide and [DOTA0,Tyr3] octreotide as carriers for somatostatin receptor-targeted scintigraphy and radionuclide therapy. *Int J Cancer*, 75, 406-411.

De Jong, M., Kwekkeboom, D., Valkema, R. & Krenning, E. P. 2003. Radiolabelled peptides for tumor therapy: current status and future directions. *Eur. J. Nucl. Med.*, 30, 463-469.

De Jong, M., Valkema, R., Jamar, F., Kvols, L. K., Kwekkeboom, D. J., Breeman, A. P. W., Bakker, W. H., Smith, C., Pauwels, S. & Krenning, E. P. 2002. Somatostatin receptor-targeted radionuclide therapy of tumors: preclinical and clinical findings. *Semin. Nucl. Med.*, 32, 133-140.

De Keizer, B., van Aken, M. O., Feelders, R. A., de Herder, W. W., Kam, B. L., van Essen, M., Krenning, E. P. & Kwekkeboom, D. J. 2008. Hormonal crises following receptor radionuclide therapy with the radiolabeled somatostatin analogue [(177)Lu-DOTA(0),Tyr (3)]octreotate. *Eur. J. Nucl. Med. Mol. Imaging*, 35, 749-755.

de Kerviler, E., Cadiot, G., Lebtahi, R., Faraggi, M., Le Guludec, D. & Mignon, M. 1994. Somatostatin receptor scintigraphy in forty-eight patients with the Zollinger-Ellison syndrome. GRESZE: Groupe d'Etude du Syndrome de Zollinger-Ellison. *Eur. J. Nucl. Med.*, 21, 1191-1197.

De Kraker, J., Hoefnagel, C. A., Caron, H., Valdés Olmos, R. A., Zsiros, J., Heij, H. A. & Voûte, P. A. 1995. First line targeted radiotherapy, a new concept in the treatment of advanced stage neuroblastoma. *Eur J Cancer*, 31A, 600-602.

Delpassand, E. S., Sims-Mourtada, J., Saso, H., Azhdarinia, A., Ashoori, F., Torabi, F., Espenan, G., Moore, W. H., Woltering, E. & Anthony, L. 2008. Safety and efficacy of radionuclide therapy with high-activity In-111 pentetreotide in patients with progressive neuroendocrine tumors. *Cancer Biother Radiopharm*, 23, 292-300.

Denoyer, D., Perek, N., Le Jeune, N., Frere, D. & Dubois, F. 2004. Evidence that ^{99m}Tc-(V)-DMSA uptake is mediated by NaPi cotransporter type III in tumour cell lines. *Eur. J. Nucl. Med. Mol. Imaging*, 31, 77-84.

Denoyer, D., Perek, N., Le Jeune, N., Cornillon, J. & Dubois, F. 2005. Correlation between ^{99m}Tc-(V)-DMSA uptake and constitutive level of phosphorylated focal adhesion kinase in an *in vitro* model of cancer cell lines. *Eur. J. Nucl. Med. Mol. Imaging,* 32, 820-827.

Drazin, B., Sherman, N., Sussman, K., Dahl, R. & Vatter, A. 1985. Internalization and cellular processing of somatostatin in primary culture of rat anterior pituitary cells. *Endocrinol.*, 117, 960-966.

DuBois, S. G., Messina, J., Maris, J. M., Huberty, J., Glidden, D. V., Veatch, J., Charron, M., Hawkins, R. & Matthay, K. K. 2004. Hematologic toxicity of high-dose iodine-131-metaiodobenzylguanidine therapy for advanced neuroblastoma. *J. Clin. Oncol.*, 22, 2452-2460.

Dwamena, B. A., Zempel, S., Klopper, J. F., Van Heerden, B., Wieland, D. & Shapiro, B. 1998. Brain uptake of iodine-131 metaiodobenzylguanidine following therapy of malignant pheochromocytoma. *Clin. Nucl. Med.*, 23, 441-445.

Edelman, M. J., Clamon, G., Kahn, D., Magram, M., Lister-James, J. & Line, B. R. 2009. Targeted radiopharmaceutical therapy for advanced lung cancer: phase I trial of rhenium Re188 P2045, a somatostatin analog. *J. Thorac. Oncol.*, 4, 1550-1554.

Eriksson, B., Bergström, M., Sundin, A., Juhlin, C., Orlefors, H., Oberg, K. & Långström, B. 2002. The role of PET in localization of neuroendocrine and adrenocortical tumors. *Ann. N. Y. Acad. Sci.,* 970, 159-169.

Esser, J. P., Krenning, E. P., Teunissen, J. J., Kooij, P. P., van Gameren, A. L., Bakker, W. H. & Kwekkeboom, D. J. 2006. Comparison of [(177)Lu-DOTA(0), Tyr(3)]octreotate and [(177)Lu-DOTA(0),Tyr(3)] octreotide: which peptide is preferable for PRRT? *Eur. J. Nucl. Med. Mol. Imaging*, 33, 1346-1351.

Fanti, S., Ambrosini, V., Tomassetti, P., Castellucci, P., Montini, G., Allegri, V., Grassetto, G., Rubello, D., Nanni, C. & Franchi, R. 2008. Evaluation of unusual neuroendocrine tumours by means of ^{68}Ga-DOTA-NOC PET. *Biomed. Pharmacother.*, 62, 667-671.

Fass, L. 2008. Imaging and cancer: A review. *Mol. Oncol.*, 2, 115-152.

Fogelman, I., Cook, G., Israel, O. & Van der Wall, H. 2005. Positron emission tomography and bone metastases. *Semin. Nucl. Med.*, 35, 135-142.

Forrer, F., Krenning, E. P., Kooij, P. P., Bernard, B. F., Konijnenberg, M., Bakker, W. H., Teunissen, J. J., de Jong, M., van Lom, K., de Herder, W. W. & Kwekkeboom, D. J. 2009. Bone marrow dosimetry in peptide receptor radionuclide therapy with [(177)Lu-DOTA (0),Tyr (3)]octreotate. *Eur. J. Nucl. Med. Mol. Imaging*, 36, 1138-1146.

Forrer, F., Mueller-Brand, J. & Maecke, H. 2005. Pre-therapeutic dosimetry with radiolabelled somatostatin analogues in patients withadvanced neuroendocrine tumors. *Eur. J. Nucl. Med. Mol.* Imaging, 32, 511-512.

Forrer, F., Riedweg, I., Maecke, H. R. & Mueller-Brand, J. 2008. Radiolabeled DOTATOC in patients with advanced paraganglioma and pheochromocytoma. *Q J Nucl Med Mol Imaging*, 52, 334-340.

Forrer, F., Waldherr, C., Maecke, H. R. & Mueller-Brand, J. 2006. Targeted radionuclide therapy with ^{90}Y-DOTATOC in patients with neuroendocrine tumors. *Anticancer Res,* 26, 703-708.

Giammarile, F., Chiti, A., Lassmann, M., Brans, B. & Flux, G. 2008. EANM procedure guidelines for ^{131}I-meta-iodobenzylguanidine (^{131}I-mIBG) therapy. *Eur. J. Nucl. Med. Mol. Imaging*, 35, 1039-1047.

Frilling, A., Weber, F., Saner, F., Bockisch, A., Hofmann, M., Mueller-Brand, J. & Broelsch, C. E. 2006. Treatment with ^{90}Y- and ^{177}Lu-DOTATOC in patients with metastatic neuroendocrine tumors. *Surgery*, 140, 968-977.

Gabriel, M., Decristoforo, C., Donnemiller, E., Ulmer, H., Rychlinski, C. W., Mather, S. J. & Moncayo, R. 2003. An Intrapatient Comparison of ^{99m}Tc-EDDA/HYNIC-TOC with ^{111}In-DTPA-Octreotide for Diagnosis of Somatostatin Receptor–Expressing Tumors. *J. Nucl. Med.,* 44, 708-716.

Gabriel, M., Froehlich, F., Decristoforo, C., Ensinger, C., Donnemiller, E., von Guggenberg, E., Heute, D. & Moncayo, R. 2004. ^{99m}Tc-EDDA/HYNIC-TOC and ^{18}F-FDG in thyroid cancer patients with negative ^{131}I whole-body scans. *Eur. J. Nucl. Med. Mol. Imaging*, 31, 330-341.

Gabriel, M., Decristoforo, C., Kendler, D., Dobrozemsky, G., Heute, D., Uprimny, C., Kovacs, P., Von Guggenberg, E., Bale, R. & Virgolini, I. J. 2007. ^{68}Ga-DOTA-Tyr3-octreotide PET in neuroendocrine tumors: comparison with somatostatin receptor scintigraphy and CT. *J. Nucl. Med.,* 48, 508-518.

Gains, J. E., Bomanji, J. B., Fersht, N. L., Sullivan, T., D'Souza, D., Sullivan, K. P., Aldridge, M., Waddington, W. & Gaze, M. N. 2011. ^{177}Lu-DOTATATE molecular radiotherapy for childhood neuroblastoma. *J. Nucl. Med.*, 52, 1041-1047.

Gambini, J. P., Lopez Lerena, J. J., Quagliata, A., Hermida, J. C., Heuguerot, C. & Alonso, O. 2008. ^{99m}Tc-HYNIC octreotide in neuroblastoma. *Ann. Nucl. Med.*, 22, 817-819.

Gambini, J. P., Núñez, M., Vila, R., Noble, J. & Alonso, O. 2009. Tc-99m hynic octreotide SPECT-MRI in brain metastasis of thyroid papillary-insular cancer. *Clin. Nucl. Med.,* 34, 920-921.

Garkavij, M., Nickel, M., Sjogreen-Gleisner, K., Ljungberg, M., Ohlsson, T., Wingardh, K., Strand, S. & Tennvall, J. 2010. ^{177}Lu-[DOTA0,Tyr3]octreotate therapy in patients with disseminated neuroendocrine tumors: analysis of dosimetry with impact on future therapeutic strategy. *Cancer*, 116(Suppl 4), 1084-2092.

Gibril, F., Reynolds, J. C., Doppman, J. L., Chen, C. C., Venzon, D. J., Termanini, B., Weber, H. C., Stewart, C. A. & Jensen, R. T. 1996. Somatostatin receptor scintigraphy: its sensitivity compared with that of other imaging methods in detecting primary and metastatic gastrinomas. A prospective study. *Ann. Int. Med.*, 125, 26-34.

Gnanasegaran, G. & Buscombe J. R. 2005. Can In-111 Pentetreotide Predict the Bio-distribution of Y-90Lanreotide? *WJNM*, 4, 11-16.

Gnanasegaran, G., Kapse, N. & Buscombe, J. R. 2005. Recent trends in radionuclide imaging and targeted radionuclide therapy of neuroendocrine tumours. *IJNM*, 20, 55-66.

Gnanasegaran, G., Buscombe, J. R., O'Rourke, E., Caplin, M. E., Purfield, D. & Hilson, A. J. W. 2005. Brehmsstrahlung imaging after intraarterial ^{90}Y-lanreotide-radionuclide therapy for carcinoid liver metastases. *Nucl. Med. Commun.*, 26, 271-295.

Gopinath, G., Buscombe, J. R., Heath, G. & Hilson, A. J. W. 2004. Biodistribution of Y-90 lanreotide and In-111 octreotide- Are they different? *Nucl. Med. Commun.*, 23, 382.

Graham, M. M. & Menda, Y. 2011. Radiopeptide imaging and therapy in the United States. *J. Nucl. Med.*, 52, 56S-63S.

Hadj-Djilani, N. L., Lebtahi, N. E., Delaloye, A. B., Laurini, R. & Beck, D. 1995. Diagnosis and follow-up of neuroblastoma by means of iodine-123 metaiodobenzylguanidine scintigraphy and bone scan, and the influence of histology. *Eur. J. Nucl. Med.*, 22, 322-329.

Haug, A. R., Auernhammer, C. J., Wangler, B., Schmidt, G. P., Uebleis, C., Goke, B., Cumming, P., Bartenstein, P., Tiling, R. & Hacker, M. 2010. ^{68}Ga-DOTATATE PET/CT for the early prediction of response to somatostatin receptormediated radionuclide therapy in patients with well differentiated neuroendocrine tumors. *J. Nucl. Med.*, 51, 1349-1356.

Hennings, J., Lindhe, O., Bergström, M., Långström, B., Sundin, A. & Hellman, P. 2006. [^{11}C]Metomidate positron emission tomography of adrenocortical tumors in correlation with histopathological findings. *J. Clin. Endocrinol. Metab.*, 91, 1410-1414.

Heute, D., Kostron, H., Guggenberg, E. V., Ingorokva, S., Gabriel, M., Dobrozemsky, G., Stockhammer, G. & Virgolini, I. J. 2010. Response of recurrent high-grade glioma to treatment with ^{90}Y-DOTATOC. J. *Nucl. Med.,* 51, 397-400.

Higgins, G. A., Recant, L. & Fischman, A. B. 1979. The glucagonoma: surgically curable diabetes. *Am. J. Surg*., 137, 142-148.

Hirano, T., Otake, H., Yoshida, I. & Endo, K. 1995. Primary lung cancer SPECT imaging with pentavalent technetium-99m-DMSA. *J. Nucl. Med.,* 36, 202-207.

Hoefnagel, C. A. 1994. Metaiodobenzylguanidine and somatostatin in oncology: Role in the management of neural crest tumours. *Eur. J. Nucl. Med.*, 21, 561-581.

Hoefnagel, C. A., Voute, P. A., de Kraker, J. & Valdes Olmos, R. A. 1991. [^{131}I]metaiodobenzylguanidine therapy after conventional therapy for neuroblastoma. *J. Nucl. Biol. Med.*, 35, 202-206.

Hofmann, M., Maecke, H., Borner, R., Weckesser, E., Schoffski, P., Oei, L., Schumacher, J., Henze, M., Heppeler, A., Meyer, J. & Knapp, H. 2001. Biokinetics and imaging with the somatostatin receptor PET radioligand (68)Ga-DOTATOC: preliminary data. *Eur. J. Nucl. Med.,* 28, 1751-1757.

Huang, S. C. 2000. Anatomy of SUV. Standardized uptake value. *Nucl. Med. Biol.*, 27, 643-646.

ICRP Publication 80 Radiation dose to patients from radiopharmaceuticals. 1998. Annals of ICRP, 28, 3, Pergamon Press, Oxford.

ICRP Publication 53 Radiation dose to patients from radiopharmaceuticals. 1987. Annals of ICRP, 18, 1-4, Pergamon Press, Oxford.

Ilias, I., Yu, J., Carrasquillo, J. A., Chen, C. C., Eisenhofer, G., Whatley, M., McElroy, B. & Pacak, K. 2003. Superiority of 6-[18F]-fluorodopamine positron emission tomography *versus* [131I]-metaiodobenzylguanidine scintigraphy in the localization of metastatic pheochromocytoma. *J. Clin. Endocrinol. Metab.,* 88, 4083-4087.

Imhof, A., Brunner, P., Marincek, N., Briel, M., Schindler, C., Rasch, H., Mäcke, H. R., Rochlitz, C., Müller-Brand, J. & Walter, M. A. 2011. Response, survival, and long-term toxicity after therapy with the radiolabeled somatostatin analogue [^{90}Y-DOTA]-TOC in metastasized neuroendocrine cancers. *J. Clin. Oncol.*, 29, 2416-2423

Iten, F., Müller, B., Schindler, C., Rochlitz, C., Oertli, D., Mäcke, H. R., Müller-Brand, J. & Walter, M. A. 2007. Response to [90Yttrium-DOTA]-TOC treatment is associated with long-term survival benefit in metastasized medullary thyroid cancer: a phase II clinical trial. *Clin Cancer Res*, 13, 6696-6702.

Jacobsson, H., Bremmer, S. & Larsson, S. A. 2003. Visualisation of the normal adrenals at SPET examination with ^{111}In-pentetreotide. *Eur. J. Nucl. Med. Mol. Imaging*, 30, 1169-1172.

Jamar, F., Barone, R., Mathieu, I., Walrand, S., Labar, D., Carlier, P., de Camps, J., Schran, H., Chen, T., Smith, M. C., Bouterfa, H., Valkema, R., Krenning, E. P., Kvols, L. K. & Pauwels, S. 2003. ^{86}Y-DOTA0)-D-Phe1-Tyr3-octreotide (SMT487)-a phase 1 clinical study: pharmacokinetics, biodistribution and renal protective effect of different regimens of amino acid co-infusion. *Eur. J. Nucl. Med. Mol. Imaging*, 30, 510–518.

Jing, H., Li, F., Chen, L., Zhang, T. & Zhao, Y. 2011. Detection of recurrent pancreatic primitive neuroectodermal tumor by Tc-99m hydrazinonicotinyl-Tyr3-octreotide scan *Clin. Nucl. Med.*, 36, 54-55.

Kaemmerer, D., Prasad, V., Daffner, W., Hörsch, D., Klöppel, G., Hommann, M. & Baum, R. P. 2009. Neoadjuvant peptide receptor radionuclide therapy for an inoperable neuroendocrine pancreatic tumor. *World J Gastroenterol,* 15, 5867-5870.

Kahn, D., Menda, Y., Kernstine, K., Bushnell, D., McLaughlin, K., Miller, S. & Berbaum, K. 2004. The utility of ^{99m}Tc depreotide compared with F-18 fluorodeoxyglucose positron emission tomography and surgical staging in patients with suspected non-small cell lung cancer. *Chest*, 125, 494-501.

Kalff, V., Shapiro, B., Lloyd, R. V., Sisson, J. C., Holland, K., Nakajo, M. & Beierwaltes WH. 1982. The spectrum of phaeochromcytoma in hypertensive patients with neurofibromatosis. *Arch. Intern. Med.,* 142, 2092-2098.

Kalkner, K. M., Janson, E. T., Nilsson, S., Carlsson, S., Oberg, K. & Westlin, J. E. 1995. Somatostatin receptor scintigraphy in patients with carcinoid tumors: comparison between radioligand uptake and tumor markers. *Cancer Res*, 55, 5801s-5804s.

Kaltsas, G. A., Mukherjee, J. J. & Grossman, A. B. 2001. The value of radiolabelled MIBG and octreotide in the diagnosis and management of neuroendocrine tumours. *Ann. Oncol.*, 12(Suppl. 2), S47-S50.

Kaltsas, G. A., Papadogias, D., Makras, P. & Grossman, A. B. 2005. Treatment of advanced neuroendocrine tumors with radiolabelled somatostatin analogues. *Endocr Relat Cancer*, 12, 683-689.

Kaltsas, G., Rockall, A., Papadogias, D., Reznek, R. & Grossman, A. B. 2004. Recent advances in radiological and radionuclide imaging and therapy of neuroendocrine tumours. *Eur. J. Endocrinol.*, 151, 15-27.

Kam, B. L. R., Teunissen, J. J. M., Krenning, E. P., de Herder, W. W., Khan, S., van Vliet, E. I. & Kwekkeboom, D. J. 2012. Lutetium-labelled peptides for therapy of neuroendocrine tumours. *Eur. J. Nucl. Med. Mol. Imaging*, 39(Suppl 1), S103–S112.

Kassis, A. I. & Adelstein, S. J. 2005. Radiobiologic principles in radionuclide therapy. *J. Nucl. Med.*, 46(Suppl), 4S-12S.

Kayani, I., Bomanji, J. B., Groves, A., Conway, G., Gacinovic, S., Win, T., Dickson, J., Caplin, M. & Ell, P. J. 2008. Functional imaging of neuroendocrine tumors with combined PET/CT using ^{68}Ga-DOTATATE (DOTA-D-Phe1,Tyr3-octreotate) and ^{18}F-FDG. *Cancer*, 112, 2447-2455.

Kennedy, A. S., Dezarn, W. A., McNeillie, P., Coldwell, D., Nutting, C., Carter, D., Murthy, R., Rose, S., Warner, R. R., Liu, D., Palmedo, H., Overton, C., Jones, B. & Salem, R. 2008. Radioembolization for unresectable neuroendocrine hepatic metastases using resin ^{90}Y-microspheres: early results in 148 patients. *Am. J. Clin. Oncol.*, 31, 271-279.

Khagaghi, F. A., Shapiro, B. M., *et al.,* 1989. Labetalol reduces I131 MIBG uptake by phaeochromocytoma and normal tissues. *J. Nucl. Med.*, 30, 481-489.

Khanna, G., Bushnell, D. & O'Dorisio, M. S. 2008. Utility of radiolabelled somatostatin receptor analogues for staging/restaging and treatment of somatostatin receptor-positive pediatric tumors. *Oncologist*, 13, 382-389.

King, J., Quinn, R., Glenn, D. M., Janssen, J., Tong, D., Liaw, W. & Morris, D. L. 2008. Radioembolization with selective internal radiation microspheres for neuroendocrine liver metastases. *Cancer*, 113, 921-929.

Konijnenberg, M. W. 2003. Is the renal dosimetry for [90Y-DOTA 0,Tyr3] octreotide accurate enough to predict thresholds for individual patients? *Cancer Biother Radiopharm*, 18, 619-625.

Koopmans, K. P., Neels, O. C., Kema, I. P., Elsinga, P. H., Sluiter, W. J., Vanghillewe, K., Nisa, L., Savelli, G. & Giubbini, R. 2011. Yttrium-90 DOTATOC therapy in GEP-NET and other SST2 expressing tumors: a selected review. *Ann. Nucl. Med.*, 25, 75-85.

Koukouraki, S., Strauss, L. G, Georgoulias, V., Schuhmacher, J., Haberkorn, U., Karkavitsas, N. & Dimitrakopoulou-Strauss, A. 2006. Evaluation of the pharmacokinetics of ^{68}Ga-DOTATOC in patients with metastatic neuroendocrine tumours scheduled for ^{90}Y-DOTATOC therapy. *Eur. J. Nucl. Med. Mol. Imaging*, 33, 460-466.

Krausz, Y., Freedman, N., Rubinstein, R., Lavie, E., Orevi, M., Tshori, S., Salmon, A., Glaser, B., Chisin, R., Mishani, E. & Gross, J. D. 2011. (68)Ga-DOTA-NOC PET/CT imaging of neuroendocrine tumors: comparison with ^{111}In-DTPA-octreotide (OctreosScan®). *Mol Imaging Biol*, 13, 583-593.

Krenning, E. P., Kwekkeboom, D. J., Bakker, W. H., Breeman, W. A., Kooij, P. P., Oei, H. Y., van Hagen, M., Postema, P. T., de Jong, M. & Reubi, J. C.1993. Somatostatin receptor scintigraphy with [^{111}lnDTPA-DPhel] and [^{123}Ityr3]octreotide: The Rotterdam experience with more than 1000 patients. *Eur. J. Nucl. Med.*, 20, 716-731.

Krenning, E. P., Kwekkeboom, D. J., Pauwels, S., Kvols, L. K. & Reubi, J. C. 1995. Somatostatin Receptor Scintigraphy. Nucl. Med. Ann. N. Y., Raven Press, 1-50.

Krenning, E. P., Bakker, W. H., Kooij, P. P., Breeman, W. A., Oei, H. Y., de Jong, M., Reubi, J. C., Visser, T. J., Bruns, C., Kwekkeboom, D. J. *et al.,* 1992. Somatostatin receptor scintigraphy with indium-111-DTPA-D-Phe-1-octreotide in man: metabolism, dosimetry and comparison with iodine-123-Tyr-3-octreotide. *J. Nucl. Med.,* 33, 652-658.

Krenning, E. P., Bakker, W. H., Breeman, W. A., Koper, J. W., Kooij, P. P., Ausema, L., Lameris, J. S., Reubi, J. C. & Lamberts, S. W. 1989. Localisation of endocrine-related tumours with radioiodinated analogue of somatostatin. *Lancet*, 1, 242-244.

Kwekkeboom, D. J., Krenning, E. P., Lebtahi, R., Komminoth, P., Kos-Kudła, B., de Herder, W. W., Ploeckinger, U., the Mallorca Consensus Conference participants. 2009. ENETS Consensus guidelines for the standards of care in neuroendocrine tumors: Peptide receptor radionuclide therapy with radiolabeled somatostatin analogs. *Neuroendocrinol.*, 90, 220-226.

Kwekkeboom, D. J., Bakker, W. H., Kam, B. L., Teunissen, J. J. M., Kooij, P. P. M., de Herder, W. W., Feelders, R. A., van Eijck, C. H., de Jong, M., Srinivasan, A., Erion, J. L. & Krenning, E. P. 2003. Treatment of patients with gastro-entero-pancreatic (GEP) tumors with the novel radiolabelled somatostatin analogue [^{177}LuDOTA(0), Tyr(3)]octreotide. *Eur. J. Nucl. Med. Mol. Imaging*, 30, 417-422.

Kwekkeboom, D. J., Bakker, W. H., Kooij, P. P., Konijnenberg, M. W., Srinivasan, A., Erion, J. L., Schmidt, M. A., Bugaj, J. L., de Jong, M. & Krenning, E. P. 2001 [^{177}Lu-DOTA^{0}Tyr^{3}]octreotate: comparison with [^{111}In-DTPA^{0}]octreotide in patients. *Eur. J. Nucl. Med.,* 28, 1319-1325.

Kwekkeboom, D. J., De Herder, W. W., Kam, B. L., van Eijck, C. H., van Essen, M., Kooij, P. P., Feelders, R. A., van Aken, M. O. & Krenning, E. P. 2008. Treatment with the radiolabeled somatostatin analog [^{177}7Lu-DOTA^{0},Tyr^{3}]octreotate: toxicity, efficacy, and survival. *J. Clin. Oncol.*, 26, 2124-2130.

Kwekkeboom, D. J., Kooij, P. P., Bakker, W. H., Macke, H. R. & Krenning, E. P. 1999. Comparison of ^{111}In-DOTA-Tyr3-octreotide and ^{111}In-DTPA-octreotide in the same patients: biodistribution, kinetics, organ and tumor uptake. *J. Nucl. Med.*, 40, 762-767.

Kwekkeboom, D. J., Krenning, E. P., Bakker, W. H., Oei, H. Y., Kooij, P. P. & Lamberts, S. W. 1993. Somatostatin analogue scintigraphy in carcinoid tumours. *Eur. J. Nucl. Med.*, 20, 283-292.

Kwekkeboom, D. J., Reubi, J. C., Lamberts, S. W., Bruining, H. A., Mulder, A. H., Oei, H. Y. & Krenning, E. P. 1993. *In vivo* somatostatin receptor imaging in medullary thyroid carcinoma. *J. Clin. Endocrinol. Metab.*, 76, 1413-1417.

Kwekkeboom, D. J., Teunissen, J. J., Bakker, W. H., Kooij, P. P., de Herder, W. W., Feelders, R. A., van Eijck, C. H., Esser, J. P., Kam, B. L. & Krenning, E. P. 2005. Radiolabeled somatostatin analog [^{177}Lu-DOTA0,Tyr3]octreotate in patients with endocrine gastroenteropancreatic tumors. *J. Clin. Oncol.*, 23, 2754-2762.

Larson, S. M., Erdi, Y., Akhurst, T., Mazumdar, M., Macapinlac, H. A., Finn, R. D., Casilla, C., Fazzari, M., Srivastava, N., Yeung, H. W., Humm, J. L., Guillem, J., Downey, R., Karpeh, M., Cohen, A. E. & Ginsberg, R. 1999. Tumor treatment response based on visual and quantitative changes in global tumor glycolysis using PET-FDG imaging. The visual response score and the change in total lesion glycolysis. *Clin Positron Imaging*, 2, 159-171.

Lassmann, M., Biassoni, L., Monsieurs, M., Franzius, C. & Jacobs, F. 2007. EANM Dosimetry and Paediatrics Committees. The new EANM paediatric dosage card. *Eur. J. Nucl. Med. Mol. Imaging*, 34, 796-798.

Lebtahi, R., Cadiot, G., Sarda, L., Daou, D., Faraggi, M., Petegnief, Y., Mignon, M. & le Guludec, D. 1997. Clinical impact of somatostatin receptor scintigraphy in the management of patients with neuroendocrine gastroenteropancreatic tumors. *J. Nucl. Med.*, 38, 853-858.

Limouris, G. S., Chatziioannou, A., Kontogeorgakos, D., Mourikis, D., Lyra, M., Dimitriou, P., Stavraka, A., Gouliamos, A. & Vlahos, L. 2008. Selective hepatic arterial infusion of In-111-DTPA-Phe1-octreotide in neuroendocrine liver metastases. *Eur. J. Nucl. Med. Mol. Imaging*, 35, 1827-1837.

Olivier, P., Colarinha, P., Fettich, J., Fischer, S., Frökier, J., Giammarile, F., Gordon, I., Hahn, K., Kabasakal, L., Mann, M., Mitjavila, M., Piepsz, A., Porn, U., Sixt, R. & Van Velzen, J. 2002. Guideline for radioiodinated MIBG scintigraphy in children. Under the Auspices of the Paediatric Committee of the European Association of Nuclear Medicine.

Maecke, H. R., Hofmann, M. & Haberkorn, U. 2005. (68)Galabeled peptides in tumor imaging. *J. Nucl. Med.*, 46(Supplement 1), 172S–178S.

Mamede, M., Carrasquillo, J. A., Chen, C. C., Del Corral, P., Whatley, M., Ilias, I., Ayala, A. & Pacak, K. 2006. Discordant localization of 2-[^{18}F]-fluoro-2-deoxy-D-glucose in 6-[^{18}F]-fluorodopamine- and [(^{123})I]-metaiodobenzylguanidine-negative metastatic pheochromocytoma sites. *Nucl. Med. Commun.*, 27, 31-36.

Marincek, N., Jörg, A. C., Brunner, P., Schindler, C., Koller, M. T., Rochlitz, C., Müller-Brand, J., Maecke, H. R., Briel, M. & Walter, M. A. 2013. Somatostatin-based radiotherapy with [^{90}Y-DOTA]-TOC in neuroendocrine tumors: long-term outcome of a phase I dose escalation study. *J. Transl. Med.,* 11, 17.

Martiniova, L., Cleary, S., Lai, E. W., Kiesewetter, D. O., Seidel, J., Dawson, L. F., Phillips, J. K., Thomasson, D., Chen, X., Eisenhofer, G., Powers, J. F., Kvetnansky, R. & Pacak, K. 2012. Usefulness of [18F]-DA and [18F]-DOPA for PET imaging in a mouse model of pheochromocytoma. *Nucl. Med. Biol.,* 39, 215-526.

McEwan, A. J., Shapiro, B., Sisson, J. C., Beierwaltes, H. W. & Ackery, D. M. 1985. Radio-iodobenzylguanidine for the scintigraphic location and therapy of adrenergic tumors. *Semin. Nucl. Med.*, 15, 132-153.

McStay, M. K., Maudgil, D., Williams, M., Tibballs, J. M., Watkinson, A. F., Caplin, M. E. & Buscombe, J. R. 2005. Large volume liver metastases from neuroendocrine tumors: hepatic intraarterial ^{90}Y-DOTA-lanreotide as effective palliative therapy. *Radiology*, 237, 718-726.

Menda, Y., O'Dorisio, M. S., Kao, S., Khanna, G., Michael, S., Connolly, M., Babich, J., O'Dorisio, T., Bushnell, D. & Madsen, M. 2010. Phase I trial of ^{90}Y-DOTATOC therapy in children and young adults with refractory solid tumors that express somatostatin receptors. *J. Nucl. Med.,* 51, 1524-1531.

Miederer, M., Henriksen, G., Alke, A., Mossbrugger, I., Quintanilla-Martinez, L., Senekowitsch-Schmidtke, R. & Essler, M. 2008. Preclinical evaluation of the alpha-particle generator nuclide ^{225}Ac for somatostatin receptor radiotherapy of neuroendocrine tumors. *Clin Cancer Res*, 14, 3555-3561.

Miederer, M., Seidl, S., Buck, A., Scheidhauer, K., Wester, H. J., Schwaiger, M. & Perren, A. 2009. Correlation of immunohistopathological expression of somatostatin receptor 2 with standardised uptake values in ^{68}Ga-DOTATOC PET/CT. *Eur. J. Nucl. Med. Mol. Imaging*, 36, 48-52.

Modlin, I. M., Latich, I., Zikusoka, M., Kidd, M., Eick, G. & Chan, A. K. 2006. Gastrointestinal carcinoids: the evolution of diagnostic strategies. *J. Clin. Gastroenterol.*, 40, 572-582.

Morgenstern, A., Bruchertseifer, F., Apostolidis, C., Giesel, F., Mier, W., Haberkorn, U. & Kratochwil, C. 2012. Synthesis of ^{213}Bi-DOTATOC for peptide receptor alpha-therapy of GEP-NET patients refractory to beta therapy. *J. Nucl. Med.,* 53(Suppl. 1), 455.

Moulder, J. E., Fish, B. L. & Cohen, E. P. 1998. Angiotensin II receptor antagonists in the treatment and prevention of radiation nephropathy. *Int. J. Radiat. Biol.*, 73, 415-421.

Moulder, J. E., Fish, B. L. & Cohen, E. P. 1998. Radiation nephropathy is treatable with an angiotensin-converting enzyme inhibitor or an angiotensin II tye-I (AT1) receptor antagonist. *Radiother. Oncol.*, 46, 307-315.

Mozley, P. D., Kim, C. K., Mohsin, J., Jat, E. & Alavi, A. 1994. The efficacy of iodine-123-MIBG as a screening test for pheochromocytoma. *J. Nucl. Med.*, 35, 1138-1144.

Murthy, R., Kamat, P., Nunez, R., Madoff, D. C., Gupta, S., Salem, R. & Yao, J. C. 2008. Yttrium-90 microsphere radioembolotherapy of hepatic metastatic neuroendocrine carcinomas after hepatic arterial embolization. *J. Vasc. Interv. Radiol.*, 19, 145-151.

Nakajo, M., Shapiro, B., Copp, J., Kalff, V., Gross, M. D., Sisson, J. C. & Beierwaltes, W. H. 1983. The normal and abnormal distribution of the adrenomedullary imaging agent I-131-metaiodobenzylguanidine (I-MIBG) in man: evaluation by scintigraphy. *J. Nucl. Med.*, 24, 672-682.

Nakajo, M., Shapiro, B., Glowniak, J. Y., Sisson, J. C. & Beierwaltes, W. H. 1983. Inverse relationship between cardiac accumulation of meta[^{131}I]iodobenzylguanidine (I-131-MIBG) and circulating catecholamines in suspected pheochromocytomas. *J. Nucl. Med.*, 24, 1127-1134.

Nomura, N., Fujii, T., Kanazumi, N., Takeda, S., Nomoto, S., Kasuya, H, Sugimoto, H., Yamada, S. & Nakao, A. 2009. Nonfunctioning neuroendocrine pancreatic tumors: our experience and management. *J Hepatobiliary Pancreat Surg,* 16, 639-647.

Nanda, P. K., Lane, S. R., Retzloff, L. B., Pandey, U. S. & Smith, C. J. 2010. Radiolabeled regulatory peptides for imaging and therapy. *Curr Opin Endocrinol Diabetes Obes, 17, 69-76.*

Norton, J. A., Kivlen, M., Li, M., Schneider, D., Chuter, T. & Jensen, R. T. 2003. Morbidity and mortality of aggressive resection in patients with advanced neuroendocrine tumors. *Arch. Surg.*, 138, 859-866.

Oeberg, K. 1998. Advances in chemotherapy and biotherapy of endocrine tumors. *Curr. Opin. Oncol.*, 10, 58-65.

Oeberg, K. 2004. Management of neuroendocrine tumors. *Ann. Oncol.,* 15, iv293-298.

O'Grady, H. L. & Conlon, K. C. 2008. Pancreatic neuroendocrine tumours. *Eur. J. Surg. Oncol.*, 34, 324-332.

Ohta, H., Yamamoto, K., Endo, K., Mori, T., Hamanaka, D., Shimazu, A., Ikekubo, K., Makimoto, K., Iida, Y., Konishi, J., Morita, R., Hata, N., Horiuchi, K., Yokoyama, A., Torizuka, K. & Kuma, K. 1984. A new imaging agent for medullary carcinoma of the thyroid. *J. Nucl. Med.*, 25, 323-325.

Orlefors, H., Sundin, A., Garske, U., Juhlin, C., Oberg, K., Skogseid, B., Langstrom, B., Bergstrom, M. & Eriksson, B. 2005. Wholebody ^{11}C-5-hydroxytryptophan positron emission tomography as a universal imaging technique for neuroendocrine tumors: comparison with somatostatin receptor scintigraphy and computed tomography. *J. Clin. Endocrinol. Metab.*, 90, 3392-3400.

Otte, A., Herrmann, R., Heppeler, A., Behe, M., Jermann, E., Powell, P., Mäcke, H. R. & Müller, J. 1999. Yttrium-90 DOTATOC first clinical results. *Eur. J. Nucl. Med.,* 26, 1439-1447.

Otte, A., Jermann, E., Behe, M., Goetze, M., Bucher, H. C., Roser, H. W., Heppeler, A., Müller-Brand, J. & Mäcke, H. R. 1997. DOTATOC: A powerful new tool for receptor mediated radionuclide therapy. *Eur. J. Nucl. Med.*, 24, 792-795.

Otte, A., Müller-Brand, J., Dellas, S., Nitzsche, E. U., Herrmann, R. & Mäcke, H. R. 1998. Yttrium-90-labelled somatostatin-analogue for cancer treatment. *Lancet*, 351, 417-418.

Pacak, K., Linehan, W. M., Eisenhofer, G., Walther, M. M. & Goldstein, D. S. 2001. Recent advances in genetics, diagnosis, localizationm and treatment of pheochromocytoma. *Ann. Intern. Med.*, 134, 315-329.

Paganelli, G., Bodei, L., Junak, D. H., Rocca, P., Papi, S., Sierra, M. L., Gatti, M., Chinol, M., Bartolomei, M., Fiorenza, M. & Grana, C. 2002. ^{90}Y-DOTA-D-Phe1-Tyr3-octreotide in therapy of neuroendocrine malignancies. *Biopolymers*, 66, 393-398.

Paganelli, G., Zoboli, S., Cremonesi, M., Bodei, L., Ferrari, M., Grana, C., Bartolomei, M., Orsi, F., De Cicco, C., Mäcke, H. R., Chinol, M. & de Braud, F. 2001. Receptor-mediated radiotherapy with 90Y-DOTA-DPhe 1-Tyr3-octreotide. *Eur. J. Nucl. Med.*, 28, 426-434.

Paganelli, G., Zoboli, S., Cremonesi, M., Maecke, H. R. & Chinol, M. 1999. Receptor-mediated radionuclide therapy with ^{90}Y-DOTA-DPhe1-Tyr3-Octreotide: preliminary report in cancer patients. *Cancer Biother Radiopharm*, 14, 477-483.

Papantoniou, V., Ptohis, N. & Tsiouris, S. 2006. Diffuse tracer uptake in scintimammography: not as nonspecific or benign as originally believed? *J. Nucl. Med.*, 47, 554-555.

Papantoniou, V., Sotiropoulou, E., Valsamaki, P., Tsaroucha, A., Sotiropoulou, M., Ptohis, N., Stipsanelli, A., Dimitrakakis, K., Marinopoulos, S., Tsiouris, S., Antsaklis, A. 2011. Breast density, scintimammographic ^{99m}Tc(V)DMSA uptake and calcitonin gene related peptide (CGRP) expression in mixed invasive ductal associated with extensive *in situ* ductal carcinoma (IDC+DCIS) and pure invasive ductal carcinoma (IDC): correlation with estrogen receptor (ER) status, proliferation index Ki-67 and histological grade. *Breast Cancer*, 18, 286-291.

Papantoniou, V., Tsiouris, S., Mainta, E., Valotassiou, V., Souvatzoglou, M., Sotiropoulou, M., Nakopoulou, L., Lazaris, D., Louvrou, A., Melissinou, M., Tzannetaki, A., Pirmettis, I., Koutsikos, J. & Zerva, C. 2005. Imaging *in situ* breast carcinoma (with or without an invasive component) with technetium-99m pentavalent dimercaptosuccinic acid and technetium-99m 2-methoxy isobutyl isonitrile scintimammography. *Breast Cancer Res*, 7, R33-R45.

Papantoniou, V., Valsamaki, P., Sotiropoulou, E., Tsaroucha, A., Tsiouris, S., Sotiropoulou, M., Marinopoulos, S., Kounadi, E., Karianos, T., Fothiadaki, A., Archontaki, A., Syrgiannis, K., Ptohis, N., Makris, N. & Limouris, G. 2011. Increased breast density correlates with the proliferation–seeking radiotracer ^{99m}Tc(V)-DMSA uptake in florid epithelial hyperplasia and in mixed ductal carcinoma *in situ* with invasive ductal carcinoma but not in pure invasive ductal carcinoma and in mild epithelial hyperplasia. *Mol Imaging*, 1, 370-376.

Papantoniou, V., Valsamaki, P. & Tsiouris, S. 2012. Scintimammography- Molecular Imaging: Value and New Perspectives with ^{99m}Tc(V)-DMSA. In: Imaging of the Breast – Technical Aspects and Clinical Implication. InTech online edns, 61-80.

Pashankar, F. D., O'Dorisio M. S. & Menda Y. 2005. MIBG and somatostatin receptor analogs in children: current concepts on diagnostic and therapeutic use. *J. Nucl. Med.*, 46, 55S-61S.

Pathirana, A. A., Vinjamuri, S., Byrne, C., Ghaneh, P., Vora, J. & Poston, G. J. 2001. (131)I-MIBG radionuclide therapy is safe and cost-effective in the control of symptoms of the carcinoid syndrome. *Eur. J. Surg. Oncol.*, 27, 404-408.

Perel, Y., Conway, J., Kletzel, M., Goldman, J., Weiss, S., Feyler, A. & Cohn, S. L. 1999. Clinical impact and prognostic value of metaiodobenzylguanidine in children with metastatic neuroblastoma. *J. Pediatr. Hematol. Oncol.*, 21, 13-18.

Pfeifer, A. K., Gregersen, T., Grønbæk, H., Hansen, C. P., Müller-Brand, J., Herskind Bruun, K., Krogh, K., Kjær, A. & Knigge, U. 2011. Peptide receptor radionuclide therapy with (90)Y-DOTATOC and (177)Lu-DOTATOC in advanced neuroendocrine tumors: results from a Danish cohort treated in Switzerland. *Neuroendocrinol.*, 93, 189-196.

Pless, M., Waldherr, C., Maecke, H., Buitrago, C., Herrmann, R. & Mueller-Brand, J. 2004. Targeted radiotherapy for small cell lung cancer using ^{90}Yttrium-DOTATOC, an Yttrium-labeled somatostatin analogue: a pilot trial. *Lung Cancer*, 45, 365-371.

Prinz, R. A., Dorsch, T. R. & Lawrence, A. M. 1981. Clinical aspects of glucagons producing islet cell tumors. *Am. J. Gastroenterol.*, 76, 125-131.

Quigley, A. M., Buscombe, J. R., Shah, T., Gnanasegaran, G., Roberts, D., Caplin, M. E. & Hilson, A. J. 2005. Intertumoural variability in functional imaging within patients suffering from neuroendocrine tumours. An observational, crosssectional study. *Neuroendocrinol.*, 82, 215-220.

Ramage, J. K., Williams, R. & Buxton-Thomas, M. 1996. Imaging secondary neuroendocrine tumours of the liver: Comparison of I-123 metaiodobenzylguanidine (MIBG) and Inlll-labelled octreotide (DTPA-octreotide). *Q. J. Med.,* 89, 539-542.

Raut, C., Kulke, M., Glickman, J., Swanson, R. S. & Ashley, S. W. 2006. Carcinoid tumors. *Curr. Probl. Surg.*, 43, 383-450.

Reubi, J. C. 2003. Peptide receptors as molecular targets for cancer diagnosis and therapy. *Endocr. Rev.*, 24, 389-427.

Reubi, J. C. & Maecke, H. R. 2008. Peptide-based probes for cancer imaging. *J. Nucl. Med.*, 49, 1735-1738.

Rinke, A., Müller, H. H., Schade-Brittinger, C., Klose, K. J., Barth, P., Wied, M., Mayer, C., Aminossadati, B., Pape, U. F., Bläker, M., Harder, J., Arnold, C., Gress, T. & Arnold, R.; PROMID Study Group. 2009. Placebo-controlled, double-blind, prospective, randomized study on the effect of octreotide LAR in the control of tumor growth in patients with metastatic neuroendocrine midgut tumors: A report from the PROMID Study Group. *J. Clin. Oncol.*, 27, 4656-4663.

Rolleman, E. J., Melis, M., Valkema, R., Boerman, O. C., Krenning, E. P. & de Jong, M. 2010. Kidney protection during peptide receptor radionuclide therapy with somatostatin analogues. *Eur. J. Nucl. Med. Mol. Imaging*, 37, 1018-1031.

Rolleman, E., Valkema, R., de Jong, M., Kooij, P. & Krenning, E. 2003. Safe and effective inhibition of renal uptake of radiolabelled octreotide by a combination of lysine and arginine. *Eur. J. Nucl. Med. Mol. Imaging*, 30, 9-15.

Safford, S. D., Coleman, R. E., Gockerman, J. P., Moore, J., Feldman, J., Onaitis, M. W., Tyler, D. S. & Olson, J. A. Jr. 2004. Iodine-131 metaiodobenzylguanidine treatment for metastatic carcinoid. Results in 98 patients. *Cancer*, 101, 1987-1993.

Saxena, A., Chua, T. C., Bester, L., Kokandi, A. & Morris, D. L. 2010. Factors predicting response and survival after yttrium-90 radioembolization of unresectable neuroendocrine tumor liver metastases: a critical appraisal of 48 cases. *Ann. Surg.*, 251, 910-916.

Shapiro, B. 1995. Ten years of experience with MIBG applications and the potential of new radiolabeled peptides: A personal overview and concluding remarks. Q. *J. Nucl. Med.*, 39(Suppl. 1-4), 150-155.

Shapiro, B., Copp, J. E., Sisson, J. C., Eyre, P. L., Wallis, J. & Beierwaltes, W. H. 1985. Iodine-131 metaiodobenzylguanidine for the locating of suspected pheochromocytoma: experience in 400 cases. *J. Nucl. Med.*, 26, 576-585.

Shapiro, B., Sisson, J. C., Wieland, D. M., Mangner, T. J., Zempel, S. M., Mudgett, E., Gross, M. D., Carey, J. E., Zasadny, K. R. & Beierwaltes, W. H. 1991. Radiopharmaceutical therapy of malignant pheochromocytoma with [131I]metaiodobenzylguanidine: results from ten years of experience. *J. Nucl. Biol. Med.*, 35, 269-276.

Shen, S., DeNardo, G. L., Yuan, A., DeNardo, D. A. & DeNardo, S. J. 1994. Planar gamma camera imaging and quantitation of yttrium-90 bremsstrahlung. *J. Nucl. Med.,* 35, 1381-1389.

Shulkin, B. L. & Shapiro, B. 1990. Radioiodinated meta-iodinated benzylguanidine in the management of neuroblastomas. In: Pochedly C, ed. Neuroblastoma. Boca Raton, FL: CRC Press, 171-198.

Shulkin, B. L. & Shapiro, B. 1998. Current concepts on the diagnostic use of MIBG in children. *J. Nucl. Med.*, 39, 679-688.

Shulkin, B. L., Shapiro, B. & Hutchinson, R. J. 1992. Iodine-131 metaiodobenzylguanidine and bone scintigraphy for the detection of neuroblastoma. *J. Nucl. Med.*, 33, 1735-1740.

Shulkin, B.L., Wienland, D.M., Shapiro, B. & Sisson, J.C. 1995. PET epinephrine studies of pheochromocytoma. *J. Nucl. Med.*, 36, 229P.

Sierra, M. L., Agazzi, A., Bodei, L., Pacifici, M., Arico, D., De Cicco, C., Quarna, J., Sansovini, M., De Simone, M. & Paganelli, G. 2009. Lymphocytic toxicity in patients after peptidereceptor radionuclide therapy (PRRT) with ^{177}Lu-DOTATATE and ^{90}Y-DOTATOC. *Cancer Biotherapy & Radiopharmaceuticals*, 24, 659-665.

Sisson, J. C. & Wieland, D. M. 1986. Radiolabelled meta-iodobenzylguanidine: Pharmacology and clinical studies. *Am. J. Phys. Imag.*, 1, 96-103.

Sisson, J. C., Shapiro, B., Beierwaltes, W. H., Glomniak, J. V., Nakajo, M., Magner, T. J., Larey, J. E., Swanson, D. P., Jean, C. E. & Wieland, D. M. 1984. Radiopharmaceutical treatment of malignant pheochromocytoma. *J. Nucl. Med.,* 25, 197-206.

Sisson, J. C., Frager, M. S., Valk, T. W., Gross, M. D., Swanson, D. P., Wieland, D. M., Tobes, M. C., Beierwaltes, W. H. & Thompson, N. W. 1981. Scintigraphy localization of pheochromocytoma. *N. Engl. J. Med.*, 305, 12-17.

Slooter, G. D., Breeman, W. A., Marquet, R. L., Krenning, E. P. & van Eijck, C. H. 1999. Anti-proliferative effect of radiolabelled octreotide in a metastases model in rat liver. *Int J Cancer*, 81, 767-771.

Solanki, K. K., Bomanji, J., Moyes, J., Mather, S. J., Trainer, P. J. & Britton, K. E. 1992. A pharmacological guide to medicines which interfere with he biodistribution of radiolabelled meta-iodobenzylguanidine (MIBG). *Nucl. Med. Commun.*, 13, 513-521.

Stabin, M. G. & Gelfand, M. J. 1998. Dosimetry of pediatric nuclear medicine procedures. Q. J. *Nucl. Med.*, 42, 93-112.

Suga, K., Ogasawara, N., Ariga, M., Motoyama, K., Hara, A., Kume, N. & Matsunaga, N. 2000. Alteration of myocardial metaiodobenzylguanidine uptake after treatment of pheochromocytoma and neuroblastoma. *Eur. J. Nucl. Med.*, 27, 574-582.

Swanson, D. P., Carey, J. E., Brown, L. E., Kline, R. C., Weiland, D. M., Thrall, J. H. & Beierwaltes, W. H. 1981. Human absorbed dose calculations for iodine-131 and iodine-123 labelled metaiodobenzylguanidine (MIBG): a potential myocardial and adrenal medulla imaging agent. In: Proceedings of the 3rd International Radiopharmaceutical Dosimetry Symposium. Health and Human Services Publication FDA 81-81-66, Oak Ridge, TN, Oak Ridge Associated Universities, Rockville, Maryland, 213-224.

Sywak, M. S., Pasieka, J. L., McEwan, A., Kline, G. & Rorstad, O. 2004. ^{131}I-meta-iodobenzylguanidine in the management of metastatic midgut carcinoid tumors. *World J Surg*, 28, 1157-1162.

Taal, B. G., Hoefnagel, C. A., Valdes Olmos, R. A. & Boot, H. 1996. Combined diagnostic imaging with ^{131}I-MIBG and "'in-pentetreotide in carcinoid tumours. *Eur J Cancer*, 32, 1924-1932.

Taal, B. G., Hoefnagel, C. A., Valdes Olmos, R. A., Boot, H. & Beijnen, J. H. 1996. Palliative effect of metaiodobenzylguanidine in metastatic carcinoid tumors. *J. Clin. Oncol.*, 14, 1829-1838.

Teunissen, J. J., Kwekkeboom, D. J. & Krenning, E. P. 2004. Quality of life in patients with gastroenteropancreatic tumors treated with [^{177}Lu-DOTA0,Tyr3]octreotate. *J. Clin. Oncol.*, 22, 2724-2729.

Teunissen, J. J. M. 2009. Effects of therapy with [^{177}Lu-DOTA0,Tyr3]octreotate on endocrine function. *Eur. J. Nucl. Med. Mol. Imaging*, 36, 1758-1766.

Teunissen, J. J. M., Kwekkeboom, D. J., Valkema, R. & Krenning, E. P. 2011. Nuclear medicine techniques for the imaging and treatment of neuroendocrine tumours. *Endocrine-Related Cancer*, 18, S27–S51.

Tonini, T., Rossi, F., Claudio, P. P. 2003. Molecular basis of angiogenesis and cancer. *Oncogene*, 22, 6549-6556.

Trampal, C., Engler, H., Juhlin, C., Bergström, M. & Långström, B. 2004. Pheochromocytomas: detection with ^{11}C hydroxyephedrine PET. *Radiology*, 230, 423-428.

Troncone, L. & Rufini, V. 2004. *MIBG in diagnosis of neuroendocrine tumors.* Nuclear Medicine in Clinical Diagnosis and Treatment, 3rd edn. Ell PJ, Gambhir SS, Eds. London: Churchill Livingstone, 83-95.

Troncone, L., Rufini, V., Montemaggi, P., Danza, F. M., Lasorella, A. & Mastrangelo, R. 1990. The diagnostic and therapeutic utility of radioiodinated metaiodobenzylguanidine (MIBG): 5 years of experience. *Eur. J. Nucl. Med.*, 16, 325-335.

Valk, T. W., Frager, M. S., Gross, M. D., Sisson, J. C., Wieland, D. M., Swanson, D. P., Mangner, T. J. & Beierwaltes, W. H. 1981. Spectrum of pheochromocytoma in multiple endocrine neoplasia. A scintigraphic portrayal using 131I-metaiodobenzylguanidine. *Ann. Intern. Med.*, 94, 762-777.

Valkema, R., De Jong, M., Bakker, W. H., Breeman, W. A., Kooij, P. P., Lugtenburg, P. J., De Jong, F. H., Christiansen, A., Kam, B. L., De Herder, W. W., Stridsberg, M., Lindemans, J., Ensing, G., Krenning, E. P. 2002. Phase I study of peptide receptor radionuclide therapy with [In-DTPA]octreotide: the Rotterdam experience. *Semin. Nucl. Med.*, 32, 110-122.

Valkema, R., Froberg, A. C., Bakker, W., Maecke, H. R., Breeman, W. A., de Jong, M. & Krenning, E. P. 2007. Peptide receptor scintigraphy (PRS) with In-111-DOTANOC and peptide receptor radionuclide therapy (PRRT) with Lu-177-DOTANOC. *J. Nucl. Med.*, 48, 394.

Valkema, R., Jamar, F., Bakker, W. H., Norenberg, J., Smith, C., Stolz, B. *et al.,* 2001. Safety and efficacy of [Y-90-DOTA, Tyr(3)]octreotide (Y-90-SMT487;OCTREOTHERTM) peptide receptor radionuclide therapy (PRRT): preliminary results of a phase-I study (abstract OS-248). *Eur. J. Nucl. Med.*, 28(Suppl), 1025P.

Valkema, R., Pauwels, S., Kvols, L. K., Barone, R., Jamar, F., Bakker, W. H., Kwekkeboom, D. J., Bouterfa, H. & Krenning, E. P. 2006. Survival and response after peptide receptor radionuclide therapy with [^{90}Y-DOTA0 Tyr3] octreotide in patients with advanced gastroenteropancreatic neuroendocrine tumors. *Semin. Nucl. Med.*, 36, 147-156.

Valkema, R., Pauwels, S. A., Kvols, L. K., Kwekkeboom, D. J., Jamar, F., De Jong, M., Barone, R., Walrand, S., Kooij, P. P., Bakker, W. H., Lasher, J. & Krenning, E. P. 2005. Long-term follow-up of renal function after peptide receptor radiation therapy with (90)YDOTA(0),Tyr(3)-octreotide and (177)Lu-DOTA(0),Tyr(3)-octreotate. *J. Nucl. Med.*, 46(Suppl 1), 83S-91S.

Valsamaki, P., Gerali, S., Arka, A., Kotsias, D., Lucchetti, S., Psarrakos, K., Zerva, C. & Gotzamani-Psarrakou, A. 2004. A patient with MEN-IIA syndrome due to *de novo* mutation and papillary thyroid carcinoma; the role of ^{99m}Tc-depreotide in diagnosing metastases and brief review of the literature. Hell. *J. Nucl. Med.*, 7, 168-173.

Valsamaki, P., Gotzamani-Psarrakou, A., Tsiouris, S., Molyvda-Athanasopoulou, E., Psarrakos, K., Papantoniou, V., Gerali, S. & Zerva, C. 2006. Tc-99m depreotide imaging of I-131-negative recurrent metastatic papillary thyroid carcinoma. *Int J Cancer,* 119, 968-970.

Van der Harst, E., De Herder, W. W., Bruining, H. A., Bonjer, H. J., De Krijger, R. R., Lamberts, S. W. J., Van De Meiracker, A. H., Boomsma, F., Stijnen, T., Krenning, E. P., Bosman, F. T. & Kwekkeboom, D. J. 2001. [^{123}I]metaiodobenzylguanidine and [^{111}In]octreotide uptake in benign and malignant pheochromocytomas. *J. Clin. Endocrinol. Metab.*, 86, 685-693.

Van Essen, M., Krenning, E. P., De Jong, M., Valkema, R. & Kwekkeboom, D. J. 2007. Peptide receptor radionuclide therapy with radiolabelled somatostatin analogues in patients with somatostatin receptor positive tumors. *Acta Oncol*, 46, 723-734.

Van Essen, M., Krenning, E. P., Kam, B. L., De Herder, W. W., Feelders, R. A. & Kwekkeboom, D. J. 2010. Salvage therapy with ^{177}Lu-octreotate in patients with bronchial and gastroenteropancreatic neuroendocrine tumors. *J. Nucl. Med.*, 51, 383-390.

Van Essen, M., Krenning, E. P., Kam, B. L., De Herder, W. W., Van Aken, M. O. & Kwekkeboom, D. J. 2008. Report on short-term side effects of treatments with ^{177}Lu-octreotate in combination with capecitabine in seven patients with gastroenteropancreatic neuroendocrine tumours. Eur. *J. Nucl. Med. Mol. Imaging*, 35, 743-748.

Virgolini, I., Britton, K., Buscombe, J., Moncayo, R., Paganelli, G. & Riva, P. 2002. In- and Y-DOTA-lanreotide: results and implications of the MAURITIUS trial. *Semin. Nucl. Med.*, 32, 148-155.

Virgolini, I., Traub-Weidinger, T. & Decristoforo, C. 2005. Nuclear medicine in the detection and management of pancreatic islet-cell tumours. *Best Practice & Research: Clin. Endocrinol. Metab.*, 19, 213-227.

Wadas, T. J., Eiblmaier, M., Zheleznyak, A., Sherman, C. D., Ferdani, R., Liang, K., Achilefu, S. & Anderson, C. J. 2008. Preparation and biological evaluation of ^{64}Cu-CB-TE$_2$A-sst$_2$-ANT, a somatostatin antagonist for PET imaging of somatostatin receptor-positive tumors. *J. Nucl. Med.*, 49, 1819-1827.

Wadsak, W. Mitterhauser, M., Rendl, G., Schuetz, M., Mien, L. K., Ettlinger, D. E., Dudczak, R., Kletter, K. & Karanikas, G. 2006. [^{18}F]FETO for adrenocortical PET imaging: a pilot study in healthy volunteers. *Eur. J. Nucl. Med. Mol. Imaging*, 33, 669-672.

Waldherr, C., Pless, M., Mäcke, H. R., Haldemann, A. & Mueller-Brand, J. 2001. The clinical value of [^{90}Y-DOTA]-D-Phe1-Tyr3-octreotide (^{90}Y-DOTATOC) in the treatment of neuroendocrine tumors: a clinical phase II study. *Ann. Oncol.*, 12, 941-945.

Waldherr, C., Pless, M., Mäcke, H. R., Schumacher, T., Crazzolara, A., Nitzsche, E. U., Haldemann, A. & Müller-Brand, J. 2002. Tumor response and clinical benefit in neuroendocrine tumors after 7.4 GBq ^{90}Y-DOTATOC. *J. Nucl. Med.*, 43, 610-616.

Wehrmann, C., Senftleben, S., Zachert, C., Müller, D. & Baum, R. P. 2007. Results of individual patient dosimetry in peptide receptor radionuclide therapy with ^{177}Lu DOTA-TATE and ^{177}Lu DOTA-NOC. *Cancer Biotherapy & Radiopharmaceuticals*, 22, 406-416.

Welchick, M. G., Alavi, A., Kressel, H. Y. & Engelman, K. 1989. Localisation of pheochromocytoma: MIBG, CT and MRI correlation. *J. Nucl. Med.*, 30, 328-336.

Westlin, J. E., Janson, E. T., Arnberg, H., Ahlstrom, H., Oberg, K. & Nilsson, S. 1993 Somatostatin receptor scintigraphy of carcinoid tumours using the [^{111}In-DTPA-D-Phe1]-octreotide. *Acta Oncol*, 32, 783-786.

Whithers, H. R. 1992. *Biologic basis of radiation therapy*, in Perez CA, Brady LW (eds): Principles and Practice of Radiation Oncology (ed 2). Philadelphia, PA, JB Lippincott Company, 64.

Wild, D., Schmitt, J. S., Ginj, M., Macke, H. R., Bernard, B. F., Krenning, E., De Jong, M., Wenger, S. & Reubi, J. C. 2003. DOTA-NOC, a high-affinity ligand of somatostatin receptor subtypes 2, 3 and 5 for labelling with various radiometals. *Eur. J. Nucl. Med. Mol. Imaging*, 30, 1338-1347.

Wild, D., Macke, H. R., Waser, B., Reubi, J. C., Ginj, M., Rasch, H., Muller-Brand, J. & Hofmann, M. 2005. ^{68}Ga-DOTANOC: a first compound for PET imaging with high affinity for somatostatin receptor subtypes 2 and 5. *Eur. J. Nucl. Med. Mol. Imaging*, 32, 724.

Win, Z., *Al*-Nahhas, A., Towey, D., Todd, J. F., Rubello, D., Lewington, V. & Gishen, P. 2007. ^{68}Ga-DOTATATE PET in neuroectodermal tumours: first experience. *Nucl. Med. Commun.*, 28, 359-363.

Yanik, G. A., Levine, J. E., Matthay, K. K., Sisson, J. C., Shulkin, B. L., Shapiro, B., Hubers, D., Spalding, S., Braun, T., Ferrara, J. L. M. &.Hutchinson R. J. 2002. Pilot study of iodine-131- metaiodobenzylguanidine in combination with myeloablative chemotherapy and autologous stem-cell support for the treatment of neuroblastoma. *J. Clin. Oncol.*, 20, 2142-2149.

Yao, J. C., Hassan, M., Phan, A., Dagohoy, C., Leary, C., Mares, J. E., Abdalla, E. K., Fleming, J. B., Vauthey, J. N., Rashid, A. & Evans, D. B. 2008. One hundred years after "carcinoid": epidemiology of and prognostic factors for neuroendocrine tumors in 35,825 cases in the United States. *J. Clin. Oncol.*, 26, 3063-3072.

Zaidi, H. & Alavi, A. 2007. Current trends in PET and combined (PET/CT and PET/MR) systems design. *PET Clinics*, 2, 109-123.

Zimmer, T., Stolzel, U., Bader, M., Koppenhagen, K., Hamm, B., Buhr, H., Riecken, E. O. & Wiedenmann, B. 1996. Endoscopic ultrasonography and somatostatin receptor scintigraphy in the preoperative localisation of insulinomas and gastrinomas. *Gut*, 39, 562-568.

Send Orders for Reprints to reprints@benthamscience.net
352 Cutting Edge Therapies for Cancer in the 21st Century, 2014, 352-386

CHAPTER 11

Using Molecular Prognostic Markers as a Basis for Designing Novel Oral Cancer Therapeutics

Faizan Alawi[1,*] and John J. Sauk[2]

[1]Department of Pathology, School of Dental Medicine, Department of Dermatology, School of Medicine, University of Pennsylvania, Philadelphia, PA, USA and [2]School of Dentistry and R. Brown Cancer Center, University of Louisville, Louisville, Kentucky, USA

Abstract: The primary objective of cancer classification is to predict a patient's response to a panel of treatment modalities, thereby guiding the development of a rational therapy and optimizing therapeutic success. However, traditional staging methods used to classify oral squamous cell carcinoma (OSCC) are marginally effective in predicting clinical outcomes. Emerging data and increasingly refined and cost-effective high-throughput technologies have the potential to advance oral cancer classification and treatment beyond the empiric towards a more molecularly-defined, individualized approach. Yet, despite an increasing appreciation of the diverse genomic, proteomic and epigenetic aberrations associated with OSCC, the promise of basing OSCC treatment decisions on molecular biomarkers has yet to be realized. Herein, we highlight a few specific examples of well-studied or intriguing prognostic biomarkers, and include a brief review of high-throughput technologies that have been used in the study of OSCC, and that could emerge as critical tools in the prediction of OSCC prognosis and in the design of novel oral cancer therapeutics. In the age of molecular therapeutics and personalized cancer medicine, this is likely to take the form of drugs or other compounds targeted to specific proteins or other cellular components, and with a minimal side effect profile.

Keywords: Oral squamous cell carcinoma, patient-tailored therapy, prognosis, cancer biomarkers, epigenetics, high-throughput technology, biomarker, hypoxia inducible factor-1A (HIF1A), MYC, RNA, microRNA, epigenetics, p16, histone modifications.

1. INTRODUCTION

Histopathology is still regarded as the "gold standard" for cancer diagnosis, and also plays a central role in the selection of treatment modalities and the

***Address correspondence to Faizan Alawi:** Department of Pathology, School of Dental Medicine, University of Pennsylvania, Philadelphia, PA USA; Tel: (215) 573-7638; E-mail: falawi@upenn.edu

predication of outcomes. However, analysis founded on histopathology, is commonly recognized as more of an art than science. Typically, pathologists describe different morphological features in tumors, nonetheless, the relative impact of each on patient outcome and tumor progression remains unclear (Bearer *et al.,* 2009). Consequently, determining the clinical predictive value from histological epidemiology continues to be inadequate. Nevertheless, the value of histopathologic analysis is that it does not rely on any single feature alone and thus obtains a comprehensive view of the entire morphological behavior of any particular tumor at the time of biopsy or excision. There is, however, a recognized need for more foretelling criteria that embrace a spectrum of treatment strategies, which has spawned the need to embrace physical and molecular parameters that incorporate diagnostic criteria that are more useful as prognostics. The literature is replete in articles related to prognostic factors, although results frequently differ on the significance of certain markers in predicting outcomes. In many instances patient data is lacking and the level of sampling is inadequate. To begin to address this problem the National Cancer Institute-European Organisation for Research and Treatment of Cancer (NCI-EORTC) First International Meeting on Cancer Diagnostics made a major recommendation of the development of guidelines for the reporting of tumor marker studies. Subsequently, reporting recommendations for tumor marker prognostic studies guidelines (REMARK) were formulated to promote the quality and reporting of results of prognostic factors in cancer; the guidelines are available at http://www.cancerdiagnosis.nci.nih.gov/assessment /progress/clinical.html (McShane *et al.,* 2006).

More recently, Halabi and Owzar (Halabi and Owzar 2010) have highlighted the importance of identifying and validating prognostic factors at the time of diagnosis or initial treatment. The authors point out that assessment of prognostic factors, which relate baseline clinical and experimental covariables to outcomes, is one of the major objectives in patient care and clinical research. They note that customarily, the incentive for the identification of prognostic factors was the necessity to correctly estimate the effect of treatment adjusting for these variables. However, it has become more apparent that the variability in outcome may be related to prognostic factors rather than to differences in treatments.

Recently, physical oncology has evolved as a discipline to address many of the above challenges and to achieve a higher level of prognostics (Deisboeck *et al.,* 2011, Lowengrub *et al.,* 2010). The goal of this approach is to provide information about tumor behavior in predictive, diagnostic, and therapeutic domains by integrating information from individual or multiple specimens across many variables. These may include: genetic alterations, mitotic rates, tumor size, and vascular parameters; and across multiple dimensions, from molecular distribution, dynamic diffusivity, cellular organelle and cell body shape and behavior, tumor growth dynamics, to whole body physiology (Bearer *et al.,* 2009, Deisboeck *et al.,* 2011, Frieboes *et al.,* 2011, Lowengrub *et al.,* 2010). To date this approach has been applied to brain tumors and some breast cancers (Frieboes *et al.,* 2011). For example, quantitative multiscale models have predicted that morphologic instability of a tumor mass, *i.e.*, morphology resulting in finger-like irregularity (Frieboes *et al.,* 2011, Michor 2008) of the tumor margin, may provide a powerful tissue-invasion mechanism since it allows tumor cells to escape growth limitations imposed by diffusion and invade the host independently of the extent of angiogenesis (Frieboes *et al.,* 2011, Harpold *et al.,* 2007). This led subsequently to find that as new clones arise, those with more survival capabilities invade the original tumor as well as adjacent tissue (Bearer *et al.,* 2009). These aggressive clones replace original tumor cells, which are more likely to die as growth rate increases and oxygen levels decrease. This sequence produces a striking level of instability and results in further disordered cellular behavior and architecture, metabolic consumption, oxygen levels, extracellular matrix fluidics, tension and/or density, and vascular permeability. Consequently, this approach to modeling revealed that oxygen and/or nutrient gradients are a major driver of malignant progression. Thus, cells which escape and survive at low oxygen tension likely have increased invasive and mitotic potential (Bearer *et al.,* 2009). Noteworthy, is that this conclusion preceded the outcomes from bevacizumab (Avastin, Genentech) therapy, where withdrawal from the drug results in rapid tumor regrowth (Frieboes *et al.,* 2011). The present review does not seek to develop a physical oncology for oral squamous cell carcinomas (OSCC) but rather examines molecular parameters that would be included in a strategy to yield a more consistent set of prognostics thereby leading to more effective and novel OSCC therapeutics.

The primary objective of cancer classification is to predict a patient's response to a panel of treatment modalities, thereby guiding the development of a rational therapy and optimizing therapeutic success. However, traditional staging methods used to classify OSCC are marginally effective in predicting clinical outcomes.

One of the key metrics used in assessing prognosis of oral cancer is the disease status of lymph nodes. It has long been apparent that presence of lymph node metastasis in OSCC may decrease the survival rate by up to 50%, in that the neck is often the point of treatment failure and recurrence of OSCC (Huang *et al.*, 2009c, Huang and O'Sullivan 2013). Since the presence of lymphatic metastasis can adversely impact prognosis and significantly affect the selection of a treatment regimen, the presence of nodal disease has been included as a vital component of the cancer staging system. However, based on current cancer taxonomy genetically heterogeneous tumors that possess distinct clinical phenotypes are often lumped together. Moreover, while most OSCCs appear histologically similar, notwithstanding the degree of differentiation, OSCCs may also be subdivided at the molecular level based upon exposure to certain risk factors (Lingen *et al.*, 2000, Ostwald *et al.*, 2000).

Several reports have identified distinct molecular differences in the pathogenesis of lung cancers in smokers and never-smokers (Kim *et al.*, 2001, Marsit *et al.*, 2005). The same may hold true for smoking-related OSCCs *versus* those that develop in non-smokers. There may even be sex-related differences between male and female smokers and non-smokers, respectively. Chronic sunlight exposure is the most important risk factor for SCC of the lower lip. To this end, p53 mutations are more prevalent in tumors of the lower lip than in OSCCs of other anatomic sites (Ostwald *et al.*, 2000). Cheong *et al.*, (Cheong *et al.*, 2009a) identified a host of genes that were differentially expressed between OSCCs derived from smokers in relation to those in betel quid chewers in a South Asian population. Finally, approximately 15-20% of OSCCs develop in patients who don't have any known risk factors. Lingen *et al.*, (Lingen *et al.*, 2000) found that overexpression of p53 in SCC of the tongue in young patients with no known risk factors was not associated with mutations in exons 5-9 (the most common sites for p53 mutations). This led to the hypothesis that OSCC in individuals under the age of 40 with no known risk factors may constitute a unique subset of OSCC. It is important to note that while human papillomavirus (HPV) is recognized as a significant risk factor for oropharyngeal squamous cell carcinoma, HPV is not a risk factor for OSCC and likely does not explain the increased prevalence of OSCC in young adults (Lingen *et al.,* 2013, O'Regan *et al.,* 2008).

Since current oral cancer therapy is dictated by the clinical stage of disease, the identification of groups of OSCCs with distinct genetic, epigenetic and/or proteomic “signatures” may provide a powerful tool in the prediction of clinical outcome for patients. Indeed, studies of other cancer types now provide compelling evidence that molecular profiling can be used to guide therapeutic decision-making and predict clinical outcomes. In a retrospective study by van ‘t Veer *et al.,* (van 't Veer *et al.,* 2003), distinct groups of genes were identified in primary breast tumors that significantly correlated with a poor clinical prognosis. The predictive power of these molecular profiles to identify patients with a poor prognosis was significantly greater than that of traditionally used approaches. The authors further determined that had molecular forecasting been available at the time of initial treatment planning, the recommended treatment for 45-65% of patients would have been combined surgery and radiotherapy. In contrast, based on the histologic and clinical guidelines available at the time, these same patients were unnecessarily advised to receive adjuvant chemotherapy, thus subjecting them to the debilitating side-effects typically associated with cytotoxic medications. Studies of other cancer types, including non-Hodgkin lymphoma and neuroblastoma, have also yielded somewhat similar findings (Cho *et al.,* 2011, Dhanasekaran *et al.,* 2001, Nutt *et al.,* 2003, Pugh *et al.,* 2012).

Despite an increasing appreciation of the diverse genomic, proteomic and epigenetic aberrations associated with OSCC, the promise of basing OSCC treatment decisions on molecular biomarkers has yet to be realized. Indeed, a tumor-derived marker does not always imply its usefulness as a tumor biomarker. Nonetheless, emerging data and increasingly refined and cost-effective, high-throughput technologies have the potential to advance oral cancer classification and treatment beyond the empiric towards a more molecularly-defined, individualized approach. Herein, we highlight a few specific examples of well-studied or intriguing prognostic biomarkers, and include a brief review of high-throughput technologies that have been used in the study of OSCC, and that could yet emerge as critical tools in the prediction of OSCC prognosis.

2. GENOMIC DNA BIOMARKERS

A variety of molecular and cytogenetic abnormalities have been identified in OSCC that may potentially contribute to the malignant phenotype and influence clinical progression. Historically, these genomic changes were identified through a variety of cumbersome techniques that were generally impractical for routine clinical usage. More recently, automatable, array-based comparative genomic hybridization (aCGH) and the use of high-density single nucleotide polymorphism (SNP) arrays, have led to a significant advance in our understanding of the genomic changes that are associated with OSCC and may hold promise as diagnostic and prognostic tools (Mei *et al.,* 2000, Peng *et al.,* 2011, Sparano *et al.,* 2006).

Comparative genomic hybridization provides a genome-wide assessment of DNA copy number variations. The advent of aCGH has enabled detection of these genomic changes at a resolution of less than 1 megabase, which is a much higher resolution than was previously possible (Sparano *et al.,* 2006). In addition to identifying regions of DNA amplification, homozygous deletions and single copy losses can be mapped across the entire genome within a single hybridization experiment. This technology has been used in the study of a wide spectrum of cancers and normal tissues, and identified genome copy variations have been catalogued in the Database of Genomic Variants (Iafrate *et al.,* 2004, Zhang *et al.,* 2006).

With increased refinement of aCGH technology, novel genome copy changes are still being discovered. Nonetheless, there are several important considerations one needs to take into account when proposing the use of aCGH for diagnostic purposes. aCGH detects copy number variations and not absolute copy number changes. Thus, a tumor harboring perfectly tetraploid cells would potentially yield data that is indistinguishable from diploid cells; aCGH does not provide information on DNA ploidy status. The use of formalin-fixed tissues or an insufficient amount of DNA available for analysis from fresh clinical samples also prove to be common technical barriers in the use of this technology. In addition,

OSCCs are genetically heterogeneous tumors. Thus, OSCCs harbor dozens of distinct chromosomal regions exhibiting either amplification or deletion (Garnis *et al.,* 2004a, Mei *et al.,* 2000, Peng *et al.,* 2011, Sparano *et al.,* 2006). Variability between the data of different studies may be a result of the types of OSCCs analyzed, the inclusion of biologically distinct oropharyngeal cancers, the array platform used (custom-designed *versus* commercially-available), or the methods by which the samples were procured and processed. In some studies, the samples were enriched for malignant epithelium either through gross dissection or laser-capture micro-dissection. In other studies, the experimental samples either included the epithelial and mesenchymal tissues for analysis, or the method by which the samples were procured was not specified. Thus, while aCGH studies have yielded a wealth of information, the cumulative findings have also yielded inconsistencies and contradictory data. Notwithstanding the experimental variability, some of the reported genomic copy changes are recurrent not only in a majority of OSCCs within a given study, but also across independent studies. Several of these genomic changes are discussed here.

Most of the early studies made use of aCGH to establish differences between OSCC and non-transformed oral mucosa (Garnis *et al.,* 2004a, Garnis *et al.,* 2004b, Garnis *et al.,* 2004c, Garnis *et al.,* 2009). More recent studies have identified genomic changes that may differentiate OSCCs based on etiology. Importantly, recurrent genome copy variations may also be associated with relevant clinical parameters, including disease-specific survival, local and regional relapse, distant metastasis, and/or the risk for second primary tumors. In particular, DNA amplifications within regions on chromosomes 3q26-27, 7p11, and 11q13, respectively, have all been individually associated with increased clinical stage, increased incidence of cervical lymph node metastasis and reduced overall survival (Chiang *et al.,* 2008, Garnis *et al.,* 2004b, Garnis *et al.,* 2009, Mei *et al.,* 2000, Peng *et al.,* 2011, Sheu *et al.,* 2009, Sparano *et al.,* 2006, Sugahara *et al.,* 2011). The link between prognostic variables and the aforementioned genome copy variants has been observed in several independent studies. Several reports suggest that amplification of epidermal growth factor receptor (EGFR) may at least partially explain the association of 7p11 amplification with increased lymph node metastasis (Chiang *et al.,* 2008, Garnis *et al.,* 2004a, Sheu *et al.,* 2009). EGFR is a cell-surface receptor kinase whose activation can be triggered by an array of different ligands. Once activated, EGFR sparks a wide-spread signal transduction cascade, thereby stimulating DNA replication, cell proliferation, cell migration, and other cellular functions that potentiate the malignant phenotype.

Several genes implicated in oral carcinogenesis and prognosis are encoded within the 11q13 amplicon (Garnis *et al.,* 2004a, Huang *et al.,* 2002, Martin *et al.,* 2008, Sugahara *et al.,* 2011). These include cyclin D1 (CCND1), cortactin (CTTN), fibroblast growth factor 3 (FGF3), FGF4, and oral cancer overexpressed protein 1A (ORAOV1). CCND1 is an important cell cycle regulatory factor and is amplified in a host of different cancer types. Overexpression of cyclin D1 in anterior tongue cancers may be associated with increased lymph node stage, increased tumor grade, and reduced disease-free and overall survival (Myo *et al.,* 2005). CTTN is commonly upregulated in SCCs of the head and neck. CTTN regulates cytoskeletal organization and cellular adhesion, and high levels promote tumor cell invasion and metastasis (Sugahara *et al.,* 2011). FGF3 and FGF4 are often co-amplified in cancers and have an array of functions that potentiate the malignant phenotype including invasion and metastasis (Hillbertz *et al.,* 2012, Sugahara *et al.,* 2011). ORAOV1 amplification has been significantly associated with poor histological differentiation, larger tumor size, lymph node metastasis, and advanced clinical stage (Hillbertz *et al.,* 2012, Huang *et al.,* 2002, Jiang *et al.,* 2009). It has been suggested that ORAOV1 may be the primary driving force behind the prognostic associations of the 11q13 amplicon (Huang *et al.,* 2002). The cellular functions of ORAOV1, which was originally described as an oral cancer marker, remain poorly understood; regulatory roles in potentiating cell growth and angiogenesis have been attributed to this putative oncogene.

A deletion of a region on 3p26 has also been strongly associated with poor prognostic outcome (Partridge *et al.,* 1996, Uchida *et al.,* 2011). Similarly, a copy number decrease at 3p14 may also be a relatively common occurrence in OSCC (Uzawa *et al.,* 2001). The fragile histidine triad (FHIT) gene is located within this genomic locus and loss of FHIT expression may be a predictor of poor outcome in tongue cancer; FHIT plays an important role in purine metabolism (Uzawa *et al.,* 2001). While the association of 3p14 deletion and prognosis has not been assessed, with further study, these and other DNA copy variations may become clinically relevant biomarkers in patients with OSCC.

Another important drawback of aCGH technology is that not all genetically-relevant changes can be identified (Sparano *et al.,* 2006). While single copy gains and losses can be detected by aCGH, large copy number variations remain much easier to detect. Hence, clinically relevant genomic aberrations may be missed or under-represented in the final analysis. Moreover, not all genome copy variations are pathologic. Some are considered naturally-occurring polymorphisms and are found within specific subsets of the general population. A cursory review of the Database of Genomic Variants (Iafrate *et al.,* 2004, Zhang *et al.,* 2006) reveals only a minority of catalogued regions that actually harbor known genes or other functional sequences. Thus, in addition to false-negatives, false-positives can also occur whereby in the absence of a patient-matched control, there is a risk for over-interpretation of copy number variations which may simply represent genomic polymorphisms. Further study is needed to determine the association between genome-level polymorphisms and risk of OSCC development and/or progression.

Similar to aCGH, SNP arrays allow for genome-wide analysis of DNA copy variations but also offer several additional advantages (Mei *et al.,* 2000, Peng *et al.,* 2011, Xu *et al.,* 2010). In particular, SNP array analysis can detect not only copy-neutral genomic variations but also other patterns of allelic imbalance, including loss of heterozygosity (LOH). LOH is an important mechanism by which tumor suppressor genes become inactivated, thereby increasing the risk for neoplastic progression. Several tumor suppressor genes, including TP53 and $p16^{INK4a}$, play important roles in oral carcinogenesis. Loss of $p16^{INK4a}$ expression is generally associated with a less favorable prognosis than OSCCs expressing high levels of $p16^{INK4a}$ (Perez-Sayans *et al.,* 2011a). $p16^{INK4a}$ is found in a region on chromosome 9p21 which is frequently deleted during the course of OSCC development. LOH at this and other genomic sites can also occur through other molecular changes, including chromosome nondisjunction, mitotic recombination, gene conversion, and others. These latter mechanisms do not result in DNA copy variations and are therefore invisible by aCGH analysis. In contrast, they would be detected by SNP array analysis.

Two recent studies suggest use of SNP array technology in the study of OSCC may have important prognostic utility. Using a commercially available SNP array, Peng *et al.,* (Peng *et al.,* 2011) reported that 61 distinct and previously unidentified copy number variations on 8q22-24 were significantly associated with extracapsular lymph node spread and disease-specific death within the first five years after OSCC diagnosis. In addition, the authors determined that patients with these amplifications were more likely to develop a second primary tumor at an earlier time than those without the amplifications. Recurrent copy number variations were also detected on several other chromosomes, but their association with clinical parameters was not assessed.

Of the genes encoded within the amplified regions on 8q22-24, the authors identified the MYC transcription factor and several additional genes that are either directly or indirectly regulated by MYC (Peng *et al.,* 2011). This supports the notion that MYC and its associated transcriptome may negatively influence the prognosis of OSCC. However, it is important to note that other studies have yielded a less convincing association between MYC amplification and oral cancer prognosis. Thus, further study is still needed before MYC can be considered a bona fide prognostic biomarker.

In addition to MYC, the authors identified twenty-four genes within the amplified genomic regions that were also shown to be individual predictors of second primary malignancies, local or regional tumor relapse, distant metastasis and/or poor survival. Importantly, 22 of the 24 genes have been previously implicated in tumorigenesis; 11 of 24 have been related to oral carcinogenesis. One of these genes, DEPTOR, encodes a regulatory inhibitor of the mammalian target of rapamycin (mTOR) complex 1 and is upregulated in various cancer types (Wang *et al.,* 2012b). High levels of DEPTOR in thyroid carcinoma are associated with locoregional tumor spread, distant metastasis, increased recurrence and poor overall survival (Wang *et al.,* 2012b). However, the actual mechanisms by which DEPTOR participates in tumor progression remain to be determined. Thus, while genome copy variations may eventually yield clinically relevant information, much study remains to be done in determining whether the actual genes encoded within these regions are prognostically relevant.

Using a commercially available SNP array that was different from the one employed by Peng *et al.,* (Peng *et al.,* 2011), Xu *et al.,* (Xu *et al.,* 2010) also identified several known and novel DNA copy number alterations within their own sample set of OSCCs. These included amplifications of 3q21-29, 20q, 8q21-24, 11q13; amplifications in these latter two loci were also reported by the Peng group. Xu *et al.,* (Xu *et al.,* 2010) also identified several deletions within regions of chromosomes 9p21, 18q11, and 22q. A true genome-wide analysis of the tumors was not performed since portions of five different chromosomes were not represented on the SNP array employed in this study. Thus, the results of these two SNP array studies cannot be directly compared. Nonetheless, both studies determined that amplification of 11q13 was significantly associated with increased lymph node metastasis and poor survival. As noted above, several independent aCGH analyses also yielded similar associations between 11q13 amplification and poor OSCC prognosis (Huang *et al.,* 2002, Sugahara *et al.,* 2011). While promising as a potential prognostic biomarker, further study is needed before 11q13 amplification can be routinely assessed in patients with OSCC.

While SNP arrays are often used to detect copy number variations, they can also identify sequence changes at the gene level. Single nucleotide chromosomal or gene variations may be enough to cause allelic imbalance, thereby significantly increasing disease susceptibility. To date, a variety of gene SNPs have been linked to OSCC susceptibility (Munoz-Guerra *et al.,* 2009, Tu *et al.,* 2008, Vaezi *et al.,* 2011, Wang *et al.,* 2012a). In contrast, prognostically relevant SNPs have been identified only within a limited number of genes; two examples are described here.

Hypoxia inducible factor-1A (HIF1A) is a transcription factor that directly and indirectly regulates the expression of several gene products that promote angiogenesis and tissue oxygenation, including vascular endothelial growth factor (VEGF), erythropoeitin (EPO) and vasodilatatory factors such as inducible nitric oxide synthase (NOS2) (Munoz-Guerra *et al.,* 2009, Perez-Sayans *et al.,* 2011c). HIF1A also enhances glucose metabolism through activation of multiple glucose transporters and glycolytic enzymes, and optimizes mitochondrial respiration to sustain tumor growth in low oxygen microenvironments. These adaptive responses confer a growth advantage to hypoxic tumor cells and promote survival.

Upregulation of HIF1A is associated with advanced clinical stage, poor overall survival and reduced disease-free survival in patients with OSCC (Munoz-Guerra *et al.,* 2009, Perez-Sayans *et al.,* 2011c). However, even in the absence of HIF1A overexpression, a G1790A polymorphism in exon 12 of HIF1A is also significantly associated with disease-relapse and shorter disease-free survival in patients with OSCC and other cancer types (Munoz-Guerra *et al.,* 2009). In contrast, C1772T, which is another commonly occurring SNP and found within the same exon as G1790A, has no apparent bearing on prognosis. The exact mechanisms by which the G1790A SNP augments HIF1A function remain unclear.

In other studies, the presence of a T309G polymorphism in the HDM2 gene promoter, in conjunction with p53 mutation, strongly associated with increased frequency of extracapsular lymph node spread and poor disease-free OSCC survival (Huang *et al.,* 2009b). Similarly, the combination of HDM2 T309G and a G72C SNP in p53 was also shown to correlate with poor disease-free and overall survival, respectively (Tu *et al.,* 2008). T309G has also been implicated in the pathogenesis and prognosis of several other cancer types. HDM2 is a direct negative regulator of p53; this important molecular pathway plays an important role in OSCC progression. These cumulative findings, together with the use of larger sample sets, validation with independent test sets and additional refinement of the technology, suggests that SNP array analysis of OSCCs may have great value in discovery-type experiments, and may hold eventual promise as a diagnostic tool to aid in the prediction of prognosis and facilitate the goal of designing patient-tailored therapies.

3. RNA BIOMARKERS

3.1. Messenger RNA

High-resolution aCGH and SNP arrays can help prioritize candidate transcripts for further studies. Yet, it is a detailed analysis of the genes and other functional sequences, including non-coding RNA, found within these variant regions, and an understanding of their respective functions in oral carcinogenesis that will likely yield the most information. Attempts at finding molecular predictors of OSCC tumor aggressiveness have resulted in the identification of relatively few candidate genes whose expression levels may show sufficient prognostic utility in OSCC. While a comprehensive analysis of each putative biomarker is beyond the scope of this review, it is apparent that these genetic changes impact multiple molecular networks (Chen *et al.,* 2008, Liu *et al.,* 2012, Ziober *et al.,* 2006).

Dysregulation of MYC which is encoded within an amplified region on 8q24 has been associated with poor prognosis (Peng *et al.,* 2011). MYC is an essential transcription factor that directly and indirectly regulates the expression of 15% of all genes, including genes encoding microRNAs. MYC controls most if not all important cellular functions, including several implicated in tumorigenesis. Thus, the clinical outcome of OSCC may be more reliably predicted by the combined influence of several genes than by any individual gene. For this reason, microarray-based gene expression profiling has significantly advanced our understanding of OSCC and holds potential promise as a prognostic tool.

The technical component of a microarray analysis can be completed over a period of a few days. Briefly, total RNA is extracted from sample tissues, and messenger RNA (mRNA) is reverse transcribed into cDNA. During this process, fluorescent-labeled nucleotides are incorporated into the cDNA. The cDNA is then fragmented and hybridized to microarrays. While most high-throughput, discovery-type studies have made use of Affymetrix (Santa Clara, CA) gene arrays, a variety of commercial platforms are available (Liu *et al.,* 2012). As many as 33,000 distinct probes may be imprinted on these chips; the probes correspond to snippets of known gene sequences. After hybridization of the fluorescent-labeled cDNA to the array, a laser scanner is then used to collect the emission of the fluorescence signals. Following a series of complex bioinformatic and statistical analyses, the final output yields a quantitative assessment of relative gene expression levels. Validation of individual gene expression is usually performed using the original source RNA and quantitative reverse-transcription polymerase chain reaction.

The benefits of microarray-based gene expression profiling lie in the specific types of analyses being performed. In some studies, investigators examined the tumor "signatures" that distinguish OSCC from non-transformed oral epithelium. As an example, we previously identified a minimal 25-gene signature that could differentiate OSCC from patient-matched normal oral mucosa (Ziober *et al.,* 2006). Interestingly, this dataset was enriched for collagen and matrix metalloproteinase genes, including COL1A1, COL3A1, COL4A, COL5A1, COL5A2, COL11, MMP1, MMP9, and MMP11. The predictive value of this gene signature was further cross-validated using three separate and independent test sets with an average of 87% accuracy. In contrast, Chen *et al.,* showed that the combined dysregulated expression of only four genes, COL1A1, COL4A1, laminin gamma2 chain (LAMC2) and peptidyl arginine deiminase (PADI1), sufficiently and reliably differentiated OSCCs from non-transformed oral epithelium (Chen *et al.,* 2008).

Microarray analyses have also led to the identification of several genes linked together through the metabolic pathways that they collectively regulate, and which could be responsible for malignant transformation (Liu *et al.,* 2012). Furthermore, gene signatures may also differentiate OSCCs based on specific etiology (Cheong *et al.,* 2009b). Collectively, these types of findings may form the rationale for the eventual development of non-invasive technologies that could be used in mass screening, diagnosis and transformation risk assessment of patients with preneoplastic oral epithelial disease. However, for patients who have already developed OSCC, the true value of microarray-based gene expression profiling lies in the potential to associate distinct patterns of gene expression with prognosis and treatment response.

Gene profiling is currently being used to guide treatment in patients with breast cancer, lymphoma and other tumor types. To this end, gene signatures may also be superior identifiers and/or predictors of OSCC behavior and patient outcome than conventional clinical criteria. Tumor signatures have been identified that may be predictive of treatment response. Several independent groups have also identified OSCC expression profiles that can reliably predict the potential for regional lymph node metastasis. O'Donnell *et al.,* (O'Donnell *et al.,* 2005) identified a 116-gene signature that reliably differentiated regionally metastatic OSCCs from non-metastatic primary tumors. In contrast, Mendez *et al.,* (Mendez *et al.,* 2011) and Pasini *et al.,* (Pasini *et al.,* 2012) identified four-gene signatures that were predictive of lymph node metastasis. The Mendez dataset included MYO5A, RFN145, FBXO32 and CTONG2002744 while the Pasini signature included CSNK1A1, SCARB1, SPRR2B, and G3BP2. Reis *et al.,* (Reis *et al.,* 2011) showed that overexpression of only four genes, MMP1, COL4A1, P4HA2 and THBS2, in histologically normal surgical margins was highly predictive of local recurrence.

In the three aforementioned studies, there was no overlap between any of the four-gene signatures. Moreover, none of these genes were identified in the 116-gene signature reported by O'Donnell *et al.,* (O'Donnell *et al.,* 2005). Herein lies one of the most important reasons why gene expression profiling has not yet reached the clinical arena for patients with OSCC. Many of these high-throughput studies have used different microarray platforms. Alternatively, the clinical parameters being assessed and sample sizes have also varied between studies. The types of samples studied and inter- and intra-tumor heterogeneity may also be important factors. For example, some studies have made use of biopsy specimens while others used surgical resection specimens but without specifying how the samples were either procured or processed. Together, this wide variability makes it challenging to directly compare the results of one study to another. Before microarray-based gene expression profiling is accepted as a means by which to predict prognosis and guide OSCC therapy, large scale, multi-institutional studies need to be performed using the same microarray platform and validated using large independent test sets. The cost and time associated with these analyses also have to be reduced. Ultimately, an integrative approach using SNP arrays to assess genome variation combined with gene expression profiling may prove to be much more informative than either analysis alone (Peng *et al.,* 2011, Xu *et al.,* 2010, Serrano *et al.,* 2012). Since coding genes produce protein, protein arrays and other high-throughput techniques, including mass spectrometry, may also be considered. However, the use of protein-centric technologies in biomarker discovery and OSCC prognostication remains in its relative infancy.

3.2. MicroRNA

DNA is transcribed into coding and non-coding RNA (ncRNA). While much effort has been expended on gene discovery and analysis of protein function, mRNA only makes up a small percentage of the total RNA within a cell. In contrast, ncRNAs make up the vast majority of the RNA pool. While ribosomal RNA is the most abundant, small ncRNAs (< 250 nucleotides), including microRNAs (miRNAs), small nucleolar RNAs, small nuclear RNAs, and other small ncRNAs, also make up a large proportion of the human transcriptome (Lipovich *et al.,* 2010). Functionality of at least some of these ncRNAs in neoplasia is inferred from the observation that they exhibit altered expression in cancers, including OSCC (Nallar and Kalvakolanu 2013, Wu *et al.,* 2011). Of the various classes of ncRNAs, miRNAs have emerged as potentially important OSCC biomarkers, and some may hold clinical value.

MiRNAs are small 21-23 nucleotide RNA molecules that directly regulate post-transcriptional gene expression. There are currently over 2000 unique, annotated human miRNAs (Wu *et al.,* 2011). Several additional miRNA-like sequences, including a subset that are embedded within and processed from small nucleolar RNAs, remain to be annotated. Thus, it is very likely that the miRNA transcriptome will continue to expand.

MiRNAs are complementary to sequences found in 3'-untranslated regions of their target mRNA, but regulation may also occur through binding to sites within 5'-untranslated regions. It is estimated that at least 30% of all human mRNAs are targeted by miRNAs. While most miRNAs repress mRNA translation, activation of translation has also been described. As such, some miRNAs have been characterized as tumor suppressors while others as oncogenes. Thus, it is not surprising that miRNAs play critical roles in an array of cellular processes, including many that directly or indirectly influence tumorigenesis. It is in this regards that some investigators hypothesize a critically important role for miRNAs in cancer development and progression.

As with gene expression profiling, miRNA microarray-based expression profiling has yielded a wealth of intriguing data (Serrano *et al.,* 2012). However, the same caveats apply to studies investigating miRNA signatures as they do to aCGH and mRNA expression profiling. Differences in sample procurement, intra- and inter-tumoral heterogeneity, the use of various miRNA microarray or PCR-ready platforms, and variations in the clinical parameters being assessed and sample sizes analyzed are just some of experimental variables that make direct comparison of data between studies a challenge. In addition, differences in the amount of time between initial diagnosis and follow-up, or in the frequency of follow-ups may also influence the experimental results. Moreover, although miRNA profiling has been widely used in the study of cancer, OSCC has received relatively little attention. Nonetheless, there is at least some consistency between the results of different studies which suggests that specific miRNAs may eventually prove to be important prognostic biomarkers.

Distinct miRNA signatures have been shown to reliably differentiate OSCCs from non-transformed oral epithelium (Cervigne *et al.,* 2009). Moreover, Lajer *et al.,* (Lajer *et al.,* 2011) identified a panel of 18 distinct miRNAs that were reliably predictive of regional lymph node metastasis. Two of these differentially expressed miRNAs, miR-21 and miR-375, are of particular interest since several other investigators have also identified and validated these same miRNAs as predictors of OSCC survival (Li *et al.,* 2009, Wu *et al.,* 2011). High levels of miR-21 have been associated with poor prognosis in SCCs of the tongue and in cancers from a variety of other anatomic sites (Li *et al.,* 2009). Conversely, downregulation of miR-375 correlates with poor survival and metastasis, and may regulate tumor invasiveness of OSCCs and other head and neck SCCs (Harris *et al.,* 2012).

A given miRNA could potentially regulate the post-transcriptional expression of hundreds if not thousands of genes. Thus, the challenge of determining the impact of a particular miRNA on prognosis is directly related to understanding the complexity of the miRNA and its target gene interactions. An appreciation of this genetic complexity led Serrano *et al.,* (Serrano *et al.,* 2012) to employ multiple high-throughput platforms to simultaneously assess DNA copy number, and mRNA and miRNA expression profiles in OSCC. This integrative analysis did not identify miR-21 or miR-375 as being prognostically relevant, but did lead to the discovery of three miRNAs, miR-140-3p, miR-29a and miR-29c, which were differentially expressed between metastatic and non-metastatic OSCCs, and which showed strong positive correlation with their DNA copy numbers and a negative correlation with the expression of their target genes. This led the authors to conclude that genome copy number changes may lead to dysregulation of not only mRNAs but also miRNAs which, in turn, could influence OSCC prognosis. While these preliminary findings are intriguing and suggest the benefits of integrative genomic approaches in the study of OSCC, the clinical usefulness of these and other putative miRNA biomarkers remains premature and will require additional study.

As with coding genes, miRNA SNPs may also eventually hold clinical value (Chu *et al.,* 2012). Overexpression of miR-146 has been observed in OSCC and several other cancer types. As an individual variable, high levels of miR-146 have not yet been attributed any prognostic significance in OSCC. However, a report by Hung *et al.,* (Hung *et al.,* 2012) suggests that a G to C polymorphism (rs2910164) within the precursor miR-146 sequence influences the functionality of the mature miRNA and promotes clinical progression of OSCC. This polymorphism was found to be significantly more prevalent in OSCC patients with lymph node involvement compared to patients without lymph node metastasis.

To date, most miRNA-based studies like the ones referenced here have employed either microarrays for genome-wide assessments or PCR-based arrays in more targeted experimental approaches. However, the advent of next-generation deep sequencing technologies also holds significant promise in small ncRNA discovery and as a potential molecular diagnostic tool (Lipovich *et al.,* 2010). Current technology is cost-prohibitive and preparation of the samples for analysis is too labor-intensive for routine clinical usage. Nonetheless, compared to PCR- or microarray-based approaches, deep sequencing is unbiased and not limited by the content of the arrays. It can also be used to measure absolute RNA abundance and has a much wider dynamic range whereby a single sample yields millions of RNA sequence reads. This will enable the identification of not just individual known and novel mRNAs and small ncRNA transcripts, but also whole classes of previously unrecognized ncRNAs – small and large. To date, a comprehensive catalogue of the identity and function of ncRNAs in OSCC pathogenesis and as comparative predictors of prognosis is lacking. However, emerging evidence suggests that small nucleolar RNAs may also play a potential role in tumorigenesis (Nallar & Kalvakolanu 2013). We have observed that specific snoRNAs are significantly upregulated in oral cancer cell lines relative to non-transformed oral keratinocytes (Alawi F & Lin P, unpublished data). The roles of these ncRNAs in oral cancer development and prognosis are currently unknown. Thus, this clearly remains an intriguing avenue of study.

4. EPIGENETIC BIOMARKERS

Epigenetic modifications are defined as chromosomal changes that arise without alterations in the DNA sequence. Depending on the specific modifications, these regulatable and sometimes not heritable changes result in either condensation or decondensation of chromatin leading to silencing or activation of gene expression. Like mRNAs, miRNA expression can also be regulated by epigenetic mechanisms. Moreover, miRNA-induced gene silencing also falls under the rubric of epigenetics. Several epigenetic changes have been linked to OSCC development, but their use as biomarkers of prognosis remain only partially characterized. For the purposes of this discussion, we will only focus on DNA methylation and histone modifications.

4.1. DNA Methylation

DNA methylation is one of the most common and well-studied epigenetic modifications that are found in OSCC. A methyl group is covalently added to cytosine residues within CpG dinucleotides (Kulis and Esteller 2010). These CpG sequences are generally grouped within larger clusters known as CpG islands. Although found in low abundance throughout the genome, CpG islands are often enriched in or within close proximity of gene promoters and other transcriptional regulatory sites. It is estimated that close to 60% of all gene promoters contain CpG islands (Kulis & Esteller 2010).

In otherwise normal physiologic states (ie during development, growth, in healthy tissues, *etc.*), CpG islands are unmethylated in transcriptionally-active promoters, and methylated in transcriptionally-silent promoters. In pathologic states, including neoplasia, DNA methylation is dysregulated. In particular, DNA hypermethylation may lead to inactivation of an array of tumor suppressor genes that are relevant in carcinogenesis and may be of prognostic significance. Indeed, loss of tumor suppressor function arises more commonly from epigenetic silencing than genetic changes (Kulis & Esteller 2010). Specific gene promoters may be hypermethylated at different stages of tumorigenesis or in tissue-specific patterns (Su *et al.,* 2010). Evidence also suggests that OSCCs may be differentiated based on DNA methylation patterns, and that this may also influence prognosis (Hasegawa *et al.,* 2002, Huang *et al.,* 2009a, Su *et al.,* 2010, Supic *et al.,* 2009, Supic *et al.,* 2011a). DNA methylation may also be used to classify OSCCs based on etiology (Smith *et al.,* 2007).

There are a variety of methods available to assay DNA methylation, including bisulfite conversion of DNA followed by quantitative pyrosequencing, methylation-specific multiplex ligation-dependent probe amplification and/or sensitive melting analysis after real-time-methylation-specific PCR (Kulis & Esteller 2010). Bisulfite treatment converts unmethylated cytosines to uracil while methylated cytosines remain unchanged. Another commonly used approach includes the use of methylation-sensitive restriction enzymes which can digest target sequences only if they are unmethylated. A more detailed review of the various methylation assays is described by Kulis and Esteller (Kulis & Esteller 2010).

There are advantages and disadvantages associated with each of these different techniques. The high cost associated with these assays remains a hindrance. The most important advantages in using DNA methylation biomarkers include: (1) the ease with which the analysis can be performed, (2) the regions which are subject to DNA methylation are defined and can be directly assayed, and (3) since tumor cells may be shed into biological fluids such as saliva, sputum, serum or urine (depending on the cancer type and site of origin), DNA methylation analysis can be performed on non-invasively derived patient samples.

Currently, the easiest and most cost-effective assay is methylation-specific PCR (Kulis & Esteller 2010). While one can conceivably assay several genes in one analysis, this is a targeted experimental approach. Therefore, one needs to have prior insight as to the prognostic utility of a specific methylated gene or genes. In most cases, the studies that have led to identification of hypermethylated genes in OSCC studies employed targeted PCR-based approaches whereby the genes chosen were typically those whose decreased expression had been previously associated with OSCC progression (Viet and Schmidt 2010). These types of gene-targeted studies may eventually prove to be useful in identifying and validating potential methylated biomarkers. However, the benefits of DNA methylation analysis in predicting OSCC prognosis are currently limited by the relative paucity of clinical data and lack of validation across independent study sets. Moreover, not all genes that are affected by promoter hypermethylation contribute directly to the malignant phenotype, and thus are not useful as biomarkers (Viet & Schmidt 2010).

Methylation of several genes, including those encoding miRNAs, has been associated with OSCC prognosis (Huang *et al.,* 2009a, Kozaki *et al.,* 2008, Su *et al.,* 2010, Supic *et al.,* 2009, Supic *et al.,* 2011a). Some studies analyzed DNA methylation in head and neck squamous cell carcinoma without discriminating between OSCC and other sites. Thus, direct applicability of these methylated genes to OSCC prognosis cannot be certain. Select genes that have been specifically analyzed in OSCC are discussed here.

Functional inactivation of $p16^{INK4a}$ is a common event during oral carcinogenesis (Perez-Sayans *et al.,* 2011b). Homozygous deletion, somatic mutation and transcriptional silencing, *via* DNA hypermethylation, of $p16^{INK4a}$ have been identified in over 80% of OSCCs. OSCCs exhibiting undetectable or low $p16^{INK4a}$ expression have a poorer prognosis than tumors with high levels of $p16^{INK4a}$ (Perez-Sayans *et al.,* 2011b). O'Regan *et al.,* (O'Regan *et al.,* 2008) detected $p16^{INK4a}$ promoter methylation more commonly in OSCCs derived from females than from males, and mostly in individuals under the age of 40 years; $p16^{INK4a}$ deletions were more common in older individuals. This is supported by other independent studies (Hasegawa *et al.,* 2002). In addition, hypermethylated $p16^{INK4a}$ was associated with a higher risk for lymph node metastasis in young patients, and distant metastasis and shortened disease-free survival in older individuals (O'Regan *et al.,* 2008). $p16^{INK4a}$ silencing was also reportedly more common in tumors from the anterior tongue rather than the posterior tongue. This suggests the possibility of an etiology-specific $p16^{INK4a}$ methylation pattern that may be related to the presence or absence of HPV 16 and that may influence prognosis. Various investigators identified HPV 16 DNA within SCCs of the tongue base but not in the anterior tongue tumors (Hasegawa *et al.,* 2002, O'Regan *et al.,* 2008).

p14^{ARF} is encoded within the same CDKN2 gene that encodes p16^{INK4a} (Kwong *et al.,* 2005, Sailasree *et al.,* 2008). p14^{ARF} negatively regulates HDM2 which is the p53 E3 ubiquitin ligase and responsible for p53 degradation. Thus, activation of p14^{ARF} results in p53 stabilization. Conversely, loss of p14^{ARF} function, as is common during tumorigenesis, results in increased p53 turnover. About 10-25% of OSCCs exhibit p14^{ARF} promoter hypermethylation; silencing of this gene has been strongly associated with lymph node metastasis and Stage III/IV cancers (Ishida *et al.,* 2005, Kwong *et al.,* 2005, Sailasree *et al.,* 2008). In addition, Ishida *et al.,* (Ishida *et al.,* 2005) showed that concurrent loss of both p16^{INK4a} and p14^{ARF} correlated significantly with increased tumor size, advanced stage OSCCs, and lymph node involvement.

Promoter hypermethylation of CDH1 (E-cadherin) is frequently identified in OSCC and several studies also suggest prognostic significance of this epigenetic silencing (Su *et al.,* 2010, Supic *et al.,* 2009). In a study examining advanced OCSC patients, Supic *et al.,* (Supic *et al.,* 2009) reported that CDH1 hypermethylation was significantly associated with lymph node metastasis, Stage III cancer, and poor overall survival. In contrast, promoter methylation of other genes, including MGMT (O(6)-methylgunanine-DNA methyl transferase), DAPK (death-associated protein kinase), and RUNX3 (Runt-related transcription factor 3) had no effect on the prognostic variables assessed (Supic *et al.,* 2009). However, a separate study by the same authors examined gene hypermethylation in cancer-free surgical margins, and found that DAPK hypermethylation in surgical margins was strongly associated with reduced overall survival (Supic *et al.,* 2011b). Upon examining only tongue cancers, Supic *et al.,* (Supic *et al.,* 2011a) observed that RUNX3 hypermethylation was significantly associated with lymph node metastasis and high tumor stage. These three studies by the same group of authors reinforce the notion that the results of any given analysis are influenced by sample procurement, the method of analysis and the clinical variables being assessed.

De Shutter *et al.,* (De Shutter *et al.,* 2009) reported silencing of MGMT and TIMP3 (tissue inhibitor of metalloproteinase 3) in at least 40% of paraffin-embedded tumor biopsies derived from patients with advanced HNSCC treated with a hybrid accelerated fractionation radiotherapy schedule. Promoter hypermethylation of these two genes was significantly associated with improved locoregional control, disease-free survival and overall survival. In contrast, Nayak *et al.*, (Nayak *et al.*, 2007) noted that while TIMP3 was hypermethylated in over 70% of their tumor samples relative to normal controls, there was no correlation with either survival or any other clinical variables. Similarly, Supic *et al.*, (Supic *et al.*, 2009, Supic *et al.*, 2011b) did not associate MGMT hypermethylation with any prognostic variables in two separate studies examining OSCCs. These analyses further suggest that data interpretation and extrapolation across different studies should be regarded with caution.

Several tumor suppressor genes within the RAS/phosphatidyl inositol 3 kinase/AKT signaling nexus are hypermethylated during tumorigenesis. Loss of function of these genes, including RASSF1A and RASSF2A (Ras association (RalGDS/AF-6) domain family member 1 and 2, respectively), leads to constitutive activation of this important signal transduction cascade, thereby driving cancer progression (Huang *et al.,* 2009a, Su *et al.,* 2010). The combined hypermethylation of RASSF1A and RASSF2A has been significantly associated with poor OSCC disease-free survival following radiotherapy but not surgery (Huang *et al.,* 2009a). RASSF1A and RASSF2A hypermethylation are also associated with poor prognosis in several other cancer types. Nonetheless, before these and other putative biomarkers can be considered for use in the clinical setting, they need to be further validated in additional, rigorously controlled, retrospective and prospective studies.

While gene-specific CpG hypermethylation is generally increased, cancers actually exhibit a global decrease in CpG methylation (Kulis & Esteller 2010, Richards *et al.,* 2009). The 'methylome' is defined as the comprehensive aggregate of DNA methylation across the genome. To assess whole genome methylation levels, one typically examines the methylation status of long interspersed elements (LINE) and short interspersed elements (SINE) (Kulis & Esteller 2010, Richards *et al.,* 2009). LINE and SINE are retrotransposons that make up as much as 40% of the entire DNA sequence. The actual function of these repetitive elements remains in question. In normal cells, retrotransposons are methylated and silenced thereby ensuring genomic integrity. In cancer cells, hypomethylation of retrotransposons triggers their activation and subsequent mobilization through an incompletely understood "copy-and-paste" mechanism. This results in integration of retrotransposons at random sites throughout the genome, thereby increasing the risk of mutagenesis and induction of genomic instability. Loss of DNA methylation can also lead to oncogene activation and may also activate cancer-promoting latent viral sequences (Kulis & Esteller 2010).

Genome hypomethylation may be predictive of tumor etiology and influence the clinical prognosis of various cancers, including OSCC (Richards *et al.,* 2009, Smith *et al.,* 2007). LINE/SINE hypomethylation was reportedly more common in HPV-negative head and neck SCCs, specifically those caused by smoking and alcohol consumption, than in HPV-positive tumors (Richards *et al.,* 2009, Smith *et al.,* 2007). In addition, Smith *et al.,* (Smith *et al.,* 2007) observed that an increasing degree of LINE/SINE hypomethylation was significantly associated with advanced tumor stage; 34% of the analyzed samples were OSCCs. The contributions of global DNA hypomethylation to OSCC progression and its association with prognostic variables remain an intriguing avenue of investigation.

4.2. Histone Modifications

Chromatin disruption has emerged as an important cause and consequence of cancer (Jithesh *et al.,* 2013, Jones 2005). Chromatin is packaged into nucleosomes. Each nucleosome is composed of approximately 146 base pairs of DNA wrapped around an octamer of small, highly basic proteins known as histones (Jones 2005). The four core histones are H2A, H2B, H3 and H4. Histone variants also exist, including H2A.X which plays an important role in the DNA damage response.

Post-transcriptional modifications of histones are fundamental to all aspects of eukaryotic biology. The most well-studied of these changes includes acetylation, methylation, phosphorylation and ubiquitination (Jithesh *et al.,* 2013). In most cases, histone acetylation, methylation and ubiquitination occurs on lysine residues. Phosphorylation typically occurs on serine or tyrosine residues. The roles of histone phosphorylation and ubiquitination on cancer development and/or prognosis remain poorly understood. In contrast, there is ample evidence suggesting that histone acetylation and methylation may predict if not impact on cancer prognosis.

Histone acetylation typically marks transcriptionally active chromatin regions (euchromatin) (Jones 2005). Histone methylation, particular tri-methylated modifications, often marks inactive chromatin (heterochromatin). Specific methylation marks may also be associated with euchromatin. Ultimately, histone acetylation and methylation are dynamically and synergistically linked with CpG methylation (Jones 2005). Together, these chromatin modifications maintain a proper balance between global gene expression and transcriptional repression.

Specific histone modifications may be associated with various histologic and clinical parameters, including tumor grade, clinical stage, metastasis and overall survival (Jones 2005). The association between specific histone modifications and OSCC prognosis remains poorly understood and requires investigation. However, at least some chromatin modulatory factors have been ascribed prognostic relevance in OSCC (Jithesh *et al.,* 2013). These include histone acetylases, histone deacetylases, and other chromatin modulatory factors.

Histone acetylases and deacetylases also directly regulate the activities of non-histone proteins. Using high resolution mass spectrometry, acetylation sites were recently identified in over 1,700 distinct human proteins, including MYC, p53 and HIF1A (Choudhary *et al.,* 2009). This suggests that dysregulated protein acetylation is implicated in an array of cellular functions that directly influence the malignant phenotype, including DNA replication, DNA transcription, cell cycle progression, differentiation, and apoptosis. To this end, overexpression of histone deacetylase 1 (HDAC1) is significantly associated with poor histopathologic grade, lymph node metastasis, young age of onset, and poor disease-free survival in patients with tongue cancer (Theocharis *et al.,* 2011). High levels of HDAC2 have been associated with large tumor size, depth of local invasion, advanced clinical stage and lymph node metastasis (Chang *et al.,* 2009, Theocharis *et al.,* 2011). HDAC6 expression levels also significantly correlate with advanced clinical stage (Sakuma *et al.,* 2006). Overexpression of other chromatin remodeling factors, including remodeling and spacing factor-1 (RSF-1), may significantly correlate with angiolymphatic invasion, metastasis, local recurrence and advanced clinical stage at initial presentation (Fang *et al.,* 2011).

An emerging strategy in cancer chemotherapy involves the use of chemical inhibition of chromatin modulatory factors, including histone deacetylases (Iglesias-Linares *et al.,* 2010). These drugs remain mostly in the experimental stages and/or in clinical trials. Nonetheless, the notion that targeted alterations in chromatin structure may be therapeutically effective highlights the importance of aberrant epigenetic modulation in the pathogenesis and prognosis of OSCC.

5. MOLECULAR-BASED APPROACHES TO THERAPY

In the past, primary surgery of locally advanced head and neck squamous cell carcinoma (HNSCC) was traditionally followed by postoperative radiotherapy (Bonner *et al.,* 2006, Bonner *et al.,* 2010). Despite such relatively aggressive bimodality treatment, this approach yielded locoregional recurrence, distant metastasis, and 5-year survival rates of 30%, 25%, and 40%, respectively (Laramore *et al.,* 1992). Improvements in survival rates after adjuvant concurrent chemoradiotherapy over radiotherapy alone for patients with advanced head and neck SCC have been reported (Furness *et al.,* 2010, Furness *et al.,* 2011, Laramore *et al.,* 1992, Murthy *et al.,* 2010, Sher *et al.,* 2011). However, it is generally accepted that there is substantial morbidity of adding chemotherapy to radiotherapy, and considerable debate exists regarding the pathologic tumor parameters that predict the need for more aggressive adjuvant treatment. In the age of molecular therapeutics and personalized cancer medicine, this is likely to take the form of drugs or other compounds targeted to specific proteins or other cellular components, and with a minimal side effect profile.

Emerging data suggests that monoclonal antibody therapy and small-molecule tyrosine kinase inhibitors aimed at suppressing EGFR kinase activity may improve outcome over primary radiotherapy alone in patients with squamous cancers of other head and neck sites (Bonner *et al.,* 2006, Bonner *et al.,* 2010). A similarly modest outcome has been observed in patients with non-small cell lung cancer and colorectal cancers (La Thangue and Kerr 2011). These EGFR-centric treatments have received regulatory approval in the United States and are now accepted therapies for both of these solid cancers. Clinical trials are ongoing in assessing the benefits of such therapy in OSCC patients. Nonetheless, despite the plethora of molecular data, very few biologic agents have been designed and effectively employed in the treatment of OSCC. Increased identification of the various genetic, genomic and epigenetic changes that characterize OSCC will enhance our understanding of disease pathogenesis and may eventually help to ensure patients with OSCC can reap the benefits of personalized medicinal approaches to therapy.

ACKNOWLEDGEMENT

Declared None.

CONFLICT OF INTEREST

The authors confirm that this chapter content has no conflict of interest.

REFERENCES

Bearer, E.L., Lowengrub, J.S., Frieboes, H.B., Chuang, Y.L., Jin, F., Wise, S.M., Ferrari, M., Agus, D.B., & Cristini, V. 2009. Multiparameter computational modeling of tumor invasion. *Cancer Res.*, 69, (10) 4493-4501 available from: PM:19366801

Bonner, J.A., Harari, P.M., Giralt, J., Azarnia, N., Shin, D.M., Cohen, R.B., Jones, C.U., Sur, R., Raben, D., Jassem, J., Ove, R., Kies, M.S., Baselga, J., Youssoufian, H., Amellal, N., Rowinsky, E.K., & Ang, K.K. 2006. Radiotherapy plus cetuximab for squamous-cell carcinoma of the head and neck. *N.Engl.J.Med.*, 354, (6) 567-578 available from: PM:16467544

Bonner, J.A., Harari, P.M., Giralt, J., Cohen, R.B., Jones, C.U., Sur, R.K., Raben, D., Baselga, J., Spencer, S.A., Zhu, J., Youssoufian, H., Rowinsky, E.K., & Ang, K.K. 2010. Radiotherapy plus cetuximab for locoregionally advanced head and neck cancer: 5-year survival data from a phase 3 randomised trial, and relation between cetuximab-induced rash and survival. *Lancet Oncol.*, 11, (1) 21-28 available from: PM:19897418

Cervigne, N.K., Reis, P.P., Machado, J., Sadikovic, B., Bradley, G., Galloni, N.N., Pintilie, M., Jurisica, I., Perez-Ordonez, B., Gilbert, R., Gullane, P., Irish, J., & Kamel-Reid, S. 2009. Identification of a microRNA signature associated with progression of leukoplakia to oral carcinoma. *Hum.Mol.Genet.*, 18, (24) 4818-4829 available from: PM:19776030

Chang, H.H., Chiang, C.P., Hung, H.C., Lin, C.Y., Deng, Y.T., & Kuo, M.Y. 2009. Histone deacetylase 2 expression predicts poorer prognosis in oral cancer patients. *Oral Oncol.*, 45, (7) 610-614 available from: PM:18951835

Chen, C., Mendez, E., Houck, J., Fan, W., Lohavanichbutr, P., Doody, D., Yueh, B., Futran, N.D., Upton, M., Farwell, D.G., Schwartz, S.M., & Zhao, L.P. 2008. Gene expression profiling identifies genes predictive of oral squamous cell carcinoma. *Cancer Epidemiol.Biomarkers Prev.*, 17, (8) 2152-2162 available from: PM:18669583

Cheong, S.C., Chandramouli, G.V., Saleh, A., Zain, R.B., Lau, S.H., Sivakumaren, S., Pathmanathan, R., Prime, S.S., Teo, S.H., Patel, V., & Gutkind, J.S. 2009a. Gene expression in human oral squamous cell carcinoma is influenced by risk factor exposure. *Oral Oncol.*, 45, (8) 712-719 available from: PM:19147396

Cheong, S.C., Chandramouli, G.V., Saleh, A., Zain, R.B., Lau, S.H., Sivakumaren, S., Pathmanathan, R., Prime, S.S., Teo, S.H., Patel, V., & Gutkind, J.S. 2009b. Gene expression in human oral squamous cell carcinoma is influenced by risk factor exposure. *Oral Oncol.*, 45, (8) 712-719 available from: PM:19147396

Chiang, W.F., Liu, S.Y., Yen, C.Y., Lin, C.N., Chen, Y.C., Lin, S.C., & Chang, K.W. 2008. Association of epidermal growth factor receptor (EGFR) gene copy number amplification with neck lymph node metastasis in areca-associated oral carcinomas. *Oral Oncol.*, 44, (3) 270-276 available from: PM:17468034

Cho, Y.J., Tsherniak, A., Tamayo, P., Santagata, S., Ligon, A., Greulich, H., Berhoukim, R., Amani, V., Goumnerova, L., Eberhart, C.G., Lau, C.C., Olson, J.M., Gilbertson, R.J., Gajjar, A., Delattre, O., Kool, M., Ligon, K., Meyerson, M., Mesirov, J.P., & Pomeroy, S.L. 2011. Integrative genomic analysis of medulloblastoma identifies a molecular subgroup that drives poor clinical outcome. *J.Clin.Oncol.*, 29, (11) 1424-1430 available from: PM:21098324

Choudhary, C., Kumar, C., Gnad, F., Nielsen, M.L., Rehman, M., Walther, T.C., Olsen, J.V., & Mann, M. 2009. Lysine acetylation targets protein complexes and co-regulates major cellular functions. *Science*, 325, (5942) 834-840 available from: PM:19608861

Chu, Y.H., Tzeng, S.L., Lin, C.W., Chien, M.H., Chen, M.K., & Yang, S.F. 2012. Impacts of microRNA gene polymorphisms on the susceptibility of environmental factors leading to carcinogenesis in oral cancer. *PLoS.One.*, 7, (6) e39777 available from: PM:22761899

De, S.H., Geeraerts, H., Verbeken, E., & Nuyts, S. 2009. Promoter methylation of TIMP3 and CDH1 predicts better outcome in head and neck squamous cell carcinoma treated by radiotherapy only. *Oncol.Rep.*, 21, (2) 507-513 available from: PM:19148529

Deisboeck, T.S., Wang, Z., Macklin, P., & Cristini, V. 2011. Multiscale cancer modeling. *Annu.Rev.Biomed.Eng*, 13, 127-155 available from: PM:21529163

Dhanasekaran, S.M., Barrette, T.R., Ghosh, D., Shah, R., Varambally, S., Kurachi, K., Pienta, K.J., Rubin, M.A., & Chinnaiyan, A.M. 2001. Delineation of prognostic biomarkers in prostate cancer. *Nature*, 412, (6849) 822-826 available from: PM:11518967

Fang, F.M., Li, C.F., Huang, H.Y., Lai, M.T., Chen, C.M., Chiu, I.W., Wang, T.L., Tsai, F.J., Shih, I., & Sheu, J.J. 2011. Overexpression of a chromatin remodeling factor, RSF-1/HBXAP, correlates with aggressive oral squamous cell carcinoma. *Am.J.Pathol.*, 178, (5) 2407-2415 available from: PM:21514451

Frieboes, H.B., Chaplain, M.A., Thompson, A.M., Bearer, E.L., Lowengrub, J.S., & Cristini, V. 2011. Physical oncology: a bench-to-bedside quantitative and predictive approach. *Cancer Res.*, 71, (2) 298-302 available from: PM:21224346

Furness, S., Glenny, A.M., Worthington, H.V., Pavitt, S., Oliver, R., Clarkson, J.E., Macluskey, M., Chan, K.K., & Conway, D.I. 2010. Interventions for the treatment of oral cavity and oropharyngeal cancer: chemotherapy. *Cochrane.Database.Syst.Rev.* (9) CD006386 available from: PM:20824847

Furness, S., Glenny, A.M., Worthington, H.V., Pavitt, S., Oliver, R., Clarkson, J.E., Macluskey, M., Chan, K.K., & Conway, D.I. 2011. Interventions for the treatment of oral cavity and oropharyngeal cancer: chemotherapy. *Cochrane.Database.Syst.Rev.* (4) CD006386 available from: PM:21491393

Garnis, C., Campbell, J., Zhang, L., Rosin, M.P., & Lam, W.L. 2004a. OCGR array: an oral cancer genomic regional array for comparative genomic hybridization analysis. *Oral Oncol.*, 40, (5) 511-519 available from: PM:15006624

Garnis, C., Chari, R., Buys, T.P., Zhang, L., Ng, R.T., Rosin, M.P., & Lam, W.L. 2009. Genomic imbalances in precancerous tissues signal oral cancer risk. *Mol.Cancer*, 8, 50 available from: PM:19627613

Garnis, C., Coe, B.P., Ishkanian, A., Zhang, L., Rosin, M.P., & Lam, W.L. 2004b. Novel regions of amplification on 8q distinct from the MYC locus and frequently altered in oral dysplasia and cancer. *Genes Chromosomes.Cancer*, 39, (1) 93-98 available from: PM:14603447

Garnis, C., Coe, B.P., Zhang, L., Rosin, M.P., & Lam, W.L. 2004c. Overexpression of LRP12, a gene contained within an 8q22 amplicon identified by high-resolution array CGH analysis of oral squamous cell carcinomas. *Oncogene*, 23, (14) 2582-2586 available from: PM:14676824

Halabi, S. & Owzar, K. 2010. The importance of identifying and validating prognostic factors in oncology. *Semin.Oncol.*, 37, (2) e9-18 available from: PM:20494694

Harpold, H.L., Alvord, E.C., Jr., & Swanson, K.R. 2007. The evolution of mathematical modeling of glioma proliferation and invasion. *J.Neuropathol.Exp.Neurol.*, 66, (1) 1-9 available from: PM:17204931

Harris, T., Jimenez, L., Kawachi, N., Fan, J.B., Chen, J., Belbin, T., Ramnauth, A., Loudig, O., Keller, C.E., Smith, R., Prystowsky, M.B., Schlecht, N.F., Segall, J.E., & Childs, G. 2012. Low-level expression of miR-375 correlates with poor outcome and metastasis while altering the invasive properties of head and neck squamous cell carcinomas. *Am.J.Pathol.*, 180, (3) 917-928 available from: PM:22234174

Hasegawa, M., Nelson, H.H., Peters, E., Ringstrom, E., Posner, M., & Kelsey, K.T. 2002. Patterns of gene promoter methylation in squamous cell cancer of the head and neck. *Oncogene*, 21, (27) 4231-4236 available from: PM:12082610

Hillbertz, N.S., Hirsch, J.M., Jalouli, J., Jalouli, M.M., & Sand, L. 2012. Viral and molecular aspects of oral cancer. *Anticancer Res.*, 32, (10) 4201-4212 available from: PM:23060540

Huang, K.H., Huang, S.F., Chen, I.H., Liao, C.T., Wang, H.M., & Hsieh, L.L. 2009a. Methylation of RASSF1A, RASSF2A, and HIN-1 is associated with poor outcome after radiotherapy, but not surgery, in oral squamous cell carcinoma. *Clin.Cancer Res.*, 15, (12) 4174-4180 available from: PM:19509163

Huang, S.F., Chen, I.H., Liao, C.T., Wang, H.M., Liou, S.H., & Hsieh, L.L. 2009b. Combined effects of MDM2 SNP 309 and p53 mutation on oral squamous cell carcinomas associated with areca quid chewing. *Oral Oncol.*, 45, (1) 16-22 available from: PM:18487080

Huang, S.H., Hwang, D., Lockwood, G., Goldstein, D.P., & O'Sullivan, B. 2009c. Predictive value of tumor thickness for cervical lymph-node involvement in squamous cell carcinoma of the oral cavity: a meta-analysis of reported studies. *Cancer*, 115, (7) 1489-1497 available from: PM:19197973

Huang, S.H. & O'Sullivan, B. 2013. Oral cancer: Current role of radiotherapy and chemotherapy. *Med.Oral Patol.Oral Cir.Bucal.*, 18, (2) e233-e240 available from: PM:23385513

Huang, X., Gollin, S.M., Raja, S., & Godfrey, T.E. 2002. High-resolution mapping of the 11q13 amplicon and identification of a gene, TAOS1, that is amplified and overexpressed in oral cancer cells. *Proc.Natl.Acad.Sci.U.S.A*, 99, (17) 11369-11374 available from: PM:12172009

Hung, P.S., Chang, K.W., Kao, S.Y., Chu, T.H., Liu, C.J., & Lin, S.C. 2012. Association between the rs2910164 polymorphism in pre-mir-146a and oral carcinoma progression. *Oral Oncol.*, 48, (5) 404-408 available from: PM:22182931

Iafrate, A.J., Feuk, L., Rivera, M.N., Listewnik, M.L., Donahoe, P.K., Qi, Y., Scherer, S.W., & Lee, C. 2004. Detection of large-scale variation in the human genome. *Nat.Genet.*, 36, (9) 949-951 available from: PM:15286789

Iglesias-Linares, A., Yanez-Vico, R.M., & Gonzalez-Moles, M.A. 2010. Potential role of HDAC inhibitors in cancer therapy: insights into oral squamous cell carcinoma. *Oral Oncol.*, 46, (5) 323-329 available from: PM:20207580

Ishida, E., Nakamura, M., Ikuta, M., Shimada, K., Matsuyoshi, S., Kirita, T., & Konishi, N. 2005. Promotor hypermethylation of p14ARF is a key alteration for progression of oral squamous cell carcinoma. *Oral Oncol.*, 41, (6) 614-622 available from: PM:15975525

Jiang, L., Yang, H.S., Wang, Z., Zhou, Y., Zhou, M., Zeng, X., & Chen, Q.M. 2009. ORAOV1-A correlates with poor differentiation in oral cancer. *J.Dent.Res.*, 88, (5) 433-438 available from: PM:19493886

Jithesh, P.V., Risk, J.M., Schache, A.G., Dhanda, J., Lane, B., Liloglou, T., & Shaw, R.J. 2013. The epigenetic landscape of oral squamous cell carcinoma. *Br.J.Cancer*, 108, (2) 370-379 available from: PM:23287992

Jones, P.A. 2005. Overview of cancer epigenetics. *Semin.Hematol.*, 42, (3 Suppl 2) S3-S8 available from: PM:16015502

Kim, D.H., Nelson, H.H., Wiencke, J.K., Zheng, S., Christiani, D.C., Wain, J.C., Mark, E.J., & Kelsey, K.T. 2001. p16(INK4a) and histology-specific methylation of CpG islands by exposure to tobacco smoke in non-small cell lung cancer. *Cancer Res.*, 61, (8) 3419-3424 available from: PM:11309302

Kozaki, K., Imoto, I., Mogi, S., Omura, K., & Inazawa, J. 2008. Exploration of tumor-suppressive microRNAs silenced by DNA hypermethylation in oral cancer. *Cancer Res.*, 68, (7) 2094-2105 available from: PM:18381414

Kulis, M. & Esteller, M. 2010. DNA methylation and cancer. *Adv.Genet.*, 70, 27-56 available from: PM:20920744

Kwong, R.A., Kalish, L.H., Nguyen, T.V., Kench, J.G., Bova, R.J., Cole, *I.E.*, Musgrove, E.A., & Sutherland, R.L. 2005. p14ARF protein expression is a predictor of both relapse and survival in squamous cell carcinoma of the anterior tongue. *Clin.Cancer Res.*, 11, (11) 4107-4116 available from: PM:15930346

La Thangue, N.B. & Kerr, D.J. 2011. Predictive biomarkers: a paradigm shift towards personalized cancer medicine. *Nat.Rev.Clin.Oncol.*, 8, (10) 587-596 available from: PM:21862978

Lajer, C.B., Nielsen, F.C., Friis-Hansen, L., Norrild, B., Borup, R., Garnaes, E., Rossing, M., Specht, L., Therkildsen, M.H., Nauntofte, B., Dabelsteen, S., & von, B.C. 2011. Different miRNA signatures of oral and pharyngeal squamous cell carcinomas: a prospective translational study. *Br.J.Cancer*, 104, (5) 830-840 available from: PM:21326242

Laramore, G.E., Scott, C.B., al-Sarraf, M., Haselow, R.E., Ervin, T.J., Wheeler, R., Jacobs, J.R., Schuller, D.E., Gahbauer, R.A., Schwade, J.G., &. 1992. Adjuvant chemotherapy for resectable squamous cell carcinomas of the head and neck: report on Intergroup Study 0034. *Int.J.Radiat.Oncol.Biol.Phys.*, 23, (4) 705-713 available from: PM:1618662

Li, J., Huang, H., Sun, L., Yang, M., Pan, C., Chen, W., Wu, D., Lin, Z., Zeng, C., Yao, Y., Zhang, P., & Song, E. 2009. MiR-21 indicates poor prognosis in tongue squamous cell carcinomas as an apoptosis inhibitor. *Clin.Cancer Res.*, 15, (12) 3998-4008 available from: PM:19509158

Lingen, M.W., Chang, K.W., McMurray, S.J., Solt, D.B., Kies, M.S., Mittal, B.B., Haines, G.K., & Pelzer, H.J. 2000. Overexpression of p53 in squamous cell carcinoma of the tongue in young patients with no known risk factors is not associated with mutations in exons 5-9. *Head Neck*, 22, (4) 328-335 available from: PM:10862014

Lingen, M.W., Xiao, W., Schmitt, A., Jiang, B., Pickard, R., Kreinbrink, P., Perez-Ordonez, B., Jordan, R.C., & Gillison, M.L. 2013. Low etiologic fraction for high-risk human papillomavirus in oral cavity squamous cell carcinomas. *Oral Oncol.*, 49, (1) 1-8 available from: PM:22841678

Lipovich, L., Johnson, R., & Lin, C.Y. 2010. MacroRNA underdogs in a microRNA world: evolutionary, regulatory, and biomedical significance of mammalian long non-protein-coding RNA. *Biochim.Biophys.Acta*, 1799, (9) 597-615 available from: PM:20951849

Liu, Z., Niu, Y., Li, C., Yang, Y., & Gao, C. 2012. Integrating multiple microarray datasets on oral squamous cell carcinoma to reveal dysregulated networks. *Head Neck*, 34, (12) 1789-1797 available from: PM:22179951

Lowengrub, J.S., Frieboes, H.B., Jin, F., Chuang, Y.L., Li, X., Macklin, P., Wise, S.M., & Cristini, V. 2010. Nonlinear modelling of cancer: bridging the gap between cells and tumours. *Nonlinearity.*, 23, (1) R1-R9 available from: PM:20808719

Marsit, C.J., Wiencke, J.K., Nelson, H.H., Kim, D.H., Hinds, P.W., Aldape, K., & Kelsey, K.T. 2005. Alterations of 9p in squamous cell carcinoma and adenocarcinoma of the lung: association with smoking, TP53, and survival. *Cancer Genet.Cytogenet.*, 162, (2) 115-121 available from: PM:16213358

Martin, C.L., Reshmi, S.C., Ried, T., Gottberg, W., Wilson, J.W., Reddy, J.K., Khanna, P., Johnson, J.T., Myers, E.N., & Gollin, S.M. 2008. Chromosomal imbalances in oral squamous cell carcinoma: examination of 31 cell lines and review of the literature. *Oral Oncol.*, 44, (4) 369-382 available from: PM:17681875

McShane, L.M., Altman, D.G., Sauerbrei, W., Taube, S.E., Gion, M., & Clark, G.M. 2006. Reporting recommendations for tumor marker prognostic studies (remark). *Exp.Oncol.*, 28, (2) 99-105 available from: PM:16837898

Mei, R., Galipeau, P.C., Prass, C., Berno, A., Ghandour, G., Patil, N., Wolff, R.K., Chee, M.S., Reid, B.J., & Lockhart, D.J. 2000. Genome-wide detection of allelic imbalance using human SNPs and high-density DNA arrays. *Genome Res.*, 10, (8) 1126-1137 available from: PM:10958631

Mendez, E., Lohavanichbutr, P., Fan, W., Houck, J.R., Rue, T.C., Doody, D.R., Futran, N.D., Upton, M.P., Yueh, B., Zhao, L.P., Schwartz, S.M., & Chen, C. 2011. Can a metastatic gene expression profile outperform tumor size as a predictor of occult lymph node metastasis in oral cancer patients? *Clin.Cancer Res.*, 17, (8) 2466-2473 available from: PM:21300763

Michor, F. 2008. Mathematical models of cancer stem cells. *J.Clin.Oncol.*, 26, (17) 2854-2861 available from: PM:18539964

Munoz-Guerra, M.F., Fernandez-Contreras, M.E., Moreno, A.L., Martin, I.D., Herraez, B., & Gamallo, C. 2009. Polymorphisms in the hypoxia inducible factor 1-alpha and the impact on the prognosis of early stages of oral cancer. *Ann.Surg.Oncol.*, 16, (8) 2351-2358 available from: PM:19449077

Murthy, V., Agarwal, J.P., Laskar, S.G., Gupta, T., Budrukkar, A., Pai, P., Chaturvedi, P., Chaukar, D., & D'Cruz, A. 2010. Analysis of prognostic factors in 1180 patients with oral cavity primary cancer treated with definitive or adjuvant radiotherapy. *J.Cancer Res.Ther.*, 6, (3) 282-289 available from: PM:21119254

Myo, K., Uzawa, N., Miyamoto, R., Sonoda, I., Yuki, Y., & Amagasa, T. 2005. Cyclin D1 gene numerical aberration is a predictive marker for occult cervical lymph node metastasis in TNM Stage I and II squamous cell carcinoma of the oral cavity. *Cancer*, 104, (12) 2709-2716 available from: PM:16265665

Nallar, S.C. & Kalvakolanu, D.V. 2013. Regulation of snoRNAs in Cancer: Close Encounters with Interferon. *J.Interferon Cytokine Res.*, 33, (4) 189-198 available from: PM:23570385

Nayak, C.S., Carvalho, A.L., Jeronimo, C., Henrique, R., Kim, M.M., Hoque, M.O., Chang, S., Jiang, W.W., Koch, W., Westra, W., Sidransky, D., & Califano, J. 2007. Positive correlation of tissue inhibitor of metalloproteinase-3 and death-associated protein kinase hypermethylation in head and neck squamous cell carcinoma. *Laryngoscope*, 117, (8) 1376-1380 available from: PM:17592394

Nutt, C.L., Mani, D.R., Betensky, R.A., Tamayo, P., Cairncross, J.G., Ladd, C., Pohl, U., Hartmann, C., McLaughlin, M.E., Batchelor, T.T., Black, P.M., von, D.A., Pomeroy, S.L., Golub, T.R., & Louis, D.N. 2003. Gene expression-based classification of malignant gliomas correlates better with survival than histological classification. *Cancer Res.*, 63, (7) 1602-1607 available from: PM:12670911

O'Donnell, R.K., Kupferman, M., Wei, S.J., Singhal, S., Weber, R., O'Malley, B., Cheng, Y., Putt, M., Feldman, M., Ziober, B., & Muschel, R.J. 2005. Gene expression signature predicts lymphatic metastasis in squamous cell carcinoma of the oral cavity. *Oncogene*, 24, (7) 1244-1251 available from: PM:15558013

O'Regan, E.M., Toner, M.E., Finn, S.P., Fan, C.Y., Ring, M., Hagmar, B., Timon, C., Smyth, P., Cahill, S., Flavin, R., Sheils, O.M., & O'Leary, J.J. 2008. p16(INK4A) genetic and epigenetic profiles differ in relation to age and site in head and neck squamous cell carcinomas. *Hum.Pathol.*, 39, (3) 452-458 available from: PM:18261630

Ostwald, C., Gogacz, P., Hillmann, T., Schweder, J., Gundlach, K., Kundt, G., & Barten, M. 2000. p53 mutational spectra are different between squamous-cell carcinomas of the lip and the oral cavity. *Int.J.Cancer*, 88, (1) 82-86 available from: PM:10962443

Partridge, M., Emilion, G., & Langdon, J.D. 1996. LOH at 3p correlates with a poor survival in oral squamous cell carcinoma. *Br.J.Cancer*, 73, (3) 366-371 available from: PM:8562343

Pasini, F.S., Maistro, S., Snitcovsky, I., Barbeta, L.P., Rotea Mangone, F.R., Lehn, C.N., Walder, F., Carvalho, M.B., Brentani, M.M., & Federico, M.H. 2012. Four-gene expression model predictive of lymph node metastases in oral squamous cell carcinoma. *Acta Oncol.*, 51, (1) 77-85 available from: PM:21985131

Peng, C.H., Liao, C.T., Peng, S.C., Chen, Y.J., Cheng, A.J., Juang, J.L., Tsai, C.Y., Chen, T.C., Chuang, Y.J., Tang, C.Y., Hsieh, W.P., & Yen, T.C. 2011. A novel molecular signature identified by systems genetics approach predicts prognosis in oral squamous cell carcinoma. *PLoS.One.*, 6, (8) e23452 available from: PM:21853135

Perez-Sayans, M., Suarez-Penaranda, J.M., Gayoso-Diz, P., Barros-Angueira, F., Gandara-Rey, J.M., & Garcia-Garcia, A. 2011a. p16(INK4a)/CDKN2 expression and its relationship with oral squamous cell carcinoma is our current knowledge enough? *Cancer Lett.*, 306, (2) 134-141 available from: PM:21411222

Perez-Sayans, M., Suarez-Penaranda, J.M., Gayoso-Diz, P., Barros-Angueira, F., Gandara-Rey, J.M., & Garcia-Garcia, A. 2011b. p16(INK4a)/CDKN2 expression and its relationship with oral squamous cell carcinoma is our current knowledge enough? *Cancer Lett.*, 306, (2) 134-141 available from: PM:21411222

Perez-Sayans, M., Suarez-Penaranda, J.M., Pilar, G.D., Barros-Angueira, F., Gandara-Rey, J.M., & Garcia-Garcia, A. 2011c. Hypoxia-inducible factors in OSCC. *Cancer Lett.*, 313, (1) 1-8 available from: PM:21959110

Pugh, T.J., Weeraratne, S.D., Archer, T.C., Pomeranz Krummel, D.A., Auclair, D., Bochicchio, J., Carneiro, M.O., Carter, S.L., Cibulskis, K., Erlich, R.L., Greulich, H., Lawrence, M.S., Lennon, N.J., McKenna, A., Meldrim, J., Ramos, A.H., Ross, M.G., Russ, C., Shefler, E., Sivachenko, A., Sogoloff, B., Stojanov, P., Tamayo, P., Mesirov, J.P., Amani, V., Teider, N., Sengupta, S., Francois, J.P., Northcott, P.A., Taylor, M.D., Yu, F., Crabtree, G.R., Kautzman, A.G., Gabriel, S.B., Getz, G., Jager, N., Jones, D.T., Lichter, P., Pfister, S.M., Roberts, T.M., Meyerson, M., Pomeroy, S.L., & Cho, Y.J. 2012. Medulloblastoma exome sequencing uncovers subtype-specific somatic mutations. *Nature*, 488, (7409) 106-110 available from: PM:22820256

Reis, P.P., Waldron, L., Perez-Ordonez, B., Pintilie, M., Galloni, N.N., Xuan, Y., Cervigne, N.K., Warner, G.C., Makitie, A.A., Simpson, C., Goldstein, D., Brown, D., Gilbert, R., Gullane, P., Irish, J., Jurisica, I., & Kamel-Reid, S. 2011. A gene signature in histologically normal surgical margins is predictive of oral carcinoma recurrence. *BMC.Cancer*, 11, 437 available from: PM:21989116

Richards, K.L., Zhang, B., Baggerly, K.A., Colella, S., Lang, J.C., Schuller, D.E., & Krahe, R. 2009. Genome-wide hypomethylation in head and neck cancer is more pronounced in HPV-negative tumors and is associated with genomic instability. *PLoS.One.*, 4, (3) e4941 available from: PM:19293934

Sailasree, R., Abhilash, A., Sathyan, K.M., Nalinakumari, K.R., Thomas, S., & Kannan, S. 2008. Differential roles of p16INK4A and p14ARF genes in prognosis of oral carcinoma. *Cancer Epidemiol.Biomarkers Prev.*, 17, (2) 414-420 available from: PM:18268126

Sakuma, T., Uzawa, K., Onda, T., Shiiba, M., Yokoe, H., Shibahara, T., & Tanzawa, H. 2006. Aberrant expression of histone deacetylase 6 in oral squamous cell carcinoma. *Int.J.Oncol.*, 29, (1) 117-124 available from: PM:16773191

Serrano, N.A., Xu, C., Liu, Y., Wang, P., Fan, W., Upton, M.P., Houck, J.R., Lohavanichbutr, P., Kao, M., Zhao, L.P., Schwartz, S.M., Chen, C., & Mendez, E. 2012. Integrative analysis in oral squamous cell carcinoma reveals DNA copy number-associated miRNAs dysregulating target genes. *Otolaryngol.Head Neck Surg.*, 147, (3) 501-508 available from: PM:22470160

Sher, D.J., Thotakura, V., Balboni, T.A., Norris, C.M., Jr., Haddad, R.I., Posner, M.R., Lorch, J., Goguen, L.A., Annino, D.J., & Tishler, R.B. 2011. Treatment of oral cavity squamous cell carcinoma with adjuvant or definitive intensity-modulated radiation therapy. *Int.J.Radiat.Oncol.Biol.Phys.*, 81, (4) e215-e222 available from: PM:21531515

Sheu, J.J., Hua, C.H., Wan, L., Lin, Y.J., Lai, M.T., Tseng, H.C., Jinawath, N., Tsai, M.H., Chang, N.W., Lin, C.F., Lin, C.C., Hsieh, L.J., Wang, T.L., Shih, I., & Tsai, F.J. 2009. Functional genomic analysis identified epidermal growth factor receptor activation as the most common genetic event in oral squamous cell carcinoma. *Cancer Res.*, 69, (6) 2568-2576 available from: PM:19276369

Smith, I.M., Mydlarz, W.K., Mithani, S.K., & Califano, J.A. 2007. DNA global hypomethylation in squamous cell head and neck cancer associated with smoking, alcohol consumption and stage. *Int.J.Cancer*, 121, (8) 1724-1728 available from: PM:17582607

Sparano, A., Quesnelle, K.M., Kumar, M.S., Wang, Y., Sylvester, A.J., Feldman, M., Sewell, D.A., Weinstein, G.S., & Brose, M.S. 2006. Genome-wide profiling of oral squamous cell carcinoma by array-based comparative genomic hybridization. *Laryngoscope*, 116, (5) 735-741 available from: PM:16652080

Su, P.F., Huang, W.L., Wu, H.T., Wu, C.H., Liu, T.Y., & Kao, S.Y. 2010. p16(INK4A) promoter hypermethylation is associated with invasiveness and prognosis of oral squamous cell carcinoma in an age-dependent manner. *Oral Oncol.*, 46, (10) 734-739 available from: PM:20729138

Sugahara, K., Michikawa, Y., Ishikawa, K., Shoji, Y., Iwakawa, M., Shibahara, T., & Imai, T. 2011. Combination effects of distinct cores in 11q13 amplification region on cervical lymph node metastasis of oral squamous cell carcinoma. *Int.J.Oncol.*, 39, (4) 761-769 available from: PM:21701773

Supic, G., Kozomara, R., Brankovic-Magic, M., Jovic, N., & Magic, Z. 2009. Gene hypermethylation in tumor tissue of advanced oral squamous cell carcinoma patients. *Oral Oncol.*, 45, (12) 1051-1057 available from: PM:19665921

Supic, G., Kozomara, R., Jovic, N., Zeljic, K., & Magic, Z. 2011a. Hypermethylation of RUNX3 but not WIF1 gene and its association with stage and nodal status of tongue cancers. *Oral Dis.*, 17, (8) 794-800 available from: PM:21819494

Supic, G., Kozomara, R., Jovic, N., Zeljic, K., & Magic, Z. 2011b. Prognostic significance of tumor-related genes hypermethylation detected in cancer-free surgical margins of oral squamous cell carcinomas. *Oral Oncol.*, 47, (8) 702-708 available from: PM:21697000

Theocharis, S., Klijanienko, J., Giaginis, C., Rodriguez, J., Jouffroy, T., Girod, A., Alexandrou, P., & Sastre-Garau, X. 2011. Histone deacetylase-1 and -2 expression in mobile tongue squamous cell carcinoma: associations with clinicopathological parameters and patients survival. *J.Oral Pathol.Med.* available from: PM:21457345

Tu, H.F., Chen, H.W., Kao, S.Y., Lin, S.C., Liu, C.J., & Chang, K.W. 2008. MDM2 SNP 309 and p53 codon 72 polymorphisms are associated with the outcome of oral carcinoma patients receiving postoperative irradiation. *Radiother.Oncol.*, 87, (2) 243-252 available from: PM:18423915

Uchida, K., Oga, A., Nakao, M., Mano, T., Mihara, M., Kawauchi, S., Furuya, T., Ueyama, Y., & Sasaki, K. 2011. Loss of 3p26.3 is an independent prognostic factor in patients with oral squamous cell carcinoma. *Oncol.Rep.*, 26, (2) 463-469 available from: PM:21617881

Uzawa, N., Akanuma, D., Negishi, A., Iwaki, H., Uzawa, Y., Amagasa, T., & Yoshida, M.A. 2001. Homozygous deletions on the short arm of chromosome 3 in human oral squamous cell carcinomas. *Oral Oncol.*, 37, (4) 351-356 available from: PM:11337267

Vaezi, A., Wang, X., Buch, S., Gooding, W., Wang, L., Seethala, R.R., Weaver, D.T., D'Andrea, A.D., Argiris, A., Romkes, M., Niedernhofer, L.J., & Grandis, J.R. 2011. XPF expression correlates with clinical outcome in squamous cell carcinoma of the head and neck. *Clin.Cancer Res.*, 17, (16) 5513-5522 available from: PM:21737503

van 't Veer, L.J., Dai, H., van de Vijver, M.J., He, Y.D., Hart, A.A., Bernards, R., & Friend, S.H. 2003. Expression profiling predicts outcome in breast cancer. *Breast Cancer Res.*, 5, (1) 57-58 available from: PM:12559048

Viet, C.T. & Schmidt, B.L. 2010. Understanding oral cancer in the genome era. *Head Neck*, 32, (9) 1246-1268 available from: PM:20187013

Wang, W.Y., Chien, Y.C., Wong, Y.K., Lin, Y.L., & Lin, J.C. 2012a. Effects of KRAS mutation and polymorphism on the risk and prognosis of oral squamous cell carcinoma. *Head Neck*, 34, (5) 663-666 available from: PM:21688344

Wang, Z., Zhong, J., Inuzuka, H., Gao, D., Shaik, S., Sarkar, F.H., & Wei, W. 2012b. An evolving role for DEPTOR in tumor development and progression. *Neoplasia.*, 14, (5) 368-375 available from: PM:22745583

Wu, B.H., Xiong, X.P., Jia, J., & Zhang, W.F. 2011. MicroRNAs: new actors in the oral cancer scene. *Oral Oncol.*, 47, (5) 314-319 available from: PM:21474366

Xu, C., Liu, Y., Wang, P., Fan, W., Rue, T.C., Upton, M.P., Houck, J.R., Lohavanichbutr, P., Doody, D.R., Futran, N.D., Zhao, L.P., Schwartz, S.M., Chen, C., & Mendez, E. 2010. Integrative analysis of DNA copy number and gene expression in metastatic oral squamous cell carcinoma identifies genes associated with poor survival. *Mol.Cancer*, 9, 143 available from: PM:20537188

Zhang, J., Feuk, L., Duggan, G.E., Khaja, R., & Scherer, S.W. 2006. Development of bioinformatics resources for display and analysis of copy number and other structural variants in the human genome. *Cytogenet.Genome Res.*, 115, (3-4) 205-214 available from: PM:17124402

Ziober, A.F., Patel, K.R., Alawi, F., Gimotty, P., Weber, R.S., Feldman, M.M., Chalian, A.A., Weinstein, G.S., Hunt, J., & Ziober, B.L. 2006. Identification of a gene signature for rapid screening of oral squamous cell carcinoma. *Clin.Cancer Res.*, 12, (20 Pt 1) 5960-5971 available from: PM:170626

Send Orders for Reprints to reprints@benthamscience.net
Cutting Edge Therapies for Cancer in the 21st Century, 2014, 387-424

CHAPTER 12

Cancer Therapy May be Improved if Diet Contains Omega 3 Fatty Acids

Johannes F. Fahrmann, Theodore R. Witte and W. Elaine Hardman*

McKown Translational Genomics Research Institute, Departments of Biochemistry and Microbiology, Joan C. Edwards School of Medicine, Marshall University, Huntington, WV, USA

Abstract: Omega-3 (n-3) and omega-6 (n-6) polyunsaturated fatty acids (FAs) are essential fats that must be obtained from the diet. The typical western diet is heavily weighted towards n-6 FAs with little n-3 intake. Recently, numerous studies have suggested that arachidonic acid (AA), an n-6 FA, and its metabolites have a significant role in tumor promotion. Inversely, n-3 fatty acids have consistently been shown to slow the growth and increase the chemo-sensitivity of various malignancies *in vitro* and *in vivo*. Clinical studies utilizing n-3 as adjuvants to therapy have shown much promise. The purpose of this chapter is to provide an overview of n-3 and n-6 fatty acids and their application to cancer. In this chapter we will be focusing on 1) the metabolism of n-3 and n-6 FA, 2) the mechanisms of action and implications in cancer and 3) the application of n-3 as promising therapies for the treatment of cancer.

Keywords: Polyunsaturated fatty acids, nutrition and cancer, fatty acids, omega-3 fatty acids, omega-6 fatty acids, eicosapetaenoic acid (EPA), alpha-linolenic acid (ALA), linoleic acid (LA), docosahexaenoic acid (DHA), arachidonic acid (AA), COX, LOX, prostaglandines, tromboxanes.

1. BACKGROUND

Omega-3 (n-3) and omega-6 (n-6) polyunsaturated fatty acids (PUFAs) are essential fatty acids (EFAs). These fats are referred to as essential because humans, like all mammals, are unable to synthesize them and thereby must obtain them from the diet. The n-6 EFA is represented by linoleic acid (LA; 18:2n-6) and n-3 EFA is represented by alpha-linolenic acid (ALA; 18:3n-3) (Fig. **1**). LA is

***Address correspondence to W. Elaine Hardman:** Department of Biochemistry and Microbiology, Translational Genomic Research Institute, Joan C. Edwards School of Medicine, Marshall University, Huntington, WV, USA; Tel: +1 304 696 7339, E-mail: hardmanw@marshall.edu

Pier Paolo Claudio and Paraskevi Vogiatzi (Eds)

primarily found in seeds of most plants, whereas, ALA is primarily found in green leafy vegetables, flax seed, and walnuts (Simopoulos, 2008). The distinction of these two essential fatty acids (FAs) is based on the location of the first double bond from the methyl (omega) end of the FA molecule located between carbon 6-7 (n-6) or 3-4 (n-3) (Fig. **1**) (Simopoulos, 2008, Simopoulos, 1991, Simopoulos, 2000, Simopoulos, 2002).

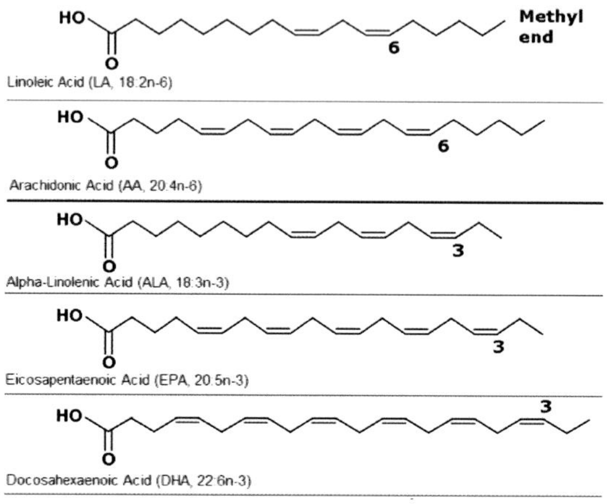

Figure 1: *Chemical Structures of Omega 3 and Omega 6 Fatty Acids*. Abbrev. X:Y- X denotes number of carbon atoms; Y denotes number of unsaturations; n-3: omega 3; n-6: omega 6. Picture modified from the European Food Information Council.

Both EFAs are capable of being metabolized in humans to their longer chain 20-carbon and 22-carbon derivatives. LA is metabolized to 20-carbon arachidonic acid (AA; 20:3n-6) and ALA is metabolized to the 20-carbon eicosapaentaenoic acid (EPA; 20:5n-3) and 22-carbon docosahexaenoic acid (DHA; 22:6n-3). This is achieved by increasing the carbon chain length and degree of unsaturation through addition of extra carbons to the carboxyl end of the fatty acid chain (Fig. **1**) and then desaturating a bond. While AA can be metabolized from its pre-cursor, LA, it can also be obtain from meats of animals that consume LA and then store AA in their meat. Similarly, EPA and DHA can be obtained from fish or fish oils (Simopoulos, 2008, Simopoulos, 1991, Simopoulos, 2000, Simopoulos, 2002).

EFAs are important components of cellular membranes and are selectively found amongst lipid classes. ALA and LA are mostly found in triglycerides, cholesterol esters with a relatively small abundance found in phospholipids. AA and EPA are found in triglycerides, cholesterol esters and phospholipids. Unlike the other n-3 FAs, DHA is predominantly found in phospholipids (Simopoulos, 2008). Furthermore, n-6 and n-3 FA compete with each other for incorporation into the cell and are substrates for the same metabolizing enzymes (reviewed in the following section). As such, consumption of n-3 such as EPA or DHA can partially displace n-6, especially AA, in the membranes of cells (Simopoulos, 2008, Simopoulos, 1991, Simopoulos, 2002, Simopoulos, 2000).

Currently, the western diet is heavily favored towards the n-6 FA with little to no n-3 FA intake. The average ratio of n-6 to n-3 in the western diet is 15-20 to 1 (Simopoulos, 2008) whereas the ideal ratio of n-6 to n-3 is 4-1:1 (Patterson, Wall, Fitzgerald, Ross and Stanton, 2012). Furthermore, mammalians lack the ability to convert n-6 to n-3 as they lack the necessary converting enzyme, omega-3 desaturase (Simopoulos, 2008). This is an important consideration; both n-6 and n-3 are integral parts of cellular membranes and are structurally similar. Yet these two classes of EFA are not interconvertible, and are metabolically and functionally distinct, often having important opposing physiological functions (Simopoulos, 2008). As such, this imbalance toward n-6 can lead to increased risk of various diseases. In support of this notion, various studies have illustrated that a high intake of n-6 and a high n-6/n-3 ratio can promote pathogenesis of many diseases including cardiovascular, autoimmune, cancer, and inflammatory disease (Simopoulos, 2008). Inversely, consumption of n-3 has been shown to have beneficial health effects and often has suppressive effects on pathogenesis (Simopoulos, 2008).

Beneficial health effects of n-3, particularly EPA and DHA, were described first in Greenland Eskimos who consumed high quantities of fish and displayed lower rates of coronary heart disease, asthma, type 1 diabetes mellitus, and multiple sclerosis (Simopoulos, 2008) than populations that consumed less fish. Since then, beneficial effects of n-3 have been extended to include cancer, inflammatory bowel disease, rheumatoid arthritis and psoriasis (Simopoulos, 2008).

The application of n-3 as potential therapeutic options for cancer is of great interest and is the principle focus of this chapter. The metabolism of PUFAs and their physiological role in humans as well as their implications on cancer will be discussed in the following sections.

2. METABOLISM

As introduced above, both LA and ALA are able to be metabolized to their longer 20-carbon and 22-carbon derivatives. This is achieved through a series of elongation and desaturation reactions mediated by specific elongase and desaturase enzymes illustrated in Fig. **2** with delta-6 desaturase being the rate limiting enzyme (Patterson, Wall, Fitzgerald, Ross and Stanton, 2012, Simopoulos, 2008). Since both n-3 and n-6 FA utilize the same enzymes their conversion to their longer derivatives can be influenced if there is a high intake of one type of EFA. For instance, a high intake of ALA can interfere with the elongation and desaturation of LA. This concept has been demonstrated in human studies which illustrated that a constant consumption of ALA with a decreasing consumption of LA led to increases in EPA in the plasma phospholipids (Liou, King, Zibrik and Innis, 2007). Additionally, the elongation and desaturation of n-3 and n-6 FA can also be hindered by the presence of *trans*-fats, which inhibit the delta-6 desaturase (Patterson, Wall, Fitzgerald, Ross and Stanton, 2012, Simopoulos, 2008). As such, the propensity of PUFAs to undergo elongations and desaturations is largely dependent on the type of fat intake of the individual.

The elongation and desaturation of LA and ALA is an important process as the bioactivity of these EFAs is thought to be predominately mediated through their longer chain metabolites. Of the various n-6 and n-3 derivatives, AA and EPA are especially important as these FAs are precursors for eicosanoid production (Haeggstrom, Rinaldo-Matthis, Wheelock and Wetterholm, 2010, Serhan and Petasis, 2011). Eicosanoids are biologically active, 20-carbon lipids which are important mediators of acute inflammation, and have been implicated in several specific diseases such as thrombosis, cancer, atherosclerosis, asthma and rhinitis (Haeggstrom, Rinaldo-Matthis, Wheelock and Wetterholm, 2010, Patterson, Wall, Fitzgerald, Ross and Stanton, 2012). These AA-derived and EPA-derived eicosanoids are produced by three major pathways: the cyclooxygenase (COX), lipoxygenase (LOX) and cytochrome P450 (CYP) pathways (Haeggstrom, Rinaldo-Matthis, Wheelock and Wetterholm, 2010, Luo and Wang, 2011,

Patterson, Wall, Fitzgerald, Ross and Stanton, 2012). Collectively, eicosanoids consist of prostaglandins (PGs), thromboxanes (TXs), leukotrienes (LTs), hydroxyeicosatetraenoic acids (HETEs), epoxyeicosatrienoic acids (EET), epoxyeicosatetraenoic acids (EETeTrs) and hydroxyeicosapentaenoic acids (HEPE) (Arnold, Konkel, Fischer and Schunck, 2010, Luo and Wang, 2011, Patterson, Wall, Fitzgerald, Ross and Stanton, 2012). The synthesis of the various eicosanoids is illustrated in Fig. **3**.

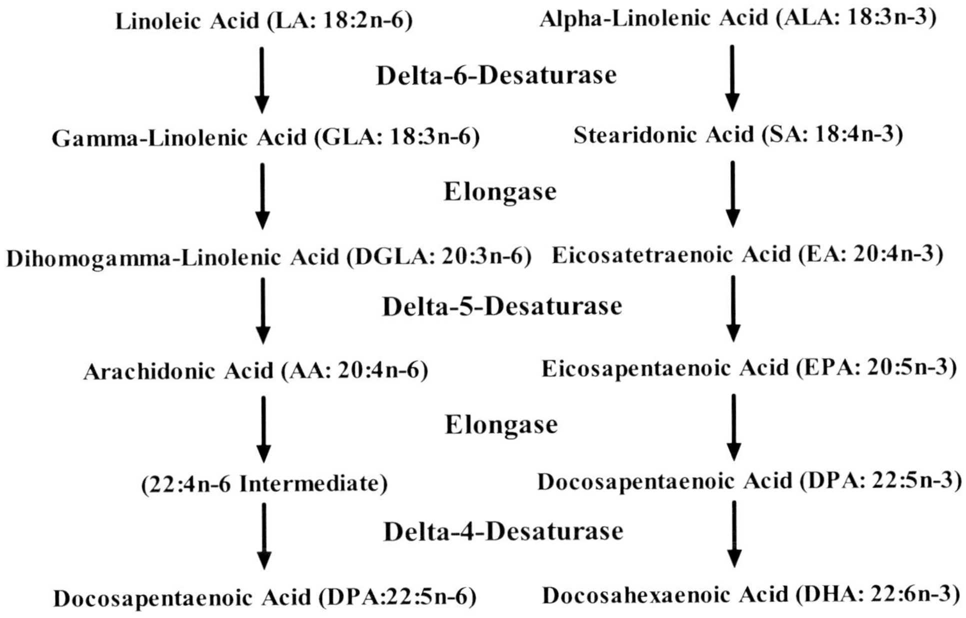

Figure 2: *Metabolism of Linoleic Acid and Alpha-Linolenic Acid to their longer-chain derivatives.* Abbrev. X:Y- X denotes number of carbon atoms; Y denotes number of unsaturations; n-3: omega 3; n-6: omega 6.

While PUFA are able to undergo enzymatic metabolism, they are also able to undergo non-enzymatic degradation. Non-enzymatic degradation of PUFA is mediated by various reactive oxygen and nitrogen species (ROS/RNS) which oxidize lipids, collectively referred to as lipid peroxidation, and yield a diverse array of products (Niki, 2009). The degree of lipid peroxidation is dependent on the number of unsaturations possessed by the FA molecule. As such, the higher the degree of unsaturation the FA molecule possesses the greater the amount of lipid peroxidation that can ensue (Niki, 2009).

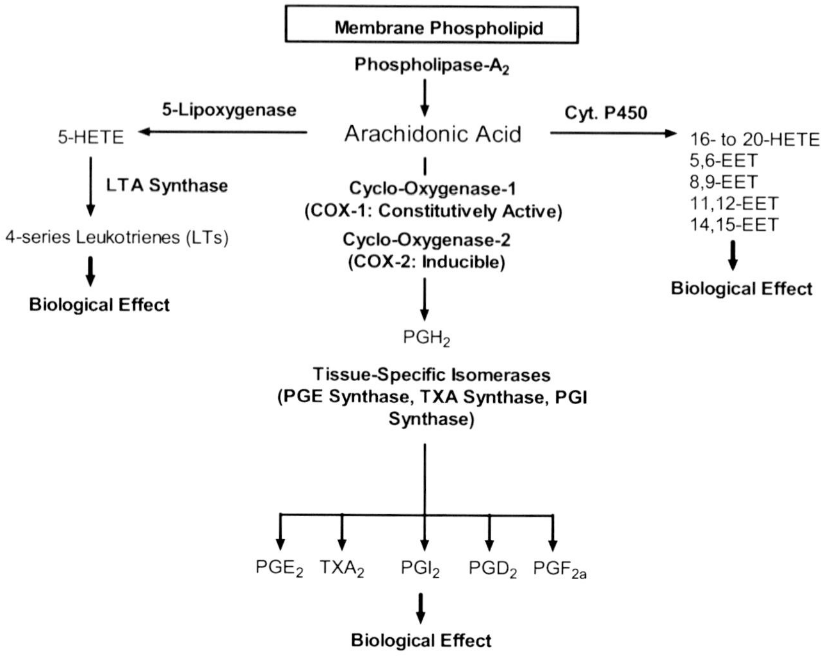

Figure 3: *Schematic of Eicosanoid Production.* Within a cell, AA or EPA is released from the membrane phospholipids by the enzyme phospholipase-A2 (PLA_2) where after they will be metabolized by the cyclo-oxygenase enzymes (COX-1, a constitutive enzyme, or COX-2, an inducible enzyme), 5-lipoxygenase (LOX) or cytochrome p450 (CYP). AA COX-derived eicosanoid PGH_2 is subsequently metabolized by a series of specific prostaglandin synthase enzymes leading to the production of the 2-series prostaglandins: PGE_2, PGI_2, PGD_2, and $PGF_{2\alpha}$ and thromboxanes A_2 and B_2. AA LOX-derived eicosanoid 5-hydroperoxyeicosatetraenoic acid (5-HPETE) is subsequently metabolized by Leukotriene Synthase to produce the 4-series of leukotrienes: LTA_4, LTB_4, LTC_4, LTD_4 and LTE_4. Metabolism of AA by CYP produces the 16- to 20-HETEs and 5,6-, 8,9-, 11,12- and 14,15-epoxyeicosatrienoic acids (EETs). In contrast, EPA can also act as a substrate for COX, LOX and CYP enzymes and give rise to an entirely different set of eicosanoids. These are the 3-series prostaglandins and thromboxanes and the 5-series leukotrienes and epoxyeicosatetraenoic acids (EETeTrs) and 19- and 20-hydroxyeicosapentaenoic acids (HEPE).

Lipid peroxidation can be mediated by free radical-mediated oxidation or free radical-independent non-enzymatic oxidation (Niki, 2009). Free radical-mediated lipid peroxidation is achieved by a chain mechanism in which one initiating free radical can oxidize many molecules of lipids (Niki, 2009). The type of free radical which oxidizes the lipid molecules is dependent on the condition of the cell (Niki, 2009). Free radical-independent non-enzymatic oxidation is mediated by singlet oxygen and ozone (Niki, 2009). Singlet oxygen oxidizes unsaturated lipids mainly by the ene-reaction to give hydroperoxide with concomitant double-bond migration, with minor side reactions such as 1,4 addition to give 1,4-endoperoxide and 1,2 addition to give dioxetane, which readily decomposes to yield carbonyl compounds (Niki, 2009).

Collectively, PUFA are substrates for a variety of enzymatic and non-enzymatic reactions. The type of PUFA, degree of unsaturation and intake all influence the rate and type of by-products that are produced aiding to the complexity of PUFA metabolism and the versatility of their actions.

3. MECHANISMS OF ACTION

The mechanisms through which PUFA exert their actions are diverse and multifaceted, a trait aided by the diversity of their by-products. However, one of the most prominent roles of PUFA is their involvement with inflammation.

Inflammation is an important physiological host defense mechanism that protects the host from infection and other insults. Inflammation initiates pathogen killing and tissue repair processes as well as restoration of homeostasis at an infected or damaged site (Niki, 2009). Under normal conditions, inflammation is tightly regulated to prevent excessive damage to the host. Regulation is often mediated through negative feedback mechanisms such as anti-inflammatory cytokines, inhibition of pro-inflammatory cascades, shedding of receptors for inflammatory mediators and through activation of regulatory cells (Niki, 2009). As such, controlled, regulated inflammatory responses are essential to remain healthy and maintain body homeostasis. However, a loss of tolerance and/or regulation of inflammatory processes can lead to excessive, irreparable damage to the host tissue leading to various pathologies, including cancer (Niki, 2009).

Eicosanoids are key mediators and regulators of inflammation (Calder, 2009, Haeggstrom, Rinaldo-Matthis, Wheelock and Wetterholm, 2010, Serhan and Petasis, 2011). As previously mentioned, the eicosanoids produced by AA are comprised of the 2-series PGs and TXs and the 4-series LTs. PGE_2 and the 4-series LTs are particularly important as these eicosanoids modulate both the intensity and duration of the inflammatory response (Calder, 2009). However, eicosanoid production is not solely derived from AA, but can also be derived from EPA. The eicosanoids produced from EPA, which includes the 3-series PGs/TXs and 5-series LTs, are functionally different from their AA-derived counterparts and often have antagonistic actions on inflammation (Table **1**) (Calder, 2009).

Prostaglandins and thromboxanes, collectively referred to as prostanoids, exert their biological effects by binding to cell-surface prostanoid receptors belonging to the family of G-protein-coupled rhodopsin receptors (GPCRs) or nuclear receptors such as the peroxisome proliferator-activated receptors (PPARs) (Cathcart, Lysaght and Pidgeon, 2011, Ricciotti and FitzGerald, 2011). The prostanoid receptor family is composed of 8 members: E prostanoid receptor (EP 1-4); D prostanoid receptor (DP1); F prostanoid receptor (FP); I prostanoid receptor (IP); and thromboxane receptor (TP) (Ricciotti and FitzGerald, 2011). These prostanoid receptors are coupled to a range of intracellular signaling pathways summarized in Table **2**.

Of particular interest are the EP receptors and PGE_2 as PGE_2 is one of the most abundant eicosanoids produced in the body (Ricciotti and FitzGerald, 2011). EP2 and EP4 activate adenylyl cyclase to generate cyclic adenosine monophosphate (cAMP) leading to activation of protein kinase A (PKA) (Alfranca, Iniguez, Fresno and Redondo, 2006, Ricciotti and FitzGerald, 2011). PKA can, in turn, inhibit glycogen synthase kinase 3 (GSK3α), thereby promoting transcription of T-cell factor (Tcf)-dependent genes such as COX-2. Additionally, EP4 specifically activates the phosphoinositide 3-kinase (PI3K)/ protein kinase B (Akt) pathway which, in some cell types, augments extracellular signal-regulated kinase (ERK) activity and mediates expression of early growth response protein 1 (EGR-1) and subsequent transcription of genes such as prostaglandin E synthase-1 (mPGES-1) (Alfranca, Iniguez, Fresno and Redondo, 2006). PGE_2 has also been shown to activate nuclear factor kappa B (NFκB), a key mediator of the inflammatory processes(Ditsworth and Zong, 2004), and hypoxia inducible factor-1 alpha (HIF-1α) (Alfranca, Iniguez, Fresno and Redondo, 2006). Additionally, PGE_2 has been shown to transactivate the epidermal growth factor receptor (EGFR) *via* activation of proto-oncogene tyrosine-protein kinase Src (c-Src), which activates EGFR directly or indirectly by inducing metalloproteinase activity that releases membrane bound transforming growth factor-alpha (TGFα) (Buchanan, Wang, Bargiacchi and DuBois, 2003, Pai, Soreghan, Szabo *et al.*, 2002). Collectively, the bioactivity of PGE_2 is diverse and cell-type specific. However, PGE_2 is typically associated with promotion of increased states of inflammation and has been implicated in various tumorigenic processes (Reader, Holt and Fulton, 2011).

Table 1: Pro-Inflammatory Effects of N-6 Fatty Acid-Derived Eicosanoids and Anti-Inflammatory Effects of N-3 Fatty Acid-Derived Eicosanoids

Pro-Inflammatory Effects of the n-6 Fatty-Acid-Derived Eicosanoids			
	Arachidonic Acid (n-6) Derived Eicosanoids	**Physiological Effect**	**Organ or Cells**
Prostaglandins	PGD_2	Bronchoconstriction Pro-inflammatory Pro-arrhythmic	Bronchi Activation of Eosinophils Vessels
	PGE_2	Induces Fever Causes Pain Increases Production of IL-6	Nociceptor Sensory Neurons
	PGF_2	Bronchoconstriction Pro-arrhythmic	Bronchi Vessels
	PGI_2	Causes Pain	Nociceptor Sensory Neurons
Thromboxanes	TXA_2/TXB_2	Pro-aggregation Vasoconstriction Bronchoconstriction	Platelets Vessels Bronchi
Leukotrienes	$LTA_4/LTB_4/LTC_4/LTD_4/LTE_4$	Pro-inflammatory Chemotaxis Release of ROS	Leukocytes Leukocytes Granulocytes
Anti-Inflammatory Effects of The n-3 Fatty-Acid-Derived Eicosanoids			
	Eicosapentaenoic Acid and Docosahexaenoic Acid (n-3) Derived Eicosanoids	Physiological Effect	Organ or Cells
Prostaglandins	$PGD_3/PGE_3/PGF_3/PGI_3$	Anti-arrhythmic	Vessels
Thromboxanes	TXA_3/TXB_3	Anti-aggregation	Platelets
Leukotrienes	$LTA_5/LTB_5/LTC_5/LTD_5/LTE_5$	Anti-inflammatory	Leukocytes
Resolvins	RVE_1	Anti-aggregation Anti-inflammatory	Platelets Dendritic Cells
	RVD	Anti-inflammatory	Dendritic Cells
Neuroprotectin	NPD_1	Anti-inflammatory Anti-apoptotic Decreases Oxidative Stress	Retina (photoreceptor cells) and Brain

Modified from Calder et al., (Calder, 2009).

While eicosanoids are primary mediators of inflammation, products of lipid peroxidation can also contribute to an inflammatory state. While the mechanisms, dynamics and products of lipid peroxidation are still under investigation, it has been shown that lipid peroxidation induces: 1) disturbances of fine structures, 2) alterations in integrity, fluidity and permeability of cell membranes leading to functional loss, 3) modifies low-density lipoproteins to pro-atherogenic and pro-inflammatory forms, and 4) can generate potentially toxic products (Greenberg, Li, Gugiu *et al.*, 2008, Niki, 2009). Despite the potential mutagenic and genotoxic effects that lipid peroxides can elicit, it has also become evident that lipid peroxidation products exert various biological functions *in vivo* such as regulation of gene expression, signaling messengers, activators of receptors and nuclear transcription factors, and inducers of adaptive responses (Niki, 2009). Recent studies have provided evidence that many products of lipid peroxidation exert opposite duel effects, depending on conditions, such as cytotoxic or cytoprotective effects, pro- and anti-atherogenic effects, pro- and anti-apoptotic effects and pro- and anti-inflammatory effects (Parthasarathy, Santanam, Ramachandran and Meilhac, 2000, Zmijewski, Landar, Watanabe *et al.*, 2005). Thus, the contribution of lipid peroxides to a pro-inflammatory state is complex and context dependent.

Table 2: Signal Transduction of AA-derived Prostanoids

Class	Subtype	G-Protein Coupled	Second Messenger(s)
PGE_2	EP1	G_q	↑IP_3
	EP2	G_s	↑cAMP
	EP3	G_i, G_{12}, G_{Rho}	↓cAMP, ↑Ca^{2+}
	EP4	G_s	↑cAMP
PGD_2	DP	G_s	↑cAMP
	CRTH2	G_i	↓cAMP, ↑Ca^{2+}
$PGF_{2\alpha}$	FP_A, FP_B	G_q, G_{Rho}	↑IP_3
PGI_2	IP-IP	G_s, G_q, G_i	↑IP_3, ↑↓cAMP
	IP-TP_α	G_s	↑cAMP
TxA_2	TP_α, TP_β	G_q, G_s (α), G_i (β), G_h, $G_{12/13}$	↑IP_3, ↑↓cAMP ↑Ca^{2+}

Modified from Alfranca et al (Alfranca, Iniguez, Fresno and Redondo, 2006).

The mechanisms of action exerted by n-6 and n-3 are diverse and multi-faceted. Typically, n-6 FAs are considered to be pro-inflammatory; whereas n-3 FAs are considered to be anti-inflammatory. This is an important consideration. States of chronic inflammation are an underlying cause for various pathologies including cancer (Balkwill and Coussens, 2004, Clevers, 2004). A diet rich in n-6 will shift the balance toward a pro-inflammatory and pro-thrombotic state and can, thereby, promote tumor promotion and progression. Inversely, the addition of n-3 can antagonize the pro-inflammatory effects of n-6 thereby providing a potential therapy for the treatment of cancer, the focal point of this chapter.

4. OMEGA-3 FATTY ACIDS AND CANCER

Recently, numerous studies have supported the notion that AA and its metabolites have a significant role in tumor promotion (Hyde and Missailidis, 2009). While the role of AA and its metabolites on tumor promotion is intricate and multi-faceted, much attention has been placed on COX-2 and PGE_2. It is clear that overexpression of COX-2 is implicated in various forms of human cancers including lung (Krysan, Dohadwala, Luo *et al.*, 2004), breast (Barnes, Haywood, Flint, Knox and Bundred, 2006), colorectal (Chan, Ogino and Fuchs, 2007), prostate (Lee, Pan, Cheng, Chi and Liu, 2001), head and neck (Tang, Lin, Chang *et al.*, 2003), and chronic lymphocytic leukemia (Ryan, Pollock, Kaur *et al.*, 2006, Secchiero, Barbarotto, Gonelli *et al.*, 2005). In conjunction, AA-COX derived eicosanoid, PGE_2, is the most abundantly formed prostaglandin (Ricciotti and FitzGerald, 2011) and has been implicated in various aspects of tumorigenesis *via* induction of cell proliferation, anti-apoptosis, angiogenesis, invasion, and metastasis (Greenhough, Smartt, Moore *et al.*, 2009). In addition, PGE_2 has also been linked to upregulation of B-cell CLL/lymphoma 2 (Bcl-2), an anti-apoptotic protein, and induction of NFκB (Wang and Dubois, 2010).

NFκB belongs to a family of transcription factors that play a pivotal role in inflammatory and stress responses as well as in tumor cell resistance to apoptosis (Balkwill and Coussens, 2004, Darnell, 2002). NFκB controls various cytokines (*e.g.* IL-1, IL-2, IL-6, IL-12, TNF-α), chemokines (*e.g.* IL-8, MIP-1α, MCP1), adhesion molecules (*e.g.* ICAM, VCAM and E-selectin) and inducible effector enzymes such as inducible nitric oxide synthase (iNOS) and COX-2 (Schmitz and

Ecker, 2008). Several studies have demonstrated that NFκB can promote oncogenesis by virtue of its ability to regulate the expression of a wide array of genes that modulate apoptosis, proliferation, inflammation, tumor metastasis, and angiogenesis(Clevers, 2004). Increased constitutively active NFκB has been observed in various solid tumors as well as hematological malignancies(Braun, Carvalho, Fabre *et al.*, 2006, Darnell, 2002, Ditsworth and Zong, 2004). Activation of NFκB has been linked to aggressive tumor growth and resistance to both chemotherapy and radiotherapy (Li and Sethi, 2010). NFκB regulates COX-2 (Schmitz and Ecker, 2008). COX-2 increases production of PGE_2 (Calder, 2009). PGE_2 in turn can stimulate various pathways associated with tumorigenesis including activation of NFκB (Ditsworth and Zong, 2004, Wang and Dubois, 2010). Thus, the relationship between NFκB, COX-2 and PGE_2 is inherently intertwined and potentially self-propagating.

N-3 and n-6 compete with each other for incorporation and metabolism. The effects of n-3 derived metabolites are antagonistic of n-6 derived metabolites. Given the involvement of AA and its metabolites in tumor promotion, the use of n-3, particularly EPA and DHA, as therapeutic options for various malignancies presents a promising avenue of research.

N-3 fatty acids have consistently been shown to slow the growth and increase the chemo-sensitivity of various malignancies *in vitro* and in animal models (Das and Madhavi, 2011, Das, Madhavi, Sravan Kumar, Padma and Sangeetha, 1998, Dekoj, Lee, Desai *et al.*, 2007, Hardman, Avula, Fernandes and Cameron, 2001). While the growth-inhibitory and chemo-sensitizing effects of n-3 are diverse, much attention has been placed on COX-2, NFκB, the "PGE_2-to-PGE_3" switch and lipid peroxidation. In the following sections, the application of n-3 as therapeutic options for the treatment of Breast Cancer, Lung Cancer, and Chronic Lymphocytic Leukemia will be explored highlighting both *in vitro* and *in vivo* studies as well as clinical studies.

4.1. Omega-3 Fatty Acids and Breast Cancer

Breast cancer is the most common cancer in women (Bray, Ren, Masuyer and Ferlay, 2013). Currently, a wide variety of treatment options exist for breast cancer including mastectomy, chemotherapy, hormonal therapy, radiation therapy, or a combination of these (Brennan, Wilcken, French, Ung and Boyages, 2005). While treatments for early stages of breast cancer have had high success rates, overall survival rates for patients who develop metastatic breast cancer (MBC) remains dismally low. This is due to a variety of factors which can influence response rates to treatment including performance status, comorbidities, burden and pace of disease, tumor subtype, prior exposure to therapy and drug resistance (Bougnoux, Hajjaji, Ferrasson *et al.*, 2009, Gogineni and DeMichele, 2012). Additionally, non-selective toxicities associated with chemotherapy treatment can result in reduced drug efficacy and dose limitations (Bougnoux, Hajjaji, Ferrasson *et al.*, 2009). As such, a therapeutic intervention that can decrease the incidence and growth of breast cancer or increase the chemo-sensitivity of malignant cells without additional adverse effects would provide clinical benefit.

Clinical, epidemiological, and mechanistic studies *in vitro* and *in vivo* suggest that the consumption of Omega-3s may decrease the incidence and growth of breast cancer, increase the response to chemotherapeutics and hormonal therapy, and improve recovery.

Numerous studies have indicated the potential involvement of COX-2 in breast cancer progression. Benign ductal carcinoma *in-situ* (DCIS) may progress to invasive cancer (14%-53%) but a large number are undiagnosed at autopsy-indicating that a large number may not progress (Erbas, Provenzano, Armes and Gertig, 2006). A meta-analysis through the course of breast cancer development showed similar levels of COX-2 expression in DCIS and invasive breast cancer. It has been suggested that the presence of COX-2 in the non-invasive tumors may contribute to the development of malignancy (Glover, Hughes, Cantwell and Murray, 2011). Perrone *et al.,* illustrated that in non-invasive DCIS COX-2 was positively correlated to vascular endothelial growth factor (VEGF) and Human Epidermal Growth Factor Receptor 2 (Her-2/Neu) expression, angiogenesis and growth factors which contribute to the development of invasiveness (Perrone, Santini, Vincenzi *et al.*, 2005). Additionally, Miglietta *et al.,* found that COX-2 over-expression in breast cancer corresponded to the degree of vascular invasion (Miglietta, Toselli, Ravarino *et al.*, 2010). Ristimaki *et al.,* indicated that COX-2 is over-expressed in a third of invasive breast tumors and is significantly associated with reduced disease free survival, axillary metastases, and tumor growth- especially in ER negative tumors (Ristimaki, Sivula, Lundin *et al.*, 2002). Similarly, Denkert *et al.,* found that elevated COX-2 expression in breast carncinomas was significantly associated with a decrease in disease-free survival and decreased overall survival in a univariate analysis, however, multivariate analysis found that COX-2 was borderline significant for disease-free survival (Denkert, Winzer, Muller *et al.*, 2003). It should also be noted that no significant associations were found between disease-free survival and overall survival and COX-1 expression in the studies by Denkert *et al.,* indicating that the association of COX with disease progression is likely to be specific for COX-2 and not COX-1 (Denkert, Winzer, Muller *et al.*, 2003).

The importance of COX-2 and inflammation in breast cancer has led to attempts to prevent progression by inhibiting COX-2 activity or otherwise decreasing the production of PGE_2. Omega-3s compete with n-6 PUFAs at all steps of metabolism to prostaglandins, effectively decreasing the production of PGE_2 (Simopoulos, 2008). Consuming n-3 PUFAs or displacing n-6 PUFAs from the diet may decrease PGE_2 synthesis, and slow tumor progression.

Increased n-3 ALA and DHA, as well as an increased n-3/n-6 ratio in mammary adipose tissue correlated to decreased risk of breast cancer (Maillard, Bougnoux, Ferrari *et al.*, 2002). Conversely, the levels of ALA, EPA, and DHA in serum are significantly lower in breast cancer patients (Lv and Yang, 2012). When the lipid compositions of malignant and adjacent normal breast tissues were compared, the malignant tissues were found to have relatively higher levels of n-6, especially long chain PUFAs, and increased PGE_2 (Pender-Cudlip, Krag, Martini *et al.*, 2013). The trend was more evident in ER- than ER+ patients (Pender-Cudlip, Krag, Martini *et al.*, 2013). High levels of LA, an n-6, in breast cancer tissue have been found to be predictive of malignancy (Lv and Yang, 2012). Urinary PGE-M, an end metabolite of PGE_2, was increased in breast cancer patients with lung metastases when compared to patients with early breast cancer (Morris, Zhou, Milne *et al.*, 2013). In a study of premenopausal women, LA consumption correlated to increased levels of 4-hydroxy estradiol and etheno-DNA adducts (Sun, Nair, Linseisen, Owen and Bartsch, 2012). The formation of 4-hydroxy estradiol in preference to 2-OH can be caused by PGE_2, demonstrated in ER+

breast cancer *in vitro* (Han, Kim, Hwang, Song and Jeong, 2010). In cultured primary adipose stromal cells PGE_2 induces aromatase, which may increase estrogen in the local tumor environment (Karuppu, Kalus, Simpson and Clyne, 2002). Besides being a plausible mechanism of initiation, 4-hydroxy estradiol has been shown to stimulate invasiveness of breast cancer *in vitro* (Paquette, Bisson, Baptiste *et al.*, 2005). Collectively, these observations suggest that increasing n-3 or displacing n-6 may slow the progression of breast cancer by decreasing PGE_2 and inflammation.

Animal and *in vitro* studies suggest that the efficacy of Tamoxifen, an anti-estrogen drug used to treat breast cancer, can be improved by fish oil consumption. Fish oil consumption led to decreased Akt activation, and decreased downstream NFκB activation (Ghosh-Choudhury, Mandal, Woodruff *et al.*, 2009). NFκB has been demonstrated to be hyperactive in malignant breast tissue and contributes to tumor survival (Vinothini and Nagini, 2010). DeGraffenried *et al.* illustrated that MCF-7 cells transfected with a constitutive active Akt plasmid were more resistant to Tamoxifen than control MCF-7 cells. Treatment with n-3, EPA, decreased Akt activation in transfected MCF-7 cells and increased the effects of Tamoxifen (DeGraffenried, Friedrichs, Fulcher *et al.*, 2003).

Omega-3 PUFAs may also enhance response to chemotherapeutic agents by increasing the apoptotic potential of transformed cells. The presence of DHA in the cellular membrane contributes to lipid peroxidation and oxidative stress, possibly enhancing therapies using these as mechanisms of cytotoxicity (Bougnoux, Germain, Chajes *et al.*, 1999). DHA additionally alters membrane fluidity and possibly receptor activity (Corsetto, Cremona, Montorfano *et al.*, 2012).

Studies by Bougnoux *et al.,* indicated that response was positively correlated with n-3 levels in breast adipose tissue in patients with localized breast carcinoma given a therapy of mitoxantrone, vindesine, cyclophosphamide, and 5-fluorouracil (Bougnoux, Germain, Chajes *et al.*, 1999). Notably, increased DHA especially stood out as a positive predictor of chemosensitivity (Bougnoux, Germain, Chajes *et al.*, 1999). In line with these observations, studies by Bougnoux *et al.,* also illustrated that supplementation with 1.8 g/daily of DHA improved the efficacy of anthracycline-based therapy against the progression of visceral metastases (Bougnoux, Hajjaji, Ferrasson *et al.*, 2009). In this study, significant increases in time to progression and median overall survival were achieved in patients with the highest plasma DHA levels as compared to the lowest plasma DHA levels (8.7 months *versus* 3.5 months and 34 months *versus* 22 months; respectively) (Bougnoux, Hajjaji, Ferrasson *et al.*, 2009). Importantly, it was also found that supplementation with DHA did not induce any additional adverse effects. It should be noted that this was a small study (n= 25) and the relationship between DHA content and metastatic cancer outcome subsequent to chemotherapy does not ensure a causality (Bougnoux, Hajjaji, Ferrasson *et al.*, 2009). However, the increase in time to progression and overall survival in the high DHA group supports the use of DHA as a chemo-sensitizing agent and warrants further exploration.

The consumption of EPA+DHA from marine fish is linked to a 25% increase in disease free survival after treatment for early stage breast cancer when comparing the highest and lowest EPA+DHA consuming quintiles respectively (Patterson, Flatt, Newman *et al.*, 2011). This effect could be attributed to increased efficiency of treatment, or the previously discussed mechanisms of prevention.

Omega-3 PUFAs may be able to reduce the side effects of treatments due to their anti-inflammatory properties. In support of this notion, Ghoreishi *et al.,* illustrated that a daily dose of 630 mg Omega-3 PUFA partially prevented paclitaxel induced peripheral neuropathy (PIPN), a dose-limiting side effect of paclitaxel therapy (Ghoreishi, Esfahani, Djazayeri *et al.*, 2012). Additionally, Heller *et al.,* indicated that the addition of 0.2g/kg/daily fish oil increased liver and pancreas function while reducing weight loss in patients recovering from major elective abdominal surgery (Heller, Rossel, Gottschlich *et al.*, 2004). Inversely, inflammation and fatigue are linked to a high n-6/n-3 consumption ratio in breast cancer survivors (Alfano, Imayama, Neuhouser *et al.*, 2012). These findings suggest the n-3 may be effective in reducing the inflammation based side effects of therapy or recovery.

4.2. Omega-3 Fatty Acids and Lung Cancer

Lung cancer is the leading cause of cancer-related deaths world-wide, and non-small cell lung cancer (NSCLC) accounts for 80% of all lung cancers (Jiang, Wang and Zhao, 2013). The overall survival rate for patients with lung cancer is less than 15% and has remained largely unchanged for the past three decades (Yang, Cartwright, Chan *et al.*, 2013). Although significant advances have been made with conventional therapies, the poor prognosis and low overall survival rates for patients continues to be problematic (Jiang, Wang and Zhao, 2013). This is largely because the majority of patients with lung cancer require multiple lines of therapy due to progressive acquired drug resistance amongst malignant cells during the course of treatment (Chang, 2011). Drug resistance remains a major obstacle for the treatment of lung cancer (Chang, 2011). Therefore, a therapeutic intervention that could slow the growth of malignant cells, is selectively cytotoxic against malignant cells or can increase/restore the sensitivity of malignant cells to anti-cancer drugs would be highly desirable.

Overexpression of COX-2 has been reported in NSCLC and has been suggested to be associated with poor survival (Jiang, Wang and Zhao, 2013, Khuri, Wu, Lee *et al.*, 2001, Ochiai, Oguri, Isobe, Ishioka and Yamakido, 1999). This notion is supported by Edelman *et al.,* who indicated that NSCLC patients who overexpressed COX-2 had drastically lower survival rates as compared to NSCLC patients who did not overexpress COX-2 (Edelman, Watson, Wang *et al.*, 2008). Additionally, Edelman *et al.,* also illustrated that NSCLC patients who overexpressed COX-2 had significantly greater overall survival rates when celecoxib, a selective COX-2 inhibitor, was added to chemo-therapy as compared to COX-2 overexpressing NSCLC patients who received chemo-therapy only (Edelman, Watson, Wang *et al.*, 2008). Inversely, patients who did not overexpress COX-2 and received celecoxib with chemo-therapy demonstrated lower overall survival rates as compared to patients who had overexpressed COX-2, although this was not statistically significant (Edelman, Watson, Wang *et al.*, 2008). Similarly, Csiki *et al.,* found that urinary levels of PGE-M, the major urinary metabolite of PGE_2, was correlated with survival of patients with recurrent NSCLC receiving celecoxib plus docetaxel (Csiki, Morrow, Sandler *et al.*, 2005). Fidler *et al.,* also found that patients with NSCLC who overexpressed COX-2 had significantly greater prolonged progression-free survival when treated with celecoxib plus Erlotinib *versus* Erlotinib alone (Fidler, Argiris, Patel *et al.*, 2008). While these studies indicate that the use of COX-2 inhibitors may only be beneficial for subgroups of patients who display high levels of COX-2, interventions which target COX-2 present promising therapeutic options for the treatment of lung cancer.

Numerous studies have suggested that chronic inflammation contributes to the process of lung carcinogenesis through activation of various pathways including NFκB (Tang, Liu, Shishodia *et al.*, 2006). *In vitro* studies in NSCLC cell lines have demonstrated that tobacco components stimulate NFκB-dependent survival (Tsurutani, Castillo, Brognard *et al.*, 2005). Additionally, inhibition of COX-2 by celecoxib suppressed NFκB p65 nuclear immunolocalization induced by various carcinogens providing further insight into the importance and relationship between NFκB and COX-2 in NSCLC (Shishodia, Koul and Aggarwal, 2004). Studies by Tang *et al.,* found that high levels of immunohistochemical expression of NFκB p65 were detected in lung cancers (Tang, Liu, Shishodia *et al.*, 2006). Interestingly, in lung adenocarcinomas the NFκB p65 expression was significantly higher in advanced TNM (tumor, lymph nodes, metastasis) stages (III-IV) than in earlier stages (I-II) suggesting that NFκB is associated with disease progression (Tang, Liu, Shishodia *et al.*, 2006). These findings are further supported by Zhang *et al.,* who also found that expression of NFκB/Rel A was higher in NSCLC tissue as compared to normal adjacent tissue and normal lung tissue (Zhang, Jin, Wang *et al.*, 2007). Additionally, there was a positive correlation between NFκB activation (nuclear translocation of Rel A) and tumor clinicopathological features such as tumor grade, and TNM staging supporting the findings by Tang *et al* (Zhang, Jin, Wang *et al.*, 2007). Zhang *et al.,* also demonstrated that nuclear Rel A binding and cytoplasmic phosphorylated-inhibitor of kappa-B-alpha (pIkB-α) were positively associated with poor prognosis (Zhang, Jin, Wang *et al.*, 2007). Furthermore, it has been shown that the apoptotic rate was lower in lung cancer cells which exhibited a high NFκB expression as compared to those with a lower NFκB expression (Zhang, Ma, Li, Sun and Wang, 2006). Within these cells, expression of NFκB was correlated with caspase-3, COX-2, and p53 expression (Zhang, Ma, Li, Sun and Wang,

2006). In light of these findings, it has also been shown that inhibition of NFκB activation through the use of dimethylaminoparthenolide (DMAPT), an NFκB inhibitor, slowed the growth of NSCLC cell lines A549 and H1299 and enhanced their sensitivity to radiotherapy (Estabrook, Chin-Sinex, Borgmann *et al.*, 2011). Given the recent findings of the importance of NFκB in lung cancer, a therapeutic intervention which targets NFκB may provide clinical benefit.

The use of n-3 as a therapeutic option for the treatment of lung cancer, particularly NSCLC, has received considerable focus. Studies by Yang *et al.,* indicated that EPA slowed the growth of NSCLC cell lines A549 (COX-2 over-expressing) and H1299 (COX-2 null) *in vitro* (Yang, Cartwright, Chan *et al.*, 2013). Interestingly, EPA inhibited 50% of growth in A549 at 6.05μM whereas almost 80μM of EPA was needed to elicit similar levels of growth-inhibition in H1299 (Yang, Cartwright, Chan *et al.*, 2013). Similarly, growth of A549 xenografts were significantly suppressed by menhaden oil, an omega-3 rich oil, but not in H1299 xenografts (Yang, Cartwright, Chan *et al.*, 2013). It should be mentioned that DHA inhibited 50% of growth in A549 at 9.7μM and H1299 at 50μM indicating a differential effect on growth-inhibition between EPA and DHA (Yang, Cartwright, Chan *et al.*, 2013). Furthermore, Yang *et al.,* indicated that the production of PGE_3 was significantly higher in A549 cells treated with EPA than in H1299 cells. Similarly the ratio of PGE_3 to PGE_2 was higher in the A549 xenograft tissue than in the H1299 xenograft tissue. Additionally, in these studies, Yang *et al.,* illustrated that PGE_2 up-regulated expression of pAkt, whereas PGE_3 down-regulated expression of pAkt (Yang, Cartwright, Chan *et al.*, 2013). Collectively, the results from Yang *et al.,* indicate that EPA has the ability to generated COX-dependent PGE_3. The production of PGE_3 was found to be important for the growth-inhibitory effects induced by EPA and mediated, in part, by suppression of the pro-survival pathway Akt (Yang, Cartwright, Chan *et al.*, 2013). It should be noted that Akt is also an activator of the non-canonical NFκB pathway (Pianetti, Arsura, Romieu-Mourez, Coffey and Sonenshein, 2001). Therefore, while it has not been shown directly, the ability of EPA to modulate Akt and COX-2 activity indicates that NFκB is likely also being influenced.

Studies by Kikawa *et al.,* indicated that DHA induced significant decreases in proliferation and colony formation while significantly increasing apoptosis and lipid peroxidation in A549 cells *in vitro* (Kikawa, Herrick, Tateo *et al.*, 2010). Furthermore, the combination of DHA and ionizing radiation provided vastly superior results on growth-inhibition and increased cell death than either alone (Kikawa, Herrick, Tateo *et al.*, 2010). It was also observed that the combination of DHA and ionizing radiation induced greater increases in lipid peroxidation than either alone. Moreover, the addition of vitamin-E, a fat soluble anti-oxidant, abrogated the increase in lipid peroxidation and attenuated the increase in cell death due to DHA and ionizing radiation (Kikawa, Herrick, Tateo *et al.*, 2010). This indicates that the enhanced effect of DHA due to ionizing radiation is, in part, mediated through increased generation of toxic lipid peroxides. In line with the observations by Kikawa *et al., in vivo* studies by Maehle *et al.,* found that a n-3 diet, predominately composed of EPA and DHA, slowed the growth of A427 lung adenocarcinoma cells in athymic nude mice (Maehle, Lystad, Eilertsen *et al.*, 1999). Conversely, it was also shown that levels of thiobarbituric acid reactive substances (TBARs, by products of lipid peroxidation) were higher in tumors of mice on the n-3 diet as compared either the control or corn (n-6) diet. The addition of vitamin E abrogated the increase in TBARs and attenuated the growth-inhibitor effects of the n-3 diet (Maehle, Lystad, Eilertsen *et al.*, 1999). It should also be noted that the growth-inhibitory effects on A427 xenografts were more pronounced with the n-3 diet as compared to the n-6 based diet (Maehle, Lystad, Eilertsen *et al.*, 1999). Studies by Serini *et al.,* illustrated that DHA induced dose-responsive apoptosis in mink lung epithelial cells (Mv1LU), A549 and human lung carcinoma cell line BEN *in vitro* (Serini, Trombino, Oliva *et al.*, 2008). In these studies, it was found that DHA increased mRNA and protein expression of MAP-kinase-phosphatase-1 (MKP-1), a regulator of MAPK, and down-regulated p-ERK1/2 and p-p38 expression. The addition of phosphatase inhibitor Na3VO4 or silencing of the MKP-1 gene abrogated the increase in apoptosis induced by DHA indicating that the ability of DHA to induce apoptosis was, in part, dependent on MKP-1 induction (Serini, Trombino, Oliva *et al.*, 2008). Collectively, these studies indicate that DHA is cytotoxic against malignant cells and has the capability of enhancing the cytotoxic effects of ionizing radiation. It has also been shown that the cytotoxic effects are, in part, mediated through increased lipid peroxidation. However, it is also apparent that the cytotoxic effects of DHA are not solely dependent on lipid peroxidation but can also be mediated through other mechanisms such as up-regulation of MKP-1 as described by Serini *et al.,* indicating that the cytotoxic effects of DHA are multi-faceted.

While numerous studies have demonstrated the potential use of n-3 FAs as therapeutic options for the treatment of lung cancer through both *in vitro* and *in vivo* models, its application towards human lung cancers remains of primary interest. Recently, studies by Murphy *et al.,* indicated that supplementation with fish oil increased the first-line chemotherapy efficacy in patients with advanced NSCLC (Murphy, Mourtzakis, Chu *et al.*, 2011). In this study, patients with clinical diagnosis of stage IIIB or IV NSCLC who were chemotherapy-naïve were either supplemented with fish oil (2.5g of EPA + DHA/day; n=15) or no fish oil (standard of care group (SOC); n=31) in conjunction with first-line platinum-based doublet chemotherapy of palliative intent consisting of either carboplatin with vinorelbine or carboplatin with gemcitabine (Murphy, Mourtzakis, Chu *et al.*, 2011). Primary endpoints of this study were response rates, defined as complete response plus partial response, and clinical benefit, defined as the sum of complete response, partial response and stable disease divided by the number of patients (Murphy, Mourtzakis, Chu *et al.*, 2011). Collectively, results from Murphy *et al.,* illustrated that patients in the fish oil group had increased response rates and greater clinical benefit compared to the SOC group (60.0% *versus* 25.8%, p-value: 0.008 and 80.0% *versus* 41.9%, p-value: 0.02, respectively) (Murphy, Mourtzakis, Chu *et al.*, 2011). It should also be noted that patients in the fish oil group had greater 1-year survival rates as compared to the SOC group (60.0% *versus* 38.7%), although this was not statistically significant (Murphy, Mourtzakis, Chu *et al.*, 2011). Furthermore, patients in the fish oil group did not display any additional toxicities associated with treatment as compared to the SOC group. Inversely, as compared to the SOC group, patients in the fish oil indicated a significantly higher number of chemotherapy cycles received (number of chemotherapy cycles received ± SD: 3.9 ± 0.9 *versus* 3.0 ± 1.4, p-value: 0.02) and indicated longer, almost significant, time on chemo-therapy (time on chemotherapy (days) ± SD: 78.9 ± 23.5 *versus* 60.3 ± 31.1, p-value: 0.05) (Murphy, Mourtzakis, Chu *et al.*, 2011). This is an interesting observation as the reason behind the increased response rates and clinical benefit in the fish oil group may be due, in part, to the fact that these patients were more capable of tolerating the chemotherapy regime as a result of fish oil consumption. In support of these observations, studies by van der Meij *et al.,* indicated that patients with stage III NSCLC who consumed oral n-3 supplements (2.02g EPA + 0.92g DHA) during multimodality treatment had significantly greater quality of life parameters, physical and cognitive function, global health status and social function, and higher physical activity as compared to the placebo group (van der Meij, Langius, Spreeuwenberg *et al.*, 2012). Similarly, Murphy *et al.,* also found that patients with NSCLC who consumed fish oil (2.2g of EPA/day) retained weight and either gained or maintained muscle mass as compared to the non-intervention group during first-line therapy (Murphy, Mourtzakis, Chu *et al.*, 2011). Thus the application of n-3 in a clinical setting has shown much promise, particularly when used as an adjuvant therapy resulting in improved quality of life and increased response rates.

4.3. Omega-3 Fatty Acids and Chronic Lymphocytic Leukemia

B-Cell Chronic Lymphocytic Leukemia (CLL) is the most common form of adult leukemia in the western world (Riches, Ramsay and Gribben, 2011). CLL is primarily a disease of the elderly with two thirds of patients being 65 years of age at the time of diagnosis (Riches, Ramsay and Gribben, 2011). CLL is often initially diagnosed in the asymptomatic stages where watchful waiting is the primary course of treatment (Riches, Ramsay and Gribben, 2011). However, approximately 50% of these patients will progress to advanced, symptomatic stages (Shanafelt and Call, 2004). Progression to symptomatic stages is associated with shortened survival and need for therapy (Shanafelt and Call, 2004). Despite the success of current treatment options, such as FCR (fludarabine, cyclophosphamide and rituximab), many patients develop drug resistance and disease relapse (Riches, Ramsay and Gribben, 2011, Shanafelt and Call, 2004, Silber, Degar, Costin *et al.*, 1994). Additionally, clinical treatment of CLL in patients who require aggressive treatment is limited due to significant side-effect profiles which are often too toxic for the elderly or those with co-morbidities (Riches, Ramsay and Gribben, 2011). As such, clinical treatment of CLL is often hindered by progressive drug resistance and drug-induced toxicities (Riches, Ramsay and Gribben, 2011). Therefore, a non-toxic therapeutic intervention that could slow the progression of asymptomatic CLL to symptomatic CLL or enhance the effects of actively used chemotherapeutic drugs in patients who require therapy would be clinically beneficial.

Various studies have reported that COX-2 is constitutively expressed in primary CLL cells and that these cells are capable of producing eicosanoids PGE_2, $PGF_{2\alpha}$, and TXA_2 (Ryan, Pollock, Kaur *et al.*, 2006, Secchiero, Barbarotto, Gonelli *et al.*, 2005). Additionally, it was found that elevated COX-2 expression was particularly found amongst a subgroup of patients who exhibited poor prognostic markers (Ryan, Pollock, Kaur *et al.*, 2006). Ryan *et al.,* illustrated that the addition of COX-1/COX-2 inhibitor indomethacin and selective COX-2 inhibitor SC-58125 reduced B-CLL proliferation and survival *in vitro* (Ryan, Pollock, Kaur *et al.*, 2006). It was also observed that the cytoprotective effects of COX in B-CLL cells were specific to COX-2 and not COX-1 (Ryan, Pollock, Kaur *et al.*, 2006). Similarly, Secchiero *et al.* illustrated that NS-398, a pharmacological inhibitor of COX-2, was selectively toxic against primary CLL cells but not normal B-lymphocytes *in vitro* supporting the notion that COX-2 is essential to the survival of CLL cells (Secchiero, Barbarotto, Gonelli *et al.*, 2005). Similar findings were reported by Pepper *et al.,* who demonstrated that COX-2 inhibitors aspirin and aspirin analogues 2HBZ and 4HBZ were selectively more cytotoxic against primary CLL cells than age matched normal B- or T-lymphocytes *in vitro* (Pepper, Mahdi, Buggins *et al.*, 2011). In agreement with Ryan *et al.,* it was also found that the sensitivity of the CLL cells to aspirin and its analogues tended to be higher in poor prognostic patients, although this was not statistically significant (Pepper, Mahdi, Buggins *et al.*, 2011). Furthermore, Seccheiro *et al.,* illustrated that pre-treatment of primary CLL cells with NS-398 followed by treatment with chlorambucil, an actively used anti-cancer drug for the treatment of CLL(Secchiero, Barbarotto, Gonelli *et al.*, 2005), induced significantly greater cytotoxic effects than either alone. However, this increase in cytotoxicity was only observed in 50% of patients (Secchiero, Barbarotto, Gonelli *et al.*, 2005). Thus, targeting COX-2 presents a promising therapeutic target for the treatment of CLL.

Given that COX-2 and NFκB are inherently intertwined, targeting NFκB activation has also come into light as a promising candidate for intervention for the treatment of CLL. NFκB is of particular interest given its ability to regulate a wide variety of genes involved with anti-apoptosis, proliferation, migration, chemo-resistance as well as genes involved in inflammation such as COX-2 (Li and Sethi, 2010). Increased constitutive activation of NFκB has been observed in primary CLL cells (Hewamana, Alghazal, Lin *et al.*, 2008, Hewamana, Lin, Jenkins *et al.*, 2008, Hewamana, Lin, Rowntree *et al.*, 2009). It has also been found that increased binding of Rel A, a subunit of NFκB which contains the transactivation domain, was positively correlated with white blood cell count, a measure of tumor burden, and lymphocyte doubling time, a measure of tumor kinetics (Hewamana, Alghazal, Lin *et al.*, 2008). Similarly, results from our laboratory found similar findings that NFκB activation was positively correlated with absolute lymphocyte counts (Fahrmann, Ballester, Ballester *et al.*, 2013). Furthermore, it has been shown that Rel A DNA binding was strongly associated with Binet staging, predictive of time to initial treatment and subsequent treatment, and predictive of overall survival (Hewamana, Lin, Rowntree *et al.*, 2009). Rel A DNA binding has also been shown to be negatively correlated with induction of spontaneous apoptosis *in vitro* suggesting that NFκB is an important mediator of survival (Hewamana, Alghazal, Lin *et al.*, 2008). This is supported by the fact that inhibition of NFκB activation, through the use of an irreversible-IKK inhibitor (LC-1), induced dose-responsive increases in apoptosis (Hewamana, Lin, Jenkins *et al.*, 2008). The addition of LC-1 was also able to overcome the cytoprotective effects of CD40L and IL-4, upstream agonists of NFκB activation, providing further support of the importance of NFκB in CLL (Hewamana, Lin, Jenkins *et al.*, 2008). Additionally, studies by Pepper *et al.,* indicated that the cytotoxic effects of aspirin and its analogues were mediated by both COX-2 inhibition as well as inhibition of Rel A DNA binding supporting the interconnected relationship between COX-2 and NFκB (Pepper, Mahdi, Buggins *et al.*, 2011). It is also important to note that in the studies by Hewamana *et al.*, inhibition of NFκB activation by LC-1 exhibited strong synergy with fludarabine, a commonly used first-line treatment in CLL (Riches, Ramsay and Gribben, 2011, Silber, Degar, Costin *et al.*, 1994), in both good prognostic CLL patients who were fludarabine-sensitive and poor prognostic CLL patients who displayed chemorefractoriness toward fludarabine (Hewamana, Lin, Jenkins *et al.*, 2008). Given the ability of NFκB to promote survival of CLL cells *in vitro* and aid in various biological processes such as proliferation, migration, inhibition of apoptosis and chemo-resistance, a therapeutic interventions which target NFκB would be of considerable interest and clinically relevant.

Arachidonic acid-derived eicosanoids are known to be pro-inflammatory and can up-regulate various pathways (such as COX-2 and NFκB) associated with promotion and progression of malignancies. Omega-3 FAs compete with n-6 for incorporation and metabolism; often exerting opposing biological effects. Given that n-6s, particularly AA, are heavily consumed in the western diet and can promote COX-2 and NFκB activation, which have been found to be vital pathways in CLL, adding n-3 to the diet presents a promising therapeutic option for the treatment of CLL.

Recently, our laboratory demonstrated that consumption of an omega-3 supplement, predominately composed of EPA and DHA, suppressed the NFκB activation in a dose-responsive manner in lymphocytes isolated from patients with early-stage CLL (Fahrmann, Ballester, Ballester *et al.*, 2013). It is interesting to note that patients who were unable or unwilling to take the highest dose (7.2 g of n-3 per day), over time either 4.8 or 2.4 g of n-3 per day also suppressed NFκB activation. This indicates that as little as 2.4 g of n-3 per day can induce beneficial effects. Additionally, mRNA analysis indicated that consumption of n-3 significantly reduced mRNA abundance of 31 genes, including known NFκB targets JMJD1C, ZNF644 and COX-2 (Fahrmann, Ballester, Ballester *et al.*, 2013). It would be expected that inhibition of NFκB activation would slow the progression of the disease; however, further studies will be needed to support this hypothesis. Furthermore, consumption of n-3 increased the *in vitro* sensitivity of lymphocytes to doxorubicin (Fahrmann, Ballester, Ballester *et al.*, 2013). In line with these observations, we have also reported that EPA and DHA selectively increases the chemo-sensitivity of CLL-derived cell lines EHEB and MEC-2 and B-Prolymphocytic-derived cell line JVM-2 to anti-cancer drugs doxorubicin, vincristine and fludarabine *in vitro* (Fahrmann and Hardman, 2013). Importantly, the chemo-sensitizing effects were predominately seen with either EPA or DHA but not with AA (Fahrmann and Hardman, 2013). Conversely, enhanced chemo-sensitization of MEC-2 to doxorubicin by DHA was associated with greater lipid peroxidation than either alone. Co-treatment of DHA pre-treated MEC-2 cells with vitamin-E and doxorubicin attenuated the increase in chemo-sensitivity and decreased the levels of lipid peroxidation (Fahrmann and Hardman, 2013). This indicates that enhanced chemo-sensitization of MEC-2 to doxorubicin by DHA is dependent, in part, on the formation of lipid peroxides. Increasing the chemo-sensitivity of malignant lymphocytes is highly desirable and would be expected to increase drug efficacy and potentially reduce drug dosage resulting in reduced drug-induced toxicities. While the number of studies exploring the use of n-3 as a therapeutic option for CLL are relatively small, the results found thus far have been very promising and warrant further exploration.

5. SUMMARY AND FUTURE DIRECTIONS

The application of n-3 as a therapeutic option for the treatment of cancer is of considerable interest and an active area of research. In this respect, it is important to establish how n-3 can potentially provide benefit to cancer patients. In this context, it should be considered that n-3 and n-6 compete with each other for incorporation and metabolism to their downstream metabolites (Patterson, Wall, Fitzgerald, Ross and Stanton, 2012, Simopoulos, 2008). AA and EPA are particularly relevant given their involvement in eicosanoid production (Haeggstrom, Rinaldo-Matthis, Wheelock and Wetterholm, 2010, Luo and Wang, 2011). Typically, AA-derived eicosanoids have been shown to have pro-inflammatory properties. Inversely, EPA-derived eicosanoids have been found to have anti-inflammatory properties (Calder, 2009). The current western diet is heavily favored towards n-6 FA with little to no n-3 intake (Simopoulos, 2008). Thus, a high n-6/n-3 ratio can promote a pro-thrombotic, pro-inflammatory state. States of chronic inflammation is an underlying theme of various pathologies including cancer (Balkwill and Coussens, 2004, Clevers, 2004). In line with this thought, various solid tumors and hematological malignancies have demonstrated overexpression of COX-2 (Barnes, Haywood, Flint, Knox and Bundred, 2006, Krysan, Dohadwala, Luo *et al.*, 2004, Lee, Pan, Cheng, Chi and Liu, 2001, Ryan, Pollock, Kaur *et al.*, 2006) and constitutively active NFκB (Braun, Carvalho, Fabre *et al.*, 2006, Hewamana, Lin, Rowntree *et al.*, 2009, Li and Sethi, 2010). Conversely, it has also been demonstrated that COX-2 and NFκB are important for the survival of malignant cells and are positively associated with disease progression (Edelman, Watson, Wang *et al.*, 2008, Fidler, Argiris, Patel *et al.*, 2008, Hewamana, Lin, Rowntree *et al.*, 2009, Li and Sethi, 2010). Similarly, the

AA-derived eicosanoid, PGE_2, has been implicated in various aspects of tumor promotion (Greenhough, Smartt, Moore *et al.*, 2009) and, importantly, can activate NFκB (Wang and Dubois, 2010). As such, COX-2, PGE_2 and NFκB are cyclic in nature and self-propagating.

Inversely, n-3, particularly EPA and DHA, have been shown to suppress COX-2 and NFκB activation (Calder, 2012, Calviello, Di Nicuolo, Gragnoli *et al.*, 2004, Fahrmann, Ballester, Ballester *et al.*, 2013, Lim, Han, Dai, Shen and Wu, 2009, Yang, Cartwright, Chan *et al.*, 2013). Furthermore, *in vitro* and *in vivo* studies have indicated that EPA can reduce levels of PGE_2 while increasing PGE_3, and that PGE_3 was important for the growth-inhibitory effects of EPA (Yang, Cartwright, Chan *et al.*, 2013). Additionally, various studies have demonstrated that the cytotoxic effects of n-3, particularly DHA, can also be mediated through the formation of toxic lipid peroxides (Begin, Ells and Horrobin, 1988, Das and Madhavi, 2011, Fahrmann and Hardman, 2013, Germain, Chajes, Cognault, Lhuillery and Bougnoux, 1998). Numerous *in vitro* and *in vivo* studies have illustrated the ability of n-3 to act as chemo-sensitizing and radio-sensitizing agents (Fahrmann and Hardman, 2013, Germain, Chajes, Cognault, Lhuillery and Bougnoux, 1998, Hardman, Avula, Fernandes and Cameron, 2001). Collectively, the use of n-3 as a therapeutic option for the treatment of various malignancies has been substantially supported *in vitro* and *in vivo*. However, the capacity of n-3 to translate into clinical benefit for patients diagnosed with various malignancies is of principal importance. Clinical studies on breast and lung cancer utilizing n-3 as adjuvants to therapy have demonstrated clinical benefit (Bougnoux, Hajjaji, Ferrasson *et al.*, 2009, Ghoreishi, Esfahani, Djazayeri *et al.*, 2012, Murphy, Mourtzakis, Chu *et al.*, 2011, van der Meij, Langius, Spreeuwenberg *et al.*, 2012). Notably, in these trials, no additional adverse effects were associated with the use of n-3. Inversely, it appears that the addition of n-3 to therapy may reduce toxicities associated with treatment and improve the quality of life for the individual receiving treatment (Bougnoux, Hajjaji, Ferrasson *et al.*, 2009, Ghoreishi, Esfahani, Djazayeri *et al.*, 2012, Murphy, Mourtzakis, Chu *et al.*, 2011). It has not been determined if the improved benefits of n-3 consumption in these trials were a result of enhanced chemo-sensitivity, reduced toxicities associated with treatment or the combination of both. Similarly, it was not determined whether the improved response of patients receiving n-3 as an adjuvant to therapy was a result of suppression of COX-2 and/or NFκB activation. However, given the importance of COX-2 and NFκB in various malignancies, it is very plausible that the improved responses where, at least in part, mediated by suppression of COX-2 and/or NFκB activation. In support of this notion, studies by our laboratory indicated that consumption of n-3 suppressed the activation of NFκB in lymphocytes isolated from patients with early stage CLL and reduced mRNA abundance of COX-2 (Fahrmann, Ballester, Ballester *et al.*, 2013). This indicates that n-3 are capable of reducing COX-2 mRNA levels and suppressing NFκB activation in humans. It should also be considered that the capability of n-3 to provide benefit is likely a culmination of multiple mechanisms of action, an attribute given to the versatility of the various metabolites and degradation products produced during enzymatic metabolism and non-enzymatic degradation of n-3.

In this chapter we have discussed and highlighted the potential use of n-3 as therapeutic options for the treatment of various malignancies. While clinical studies thus far have demonstrated promising results, certain considerations should be acknowledged prior to conducting or interpreting results of new or old clinical trials. It should be considered that the application of n-3 is likely context dependent. The type of n-3 consumed, dosage of n-3 given, basal diet of the patient, gender, metabolic potential and the "n-6 to n-3" ratio can all influence the potential benefit or harm of n-3 as therapeutic options.

For instance, ALA can be elongated to EPA effectively; however, the formation of DHA proceeds with poor efficiency (<4%), and can be inhibited by the presence of AA (Gerster, 1998). Because DHA is not efficiently produced by the body or greatly stored in certain tissues, such as adipose tissue, supplementation may be the only effective way to increase DHA levels in the tissues (Arterburn, Hall and Oken, 2006). High doses of n-3 can also be potentially harmful. Studies by Burns *et al.,* indicated that patients suffering from cancer cachexia were able to tolerate a maximum dose of 0.3 g/kg of EPA + DHA per day before displaying dose-limiting toxicities (Burns, Halabi, Clamon *et al.*, 1999).

Studies by Yee *et al.,* indicated that a dose of ~2.5g/day EPA+DHA achieved the maximum possible elevation of concentrations in mammary tissue and blood in a supplementation study (Yee, Lester, Cole *et al.*, 2010). Consistent with studies by

Yee *et al.*, we found that there was no appreciable difference in plasma concentrations of EPA or DHA between 4.8 g or 7.2 g/day EPA + DHA (Fahrmann, Ballester, Ballester *et al.*, 2013). Similarly, Arterburn *et al.,* indicated that supplementation with 2g/day DHA resulted in tissue saturation and appreciably lowered AA concentrations (Arterburn, Hall and Oken, 2006). Retention time of n-3 also appears to be FA-type specific. After discontinuation of n-3 consumption for a period of 3 months, plasma concentrations of EPA and DPA (docosapentaenoic acid) returned to levels comparable to those observed at baseline. Plasma concentrations of DHA decreased following discontinuation, however, remained significantly higher than those observed at baseline. This would indicate that the retention time of DHA is longer as compared to EPA (Fahrmann, Ballester, Ballester *et al.*, 2013).

Diet also plays an important role. Given that n-3 and n-6 compete with each other for incorporation and metabolism, a high intake of n-6 in conjunction with n-3 supplementation may reduce the potential benefit from n-3 and confound potential results. Similarly, high intake of saturated fats or *trans*-fats can prevent PUFA incorporation and metabolism to the longer-chain PUFA (Simopoulos, 2008). A low intake of n-3 may also provide inadequate levels of n-3 to provide benefit and should be considered.

Additionally, gender may play a potential role in the benefit from n-3. Studies by Shapira *et al.,* have suggested that increased synthesis of long-chain PUFA from PUFA may cause women to be more sensitive than men to the overabundance of n-6 in the diet, possibly explaining disparities between male and female cancer rates (Shapira, 2012). Because of this, women may be more susceptible to the effects of excessive n-6 consumption, or n-3 deficiency – and therefore may receive more benefit from n-3 supplementation.

It is also evident that it must be determined whether consumption of n-3 leads to incorporation. The inability of a patient to incorporate n-3 would prevent the patient from receiving potential benefit and may lead to confounding results if not taken into account. For instance, studies by Bougnoux *et al.,* indicated that only patients with metastatic breast cancer who had high-DHA incorporation displayed improved outcome during anthracyline-based therapy as compared to those patients who had low-DHA incorporation rates (Bougnoux, Hajjaji, Ferrasson *et al.*, 2009).

With respect to these considerations, the ratio of n-6 and n-3 is of particular importance. Certain commonalities exist in large case studies which support the theory that the general population consumes insufficient n-3 or excess n-6. A study in France found decreased breast cancer risk in the highest n-3/n-6 consumption quintile when compared the lowest, and decreased risk was also associated with total ALA consumption from fruit and vegetable sources (Thiebaut, Chajes, Gerber *et al.*, 2009). In the Shanghai Women's Health Study a significant reduction in breast cancer risk was only found when comparing the highest marine n-3 (EPA+DHA) consumption tertile to the highest n-6 tertile (Murff, Shu, Li *et al.*, 2011). In postmenopausal Korean women a significant reduction in risk occurred at consumption of an estimated.3g EPA+DHA, but in post menopausal subjects a significant reduction in risk only existed in comparisons of highest and lowest EPA+DHA quartiles (Kim, Lim, Shin *et al.*, 2009). Thus, the ratio of n-3/n-6 should be taken into account. Currently, it is suggested that the ideal ratio of n-3 to n-6 be between 4-1:1 within healthy individuals (Patterson, Wall, Fitzgerald, Ross and Stanton, 2012).

The application of n-3 as a therapeutic option for the treatment of various malignancies is very promising and presents several advantages over conventional therapy. N-3 are non-toxic (dose-dependent) and have the potential of slowing the growth of cancer, increasing the chemo-sensitivity of malignant cells to chemo- and radio-therapy and reducing toxicities. Slowing the growth of cancer would prolong the time before treatment is required and improve the quality of life for the individual. Increased chemo-sensitivity would lead to increased drug efficacy and potential decreases in drug dosage thereby leading to reduced drug-induced toxicities. Similarly, reducing therapy-induced toxicities by n-3 can lead to potential increases in the number of cycles a patient can tolerate, thereby increasing the likelihood of receiving a response. Therefore, the use of n-3 as therapeutic options warrants further attention and presents a novel therapeutic approach. However, it should be stressed that proper design is critical in evaluating the potential use of n-3 as therapeutic options and that the considerations in this chapter should be taken into account when conducting future clinical trials.

ACKNOWLEDGEMENTS

The authors would like to gratefully acknowledge the grant support of the National Cancer Institute, RO1CA114018, the Department of Defense Breast Cancer Research Program, W81XWH-10-1-0697, and the American Institute for Cancer Research, MG07A001.

CONFLICT OF INTEREST

The authors confirm that this chapter content has no conflict of interest.

REFERENCES

Alfano, C. M., Imayama, I., Neuhouser, M. L., Kiecolt-Glaser, J. K., Smith, A. W., Meeske, K., McTiernan, A., Bernstein, L., Baumgartner, K. B., Ulrich, C. M., and Ballard-Barbash, R. 2012. Fatigue, inflammation, and omega-3 and omega-6 fatty acid intake among breast cancer survivors. *J. Clin. Oncol.*, 30, 1280-1287.

Alfranca, A., Iniguez, M. A., Fresno, M., and Redondo, J. M. 2006. Prostanoid signal transduction and gene expression in the endothelium: role in cardiovascular diseases. *Cardiovasc. Res.*,70, 446-456.

Arnold, C., Konkel, A., Fischer, R., and Schunck, W. H. 2010. Cytochrome P450-dependent metabolism of omega-6 and omega-3 long-chain polyunsaturated fatty acids. *Pharmacol. Rep.*, 62, 536-547.

Balkwill, F. and Coussens, L. M. 2004. Cancer: an inflammatory link. *Nature.*, 431, 405-406.

Arterburn, L. M., Hall, E. B., and Oken, H. 2006. Distribution, interconversion, and dose response of n-3 fatty acids in humans.Am. *J. Clin. Nutr.*, 83, 1467S-1476S.

Barnes, N., Haywood, P., Flint, P., Knox, W. F., and Bundred, N. J. 2006. Survivin expression in *in situ* and invasive breast cancer relates to COX-2 expression and DCIS recurrence. *Br. J. Cancer.*, 94, 253-258.

Begin, M. E., Ells, G., and Horrobin, D. F. 1988. Polyunsaturated fatty acid-induced cytotoxicity against tumor cells and its relationship to lipid peroxidation. *J. Natl. Cancer Inst.*, 80, 188-194.

Bougnoux, P., Germain, E., Chajes, V., Hubert, B., Lhuillery, C., Le, Floch O., Body, G., and Calais, G. 1999. Cytotoxic drugs efficacy correlates with adipose tissue docosahexaenoic acid level in locally advanced breast carcinoma. *Br. J. Cancer.*, 79, 1765-1769.

Bougnoux, P., Hajjaji, N., Ferrasson, M. N., Giraudeau, B., Couet, C., and Le, Floch O. 2009. Improving outcome of chemotherapy of metastatic breast cancer by docosahexaenoic acid: a phase II trial. *Br. J. Cancer.*, 101, 1978-1985.

Braun, T., Carvalho, G., Fabre, C., Grosjean, J., Fenaux, P., and Kroemer, G. 2006. Targeting NF-kappaB in hematologic malignancies. *Cell Death. Differ.*, 13, 748-758.

Bray, F., Ren, J. S., Masuyer, E., and Ferlay, J. 2013. Global estimates of cancer prevalence for 27 sites in the adult population in 2008. *Int. J. Cancer.*, 132, 1133-1145.

Brennan, M., Wilcken, N., French, J., Ung, O., and Boyages, J. 2005. Management of early breast cancer--the current approach. *Aust. Fam. Physician.*, 34, 755-760.

Buchanan, F. G., Wang, D., Bargiacchi, F., and DuBois, R. N. 2003. Prostaglandin E2 regulates cell migration *via* the intracellular activation of the epidermal growth factor receptor. *J. Biol. Chem.*, 278, 35451-35457.

Burns, C. P., Halabi, S., Clamon, G. H., Hars, V., Wagner, B. A., Hohl, R. J., Lester, E., Kirshner, J. J., Vinciguerra, V., and Paskett, E. 1999. Phase I clinical study of fish oil fatty acid capsules for patients with cancer cachexia: cancer and leukemia group B study 9473. *Clin. Cancer Res.*, 5, 3942-3947.

Calder, P. C. 2009. Polyunsaturated fatty acids and inflammatory processes: New twists in an old tale. *Biochimie.*, 91, 791-795.

Calder, P. C. 2012. Mechanisms of action of (n-3) fatty acids. *J. Nutr.*, 142, 592S-599S.

Calviello, G., Di, Nicuolo F., Gragnoli, S., Piccioni, E., Serini, S., Maggiano, N., Tringali, G., Navarra, P., Ranelletti, F. O., and Palozza, P. *2004*. n-3 PUFAs reduce VEGF expression in human colon cancer cells modulating the COX-2/PGE2 induced ERK-1 and -2 and HIF-1alpha induction pathway. *Carcinogenesis.*, 25, 2303-2310.

Cathcart, M. C., Lysaght, J., and Pidgeon, G. P. 2011. Eicosanoid signalling pathways in the development and progression of colorectal cancer: novel approaches for prevention/intervention. *Cancer Metastasis Rev.*, 30, 363-385.

Chan, A. T., Ogino, S., and Fuchs, C. S. 2007. Aspirin and the risk of colorectal cancer in relation to the expression of COX-2. *N. Engl. J. Med.*, 356, 2131-2142.

Chang, A. 2011. Chemotherapy, chemoresistance and the changing treatment landscape for NSCLC. *Lung Cancer.*, 71, 3-10.

Clevers, H. 2004. At the crossroads of inflammation and cancer. *Cell.*, 118, 671-674.

Corsetto, P. A., Cremona, A., Montorfano, G., Jovenitti, I. E., Orsini, F., Arosio, P., and Rizzo, A. M. 2012. Chemical-physical changes in cell membrane microdomains of breast cancer cells after omega-3 PUFA incorporation. *Cell Biochem. Biophys.*, 64, 45-59.

Csiki, I., Morrow, J. D., Sandler, A., Shyr, Y., Oates, J., Williams, M. K., Dang, T., Carbone, D. P., and Johnson, D. H. 2005. Targeting cyclooxygenase-2 in recurrent non-small cell lung cancer: a phase II trial of celecoxib and docetaxel. *Clin. Cancer Res.*, 11, 6634-6640.

Darnell, J. E., Jr. 2002. Transcription factors as targets for cancer therapy. *Nat. Rev. Cancer.*, 2, 740-749.

Das, U. N. and Madhavi, N. 2011. Effect of polyunsaturated fatty acids on drug-sensitive and resistant tumor cells *in vitro*. *Lipids Health Dis.*,10:159.

Das, U. N., Madhavi, N., Sravan, Kumar G., Padma, M., and Sangeetha, P. 1998. Can tumour cell drug resistance be reversed by essential fatty acids and their metabolites? *Prostaglandins Leukot. Essent. Fatty Acids.*, 58, 39-54.

DeGraffenried, L. A., Friedrichs, W. E., Fulcher, L., Fernandes, G., Silva, J. M., Peralba, J. M., and Hidalgo, M. 2003. Eicosapentaenoic acid restores tamoxifen sensitivity in breast cancer cells with high Akt activity. *Ann. Oncol.*,14, 1051-1056.

Dekoj, T., Lee, S., Desai, S., Trevino, J., Babcock, T. A., Helton, W. S., and Espat, N. J. *2007.* G2/M cell-cycle arrest and apoptosis by n-3 fatty acids in a pancreatic cancer model. *J. Surg. Res.*, 139, 106-112.

Denkert, C., Winzer, K. J., Muller, B. M., Weichert, W., Pest, S., Kobel, M., Kristiansen, G., Reles, A., Siegert, A., Guski, H., and Hauptmann, S. 2003. Elevated expression of cyclooxygenase-2 is a negative prognostic factor for disease free survival and overall survival in patients with breast carcinoma. *Cancer.*, 97, 2978-2987.

Ditsworth, D. and Zong, W. X. 2004. NF-kappaB: key mediator of inflammation-associated cancer. *Cancer Biol. Ther.*, 3, 1214-1216.

Edelman, M. J., Watson, D., Wang, X., Morrison, C., Kratzke, R. A., Jewell, S., Hodgson, L., Mauer, A. M., Gajra, A., Masters, G. A., Bedor, M., Vokes, E. E., and Green, M. J. 2008. Eicosanoid modulation in advanced lung cancer: cyclooxygenase-2 expression is a positive predictive factor for celecoxib + chemotherapy--Cancer and Leukemia Group B Trial 30203. *J. Clin. Oncol.*, 26, 848-855.

Erbas, B., Provenzano, E., Armes, J., and Gertig, D. 2006. The natural history of ductal carcinoma *in situ* of the breast: a review. *Breast Cancer Res. Treat.*, 97, 135-144.

Estabrook, N. C., Chin-Sinex, H., Borgmann, A. J., Dhaemers, R. M., Shapiro, R. H., Gilley, D., Huda, N., Crooks, P., Sweeney, C., and Mendonca, M. S. 2011. Inhibition of NF-kappaB and DNA double-strand break repair by DMAPT sensitizes non-small-cell lung cancers to X-rays. *Free Radic. Biol. Med.*, 51, 2249-2258.

Fahrmann, J. F., Ballester, O. F., Ballester, G., Witte, T. R., Salazar, A. J., Kordusky, B., Cowen, K. G., Ion, G., Primerano, D. A., Boskovic, G., Denvir, J., and Hardman, W. E. 2013. Inhibition of nuclear factor kappa B activation in early-stage chronic lymphocytic leukemia by omega-3 fatty acids. *Cancer Invest.*, 31, 24-38.

Fahrmann, J. F. and Hardman, W. E. 2013. Omega 3 fatty acids increase the chemo-sensitivity of B-CLL-derived cell lines EHEB and MEC-2 and of B-PLL-derived cell line JVM-2 to anti-cancer drugs doxorubicin, vincristine and fludarabine. *Lipids Health Dis.*, 12:36.

Fidler, M. J., Argiris, A., Patel, J. D., Johnson, D. H., Sandler, A., Villaflor, V. M., Coon, J., Buckingham, L., Kaiser, K., Basu, S., and Bonomi, P. 2008. The potential predictive value of cyclooxygenase-2 expression and increased risk of gastrointestinal hemorrhage in advanced non-small cell lung cancer patients treated with erlotinib and celecoxib. *Clin. Cancer Res.*, 14, 2088-2094.

Germain, E., Chajes, V., Cognault, S., Lhuillery, C., and Bougnoux, P. 1998. Enhancement of doxorubicin cytotoxicity by polyunsaturated fatty acids in the human breast tumor cell line MDA-MB-231: relationship to lipid peroxidation. *Int. J. Cancer.*, 75, 578-583.

Gerster, H. 1998. Can adults adequately convert alpha-linolenic acid (18:3n-3) to eicosapentaenoic acid (20:5n-3) and docosahexaenoic acid (22:6n-3)? *Int. J. Vitam. Nutr. Res.*, 68, 159-173.

Ghoreishi, Z., Esfahani, A., Djazayeri, A., Djalali, M., Golestan, B., Ayromlou, H., Hashemzade, S., Asghari, Jafarabadi M., Montazeri, V., Keshavarz, S. A., and Darabi, M. 2012. Omega-3 fatty acids are protective against paclitaxel-induced peripheral neuropathy: a randomized double-blind placebo controlled trial. *BMC. Cancer.*, 12: 355.

Ghosh-Choudhury, T., Mandal, C. C., Woodruff, K., St, Clair P., Fernandes, G., Choudhury, G. G., and Ghosh-Choudhury, N. 2009. Fish oil targets PTEN to regulate NFkappaB for downregulation of anti-apoptotic genes in breast tumor growth. *Breast Cancer Res. Treat.*, 118, 213-228.

Glover, J. A., Hughes, C. M., Cantwell, M. M., and Murray, L. J. 2011. A systematic review to establish the frequency of cyclooxygenase-2 expression in normal breast epithelium, ductal carcinoma *in situ*, microinvasive carcinoma of the breast and invasive breast cancer. *Br. J. Cancer.*, 105, 13-17.

Gogineni, K. and DeMichele, A. 2012. Current approaches to the management of Her2-negative metastatic breast cancer. *Breast Cancer Res.*, 14, 205.

Greenberg, M. E., Li, X. M., Gugiu, B. G., Gu, X., Qin, J., Salomon, R. G., and Hazen, S. L. 2008. The lipid whisker model of the structure of oxidized cell membranes. *J. Biol. Chem.*, 283, 2385-2396.

Greenhough, A., Smartt, H. J., Moore, A. E., Roberts, H. R., Williams, A. C., Paraskeva, C., and Kaidi, A. 2009. The COX-2/PGE2 pathway: key roles in the hallmarks of cancer and adaptation to the tumour microenvironment. *Carcinogenesis.*, 30, 377-386.

Haeggstrom, J. Z., Rinaldo-Matthis, A., Wheelock, C. E., and Wetterholm, A. 2010. Advances in eicosanoid research, novel therapeutic implications. *Biochem. Biophys. Res. Commun.*, 396, 135-139.

Han, E. H., Kim, H. G., Hwang, Y. P., Song, G. Y., and Jeong, H. G. 2010. Prostaglandin E2 induces CYP1B1 expression *via* ligand-independent activation of the ERalpha pathway in human breast cancer cells. *Toxicol. Sci.*, 114, 204-216.

Hardman, W. E., Avula, C. P., Fernandes, G., and Cameron, I. L. 2001. Three percent dietary fish oil concentrate increased efficacy of doxorubicin against MDA-MB 231 breast cancer xenografts. *Clin. Cancer Res.*, 7, 2041-2049.

Heller, A. R., Rossel, T., Gottschlich, B., Tiebel, O., Menschikowski, M., Litz, R. J., Zimmermann, T., and Koch, T. 2004. Omega-3 fatty acids improve liver and pancreas function in postoperative cancer patients. *Int. J. Cancer.*, 111, 611-616.

Hewamana, S., Alghazal, S., Lin, T. T., Clement, M., Jenkins, C., Guzman, M. L., Jordan, C. T., Neelakantan, S., Crooks, P. A., Burnett, A. K., Pratt, G., Fegan, C., Rowntree, C., Brennan, P., and Pepper, C. 2008. The NF-kappaB subunit Rel A is associated with *in vitro* survival and clinical disease progression in chronic lymphocytic leukemia and represents a promising therapeutic target. *Blood.*, 111, 4681-4689.

Hewamana, S., Lin, T. T., Jenkins, C., Burnett, A. K., Jordan, C. T., Fegan, C., Brennan, P., Rowntree, C., and Pepper, C. 2008. The novel nuclear factor-kappaB inhibitor LC-1 is equipotent in poor prognostic subsets of chronic lymphocytic leukemia and shows strong synergy with fludarabine. *Clin. Cancer Res.*, 14, 8102-8111.

Hewamana, S., Lin, T. T., Rowntree, C., Karunanithi, K., Pratt, G., Hills, R., Fegan, C., Brennan, P., and Pepper, C. 2009, Rel a is an independent biomarker of clinical outcome in chronic lymphocytic leukemia. *J. Clin. Oncol.*, 27, 763-769.

Hyde, C. A. and Missailidis, S. 2009. Inhibition of arachidonic acid metabolism and its implication on cell proliferation and tumour-angiogenesis. *Int. Immunopharmacol.*, 9, 701-715.

Jiang, H., Wang, J., and Zhao, W. 2013. Cox-2 in non-small cell lung cancer: a meta-analysis. *Clin. Chim. Acta.*,419: 26-32.

Karuppu, D., Kalus, A., Simpson, E. R., and Clyne, C. 2002. Aromatase and prostaglandin inter-relationships in breast adipose tissue: significance for breast cancer development. *Breast Cancer Res. Treat.*, 76, 103-109.

Khuri, F. R., Wu, H., Lee, J. J., Kemp, B. L., Lotan, R., Lippman, S. M., Feng, L., Hong, W. K., and Xu, X. C. 2001. Cyclooxygenase-2 overexpression is a marker of poor prognosis in stage I non-small cell lung cancer. *Clin. Cancer Res.*, 7, 861-867.

Kikawa, K. D., Herrick, J. S., Tateo, R. E., Mouradian, M., Tay, J. S., and Pardini, R. S. 2010. Induced oxidative stress and cell death in the A549 lung adenocarcinoma cell line by ionizing radiation is enhanced by supplementation with docosahexaenoic acid. *Nutr. Cancer.*, 62, 1017-1024.

Kim, J., Lim, S. Y., Shin, A., Sung, M. K., Ro, J., Kang, H. S., Lee, K. S., Kim, S. W., and Lee, E. S. 2009. Fatty fish and fish omega-3 fatty acid intakes decrease the breast cancer risk: a case-control study. *BMC. Cancer.*, 9:216-219.

Krysan, K., Dohadwala, M., Luo, J., Lin, Y., Zhu, L., Heuze-Vourc'h, N., Goodglick, L., Merchant, F., Seligson, D., Pold, M., Strieter, R., Sharma, S., and Dubinett, S. 2004. Cyclooxygenase-2-dependent expression of survivin in non-small cell lung cancer. *Chest.*, 125, 140S.

Lee, L. M., Pan, C. C., Cheng, C. J., Chi, C. W., and Liu, T. Y. 2001. Expression of cyclooxygenase-2 in prostate adenocarcinoma and benign prostatic hyperplasia. *Anticancer Res.*, 21, 1291-1294.

Li, F. and Sethi, G. 2010. Targeting transcription factor NF-kappaB to overcome chemoresistance and radioresistance in cancer therapy. *Biochim. Biophys. Acta.*, 1805,167-180.

Lim, K., Han, C., Dai, Y., Shen, M., and Wu, T. 2009. Omega-3 polyunsaturated fatty acids inhibit hepatocellular carcinoma cell growth through blocking beta-catenin and cyclooxygenase-2. *Mol. Cancer Ther.*, 8, 3046-3055.

Liou, Y. A., King, D. J., Zibrik, D., and Innis, S. M. 2007. Decreasing linoleic acid with constant alpha-linolenic acid in dietary fats increases (n-3) eicosapentaenoic acid in plasma phospholipids in healthy men. *J. Nutr.* 137, 945-952.

Luo, P. and Wang, M. H. 2011. Eicosanoids, beta-cell function, and diabetes. *Prostaglandins Other Lipid Mediat.* 95, 1-10.

Lv, W. and Yang, T. 2012. Identification of possible biomarkers for breast cancer from free fatty acid profiles determined by GC-MS and multivariate statistical analysis. *Clin. Biochem.*, 45, 127-133.

Maehle, L., Lystad, E., Eilertsen, E., Einarsdottir, E., Hostmark, A. T., and Haugen, A. 1999. Growth of human lung adenocarcinoma in nude mice is influenced by various types of dietary fat and vitamin E. *Anticancer Res.*, 19, 1649-1655.

Maillard, V., Bougnoux, P., Ferrari, P., Jourdan, M. L., Pinault, M., Lavillonniere, F., Body, G., Le, Floch O., and Chajes, V. 2002. N-3 and N-6 fatty acids in breast adipose tissue and relative risk of breast cancer in a case-control study in Tours, France. *Int. J. Cancer.*, 98, 78-83.

Miglietta, A., Toselli, M., Ravarino, N., Vencia, W., Chiecchio, A., Bozzo, F., Motta, M., Torchio, B., and Bocca, C. 2010. COX-2 expression in human breast carcinomas: correlation with clinicopathological features and prognostic molecular markers. *Expert. Opin. Ther. Targets.*, 14, 655-664.

Morris, P. G., Zhou, X. K., Milne, G. L., Goldstein, D., Hawks, L. C., Dang, C. T., Modi, S., Fornier, M. N., Hudis, C. A., and Dannenberg, A. J. 2013. Increased levels of urinary PGE-M, a biomarker of inflammation, occur in association with obesity, aging, and lung metastases in patients with breast cancer. *Cancer Prev. Res.* (Phila)., 6, 428-436.

Murff, H. J., Shu, X. O., Li, H., Yang, G., Wu, X., Cai, H., Wen, W., Gao, Y. T., and Zheng, W. 2011. Dietary polyunsaturated fatty acids and breast cancer risk in Chinese women: a prospective cohort study. *Int. J. Cancer.*, 128, 1434-1441.

Murphy, R. A., Mourtzakis, M., Chu, Q. S., Baracos, V. E., Reiman, T., and Mazurak, V. C. 2011. Nutritional intervention with fish oil provides a benefit over standard of care for weight and skeletal muscle mass in patients with nonsmall cell lung cancer receiving chemotherapy. *Cancer.*, 117, 1775-1782.

Murphy, R. A., Mourtzakis, M., Chu, Q. S., Baracos, V. E., Reiman, T., and Mazurak, V. C. 2011. Supplementation with fish oil increases first-line chemotherapy efficacy in patients with advanced nonsmall cell lung cancer. *Cancer.*, 117, 3774-3780.

Niki, E. 2009. Lipid peroxidation: physiological levels and dual biological effects. *Free Radic. Biol. Med.*, 47, 469-484.

Ochiai, M., Oguri, T., Isobe, T., Ishioka, S., and Yamakido, M. 1999. Cyclooxygenase-2 (COX-2) mRNA expression levels in normal lung tissues and non-small cell lung cancers. *Jpn. J. Cancer Res.*, 90, 1338-1343.

Pai, R., Soreghan, B., Szabo, I. L., Pavelka, M., Baatar, D., and Tarnawski, A. S. 2002. Prostaglandin E2 transactivates EGF receptor: a novel mechanism for promoting colon cancer growth and gastrointestinal hypertrophy. *Nat. Med.*, 8, 289-293.

Paquette, B., Bisson, M., Baptiste, C., Therriault, H., Lemay, R., and Cantin, A. M. 2005. Invasiveness of breast cancer cells MDA-MB-231 through extracellular matrix is increased by the estradiol metabolite 4-hydroxyestradiol. *Int. J. Cancer,* 113, 706-711.

Parthasarathy, S., Santanam, N., Ramachandran, S., and Meilhac, O. 2000. Potential role of oxidized lipids and lipoproteins in antioxidant defense. *Free Radic. Res.*, 33, 197-215.

Patterson, E., Wall, R., Fitzgerald, G. F., Ross, R. P., and Stanton, C. 2012. Health implications of high dietary omega-6 polyunsaturated Fatty acids. *J. Nutr. Metab.*, 2012: 539426.

Patterson, R. E., Flatt, S. W., Newman, V. A., Natarajan, L., Rock, C. L., Thomson, C. A., Caan, B. J., Parker, B. A., and Pierce, J. P. 2011. Marine fatty acid intake is associated with breast cancer prognosis. *J. Nutr.*, 141, 201-206.

Pender-Cudlip, M. C., Krag, K. J., Martini, D., Yu, J., Guidi, A., Skinner, S. S., Zhang, Y., Qu, X., He, C., Xu, Y., Qian, S. Y., and Kang, J. X. 2013. Delta-6-desaturase activity and arachidonic acid synthesis are increased in human breast cancer tissue. *Cancer Sci.*, 104, 760-764.

Pepper, C., Mahdi, J. G., Buggins, A. G., Hewamana, S., Walsby, E., Mahdi, E., Al-Haza'a, A., Mahdi, A. J., Lin, T. T., Pearce, L., Morgan, L., Bowen, I. D., Brennan, P., and Fegan, C. 2011. Two novel aspirin analogues show selective cytotoxicity in primary chronic lymphocytic leukaemia cells that is associated with dual inhibition of Rel A and COX-2. *Cell Prolif.*, 44, 380-390.

Perrone, G., Santini, D., Vincenzi, B., Zagami, M., La, Cesa A., Bianchi, A., Altomare, V., Primavera, A., Battista, C., Vetrani, A., Tonini, G., and Rabitti, C. 2005. COX-2 expression in DCIS: correlation with VEGF, HER-2/neu, prognostic molecular markers and clinicopathological features. *Histopathology.*, 46, 561-568.

Pianetti, S., Arsura, M., Romieu-Mourez, R., Coffey, R. J., and Sonenshein, G. E. 2001. Her-2/neu overexpression induces NF-kappaB *via* a PI3-kinase/Akt pathway involving calpain-mediated degradation of IkappaB-alpha that can be inhibited by the tumor suppressor PTEN. *Oncogene.*, 20, 1287-1299.

Reader, J., Holt, D., and Fulton, A. 2011. Prostaglandin E2 EP receptors as therapeutic targets in breast cancer. *Cancer Metastasis Rev.*, 30, 449-463.

Ricciotti, E. and FitzGerald, G. A. 2011. Prostaglandins and inflammation. *Arterioscler. Thromb. Vasc. Biol.*, 31, 986-1000.

Riches, J. C., Ramsay, A. G., and Gribben, J. G. 2011. Chronic lymphocytic leukemia: an update on biology and treatment. *Curr. Oncol. Rep.*, 13, 379-385.

Ristimaki, A., Sivula, A., Lundin, J., Lundin, M., Salminen, T., Haglund, C., Joensuu, H., and Isola, J. 2002. Prognostic significance of elevated cyclooxygenase-2 expression in breast cancer. *Cancer Res.*, 62, 632-635.

Ryan, E. P., Pollock, S. J., Kaur, K., Felgar, R. E., Bernstein, S. H., Chiorazzi, N., and Phipps, R. P. 2006. Constitutive and activation-inducible cyclooxygenase-2 expression enhances survival of chronic lymphocytic leukemia B cells. *Clin. Immunol.*, 120, 76-90.

Schmitz, G. and Ecker, J. 2008. The opposing effects of n-3 and n-6 fatty acids. *Prog. Lipid Res.*, 47, 147-155.

Secchiero, P., Barbarotto, E., Gonelli, A., Tiribelli, M., Zerbinati, C., Celeghini, C., Agostinelli, C., Pileri, S. A., and Zauli, G. 2005. Potential pathogenetic implications of cyclooxygenase-2 overexpression in B chronic lymphoid leukemia cells. *Am. J. Pathol.*, 167, 1599-1607.

Serhan, C. N. and Petasis, N. A. 2011. Resolvins and protectins in inflammation resolution. *Chem. Rev.*, 111, 5922-5943.

Serini, S., Trombino, S., Oliva, F., Piccioni, E., Monego, G., Resci, F., Boninsegna, A., Picci, N., Ranelletti, F. O., and Calviello, G. 2008. Docosahexaenoic acid induces apoptosis in lung cancer cells by increasing MKP-1 and down-regulating p-ERK1/2 and p-p38 expression. *Apoptosis.*, 13, 1172-1183.

Shanafelt, T. D. and Call, T. G. 2004. Current approach to diagnosis and management of chronic lymphocytic leukemia. *Mayo Clin. Proc.*, 79, 388-398.

Shapira, N. 2012. Women's higher risk with N-6 PUFA *vs.* men's relative advantage: an "N-6 gender nutrition paradox" hypothesis. *Isr. Med. Assoc. J.*, 14, 435-441.

Shishodia, S., Koul, D., and Aggarwal, B. B. 2004. Cyclooxygenase (COX)-2 inhibitor celecoxib abrogates TNF-induced NF-kappa B activation through inhibition of activation of I kappa B alpha kinase and Akt in human non-small cell lung carcinoma: correlation with suppression of COX-2 synthesis. *J. Immunol.*, 173, 2011-2022.

Silber, R., Degar, B., Costin, D., Newcomb, E. W., Mani, M., Rosenberg, C. R., Morse, L., Drygas, J. C., Canellakis, Z. N., and Potmesil, M. 1994. Chemosensitivity of lymphocytes from patients with B-cell chronic lymphocytic leukemia to chlorambucil, fludarabine, and camptothecin analogs. *Blood.*, 84, 3440-3446.

Simopoulos, A. P. 1991. Omega-3 fatty acids in health and disease and in growth and development. *Am. J. Clin. Nutr.*, 54, 438-463.

Simopoulos, A. P. 2000. Human requirement for N-3 polyunsaturated fatty acids. *Poult. Sci.*, 79, 961-970.

Simopoulos, A. P. 2002. The importance of the ratio of omega-6/omega-3 essential fatty acids. *Biomed. Pharmacother.*, 56, 365-379.

Simopoulos, A. P. 2008. The importance of the omega-6/omega-3 fatty acid ratio in cardiovascular disease and other chronic diseases. *Exp. Biol. Med.* (Maywood.)., 233, 674-688.

Sun, X., Nair, J., Linseisen, J., Owen, R. W., and Bartsch, H. 2012. Lipid peroxidation and DNA adduct formation in lymphocytes of premenopausal women: Role of estrogen metabolites and fatty acid intake. *Int. J. Cancer.*, 131, 1983-1990.

Tang, D. W., Lin, S. C., Chang, K. W., Chi, C. W., Chang, C. S., and Liu, T. Y. 2003. Elevated expression of cyclooxygenase (COX)-2 in oral squamous cell carcinoma--evidence for COX-2 induction by areca quid ingredients in oral keratinocytes. *J. Oral Pathol. Med.*, 32, 522-529.

Tang, X., Liu, D., Shishodia, S., Ozburn, N., Behrens, C., Lee, J. J., Hong, W. K., Aggarwal, B. B., and Wistuba, I. I. 2006. Nuclear factor-kappaB (NF-kappaB) is frequently expressed in lung cancer and preneoplastic lesions. *Cancer.*, 107, 2637-2646.

Thiebaut, A. C., Chajes, V., Gerber, M., Boutron-Ruault, M. C., Joulin, V., Lenoir, G., Berrino, F., Riboli, E., Benichou, J., and Clavel-Chapelon, F. 2009. Dietary intakes of omega-6 and omega-3 polyunsaturated fatty acids and the risk of breast cancer. *Int. J. Cancer.*, 124, 924-931.

Tsurutani, J., Castillo, S. S., Brognard, J., Granville, C. A., Zhang, C., Gills, J. J., Sayyah, J., and Dennis, P. A. 2005. Tobacco components stimulate Akt-dependent proliferation and NFkappaB-dependent survival in lung cancer cells. *Carcinogenesis.*, 26, 1182-1195.

van der Meij, B. S., Langius, J. A., Spreeuwenberg, M. D., Slootmaker, S. M., Paul, M. A., Smit, E. F., and van Leeuwen, P. A. 2012. Oral nutritional supplements containing n-3 polyunsaturated fatty acids affect quality of life and functional status in lung cancer patients during multimodality treatment: an RCT. *Eur. J. Clin. Nutr.*, 66, 399-404.

Vinothini, G. and Nagini, S. 2010. Correlation of xenobiotic-metabolizing enzymes, oxidative stress and NFkappaB signaling with histological grade and menopausal status in patients with adenocarcinoma of the breast. *Clin. Chim. Acta.*, 411, 368-374.

Wang, D. and DuBois, R. N. 2010. Eicosanoids and cancer. *Nat. Rev. Cancer.*, 10, 181-193.

Yang, P., Cartwright, C., Chan, D., Ding, J., Felix, E., Pan, Y., Pang, J., Rhea, P., Block, K., Fischer, S. M., and Newman, R. A. 2013. Anticancer activity of fish oils against human lung cancer is associated with changes in formation of PGE(2) and PGE(3) and Alteration of Akt Phosphorylation. *Mol. Carcinog.*, doi: 10.1002/mc.22008. [Epub ahead of print]

Yee, L. D., Lester, J. L., Cole, R. M., Richardson, J. R., Hsu, J. C., Li, Y., Lehman, A., Belury, M. A., and Clinton, S. K. 2010. Omega-3 fatty acid supplements in women at high risk of breast cancer have dose-dependent effects on breast adipose tissue fatty acid composition. *Am. J. Clin. Nutr.*, 91, 1185-1194.

Zhang, D., Jin, X., Wang, F., Wang, S., Deng, C., Gao, Z., and Guo, C. 2007. Combined prognostic value of both RelA and IkappaB-alpha expression in human non-small cell lung cancer. *Ann. Surg. Oncol.*, 14, 3581-3592.

Zhang, Z., Ma, J., Li, N., Sun, N., and Wang, C. 2006. Expression of nuclear factor-kappaB and its clinical significance in nonsmall-cell lung cancer. *Ann. Thorac. Surg.*, 82, 243-248.

Zmijewski, J. W., Landar, A., Watanabe, N., Dickinson, D. A., Noguchi, N., and Darley-Usmar, V. M. 2005. Cell signalling by oxidized lipids and the role of reactive oxygen species in the endothelium. *Biochem. Soc. Trans.*, 33, 1385-1389.

Send Orders for Reprints to reprints@benthamscience.net
425 *Cutting Edge Therapies for Cancer in the 21st Century*, 2014, 425-512

CHAPTER 13

Ultrasound Contrast Agents in Cancer Therapy

Rounak Nande and Pier Paolo Claudio*

McKown Translational Genomics Research Institute, Departments of Biochemistry and Microbiology & Department of Surgery, Joan C. Edwards School of Medicine, Marshall University, Huntington, WV, USA

Abstract: The field of ultrasound has expanded since the discovery of ultrasound contrast agents (UCAs) from diagnostics to therapeutic use. UCAs are known as microbubbles (MBs), which can be chemically and physically manipulated to improve their therapeutic potential. MBs can be tailored to bind to specific diseased tissues and act as carriers of different chemo-drugs and genetic materials. These engineered MBs can behave differently to ultrasound intensities resulting in different cavitation methods. Though the underlying mechanism is yet to be fully understood, there is evidence to suggest that mechanical pore formation of cellular membranes allows for the temporary uptake of drugs. The cavitation of MBs can induce temporary and reversible enhancement in the permeability of both individual cells as well as the endothelium including the blood brain barrier. There are too many side-effects and immune responses to current cancer and diseased treatments. MBs protect the immunogenic drugs from eliciting a detrimental response when delivered through the vasculature. They also help reduce the drug dosage by improving drug targeting and drug response. Thus, MBs can be used as vehicles for localized drug delivery and gene therapy allowing us to further develop the potential of curing cancer and other diseases.

Keywords: Microbubbles, ultrasound, ultrasound contrast agent, chemotherapy, adenovirus, polyethylene glycol, perfluropentane, phospholipid, sonoporation, cavitation, Blood Brain Barrier (BBB), gene therapy, chemotherapy, DNA, RNA, protein, siRNA, miRNA, drug delivery.

1. HISTORICAL OVERVIEW

Ultrasound (US) is the most widely used diagnostic imaging modality. This modality provides a safe, non-invasive, and portable real-time imaging at a low

***Address correspondence to Pier Paolo Claudio:** Department of Biochemistry and Microbiology & Department of Surgery, Translational Genomic Research Institute, Joan C. Edwards School of Medicine, Marshall University, Huntington, WV, USA; Tel: +1 304 696 3516, E-mail: claudiop@marshall.edu

Pier Paolo Claudio and Paraskevi Vogiatzi (Eds)

cost (Hernot and Klibanov, 2008). US sound waves have a frequency between 20 Hz to 20 kHz that is inaudible to the human ear (Liu, Miyoshi and Nakamura, 2006). Typically, in ultrasonography the diagnostic frequency ranges from 1-10 MHz (Zagzebski, 1996). To produce a US image a transducer that broadcasts the US wave pulses is placed on the skin or inside the body. These waves are reflected by the interfaces between different tissues or structures in the body. The imaging software system converts these reflected waves into electrical pulses and digitizes them (Hernot and Klibanov, 2008). Imaging is possible because the speed of sound in the tissue (~1500m/s) is known (Klibanov, 2007). Biological tissues (except lung or bone) mainly consist of water, which has low compressibility, and sound waves propagate without significant scattering or reflection (Klibanov, 2007). Thus the backscatter energy from tissue contains less or no harmonics (Faez, Emmer, Kooiman *et al.*, 2013). Blood, a liquid phase material has low compressibility and scatters US poorly. But the infusion of ultrasound contrast agents (UCAs) or microbubbles (MBs) can increase the scattering and reflection of the ultrasonic waves (Hernot and Klibanov, 2008). Thus, harmonics can be used to differentiate between blood flow with UCAs and the surrounding tissue (Faez, Emmer, Kooiman *et al.*, 2013).

The discovery of microbubble (MB) agents came from an accidental observation by Dr. Charles Joiner, a cardiologist in the late 1960s. Dr. Joiner performed an M-mode echocardiogram by injecting a patient with indocyanine green through the left ventricle to measure cardiac output. He observed a transient increase in the US signal from the ventricle after each injection (Calliada, Campani, Bottinelli, Bozzini and Sommaruga, 1998, Gramiak and Shah, 1968). It was later shown that small bubbles forming at the catheter tip caused the increase in the signal. But subsequent research into duplicating the results was not successful (Calliada, Campani, Bottinelli, Bozzini and Sommaruga, 1998). In 1968, Gramiak and colleagues observed a cloud of echoes after the injection of agitated saline in the aortic root (Gramiak and Shah, 1968). They showed that US backscatter for the blood pool can be increased by adding gas bubbles that exist in agitated saline (Faez, Emmer, Kooiman *et al.*, 2013, Gramiak and Shah, 1968). Thus, agitated saline is still used for the detection of right to left shunts in the heart (Soliman, Geleijnse, Meijboom *et al.*, 2007). But these bubbles were large and unstable.

They had a short half-life and did not persist in the blood for long periods of time which limited their use (Faez, Emmer, Kooiman *et al.*, 2013). Only right heart imaging was achieved because the first generation of UCAs that entrapped air and carbon dioxide in agitated saline and hydrogen peroxide could not pass through the pulmonary circulation (Xu, 2009).

Mixing some of the patient's blood with saline was found to markedly increase and prolong the stability of the bubbles (Calliada, Campani, Bottinelli, Bozzini and Sommaruga, 1998). Dr. Feinstein (Feinstein, Ten Cate, Zwehl *et al.*, 1984) found that albumin was the blood component improving MB stability (Calliada, Campani, Bottinelli, Bozzini and Sommaruga, 1998). Later on Feinstein developed the sonication method that produced more stable MBs, whose size could be controlled (Wiencek, Feinstein, Walker and Aronson, 1993). In 1994, Albunex (Molecular Biosystems, San Diego, CA) became the first commercially available contrast agent approved for human use in the United States. Albunex has a coating made of human serum albumin (Faez, Emmer, Kooiman *et al.*, 2013). This resulted in the stabilization of MBs with different substances such as phospholipid, albumin, or polymers. These formed the second generation UCAs that had a mean diameter less than 8 μm, which guarantees that UCA could pass through the pulmonary circulation and reach various organs. They survived longer in the blood stream due to their lower solubility in water and had a strong harmonic response (Xu, 2009).

The making of more stable, more effective UCAs revolutionized the pharmaceutical industry. The second commercially available contrast agent, Levovist, became available in Europe and Japan in 1996. Levovist like its forerunner Echovist (Calliada, Campani, Bottinelli, Bozzini and Sommaruga, 1998) (Bayer Schering Pharma AG, Berlin, Germany) consists of galactose microcrystals whose surfaces provide absorption sites on which air bubbles form when suspended in water (Faez, Emmer, Kooiman *et al.*, 2013). Echovist performed poorly in the right heart because its intravenous (IV) injected MBs were not stable and failed to cross the lung capillaries (Calliada, Campani, Bottinelli, Bozzini and Sommaruga, 1998). Levovist MBs were further stabilized with a trace amount of palmitic acid (Faez, Emmer, Kooiman *et al.*, 2013). Thus making it stable in the blood for 1-4 min which increased the US signal by ~20 dB

(Calliada, Campani, Bottinelli, Bozzini and Sommaruga, 1998). Levovist MBs formed in the blood flow while EchoGen® (Abbot Laboratories, Chicago, IL, USA) achieves MB formation through a totally different mechanism. It consists essentially of a perfluoro-compound (perfluoropentane), which is liquid at room temperature but becomes a gas at body temperature. EchoGen® is prepared as an aqueous emulsion with surfactants that change to gas on injection, with the formation of MBs as small as 2–8 microns (Calliada, Campani, Bottinelli, Bozzini and Sommaruga, 1998).

Since 1997, contrast agents (CAs) are further stabilized by replacing the air core with high-molecular-weight inert gases such as perfluorocarbons, which have a lower solubility and diffusivity in aqueous liquids compared with air (Faez, Emmer, Kooiman *et al.*, 2013). Clinically proven agents based on this principle include SonoVue (SF6 gas), Definity/Luminity (C3F8), Imagent (C6H14), Sonazoid (C4F10) (these materials possess a lipid stabilizer shell), and Optison (C3F8 has a shell of denatured human serum albumin (Klibanov, 2007). These became the third generation of UCAs.

The history of UCAs development has been long and difficult. Luck and astute observations helped develop and make US imaging the most cost effective technology available in the world. UCAs have opened up new opportunities in molecular imaging (Klibanov, 2007), drug delivery systems, high focused US (HIFU) surgery (Azmin, Harfield, Ahmad, Edirisinghe and Stride, 2012), and atherosclerosis (Sutton, Haworth, Pyne-Geithman and Holland, 2013).

2. ULTRASOUND CONTRAST AGENTS OR MICROBUBBLES

Ultrasound contrast agents are also known as microbubbles (MBs). MBs enhance the quantification of perfusion and blood flow (Cavalieri, Zhou and Ashokkumar, 2010). They are very echogenic and they resonate like a musical instrument (Calliada, Campani, Bottinelli, Bozzini and Sommaruga, 1998). The physical and chemical design of contrast agents (CAs) are manipulated such that synthetic surfactant, tuning of size, composition, degradability, surface properties and bio-functionality make them very echogenic (Cavalieri, Zhou and Ashokkumar, 2010). Typically, they are comprised of surfactant shell made from proteins, lipid and biodegradable polymers with an inner gas core, either of air or inert gases (Fig. **1**). MB have an average diameter of ~2 to 3μm, and the combined mass of the shell and gas core (Fig. **1**) of each MB does not exceed a pictogram (Klibanov, 2007).

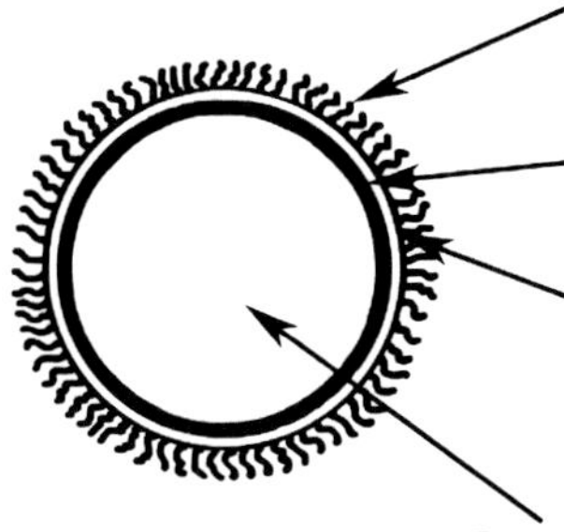

Figure 1: Schematic representation of a coated microbubble.

The particle size of MBs for intravenous injection plays a significant role and needs to be carefully controlled. MBs must be small enough to cross the capillary bed (7.5 micron). Indeed, large bubbles are unable to pass through the capillaries, whereas small bubbles are considerably less effective scatterers (Cavalieri, Zhou and Ashokkumar, 2010). It is now accepted that the size must be in the range of 1-7μm preferably around 3μm with as narrow size distribution as possible. The critical resonance frequency required to destroy the bubble depends on the diameter (Calliada, Campani, Bottinelli, Bozzini and Sommaruga, 1998). The rigidity of the shell determined by the thickness of the surfactant would also determine its resonating potency and its echogenicity. It has been determined that US reflectivity is proportional to the fourth power of a particle diameter, but also directly proportional to the concentration of the particles themselves. The resonance frequency of MBs 1–7μm in diameter lies within the 2–15 MHz range, which is the US frequency used for clinical diagnosis (Calliada, Campani, Bottinelli, Bozzini and Sommaruga, 1998).

Echogenic liposomes and various nanoparticle (NP) dispersions are being evaluated as CAs. Most liposomes have a multi-lamellar structure with embedded air pockets that are responsible for acoustic backscatter signal (Alkan-Onyuksel, Demos, Lanza *et al.*, 1996, Huang, Hamilton, Pozharski *et al.*, 2002). Without an enclosed gas core the US signal from these particles are low. NPs dispersions are mostly liquid perfluorocarbon-based emulsions (Wickline and Lanza, 2003). These NPs are also characterized as contrast agents for MRI, optical imaging, and drug delivery. US imaging using these materials require a high frequency (multi-MHz) or high degree of target surface coverage with a CA (Klibanov, 2007, Wickline, Hughes, Ngo *et al.*, 2002).

MBs do not diffuse across the endothelium and thus there is no interstitial enhancement. Essentially, MBs act as blood pool markers, or markers of any other body space into which they have been injected and their behavior is, in many respects, similar to that of labeled red blood cells. Vascular enhancement usually lasts a few minutes and the MBs are then dissolved. However, this model is complicated by evidence that some MBs are taken up by the reticuloendothelial systems (Calliada, Campani, Bottinelli, Bozzini and Sommaruga, 1998).

Single-bubble detection is possible *in vitro* in normal saline or blood with older imaging equipment. However, echoes from normal tissue can be nonlinear with non-fundamental frequency. To reduce these signals from tissues multi-pulse techniques such as phase inversion and power modulation are applied (Klibanov, 2007). However, to detect MB vibration current imaging systems use harmonic imaging, both in free-flow conditions (Klibanov, Rasche, Hughes *et al.*, 2002) and when attached to a solid target (Klibanov, 2007, Klibanov, Rasche, Hughes *et al.*, 2004). MBs are known to emit US at different frequencies such as sub-harmonic, second and third harmonic frequencies. This large discrepancy in the echoes between MBs and tissue allows for enhanced imaging with quantification of perfusion, blood flow, tumor and tissue vascularization (Cavalieri, Zhou and Ashokkumar, 2010). Thus MBs are essential for diagnosing modality.

MBs are used not only for diagnostic applications but also for molecular imaging and therapeutic applications (Bohmer, Klibanov, Tiemann *et al.*, 2009, Gessner and Dayton, 2010, Hernot and Klibanov, 2008, Lindner, 2009). Molecular imaging targets the molecular changes associated with diseases and improves the efficiency of *in vivo* imaging (Faez, Emmer, Kooiman *et al.*, 2013). However, in this chapter we will focus on its therapeutic applications in treating cancer. Initial applications of MBs depended on the rate of bubble collapse and their bio-effects such as inducing cell damage, vascular injury (Skyba, Price, Linka, Skalak and Kaul, 1998), and the lysis of thrombus (Tachibana and Tachibana, 1995). Interestingly, oscillating MBs can increase membrane permeability and open tight junctions in endothelial cells (Juffermans, van Dijk, Jongenelen *et al.*, 2009, Kooiman, Emmer, Foppen-Harteveld, van Wamel and de Jong, 2010, Meijering, Juffermans, van Wamel *et al.*, 2009, Sheikov, McDannold, Sharma and Hynynen, 2008, van Wamel, Kooiman, Harteveld *et al.*, 2006). Thus the therapeutic potential of drug delivery and drug action is increased. Based on chemical and physical nature of drugs, some MBs are known to have drugs encapsulated in liposomes, polymeric micelles, hollow particles and emulsion droplets with the aim to reduce non-specific drug resistance and side-effects associated with traditional cancer therapies (Cavalieri, Zhou and Ashokkumar, 2010).

3. TYPES OF MICROBUBBLES

MBs can be divided into several categories depending on their physical and chemical properties which are crucial in the design of a contrast agent for US guided drug delivery (Cavalieri, Zhou and Ashokkumar, 2010). There are a few characteristic that are important when designing an MB. Firstly, the intensity of the backscatter or echo caused by the MB is determined by Rayleigh scattering regime (Cavalieri, Zhou and Ashokkumar, 2010, Morse, 1968). This depends on the surface properties or shell material, gas content and colloidal properties of MBs (Cavalieri, Zhou and Ashokkumar, 2010, Cavalieri, Zhou, Tortora, Lucilla and Ashokkumar, 2012). Shell and gas components (Fig. **1**) should be biodegradable *i.e.* readily metabolized and/or excreted with minimal side-effects (Cavalieri, Zhou and Ashokkumar, 2010). Additionally, MBs shouldn't aggregate into large clusters which could result in non-specific and undesired adhesion to cells (Cavalieri, Zhou, Tortora, Lucilla and Ashokkumar, 2012). MBs should be effective at low doses (Cavalieri, Zhou and Ashokkumar, 2010). For instance, the typical US Food and Drug Administration (FDA) approved dose of MBs for a patient is approximately 10^9-10^{10} MBs given for a 1-2 mL bolus intravenous injection (Cavalieri, Zhou, Tortora, Lucilla and Ashokkumar, 2012). Additionally, pre-formed drug loaded MBs or MBs alone should be sterilizable and stable with a shelf-life of two years (Cavalieri, Zhou and Ashokkumar, 2010, Cavalieri, Zhou, Tortora, Lucilla and Ashokkumar, 2012). Other requirements include backscattering proficiency, fragility and cavitation properties of

MBs (Cavalieri, Zhou and Ashokkumar, 2010). US or acoustic pressure required to cause cavitation is measured as mechanical index (MI), a relative quotient computed as a peak negative acoustic pressure divided by the square root of the frequency (Klibanov, 2007). MBs behave differently at various acoustic pressures. For example, at MI >0.2 MBs behave in a nonlinear manner that allows to detect smaller MBs (Klibanov, 2007). At higher pressures (MI >0.4 and up to 1-1.9, depending on the frequency), MBs are completely destroyed (Klibanov, Rasche, Hughes *et al.*, 2002). Acoustic pressure depends on the diameter of the shell and its material. For example, thin lipid monolayered bubbles are flexible and vibrate in response to low-pressure US (*e.g.*, MI = 0.06) (Klibanov, 2007). Whereas, thick-shelled polymer bubbles don't crack unless at critical pressure, or vibrate resulting in low acoustic echo response (Postema, Bouakaz, Versluis and de Jong, 2005).

3.1. Agitated Gas Microbubbles (First Generation)

First generation MBs were prepared at patient bedside with two syringes connected *via* a stopcock valve, that contained air and saline (Seward, Tajik, Hagler and Ritter, 1977). When liquid and gas are rapidly transferred from one medium to another the resulting high shear flow causes air bubbles to form of varying sizes (Klibanov, 2007). These bubbles produced by agitation are called agitated-saline and are both large and unstable (Faez, Emmer, Kooiman *et al.*, 2013, Klibanov, 2007). The surface tension between the gas core and surrounding liquid causes the gas to diffuse into the surrounding liquid decreasing the size of the bubble (Klibanov, 2007). It requires a stabilizer shell to prolong its circulation time. The rate can be calculated using the equation by Epstein and Plesset (Epstein, 1950) and Chen *et al.,* (Chen, Matula and Crum, 2002) that an air bubble with a diameter of 5μm in air-saturated water disappears in approximately 125 ms and an air bubble with a diameter of 3 μm disappears in approximately 32 ms at room temperature and ambient pressure (Faez, Emmer, Kooiman *et al.*, 2013).

There are several limitations in using these bubbles such as the size of bubble, circulation time and gas core. These bubbles are effectively removed by the lungs (Faez, Emmer, Kooiman *et al.*, 2013). Additionally, these bubbles have a size greater than 10μm and are unable to traverse the pulmonary circulation (Hernot and Klibanov, 2008). MBs larger than 6-8μm are trapped in the lung capillaries and bubbles smaller than 1 μm are less stable and less ultrasound responsive (Cavalieri, Zhou and Ashokkumar, 2010). These bubbles need to be administered by intracoronary or aortic root injection to visualize the left cardiac chambers (Faez, Emmer, Kooiman *et al.*, 2013). Additionally, because it takes at least 12 sec for a contrast agent to pass from a peripheral vein (*i.e.*, the site of injection) to the end-organ (Barry B. Goldberg, 2001), to be useful these bubbles need to persist for several minutes (Faez, Emmer, Kooiman *et al.*, 2013). In 1984, Feinstein *et al.,* introduced the use of sonication to create MBs that were stable and small enough to transit through the pulmonary microcirculation from right to left heart (Feinstein, Ten Cate, Zwehl *et al.*, 1984).

Since the introduction of saline MBs, other agitated contrast agents (hydrogen peroxide, dextrose, indocyanine green dye, iodinated contrast) have been used (Hernot and Klibanov, 2008).

3.2. Coated Microbubbles filled with Air (Second Generation)

The biggest dilemma facing scientist was the circulation time of bubbles. It was found empirically that a small admixture of the patient's blood to the saline improves the stability and effectiveness of the agitated saline as a contrast agent (Blomley, Claudon and Cosgrove, 2007). Surfactants from the blood form a coating around the gas core and promote the lifetime of the MB by greatly reducing the surface tension at the interface (Faez, Emmer, Kooiman *et al.*, 2013). The first stable MB marketed was Albunex (Table **1**). Albunex had a short shelf-life after intravenous injection (tens of seconds) (Klibanov, 2007).

An encapsulating shell is necessary to sustain the gas cavity and to reduce both the diffusion of gas leaving the core and the surface tension (Cavalieri, Zhou and Ashokkumar, 2010). This increases the shelf-life (days to months) of the bubbles. The albumin coating forms an elastic solid shell around the gas core and is relatively stiff. It enhances the bubble's stability by supporting a strain to counter the effect of the surface tension (Faez, Emmer, Kooiman *et al.*, 2013). The transpulmonary passage of contrast particles became possible only after the addition of a MB shell, *i.e.*, a surfactant (lipid, protein *e.g.* denatured albumin or polymer *e.g.* poly-butyl-cyanoacrylate (Liu, Miyoshi and Nakamura, 2006)) coat, which stabilized the bubbles so that they did not attach to the extensive surface of lung endothelium capillaries (Keller, Feinstein and Watson, 1987, Klibanov, 2007). Bubble size is a critical parameter that must be controlled in the range of 1-7μm preferably around 3μm (Cavalieri, Zhou and Ashokkumar, 2010). At that point, intravenous administration of contrast became a feasible option for delivering contrast to left heart chambers (Keller, Feinstein and Watson, 1987), with some contrast reaching the myocardium vasculature. To circulate freely and avoid entrapment in the microvasculature, MB particles need to be smaller than red blood cells (typically <4.5μm in mean diameter) (Klibanov, 2007).

The compressibility of gaseous particles is many orders of magnitude higher than that of liquids and solids. As a result, the scattering efficiency from gaseous particles is many orders of magnitude higher than that from other objects. According to Rayleigh scattering the intensity of MB increases as the fourth power of frequency (Cavalieri, Zhou and Ashokkumar, 2010). For such small MBs, the surface-to-volume ratio is high, and air can easily escape and dissolve in the surrounding medium (as a result, ultrasound contrast is lost). Therefore, transpulmonary air-filled MBs with these first-generation shells did not circulate long after intravenous injection (tens of seconds) (Klibanov, 2007). Air consists mostly of nitrogen that is able to move easily out of the thin-shelled bubbles, especially in cases of oxygen inhalation that had reduced blood levels of dissolved nitrogen (Geiser, Buss, Wible *et al.*, 1996, Porter and Xie, 1995). In physiological conditions, the blood is saturated with air under atmospheric pressure, whereas the air pressure inside the bubbles is larger than atmospheric pressure due to Laplace pressure. When air-filled MBs are infused intravenously they dissolve spontaneously (Cavalieri, Zhou, Tortora, Lucilla and Ashokkumar, 2012). Surfactant such as lipid (~3nm thick), protein (15-150nm thick) or polymeric shell (200-500nm thick) eliminates the driving force for dissolution of MBs in saturated media as the elastic response of the interface arrests the shrinkage of the gas core (Cavalieri, Zhou, Tortora, Lucilla and Ashokkumar, 2012, Sirsi and Borden, 2009). To improve MBs' stability, currently used strategy is to fill them with a sparingly water soluble gas (perfluorocarbons act as osmotic agent) instead of air (Schutt, Klein, Mattrey and Riess, 2003).

At present Levovist (Table **1**) is the most widely studied MB contrast agent and the only one commercially available in several countries. Levovist (Table **1**), like its forerunner Echovist (Table **1**) (also by Schering), is made of galactose microcrystals generating air in the vial (Calliada, Campani, Bottinelli, Bozzini and Sommaruga, 1998). Adding water to the galactose powder forms a suspension in which air MBs adhere to the fine irregularities of the surface of the microcrystals remaining in the solid state, which however, dissolve after injection, releasing the gas MBs into the blood. Levovist and Sonovue (Table **1**) have a half-lives of 78 seconds and 5 minutes, respectively (Cavalieri, Zhou and Ashokkumar, 2010).

MBs are manufactured by two general techniques: self-assembly stabilization of dispersed gas particles, and double-emulsion preparation with core extraction. The first technique is for lipid or protein-based bubbles. Gases (air or fluorinated gas with low solubility) are dispersed in the aqueous medium that contains a lipid or surfactant micellar mixture or a protein that is denatured by sonication. Those components are deposited on the gas-liquid interface and stabilize the MB. Some preparations are stable on storage in the aqueous phase for many months. Alternatively, MBs can be rapidly frozen and lyophilized for extended storage in dry state. The addition of water results in a reformation of the MB aqueous dispersion immediately before use (Faez, Emmer, Kooiman *et al.*, 2013).

Table 1: Comparison of Commercially Available Contrast Agents

Agent	**Bubble Size Mean (Range)**	**Gas**	**Shell Composition**
Albunex	4.5μm (1-10μm)	Air	Albumin
Levovist	2-3μm (2-8μm)	Air	Galactose/ palmitic acid
Echovist	-	Air	D-galactose
EchoGen	2-5μm (1-30μm)	Dodecafluoropentane	Stabilized surfactant
Sonogen	2-5μm (1-30μm)	Perfluoropentane	Anionically charged surfactant
Optison	4.7μm(1-10μm)	Octafluoropropane	Albumin N-acetyltrytophan, Caprylic acid
Definity	1.5μm(1-10μm)	Octafluoropropane	Lipids: DPPA, DPPC, MPEG5000 DPPE
Imagent	6μm	Perfluorohexane	Lipid: DMPC
Sonozoid	2.4-3.6 μm (3.4μm)	Perfluorobutane	Phospholipids

Agent	Bubble Size Mean (Range)	Gas	Shell Composition
Sonovist	1-2 µm	Air	Cyanoacrylate (polymer)
Sonovue	2.5µm(1-10µm)	Sulfur hexafluoride	Lipids: Macrogol 4000, DSPC, DPPG, Palmitric acid
Sonidel MB101	2.7 µm	Perfluorocarbon	Stabilized Lipid
BG1135	2.9µm(1-8µm)	Air	Polymer
BR14	2.5-3 µm	Perfluorobutane	Lipid
BR38	<10µm	Perfluorobutane	Phospholipids
PB 127	4.0µm(3-5µm)	Nitrogen	Biodegradable polymer bilayer
PESDA	4.7 µm	Perfluorocarbon	Albumin
Artenga	2.5 µm	Variable	Lipid
AI-700	2µm	Perfluorocarbon	Poly-L-lactide co glycolide
Cardiosphere/Bisphere	4µm	Nitrogen	Polylactide/Albumin
Targeson	2.5 µm	Perfluorocarbon	Surface-modified Lipid

(Adapted from Liu, Y. *et al.*, 2006 (Liu, Miyoshi and Nakamura, 2006), Alzaraa, A. *et al.*, 2012 (Alzaraa, Gravante, Chung *et al.*, 2012) and Nomikou, N. *et al.*, 2010 (Nomikou and McHale, 2010)).

3.3. Coated Microbubbles filled with Inert Gases (Third Generation)

Since 1997, contrast agents have been further stabilized by replacing the air core with high-molecular-weight inert gases or water soluble fluorinated gases (Klibanov, 2007) such as perfluorocarbons (Faez, Emmer, Kooiman *et al.*, 2013) and sulfur hexafluoride (Hernot and Klibanov, 2008) which have a lower solubility and diffusivity in aqueous liquids compared with air (Barry B. Goldberg, 2001). Perflurocarbons act as osmotic agent and would dilute the other gases inside the bubbles thereby also reducing their partial pressure (Cavalieri, Zhou and Ashokkumar, 2010, Van Liew and Burkard, 1995). This effect counterbalances the Laplace pressure and blood pressure (Cavalieri, Zhou and Ashokkumar, 2010).

The gas core is generally surrounded by a protein (albumin), lipid, surfactant, or biocompatible polymer surfactant with a diameter ranging from 2 to 500nm. This shell improves stability against gas loss, dissolution, and MB coalescence, and produces a more standard size distribution (Hernot and Klibanov, 2008). The gases such as perfluorocarbons are exhaled through the lungs. Examples of this kind of agent are Optison (GE Healthcare, Chalfont St Giles, UK), which contains octafluoropropane and an albumin shell; SonoVue (Bracco, Milan, Italy), which has a sulfur hexafluoride core and a phospholipid coating (Faez, Emmer, Kooiman *et al.*, 2013); Definity/Luminity (C3F8), Imagent (C6H14), Sonazoid (C4F10) which possess a lipid stabilizer shell (Klibanov, 2007) (Table **1**).

3.4. Different types of Coated Microbubbles

Shell coating is critical for stabilizing MBs because the configuration and conformation of the shell material determines its stiffness which increases its resistance to rupture by US as well as its clearance efficiency by the reticuloendothelial system (Hernot and Klibanov, 2008). The shell can be stiff with albumin, lysozyme and polymers or more flexible with lipid or phospholipid. Its thickness can vary from 10 to 600nm (Cavalieri, Zhou and Ashokkumar, 2010). Surface tension, shell viscoelasticity and permeability, surface charge density, biodegradability, ligand density and payload capacity are properties that largely depend on the choice of the surface-active agent, *i.e.* lipid, protein or synthetic polymer. MBs surface properties and size play a crucial role in prolonging the circulation life of MBs as phagocytic uptake depends on surface opsonization (Moghimi, 2009) and particles size. The larger sized MBs are eliminated more rapidly. Dendritic cells and macrophages are assigned to the clearance of MBs in the bloodstream (Cavalieri, Zhou, Tortora, Lucilla and Ashokkumar, 2012). The study of MBs' biodistribution carried out by Tartis *et al.*, (Tartis, Kruse, Zheng *et al.*, 2008) using PET showed that MB shell material accumulates in the spleen through size dependent filtration mechanisms. Immunogenicity, targeting efficiency, availability, potential for imaging and drug release upon ultrasound irradiation are functional properties consequently correlated with MBs structural features (Cavalieri, Zhou, Tortora, Lucilla and Ashokkumar, 2012).

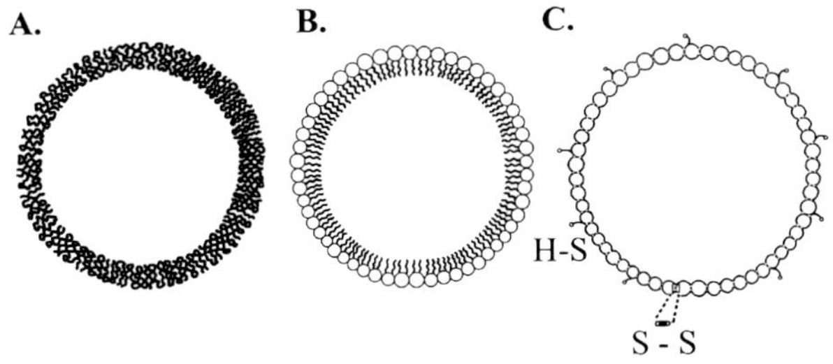

Figure 2: Schematic representation of different coated microbubbles. A) Polymer coated microbubbles. B) Phospholipid coated microbubbles. C) Protein coated microbubbles.

3.4.1. Polymer Coated Microbubbles

UCAs with polymer shells were introduced in 1990 by Wheatley *et al.,* (Wheatley, Schrope and Shen, 1990). Polymer-based contrast agents (Fig. **2a**) need to be biodegradable or disassemble into low molecular weight polymer chains in order to facilitate their ultimate elimination from the body which generally occurs predominantly *via* the kidney (Duncan, Vicent, Greco and Nicholson, 2005). The polymer shell is typically very stiff and does not vibrate significantly when insonified at low acoustic pressures (<200 kPa) (Faez, Emmer, Kooiman *et al.*, 2013). The polymer UCA (Fig. **2a**) is activated once the acoustic pressure is high enough to crack the shell and thereby releases the gas content of the bubble (Bouakaz, Versluis and de Jong, 2005). Once the shell is cracked the bubble releases debris (Chen, Matula, Brayman and Crum, 2003) and broken shell fragments that need to be eliminated. Thus, it is important to understand the long term effects of the synthetic polymers (Cavalieri, Zhou, Tortora, Lucilla and Ashokkumar, 2012). In this context phospholipid, carbohydrate and protein shells are non-immunogenic and offer better safety profile than polymer UCAs.

One can manipulate the design of polymer MBs with the chemical and physical moieties of the polymer chains on the surface of the bubbles. This can avoid the aggregation of bubbles, which could result in larger bubbles with non-specific and undesired binding. Polymer MBs' (Fig. **2a**) surface properties and colloidal stability provides a greater degree of control over its destruction threshold for some therapeutic applications. (Cavalieri, Zhou and Ashokkumar, 2010). Previously, synthetic polymers such as poly(D,L-lactide-coglycolide) (Narayan, 1999) (PLGA), polyvinylalcohol (Cavalieri, El Hamassi, Chiessi and Paradossi, 2005) (PVA), poly(methacrylic acid) (Cavalieri, Zhou, Caruso and Ashokkumar, 2011) (PMA), and thiolated poly(methacrylic acid) (Cavalieri, Zhou, Tortora, Lucilla and Ashokkumar, 2012) (PMASH) have been used as encapsulating material to prepare gas-filled microballoons. The microballoons are normally prepared by emulsion techniques using high speed stirring to deposit the polymer around air/gas core or droplets of a volatile liquid, (water-in oil-in water emulsions) which is subsequently evaporated (Cavalieri, Zhou and Ashokkumar, 2010). Then palmitic acid was suspended into the phospholipids' mixture. For example, block copolymer (PEG-PLLA or PEG-PCL) are used to stabilize the contrast agent in perfluropentane (PFP) nanoemulsions that converts into MBs under ultrasound irradiation have also been recently prepared (Rapoport, Kennedy, Shea, Scaife and Nam, 2009).

PLGA has become one of the most studied diblock copolymer biomaterials for drug encapsulation and is present in several commercially available pharmaceutical products (Bekeredjian R., Kroll R.D., Fein E., *et al.,* 2007). PLGA microparticles degrade and release the encapsulated drugs within 2-6 weeks (Wischke and Schwendeman, 2008). Previously, Wheatley and coworkers have shown that ultrasound frequency (5 and 10 MHz) degrades the PLGA shelled MBs (El-Sherif, Lathia, Le and Wheatley, 2004).

PVA particles are water-soluble and approved for general catheter embolization by the FDA. PVA particles tend to aggregate and may clump within vessels after injection blocking blood flow (Shomura, Tanigawa, Shibutani *et al.*, 2011). No studies are available on the safety and applicability of crosslinked PVA shelled-MBs for *in vivo* parenteral administration. Hence the *in vivo* biocompatibility and biodistribution of PVA MBs must be investigated (Cavalieri, Zhou, Tortora, Lucilla and Ashokkumar, 2012).

The use of synthetic thiolated poly(methacrylic acid), PMASH, macromolecules as the shell material offers control over size, morphology and functionality of the MBs. The hydrophobic features and thiols content of PMASH affect the morphology and size distribution of the MBs. This approach affords PMA-functionalized MBs that can be subsequently further modified exploiting the carboxyl and/or thiol moieties. PMASH MBs are echogenic and can be used as ultrasound contrast agents. The intracellular and blood glutathione (reducing agent) is able to de-crosslink the PMASH polymer shell into soluble low molecular weight polymer chains that can be eliminated by renal or *via* bilary excretion (Cavalieri, Zhou, Caruso and Ashokkumar, 2011, Cavalieri, Zhou, Tortora, Lucilla and Ashokkumar, 2012).

Perfluoropentane (PFP) nanoemulsions are stabilized by block copolymers (PEG-PLLA or PEG-PCL) that convert into MBs under US irradiation have been recently prepared (Rapoport, Kennedy, Shea, Scaife and Nam, 2009). These sound-activated nanoemulsions/MBs have been loaded with paclitaxel and systemically injected in a mouse bearing ovarian, breast, and pancreatic tumors. US imaging can be used to monitor the accumulation of nanoemulsions in tumor cells. US (1-MHz CW, nominal output power density 3.4 W/cm2, exposure duration 1 min-30 s) was applied 4hrs after the injection of the drug formulation. Three weeks after the treatment with nanodroplet encapsulated paclitaxel, a dramatic regression of tumors was observed in tumor therapy through US-triggered drug release from tumor accumulated nanobubbles. Interestingly, at the US intensities used in this study, the nanodroplets/MBs ultrasound formulation suppressed tumor metastasis (Cavalieri, Zhou, Tortora, Lucilla and Ashokkumar, 2012).

3.4.2. Lipid Coated Microbubbles

Lipid MBs (Fig. **2b**) are mostly surrounded by a monolayer of phospholipids (Cavalieri, Zhou and Ashokkumar, 2010). The monolayer of phospholipids is much thinner (1 to 2 nm) than the albumin shells. The shell is more flexible than albumin coating allowing for higher oscillation amplitudes to be used (Faez, Emmer, Kooiman *et al.*, 2013). Lipid shelled MBs (Fig. **2b**) typically comprise two main components: a phospholipid forming the monolayer (~4 nm) (Garstecki, 2004) and an emulsifying lipid. Multicomponent mixtures of lipid hydrophilic head groups and hydrophobic tail groups offer a vast parameter space over which to manipulate the shell composition. The structure of the lipid shelled MBs (Fig. **2b**) was extensively studied by Borden *et al.,* (Farook, Zhang, Edirisinghe, Stride and Saffari, 2007). There are several commercially available lipid-coated MB formulations approved for clinical use in the US and Europe, including Definity (Lantheus Medical Imaging), Sonovue® (Bracco Diagnostics) and Optison (GE Healthcare, Princeton, NJ, USA) (Table **1**) (Cavalieri, Zhou and Ashokkumar, 2010).

Non-drug loaded, normal MBs (NMBs) are prepared by mixing tert-butyl alcohol and purified water that is subsequently added to precise amounts of DPPG-Na and DSPC into the mother liquid to prepare the phospholipids' mixture. To produce a Docetaxel (DOC) loaded MBs, a DOC solution is prepared in tert-butyl solution. DOC solution and PEG4000 are added to the NMB mixture and stirred for

20mins. The last mixtures of 1 mL were equally transferred into each 10 mL-cylindroid vial, and then lyophilized by freezer dryer while SF6 gas is added after the lyophilization (Ren, Liao, Kang *et al.*, 2013). In another way, PFH/air mixture filled MBs can be prepared by allowing liquid PFH to evaporate into an air filled syringe. This gaseous mixture is mixed in with a lipid solution. The sonicator probe is dipped into the lipid solution and turned on. The resulting mixture creates MBs coated with lipids containing a PFH gas core in solution (Fig. **3**) (Ibsen, Benchimol, Simberg *et al.*, 2011).

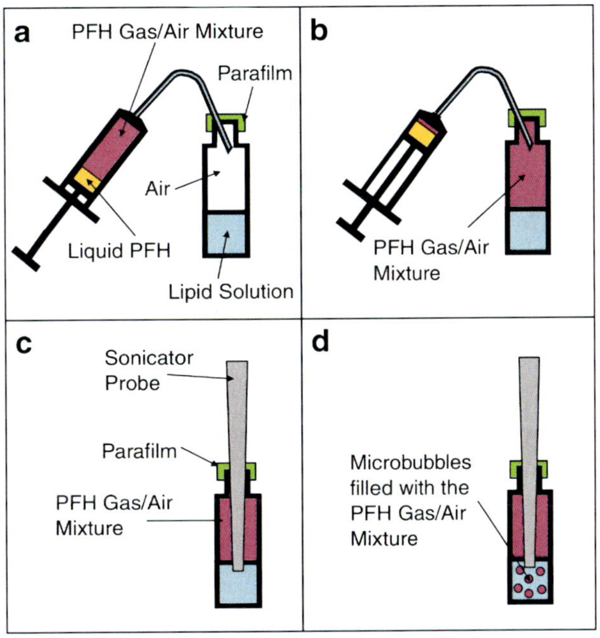

Figure 3: *Schematic representation of the manufacturing process for the PFH/air mixture filled microbubbles.* (**a**) A 5 mL syringe is filled with 0.5 mL of liquid PFH. The PFH is allowed to evaporate and mix with the air in the syringe until it reaches equilibrium. The top of the glass vial containing the lipid solution is covered with parafilm to reduce gas exchange from within the vial to the atmosphere (**b**) The PFH/air mixture is injected into the head space of the vial containing the lipid solution. Care is taken to prevent injection of any liquid PFH. The original air that was in the vial is displaced through the needle track hole made in the parafilm (**c**) The probe sonicator tip is inserted through the parafilm into the vial and the tip is positioned 1 mm below the surface of the lipid solution. (**d**) The probe sonicator is turned on and creates microbubbles which incorporate the PFH/air gas mixture in the headspace. These microbubbles are coated with the lipids from the solution. (Reprinted from Journal of Controlled Release, Vol.155, Issue 3, Ibsen, Benchimol, Simberg *et al.*, A novel nested liposome drug delivery vehicle capable of ultrasound triggered release of its payload, Pages No. 358-366, Copyright (2011), with permission from Elsevier (Ibsen, Benchimol, Simberg *et al.*, 2011)).

The emulsifying lipid containing PEG groups are essential to prevent MB coalescence to form macrobubbles within a few minutes. Pegylated lipids are also necessary to provide a steric brush to the "stealth" MBs that minimizes lipid shell interactions with blood components (opsonins) and consequently their clearance *via* the reticuloendothelial system (RES). Ligands can be covalently attached to the distal end of PEG for targeting purposes (Fig. **5**) (Klibanov, 2005). Alternatively, a ligand attached to a MB can be hidden from the surrounding medium by being buried by the PEG overbrush (Borden, Zhang, Gillies, Dayton and Ferrara, 2008). This way ligand binding to serum proteins and nonspecific adhesion (opsonins and phagocytes) are avoided (Cavalieri, Zhou, Tortora, Lucilla and Ashokkumar, 2012). These ligands can be revealed during low amplitude oscillations near the MB resonance frequency. For example, efficient adhesion of echistatin-targeted MBs to angiogenic vasculature in a fibroblast-growth-factor stimulated matrigel plug in the direction of the propagating acoustic wave is shown (Ferrara, Borden and Zhang, 2009).

At high acoustic pressure (>150 kPa), the lipid-coated bubble may lose gas and lipids because of gas diffusion and lipid shedding. The resulting bubbles persevere with a smaller diameter (Borden, Kruse, Caskey *et al.*, 2005). Guidi *et al.,* (Guidi, Vos, Mori, de Jong and Tortoli, 2010) showed that deflation of lipid-coated bubbles is an interesting phenomenon, which can be useful for bubble characterization. This deflation of lipid-coated bubbles by acoustic pressure is different from the destruction mechanism of albumin-coated bubbles (Faez, Emmer, Kooiman *et al.*, 2013). Lipid shells can readily expand, rupture, reseal, compress, buckle, or respread for each acoustic cycle (Dayton, Morgan, Klibanov, Brandenburger and Ferrara, 1999, Morgan, Allen, Dayton *et al.*, 2000).

Thin lipid shelled MBs that are active and could be destroyed at low acoustic pressures may be most useful for targeted imaging uses. Generally, lipid and protein monolayer shells (5-50nm) are considered to be too thin to hold a sufficient amount of drug cargo (Ferrara, Pollard and Borden, 2007). Drugs, nucleic acids (Hernot and Klibanov, 2008) and viruses can be loaded onto the surface of MBs through electrostatic interactions. This was first demonstrated with transfection of DNA delivered by cationically charged lipid MBs (Christensen, 2002). The drug payload into the monolayer phospholipid shell is rather limited. Thus a multilayer construction onto lipid-coated MBs was recently reported to be effective in increasing DNA loading (Borden, Caskey, Little, Gillies and Ferrara, 2007). A novel lipid MB to which PEGylated lipoplexes are attached *via* biotin-avidin-biotin linkages have been recently designed (Lentacker, 2009, Lentacker, 2009). Upon exposure to ultrasound, unaltered lipoplexes (DNA-lipid complexes) are released from these lipoplex-loaded MBs. The lipoplex loaded MBs have a much higher gene transfer capacity than either "free" PEGylated lipoplexes or naked DNA used in combination with MBs and US (Lentacker, Vandenbroucke, Lucas *et al.*, 2008). In addition, the lipoplex-loaded MBs only transfect cells when exposed to ultrasound, which presents a unique approach for space- and time-controlled gene transfer (Cavalieri, Zhou and Ashokkumar, 2010). The development of MBs carrying doxorubicin-liposome at their surface was recently reported for successful delivery of the antineoplastic drug to melanoma cells (Cavalieri, Zhou, Tortora, Lucilla and Ashokkumar, 2012).

3.4.3. Protein Coated Microbubbles

Albumin coating is the foremost for all protein coated MBs (Fig. **2c**) that consists of denatured albumin that is approximately 15 nm thick (Chomas, Dayton, Allen, Morgan and Ferrara, 2001) and forms a stiff structure around the gas core (Faez, Emmer, Kooiman *et al.*, 2013). Protein shelled MBs offer the advantage of being biocompatible and biodegradable (Cavalieri, Zhou, Tortora, Lucilla and Ashokkumar, 2012). Thick-shelled MBs that have a large cargo space to carry therapeutic agents and disrupt only at high acoustic pressures may be better suited for localized drug delivery. Thick-shelled MBs have also a larger surface area available for ligand conjugation. The lifetime of albumin shelled MBs is short (a few hours) because air diffuses rapidly out of the MBs (Cavalieri, Zhou and Ashokkumar, 2010). The albumin coating cracks when the bubble is insonified and exhibits static diffusion with a dissolution rate comparable to that of an uncoated bubble (Chomas, Dayton, May and Ferrara, 2001).

Albumin (Christiansen, 1994) and lysozyme (Cavalieri, Ashokkumar, Grieser and Caruso, 2008) shelled MBs are made mostly by sonication, which disperses gas in liquid suspension of a suitable coating material using high intensity ultrasound around 20 KHz. Additionally, protein shelled MBs can also make a combination of two ultrasound induced phenomena: emulsification and cavitation (Grinstaff and Suslick, 1991). Albumin shelled MBs are mostly stabilized by protein dimerization and hydrophobic interactions. It has also been suggested that thiols containing proteins like bovine serum albumin (BSA), human serum albumin (HAS) and haemoglobin (Hb) cross-link with cysteine residues through disulphide bond formation by the superoxide radicals generated under sonication conditions (Cavalieri, Zhou, Tortora, Lucilla and Ashokkumar, 2012). Ultrasonically synthesized serum albumin shelled MBs have a wide size distribution with a diameter ranging from 1 to 15μm (Christiansen, 1994). However, size distribution can be further controlled by sonicating at 355kHz (Cavalieri, Zhou, Tortora, Lucilla and Ashokkumar, 2012). Biodistribution studies carried out using albumin-shelled MBs showed that the protein shells are cleared from the blood stream in 3 min and accumulate in the liver, lung, and spleen of rats and pigs (Walday, Tolleshaug, Gjoen *et al.*, 1994).

Lysozyme MBs are more stable because of thicker (500nm) shell and cross-linked polymer shell (Cavalieri, Zhou and Ashokkumar, 2010). Lysozyme shell is partially arranged in amyloids fibrils with β-sheet internal structure similar to the Maltese-cross pattern obtained using cross-polarization microscopy (Yagi, Ohta and Matsuo, 2009). They are prepared by applying high-intensity ultrasound using a microtip horn (3 mm diameter) to the chemically denatured lysozyme solution. Additionally, hen egg white lysozyme contains four intramolecular disulphide bonds that can be partly broken using reducing agents, such as dithiothreitol (Zhou, 2011). Upon sonication, new intermolecular disulphide linkages are formed by the HO2 radicals generated during the cavitation process, leading to the formation of lysozyme MBs with a thick and elastic (150-200nm) protein shell (Cavalieri, Zhou, Tortora, Lucilla and Ashokkumar, 2012). Interestingly the stability of lysozyme crosslinked shell prevents Ostwald ripening endowing MBs with a relatively narrow size distribution. The size distribution (2.7±0.5μm) can be controlled using different ultrasonic experimental conditions and post treatment of MB suspension (Cavalieri, Zhou, Tortora, Lucilla and Ashokkumar, 2012). These MBs are extremely stable (up to 1 year) compared to the air-filled BSA MBs and retain the antimicrobial enzymatic activity of lysozyme (Zhou,

2011). Lysozyme is a non-toxic protein that biodegrades at proteolytic conditions under physiological condition and its use has been approved for pharmacological and therapeutic applications (Cavalieri, Zhou, Tortora, Lucilla and Ashokkumar, 2012).

Unlike albumin MBs, lysozyme MBs are positively charged colloidal particles and provide a good template for assembly of negatively charged biomolecules such as, nucleic acids, peptides and proteins (Melino, Zhou, Tortora *et al.*, 2012). Numerous therapeutic agents can be potentially conjugated to the lysozyme MBs shell exploiting hydrophobic interactions and covalent coupling to the protein amines, carboxyl and thiols functional moieties (Cavalieri, Zhou, Tortora, Lucilla and Ashokkumar, 2012). For instance doxorubicin uptake into lysozyme shell is driven by hydrophobic interactions whereas BSA coating of MBs surface is accomplished *via* both electrostatic interactions and disulfide bonds formation (Cavalieri, Zhou, Tortora, Lucilla and Ashokkumar, 2012).

4. LIGAND ATTACHMENT

Ligand attachment to a MB is essential if these bubbles are to bind to a specific receptor in the human body. Ligand-decorated bubbles move through the vasculature with the blood flow; a (small) fraction of the bubbles bumps into objects such as an endothelial cell, leukocyte, or blood clot that carries specific receptors (Klibanov, 2007) (Fig. **4**). Initial MB targeting experiments (Klibanov, Hughes, Marsh *et al.*, 1997, Klibanov, Hughes, Wojdyla *et al.*, 1998, Villanueva, Jankowski, Klibanov *et al.*, 1998) were performed in static conditions. Bubbles were brought in contact with the target surface (Figs. **4** & **5A**) (usually by inversion), and incubated for several minutes. The residual free bubbles were washed off. The retained MBs were counted and acoustic response was measured. However, this is not a good model as it does not account for blood flow within the vasculature. In order to best understand the targeting of MBs, experiments can be performed using parallel plate flow chambers as *in vitro* studies with known flow rates, and ligand and receptor densities (Klibanov, Hughes, Villanueva *et al.*, 1999, Takalkar, Klibanov, Rychak, Lindner and Ley, 2004, Weller, Villanueva, Klibanov and Wagner, 2002).

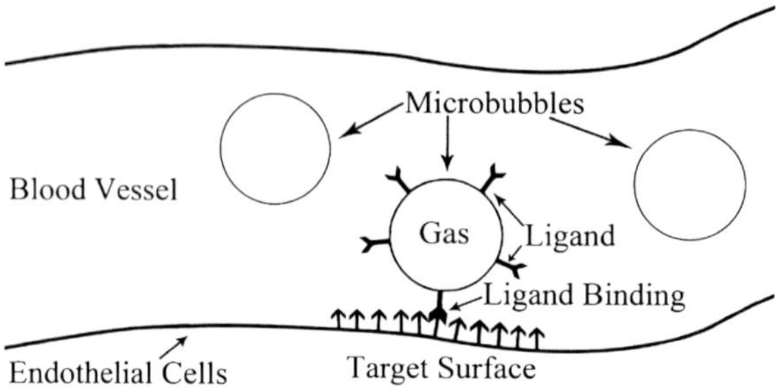

Figure 4: Schematic representation of targeted microbubbles travelling in the blood vessels that bind to the targeted surface through ligand binding.

Binding to the target depends on several factors such as specificity of ligand-receptor binding, detachment kinetics, surface densities of the ligand and receptor, blood flow, and wall shear conditions. Binding may be transient (in a fraction of a second) or permanent (for seconds or minutes), depending on how many firm bonds are formed during the initial contact (Klibanov, 2007). During MBs travel through the target vessels they may stay away from the vessel periphery further reducing the chances of reaching and selectively binding to the endothelial surface (Fig. **4** & **5A**). As such, US radiation can be applied perpendicular to the flows direction. This diverts particles toward the target area forcing them to arrest at the vessel wall which allows for a better chance for the MBs to bind to the target and stay attached to the target antigen after insonation is stopped (Fig. **5A**) (Dayton, Klibanov, Brandenburger and Ferrara, 1999, Lum, Borden, Dayton *et al.*, 2006).

The choice of attachment strategy is mostly determined by the nature of the ligand (Liu, Miyoshi and Nakamura, 2006). Coupling can be achieved through covalent and non-covalent means. If the ligand does not inactivate during the harsh conditions of bubble manufacturing they can be simply added (Klibanov, Hughes, Marsh *et al.*, 1997). For example, the protein avidin can be co-incorporated into the bubble shell during sonication (Korpanty, Grayburn, Shohet and Brekken, 2005) while retaining its activity. Additionally a carbohydrate ligand, short peptide or peptide mimetic can also easily tolerate the harsh conditions (Liu, Miyoshi and Nakamura, 2006). Many biotinylated ligands also attach non-covalently simply by adding them to the avidin or streptavidin coated bubbles (Fig. **5B**) (Klibanov, 2007, Liu, Miyoshi and Nakamura, 2006).

Alternatively, protein ligands (such as antibodies) that are not going to survive MB preparation can be covalently attached to the pre-formulated bubbles by amide bond formation (Villanueva, Jankowski, Klibanov *et al.*, 1998). The thiols and amines on the ligands can be attached covalently (Klibanov, 2005). Flow cytometry has indicated that more than 30,000 antibodies can be conjugated to each 2 to 4 μm MBs (Lindner, 2002). It is possible to insert a long flexible polymer spacer arm, for *e.g.* poly-ethylene glycol (PEG) between the anchor molecule and the ligand (Fig. **5C**) (Liu, Miyoshi and Nakamura, 2006). PEG, can be used to protrude the ligand from the MB surface, thereby increasing MB affinity and decreasing steric hindrance (Cavalieri, Zhou and Ashokkumar, 2010). Such a 'tether' can be 10 nm or even longer (Liu, Miyoshi and Nakamura, 2006) and might also diminish complement-mediated events (Cavalieri, Zhou and Ashokkumar, 2010). Thus PEG is now considered as essential as the shell coating.

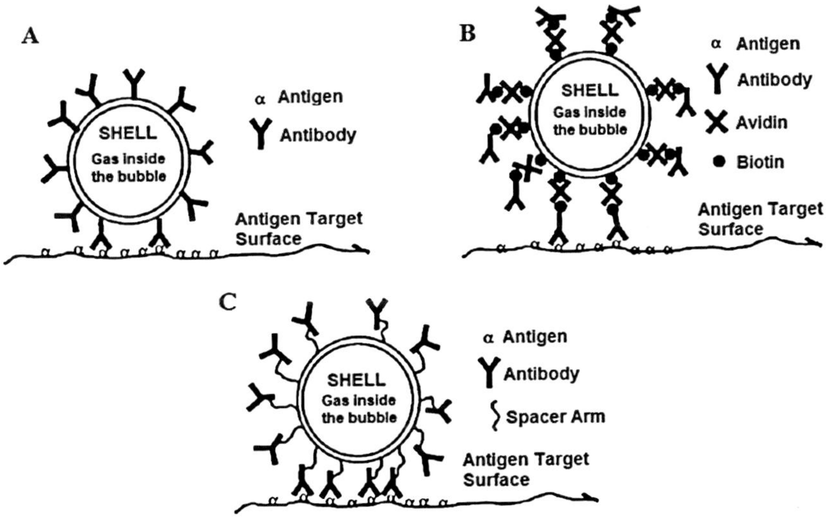

Figure 5: *Attachment of ligands to microbubble surface*: (**A**) direct, (**B**) *via* avidin bridge, (**C**) *via* a flexible spacer arm. Targeting of these microbubbles to a receptor coated surface. (Reprinted from Advanced Drug Delivery Reviews, Vol.37, Issue 1-3, Klibanov, Targeted delivery of gas-filled microspheres, contrast agents for ultrasound imaging, Pages No.139-157, Copyright (1999), with permission from Elsevier (Klibanov, 1999)).

In a flow-through situation, the ligand on the MB particle has a very limited time to bind to the receptor. For example, productive binding has to occur within 1 nanosecond in a large vessel with a blood flow of 1 m/s (Klibanov, 2007). This is an extremely short period of time beyond the ability of most antibodies. However, nature has evolved many fast-binding ligands that binds to leukocytes and tether to endothelial cells. For example, Pselectin glycoprotein ligand-1 (PSGL-1) binds on the leukocyte surface and endothelial cells expressing Pselectin (Klibanov, 2007). Inspired by the N-terminus of the PSGL-1 protein a Glycosulfopeptides, such as 2-GSP-6, carrying several sulfated tyrosines and a carbohydrate residue, were put on a MB surface which successfully adhered to selectin in high shear flow conditions (~4 dyn/cm2 wall shear stress) (Rychak, Li, Acton *et al.*, 2006). A polymeric version of sialyl Lewisx (a carbohydrate component of PSGL-1) on MBs was as successful in fast flow, as the synthetically challenging 2-GSP-6 (Klibanov, Rychak, Yang *et al.*, 2006). MBs have also been conjugated with ligands for different vascular biomarkers that have been implicated in angiogenesis such as integrins (Villanueva, Lu, Bowry *et al.*, 2007), the activated platelets in clots such as glycoprotein IIb/IIIa receptor (Kaufmann, Sanders, Davis *et al.*, 2007) and atherosclerotic lesions such as ICAM-1 and VCAM-1 (Cho, 2006, Klibanov, 2007).

5. INTERACTION OF ULTRASOUND AND MICROBUBBLE

Acoustic signals from MBs is dependent on the compressibility of the gas, bubble size, shell thickness, shell viscosity, shell density, properties of the surrounding medium, US frequency and power of the applied ultrasound (de Jong, Hoff, Skotland and Bom, 1992, Lindner, 2002).

MBs owe their functionality to the gas core, which can compress and expand easily in response to the acoustic pressure change (Fig. **8**) (Faez, Emmer, Kooiman *et al.*, 2013). This change can result in 100-fold volume change and 4-5 fold diameter change (Klibanov, 2007). Thus, when exposed to an ultrasound field, a gas bubble will undergo volumetric oscillations in response to the varying pressure (Fig. **8**) (Calliada, Campani, Bottinelli, Bozzini and Sommaruga, 1998, Postema and Schmitz, 2007). This also results in a high backscattering of the ultrasound wave. The amplitude of these oscillations will be much larger than those of a very weakly compressible body such as a red blood cell (Azmin, Harfield, Ahmad, Edirisinghe and Stride, 2012). Thus, despite their similarity in size, the MB will produce much stronger US echoes (Calliada, Campani, Bottinelli, Bozzini and Sommaruga, 1998, Postema and Schmitz, 2007). Moreover, the MBs can act as resonant systems with resonant frequencies within the same range as medical ultrasound frequencies (Faez, Emmer, Kooiman *et al.*, 2013).

Eventually, by increasing US pressure the MBs will undergo violent collapse, releasing a shock wave and often fragmenting into smaller bubbles (Figs. **6**, **7** & **8B**) (Lauterborn, 2010). This process is variously referred to as inertial, unstable, or transient cavitation (Fig. **9B**). Transient and unstable are both slightly misleading terms since a bubble can collapse repeatedly (Church, 2001) without fragmenting. But, inertial cavitation means the collapse of a gas cavity with significant amounts of energy being released (Fig. **8B**) (Faez, Emmer, Kooiman *et al.*, 2013). Broadband emissions are generated during inertial cavitation where bubbles undergo large radial oscillations that are dominated by the inertia of the surrounding liquid (Holland, Roy, Apfel and Crum, 1992). During compression of MB there is a rise in pressure and temperature within the bubble. But, during an inertial collapse the temperature may reach several thousand degrees centigrade or more (McNamara W.B., 1999). These extreme conditions are confined to the center of the bubble. However, bubble will have expanded again before any significant heat transfer can occur. Highly reactive chemical species may be produced such as free radicals and toxic chemicals such as hydrogen peroxide (H_2O_2) (Suslick, 1990) at relatively high intensities (Riesz and Kondo, 1992).

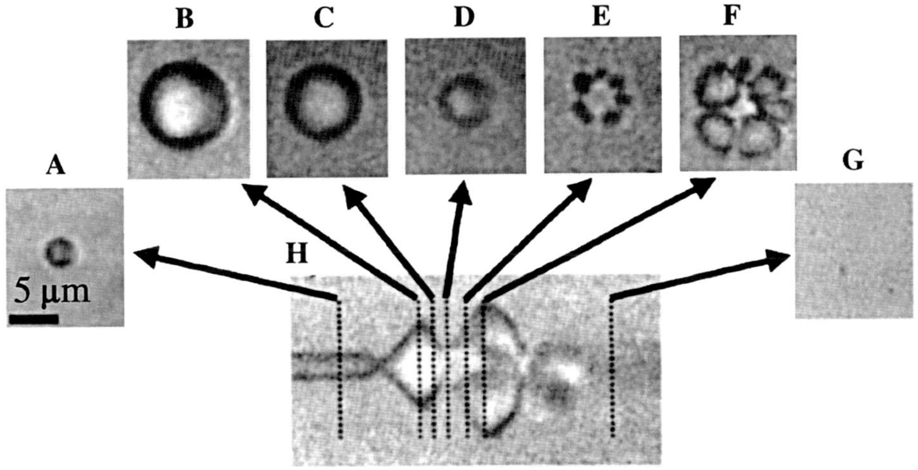

Figure 6: *Optical frame images and streak image of ultrasound contrast agents.* Optical frame images and streak image corresponding to the oscillation and fragmentation of a contrast agent microbubble, where fragmentation occurs during compression. The bubble has an initial diameter of 3 µm, shown in **A**. The streak image in h shows the diameter of the bubble as a function of time, and dashed lines indicate the times at which the two-dimensional frame images in **A–G** were acquired relative to the streak image. (Reprinted with permission from Chomas *et al.,* (Chomas, 2000) Copyright, 2000, American Institute of Physics).

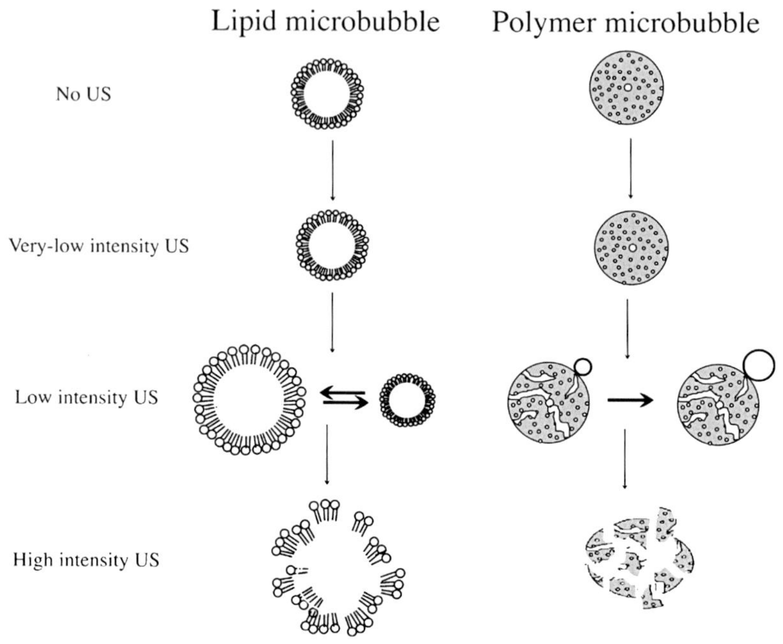

Figure 7: Schematic representation of lipid (left column) and polymer (right column) microbubble interaction with ultrasound of increasing intensity (top to bottom). (Reprinted from Advanced Drug Delivery Reviews, Vol. 60, Isssue 10, Hernot and Klibanov, Microbubbles in ultrasound-triggered drug and gene delivery, Pages No.1153-1166, Copyright (2008), with permission from Elsevier (Hernot and Klibanov, 2008)).

In addition to a temperature rise, "streaming" currents may also be set up as ultrasound propagates through a liquid as a result of momentum transfer (Hill, 2004). A similar effect can occur on a correspondingly smaller scale around MBs undergoing stable oscillations (Fig. **8A**) (Elder, 1956). If the bubble is sufficiently close to a surface, such as a cell membrane, these circulating flows may give rise to shearing stresses which have been hypothesized as the means by which uptake of therapeutic components is enhanced (Marmottant, 2008). Micro-streaming (Fig. **8A**) will also contribute to circulating material in the target region, which is extremely important in the context of therapeutic applications (Datta, Coussios, McAdory *et al.*, 2006). At higher amplitudes of oscillation, micro-streaming can cause significant damage to cells and produce mechanical erosion (Azmin, Harfield, Ahmad, Edirisinghe and Stride, 2012, Marmottant and Hilgenfeldt, 2003, Rooney, 1970). In addition when a bubble rapidly collapses near a boundary, this collapse is asymmetrical. A high-speed liquid jet may form projecting through the bubble towards the boundary. This phenomenon is known as microjetting (Fig. **8C**) (Cavalieri, Zhou and Ashokkumar, 2010). Microstreming and microjetting generate moderate shear stress on inducing hyperpolarization of the cell membrane by modifying the electrophysiologic cell activities and enhancing the cell's permeability (Fig. **8**) (Tran, 2006). For drug-loaded MBs, microjetting would be the ideal release mechanism (Fig. **8C**), since it effectively produces small holes within a cell membrane (sonoporation) which facilitates the drug uptake (Ward, Wu and Chiu, 1999). The rupture size is large enough to allow the passage of non-deformable particles up to 0.5μm in diameter, that depends on several parameters including the MB size, shell composition, acoustic pressure, and intravascular pressure (Cavalieri, Zhou and Ashokkumar, 2010).

MBs and ultrasonic waves undergo a scattering interaction by absorbing the acoustic energy (Cavalieri, Zhou and Ashokkumar, 2010). MBs in a liquid are forced to oscillate with only a relatively small to moderate increase and decrease of radius. The mechanical biological effect is estimated by certain ultrasound parameters and is called mechanical index (MI). At low MI<0.1, MBs undergo alternate equal expansion and contractions symmetrically and in a linear manner (Cavalieri, Zhou and Ashokkumar, 2010). At a slightly higher MI of 0.1 to 0.3, the bubble becomes somewhat resistant to compression than to expansion which results in stable or non-inertial cavitation (Fig. **8A** & **B**) and leads to non-linear oscillations and backscatter at a variety of frequencies (harmonics, sub-harmonics and ultra-harmonics) (Hernot and Klibanov, 2008, Sutton, Haworth, Pyne-Geithman and Holland, 2013). When the bubbles are collapsing the kinetic energy of the bubble surpasses its surface energy and fragments into a number of smaller bubbles. Fragmentation (Figs. **6**, **7** & **8B**) has been exclusively observed with contrast agents with thin, elastic shells (Bloch, 2004). At even higher acoustic pressures (MI 0.3–0.6), MBs undergo forced expansion and compression that leads to its destruction by different methods such as outward diffusion of the gas during the compression phase, diffusion *via* large shell defects, or complete fragmentation of the shell and the gas core (Figs. **6**, **7** & **8B**) (Chomas, 2000, Chomas, Dayton, Allen, Morgan and Ferrara, 2001). MBs fragmentation can instead produce violent effects which causes cell membrane permeability (Lawrie, Brisken, Francis *et al.*, 2000) and lysis (Ward, Wu and Chiu, 1999) (Fig. **8B**). Acoustical experiments are performed on a population of MBs therefore they do not show how individual MBs respond in an acoustic field. Experimental evidence is obtained with high-speed camera microscopy of insonated bubbles (Hernot and Klibanov, 2008). These optical frame or streak images show the oscillating and fragmentation changes of a 3μm MB (Fig. **6**) (Chomas, 2000).

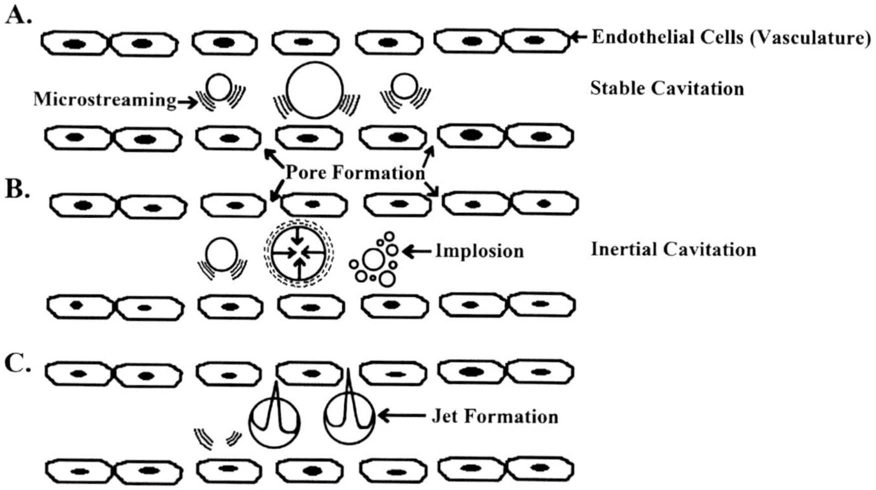

Figure 8: Schematic representation of ultrasound causing microbubbles to behave in different ways that leads to endolethelial pore formation and increase vascular permeability. **A**) Stable cavitation leads to expansion and contraction of microbubble that generates shear stress known as microstreaming. **B**) Inertial cavitations leads to implosion of the microbubbles that allows for the release of the bubble contents or fragment into smaller microbubbles. **C**) Bubbles generate microjets when the resonance diameter is larger than the blood vessels that damage the endothelial lining.

Coated MBs undergo damping as dissipation of viscous energy. Damping reduces the amplitude of the bubble oscillations and it widens the resonance curve of the bubble (Faez, Emmer, Kooiman *et al.*, 2013). MB shell material and stiffness also plays a major role in determining the type of explosion or implosion that may occur when exposed to acoustic energy. Lipid or protein MBs and polymer MBs behave differently and depend on the amplitude of ultrasound to which they are exposed (Bloch, 2004, Hernot and Klibanov, 2008). The regime of phospholipid coated MBs depends on bubble radius and the concentration of phospholipid molecules. Phospholipid MBs exist in buckled, elastic and ruptured regime. The bubble is compressed when the coating is condensed which leads to buckling, and with the bubble coating in such a tensionless state, the resulting surface tension is zero (Fig. **6D**) (Faez, Emmer, Kooiman *et al.*, 2013). When the bubble is expanded (Fig. **6B**), the coating may be ruptured and the gas core will be exposed to the surrounding liquid changing the surface tension of the gas–liquid interface. In the intermediate elastic regime, the coating is assumed to behave elastically where it is relatively stiff. During the elastic regime, its resonance frequency is high and it will not easily oscillate when driven below resonance (de Jong, 1994). An increasing acoustic pressure can modify the concentration of lipid molecules on the bubble's surface, forcing the bubble into the buckling regime, which suddenly reduces its stiffness (Faez, Emmer, Kooiman *et al.*, 2013).

An oscillating phospholipid MB would most likely lead to stable or non-inertial cavitation (Fig. **8A** & **B**). For MBs with a thin shell such as Optison (albumin shelled MBs) fragmentation is the major mechanism for bubble destruction (de Jong, Hoff, Skotland and Bom, 1992). Microjets (Fig. **8C**) are also generated during cavitation of thin-shelled MBs (Skyba, Price, Linka, Skalak and Kaul, 1998) which produce vessel wall ruptures *in vivo* and extravasation of nanoparticles into the interstitial space. Polymeric shells are stiff and will not oscillate actively at low US intensity (Fig. **7**). The shell cracks as US pressure is increased above the threshold value resulting in the escape of the encapsulated gas (Fig. **7**) (Hernot and Klibanov, 2008). This type of MB destruction is called sonic cracking (Fig. **7**). However, thick shelled rigid albumin MBs also undergo sonic cracking (de Jong and Hoff, 1993, de Jong, Hoff, Skotland and Bom, 1992). For bubbles containing drugs in the gas phase (anesthetic gases, nitric oxide, oxygen) (Cavalieri, 2008, Unger, Porter, Culp *et al.*, 2004), sonic cracking is a suitable mechanism. Fragmentation (Fig. **7**), microjetting (Fig. **8**) and sonic cracking (Fig. **7**) can be effective mechanisms in drug delivery and therefore their occurrence should be finely predicted and tuned (Cavalieri, Zhou and Ashokkumar, 2010, Postema, 2004).

6. BIO-EFFECTS

US assisted drug delivery is a very complex process that relies on biochemical and mechanical processes that occurs during sonoporation which is defined as mechanical disruption of the plasma membrane (Cavalieri, Zhou and Ashokkumar, 2010, Sutton, Haworth, Pyne-Geithman and Holland, 2013) (Fig. **9**).

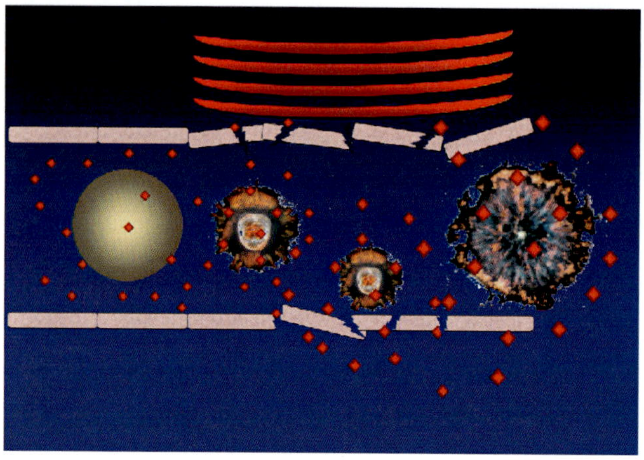

Figure 9: Ultrasound interacts with the microbubble, causing oscillation and eventual destruction, leading to the release of genetic material. The accompanying cavitation produces a local shockwave that increases cellular permeability, allowing transcapillary passage of macromolecules through small endothelial perforations. (Image courtesy of C.R. Merritt, MD, Thomas Jefferson University Hospital, Philadelphia, PA.) (Reprinted from Applied Radiology, Vol. 33, First Author (C, Howard) *et al.*, The role of ultrasound agents in gene therapy, pages 126-138, Copyright 2004, with permission from Andercon Publishing Ltd. (Howard, 2004)).

US energy can penetrate or "push" materials into skin, blood clots or other tissues (Smith, Lee, Maione *et al.*, 2003). Shear stress can be generated on the membrane of an endothelial cell through the destruction of MBs that causes high-energy microstreams and microjets which increases the permeability of blood vessels promoting the extravasation (Fig. **10**) of high molecular weight drugs (Cavalieri, Zhou, Tortora, Lucilla and Ashokkumar, 2012). This increase in permeability is probably due to transient holes in the plasma membrane and possibly the nuclear membrane (Liu, Miyoshi and Nakamura, 2006). Thus, acoustic cavitation is a pre-requisite in promoting the physical or chemical release of drugs from carriers (MBs), or in promoting the transport of drugs into cells (Fig. **10**). US-induced passage of materials from the luminal to the adventitial side of vascular tissue (Figs. **9** & **10**) have been proposed in the literature such as paracellular widening of inter-endothelial clefts and tight junctions, free passage through injured endothelial lining and transcytosis *via* fenestration and channel formation (Sheikov, McDannold, Sharma and Hynynen, 2008) (Fig. **11**).

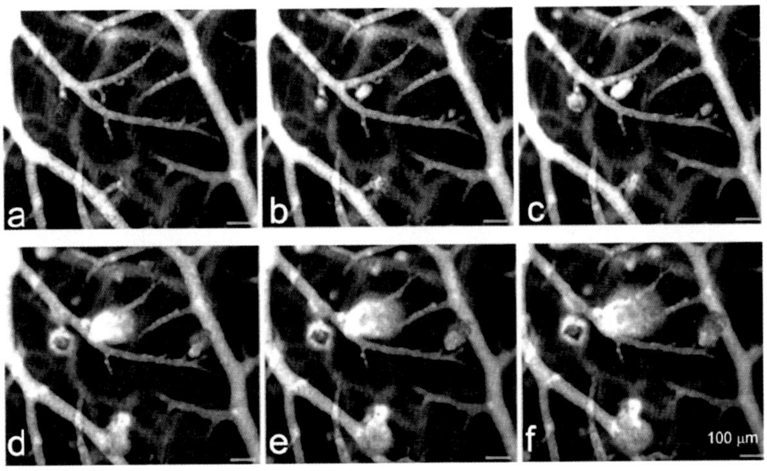

Figure 10: *Enhanced drug and gene delivery achieved with the combination of particles and ultrasound.* Isonation of circulating microbubbles in the chorioallantoic membrane model results in small vascular defects, through which a fluorescent dye is transported, reproduced with permission from (27). (**a**)–(**f**) are a sequence of images acquired from 1.00-MHz center frequency insonation at a peak negative pressure of 1.3 MPa. (**a**) was acquired before insonation, (**b**)–(**f**) were acquired 0.06, 0.12, 1.24, 2.24 and 3.24 seconds after insonation began, respectively, demonstrating the transport of the fluorescent probe from the vasculature to the tissue interstitium.(Reprinted with permission from Ferrara *et al.*, (Ferrara, Borden and Zhang, 2009) Copyright (2009) American Chemical Society).

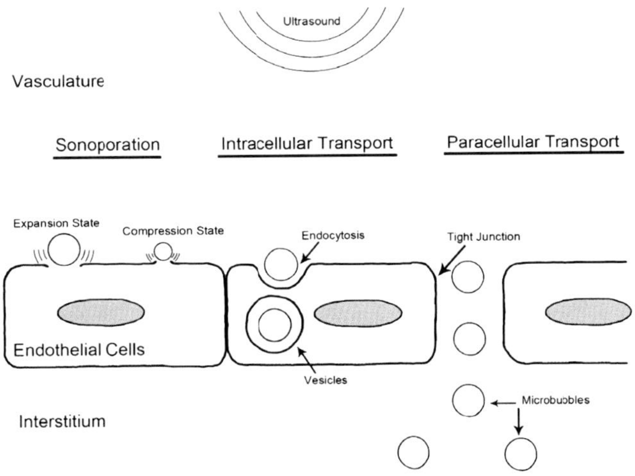

Figure 11: Ultrasound mediated drug delivery through different means of transport. Sonoporation allows for the mechanical disruption of the endothelial cell membrane. Intracellular trasnsport allows for the uptake of microbubbles through endocytosis that transports the microbubble through to the interstitium. Paracellular transport allows for the opening of the tight junctions or separation of bonds that hold the endothelial cells together which causes pore formation in the blood vessel wall.

In vivo studies suggest that a MI of 0.4 has been shown to be detrimental to the plasma membrane and microvasculature (ter Haar, 2009). However, low intensity stable cavitation may not be adequately effective in triggering the drug delivery (Cavalieri, Zhou and Ashokkumar, 2010). Reported bio-effects *in vivo* include hemolysis, damage to the microvasculature, opening of the blood brain barrier, effects on cardiac rhythm and thrombolysis (Dalecki, 2007). The vessel wall structure has also been found to influence the degree of rupture (Price, Skyba, Kaul and Skalak, 1998). The fore mentioned mechanisms have been proposed for the blood brain barrier (BBB)(Choi, Pernot, Small and Konofagou, 2007), but are also supported by studies in other tissue beds, including renal (Wible, Galen, Wojdyla *et al.*, 2002), prostate (Li, Liu, Li *et al.*, 2012) and skeletal muscle (Price, Skyba, Kaul and Skalak, 1998) tissues.

6.1. Sonoporation

Sonoporation refers to the localized, mechanical disruption of plasma membrane (Fig. **11**) (Sutton, Haworth, Pyne-Geithman and Holland, 2013). van Wamel *et al.,* (van Wamel, Kooiman, Emmer *et al.*, 2006) using high speed imaging showed transport of propidium iodide (PI) against endothelial cells as a direct correlation between cell deformation and resulting cell membrane permeability with *in vitro* studies. According to van Wamel *et al.,* (van Wamel, Kooiman, Harteveld *et al.*, 2006) poration is a transition of hydrophobic to hydrophilic pores. This transition creates cylindrical pores when a rotation of the polar heads brings a hydrophilic surface to the pore (Fig. **12**). When US is applied, the adhered MBs on the transmembrane generates a critical 'shear' force, which leads to formation of pores once the membrane breakdown force is exceeded. Rapidly oscillating MBs undergoes rapid expansion and compression (Fig. **12**) due to changes in the volume of the gases inside the bubble. This generates fluid flow over the cell surface and is termed as microstreaming (Fig. **13**), which is responsible for the disruption of cell membrane by tearing the lipid bilayer membrane open (Marmottant and Hilgenfeldt, 2003). Cells can withstand compression better than elongation, which may act as the main component that determines pore formation. Scanning electron microscopy studies have already shown that membrane poration occurs after US and MBs treatment (Mehier-Humbert, Bettinger, Yan and Guy, 2005). Mehier-Humbert *et al.,* (Mehier-Humbert, Bettinger, Yan and Guy, 2005) showed an efficient delivery

FITC-dextran (77-164 KDa) or particles of 25nm. They showed cell membranes with a pore size distribution up to 75nm with ~60% of cells being positive for delivery of the particle. This allows for direct transfer of molecules into the cytoplasm. van Wamel *et al.,* (van Wamel, Kooiman, Emmer *et al.*, 2006) have also shown that PI does not enter a cell 1 min after the US exposure. These results support the general idea that the pores reseal quickly upon termination of US. Mehier-Humbert *et al.,* (Mehier-Humbert, Bettinger, Yan and Guy, 2005) showed that almost all the routes of entry had closed 5 seconds after termination of US. The action of MBs on cells is a mechanical one and can be as important as chemical stimuli in determining vascular fate or pathological state. The most important biomedical application of the sonoporation technique is that it allows the introduction of membrane-impermeable xenomolecules (synthetic molecules) such as dyes, hormones, proteins, plasmids, *etc.* into living cells (van Wamel, Kooiman, Harteveld *et al.*, 2006).

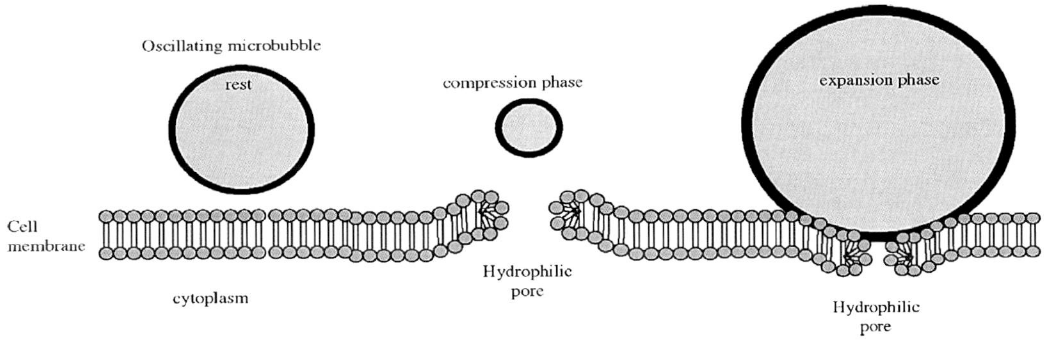

Figure 12: *Proposed model of the oscillating microbubble enforced pore formation in the cell membrane.* The pushing and pulling behavior of the microbubble causes rupture of the cell membrane creating a hydrophilic pore allowing *trans*-membrane flux of fluid and macromolecules. (Reprinted from J Control Release, Vol. 112, van Wamel, Kooiman, Harteveld *et al.*, Vibrating microbubbles poking individual cells: drug transfer into cells *via* sonoporation. Pages No. 149-55, Copyright (2006), with permission from Elsevier (van Wamel, Kooiman, Harteveld *et al.*, 2006)).

6.2. Paracellular Transport

Drugs can be delivered by paracellular transport between functional endothelial cells with MBs. Transport by low-frequency US is strongly supported in the literature (Fan, 2011). When a sound wave is propagated through a liquid medium, steady currents (Fig. **13**) are set up in the direction of beam as a result of momentum transfer (Hill, 2004). This acoustic streaming (Fig. **13**) occurs around MBs undergoing stable bubble oscillations (Fig. **13**) within the US field growing in size *via* rectified diffusion (Hsieh, 1961). These eddying flows may, in turn, impose shear stresses on nearby surfaces, such as cell membranes, and it is thought that this may promote the uptake of therapeutic components (Marmottant, 2008, Marmottant and Hilgenfeldt, 2003). When a MB oscillates near a vessel wall (Fig. **13**), its shell is estimated to travel at speeds on the order of 250 m/s (Allen, May and Ferrara, 2002), either by directly perturbing nearby structures or by causing local fluid convection (Collis, Manasseh, Liovic *et al.*, 2010). The acoustic radiation forces causes bubbles to move in the direction of the wave propagation by bringing them in contact with vessel endothelium (Leighton, 1994). Radiation pressure may be involved in Focused US + MBs-based blood brain barrier opening through activating the stretch-sensitive or mechanosensitive (MS) ion channels in the vascular endothelium (Vykhodtseva, McDannold and Hynynen, 2008). Mechanosensation (MS) channels are now known to be implicated in many basic cell functions (Hamill, 2006). During localized elongation of cell membranes the MS channels are activated by the conformational changes (Mihran, Barnes and Wachtel, 1990, Mihran, Barnes and Wachtel, 1990). The resulting openings are reversible (Yang, Lin, Kang and Chao, 2011).

Endothelial cell morphology can vary significantly between normal and diseased organs. The tissue microenvironment surrounding blood vessels seems to control the endothelial cell phenotype *in vivo* (Schnitzer, 1997). Thus the blood vessels or microvasculature in the brain differs from other organs. BBB is known to restrict the paracellular translocation of large hydrophilic macromolecules and toxic compounds into the brain *via* specific membrane located transport systems (Deli, 2009). When MB oscillations occur in the cerebral microcirculation, the BBB is disrupted, causing drug extravasation due to breakdown of transmembrane tight junction proteins that regulate the paracellular permeability of the endothelial cell layer (Jalali, 2010).

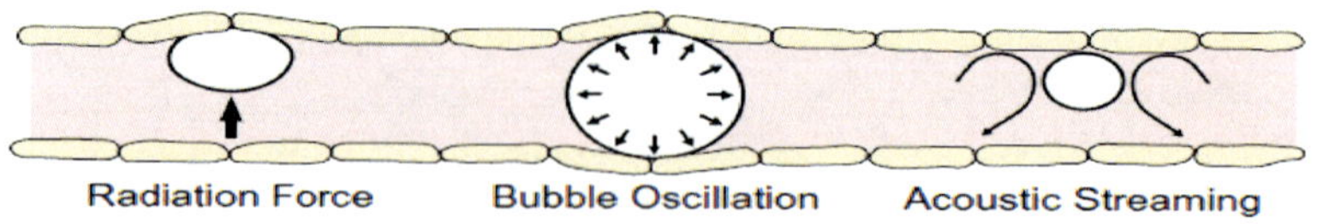

Figure 13: *Possible mechanisms for blood–brain barrier disruption via ultrasound + microbubbles*. Assuming that the effect is not due to bubble collapse (inertial cavitation), possible effects include stimulation of the endothelial cells *via* radiation force on the bubbles, bubble oscillation or from microstreaming of the fluid around the bubbles. (Reprinted from Ultrasonics, Vol 48, Vykhodtseva, McDannold and Hynynen, Progress and problems in the application of focused ultrasound for blood–brain barrier disruption, Pages No. 279-296, Copyright (2008), with permission from Elsevier (Vykhodtseva, McDannold and Hynynen, 2008)).

6.2.1. Blood Brain Barrier (BBB)

An almost impenetrable blood-brain barrier protects the central nervous system, CNS, and bars the entry of foreign susbstances. This is known to hamper the delivery of effective diagnostic or therapeutic agents and complicates the treatment of CNS diseases such as malignant brain tumors, metastatic brain tumors, Alzheimer's and Parkinson's disease (Cavalieri, Zhou, Tortora, Lucilla and Ashokkumar, 2012).

A major limitation is the poor penetration of US through the skull. US wave is poorly distorted by the skull and can be corrected by arranging the US transducers in a phase-array configuration (Clement and Hynynen, 2002) and computed tomography scans (Aubry, Tanter, Pernot, Thomas and Fink, 2003). Kinoshita *et al.,* (Kinoshita, McDannold, Jolesz and Hynynen, 2006) showed that *in situ* acoustic pressure of the mouse brain is estimated to be 87 ± 7% of that measured in water. The acoustic pressure of a 0.6MPa sonication is estimated to deliver a power of about 0.086 W cm^2 while for a 0.8MPa sonication is said to be about 0.152 W cm^2 (Kinoshita, McDannold, Jolesz and Hynynen, 2006). Recent studies have shown that with focused and pulsed US irradiation, the BBB can be disrupted locally to deliver chemotherapeutics (BCNU) and UCAs into the brain without inducing neuronal damage (Hynynen, McDannold, Vykhodtseva *et al.*, 2006, Liu, 2010). Injection of UCAs consisting of commercialized lipid and protein shelled MBs have been used in conjunction with pulsed sonication to delivery chemotherapy agents (liposomal Doxorubicin and Herceptin) and genes (packaged in Herpes Simplex Virus (HSV)) locally to the brain (Hynynen, 2008). US intensity is reduced by a factor of two and still BBB disruption (BBBD) can be observed while leaving the neurons unharmed. Acoustic energy is delivered transcranially (Fig. **14A**) focused to a focal spot with a diameter of a few millimeters (~2-3 mm) to target a small tissue volume (for *e.g.* right hemisphere) (Kinoshita, McDannold, Jolesz and Hynynen, 2006). This allows for the delivery of drugs with a molecular weight greater than 400Da (Cavalieri, Zhou, Tortora, Lucilla and Ashokkumar, 2012). Previous BBBD involved the use of convection where a catheter insertion into the brain was needed (Kinoshita, McDannold, Jolesz and Hynynen, 2006).

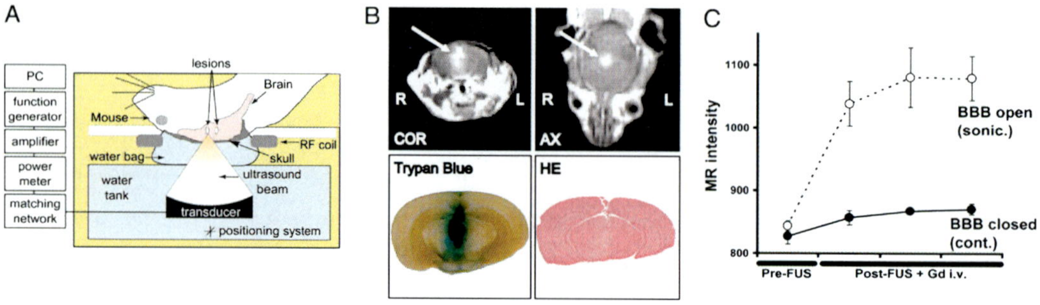

Figure 14: *Experimental settings and BBB disruption in mice by MRI-guided focused ultrasound.* (**A**) Diagram and protocol for BBB opening used in this experiment. Mice in the supine position were placed on the sonication table in the MR scanner. The ultrasound beam was focused through the intact skull on the target in the brain. (**B** and **C**) MR monitoring of BBB disruption and photographs of harvested brains showing BBB disruption induced by focused ultrasound. (**B**) Representative example with BBB disruption achieved by 0.6-MPa (peak negative-pressure amplitude) focused ultrasound exposure. (Upper) The BBB opening was easily monitored by leakage of the MR contrast agent into the brain parenchyma on axial (AX) and coronal (COR) MR images (arrows). (Lower Left) The location of the BBB opening was confirmed by trypan blue staining of the affected area. (Lower Right) No apparent macroscopic damage related to BBB disruption can be seen. (**C**) Magnitude of BBB disruption in the animal presented in B monitored by the MR-intensity change. Absolute values of the MR intensity of the sonicated target (○) and the contralateral side (control; ●) are plotted for repeated image acquisitions after sonication. Data are presented as the mean ± SD of four voxels. (Reproduced with permission from Kinoshita M *et al.,* (Kinoshita, McDannold, Jolesz and Hynynen, 2006). PNAS, Copyright (2006) National Academy of Sciences, U.S.A).

Studies showed that in rabbits a 1.63-MHz sonication allowed for a BBB opening. During the opening, a temperature elevation of 0.025°C was observed in the targeted tissues. This rise in temperature is not significant and thus an unlikely contributor to BBB leakage (Hynynen, McDannold, Vykhodtseva and Jolesz, 2001). Several studies show that opening the BBB is may be the result of interaction between the ultrasound wave and the MBs. Firstly, US wave causes the MBs to expand and contract in the capillaries resulting in mechanical stretching of the vessel wall and consequently opening of the tight junctions. This was confirmed by Kinoshita *et al.,* (Kinoshita, McDannold, Jolesz and Hynynen, 2006) by the leakage of trypan blue through the BBB into the brain parenchyma after 0.6- and 0.8-MPa sonication with a focused a 0.69 MHz US transducer and injection of Optison MBs (Fig. **14B**). The magnitude of BBB disruption in the animal presented in Fig. **14B** is monitored by the MR-intensity change and plotted as a line graph in Fig. **14C**. Secondly, US known to induce MB oscillations may also reduce the local blood flow and induce transient ischemia, which can trigger

BBB opening. Lastly, MBs that collapse during sonication can cause highly localized shock waves and fluid jets resulting in mechanical opening of the BBB (McDannold, Vykhodtseva and Hynynen, 2006).

The endothelial cells that line the microvasculature of the brain are sealed together by tight junctions thus restricting the diffusion of water-soluble substances and particularly of high molecular weight therapeutic agents (~150 kDa) such as antibody-based anticancer agents (Herceptin) (Baselga, 2000) or antibodies that showed efficacy against amyloid B reversing cognitive deficits in early Alzheimer disease (Klyubin, Walsh, Lemere *et al.*, 2005). Low frequency US irradiation has shown to decrease the expression and distributions of tight junction associated protein such as zonula occludens (ZO-1), occludin, and claudin-5 (Jalali, 2010). Occuldin is known to play a key role in the tightness of the endothelial cells (Hirase, 1997) and ZO-1 is known to anchor the transmembrane proteins to the cytoskeleton (González-Mariscal, 2000). While, claudin-5 is believed to be one of the principal elements with regards to the structure and function of BBB (Ohtsuki, 2007). Shang *et al.,* (Shang, 2011) quantified three tight junction proteins (claudin-5, occludin and ZO-1) at the blood-tumor barrier and found mRNA and protein levels before, during and after a three hour exposure to 1-MHz US, in the presence or absence of Optison MBs. The three tight junction components were significantly reduced (compared with control) by 1-MHz US at three and six hours post-exposure. However, twelve hours after exposure the protein expression and presence at the blood--tumor barrier had returned to normal levels (Shang, 2011). VEGF is expressed in vascular endothelial cells in response to shear stress, mechanical disruption and response to immune cytokines in the circulation, or adjacent extravascular tissue (Wood, 2012). Temporary opening of the endothelial junctions *via* VEGF signaling is known as an intercellular route for molecule transport (Komarova, 2010).

6.3. Damage-Induced Transport

The most disruptive mechanism is the passage of molecules through a compromised endothelium (Sutton, Haworth, Pyne-Geithman and Holland, 2013). This means of transport is mostly associated with microjetting that may lead to tissue damage as observed during *in vitro* conditions by MBs. Microjets can easily puncture a cell membrane and this effect has been observed extensively with CAs near cell monolayers (Prentice, 2005). Electron microscopy has shown that insonation with 1 MHz US and a peak transmission pressure of 1.3 MPa could increase the vascular permeability in the vessels by causing pores with a diameter of up to 55μm suggesting microjetting as the cause. These parameters are also known to expand 1.8μm UCAs to 20μm (Stieger, 2007). At the same acoustic power Yang *et al.,* (Yang, Lin, Kang and Chao, 2011) has shown that the extravasation caused by leakage of Evans Blue (EB) into the brain was found to be dependent on the applied sonication time. They also showed that BBB tends to return to normal at about 40 min following a single sonication (Yang, Lin, Kang and Chao, 2011). Thus, the reversibility of pore formation in the BBB is strength and exposure length dependent.

Skyba *et al.,* (Skyba, Price, Linka, Skalak and Kaul, 1998) were the first to visualize Optison MBs destruction resulting in microvessel (mostly capillaries ≤7μm) rupture in rat spinotrapezius muscle. This led to extravasation of RBCs into the nearby interstitial rupture. They also observed a number of nonviable cells at the microvessel rupture proportional to the MI applied. After US application, convective transport of an 8.5nm diameter of fluorescein isothiocyanate labeled dextran has been observed through micron-sized openings with a mean fluid velocity of 188.6 μm/sec at low frequency and 326.5μm/sec at high frequency in a chorioallantoic membrane (CAM) model (Stieger, Caskey, Adamson *et al.*, 2007). Similarly, a recent *ex vivo* study (Wood, 2012) demonstrated that aortic smooth muscle exposed to pulsed color-Doppler and Optison MBs induced loss of receptor-mediated contractility along with endothelium mediated relaxation. Histological studies showed the loss of endothelium and endothelial cell apoptosis (Sutton, Haworth, Pyne-Geithman and Holland, 2013). These observations were only seen in tissues treated with US and Optison (UCA), implying that smooth muscle function was impaired (Wood, 2012). Chen *et al.,* (Chen, Brayman, Kreider, Bailey and Matula, 2011) performed ultra-high speed microscopy experiments in *ex vivo* mesenteries to observe the Definity MBs oscillations in venules exposed to short US pulses (2μs). The MBs appears to be flattened when in contact with the vessel wall, during the initial expansion phase. The microjets, which may start to form during the collapse or re-expansion phase of the MBs, is clearly visible during the re-expansion phase and is directed away from the contact site (Chen, Brayman, Kreider, Bailey and Matula, 2011). MBs whose diameter is smaller than the microjet lengths, in smaller compliant microvessels, can cause considerable invagination on the opposite vessel wall and partial endothelial desquamation (Chen, Brayman, Kreider, Bailey and Matula, 2011, Sutton, Haworth, Pyne-Geithman and Holland, 2013).

Thus, liquid jets caused by the cavitation of MBs can contribute to vessel rupture (Chen, Brayman, Bailey and Matula, 2010) leading to capillary extravasation of cells, dyes and other particles, supporting its therapeutic potential for triggering localized, reversible endothelial permeability (Sutton, Haworth, Pyne-Geithman and Holland, 2013).

6.4. Transcytosis/Intracellular Transport

MB cavitation can also provoke drug transport through a vascular endothelial cell. Transcytosis or intracellular transport (Fig. **11**), in the context of drug delivery, consists of the drug being endocytosed at the luminal surface of the endothelial cell membrane (Sutton, Haworth, Pyne-Geithman and Holland, 2013). This can be achieved through either a receptor-mediated fashion (Ghitescu, Fixman, Simionescu and Simionescu, 1986) or by invagination caused by cavitation with US (Chen, Brayman, Bailey and Matula, 2010). Ghitescu *et al.,* (Ghitescu, Fixman, Simionescu and Simionescu, 1986) showed specific adsorptive binding of albumin complexes to plasmalemmal vesicles and clustering in uncoated pits. Plasmalemmal vesicles allow endothelial cells to transport molecules such as proteins from the blood that are too large to diffuse through cell junctions or fenestrae and this transport takes place both by vectorial transcytosis (vesicles) and by connective transcytosis (channels) (Fig. **11**). Ghitescu *et al.,* (Ghitescu, Fixman, Simionescu and Simionescu, 1986), also demonstrated that albumin can stimulate endocytosis and transcytosis (Fig. **11**) in mouse pulmonary and myocardial endothelium. Thus, albumin coated MBs could potentially go through a similar process. Subsequent transportation through several intracellular compartments and secretion from the cell at the basolateral aspect (Niles and Malik, 1999) results in delivery to vascular tissue. Transcytosis or endocytosis *via* caveolar, an alternative pathway for targeted drug delivery (Schnitzer, Oh, Pinney and Allard, 1994). This is a receptor-mediated process *via* receptor-targeted drug vesicles (McIntosh, Tan, Oh and Schnitzer, 2002, Sutton, Haworth, Pyne-Geithman and Holland, 2013).

According to Chen *et al.,* (Chen, Brayman, Bailey and Matula, 2010), invagination occurs when bubbles collapsed near the vessel wall that results in the vessel wall being pulled inward toward the lumen. Invagination causes higher strain on the vessel wall than distention resulting in vessel rupture (Chen, Brayman, Bailey and Matula, 2010). These localized mechanical destruction of the endothelial membrane results in endocytosis and subsequent transcytosis (Fig. **12**). Cavitating MBs near the cell membrane can create a pore for increased membrane permeability to macromolecules, genes such as wt-p53 (plasmid vector) (Taniyama, Tachibana, Hiraoka *et al.*, 2002) and extracellular ions such as Ca^{+2} (Fan, Liu, Mayer and Deng, 2012), which is repaired by cellular mechanisms within seconds (Deng, Sieling, Pan and Cui, 2004). Meijering *et al.,* (Meijering, Juffermans, van Wamel *et al.*, 2009) demonstrated that endocytosis plays a key role in UMTD of macromolecules sized between 4 and 500 kDa. Dextran molecules of 155 and 500 kDa were mainly localized in vesicle-like structures after UMTD are a result of macropinocytosis, clathrin-mediated and caveolin-mediated endocytosis. They also showed increased membrane permeability to extracellular ions is upregulated by endocytosis due to the calcium flux into the cell (Meijering, Juffermans, van Wamel *et al.*, 2009). The types of MB oscillations required to observe these effects have also been investigated. Inertially cavitating MBs near the cell membrane form 1 - 200 nm pores due to localized tensions (Zhou, Cui and Deng, 2008). These pores are capable of resealing bifunctionally by either rapid phospholipid rearrangement or gradual, exocytosis-mediated membrane tension changes, which restores membrane integrity (Fan, Liu, Mayer and Deng, 2012). Thus, US enhanced endocytosis is an important pathway for targeting drug delivery by UTMD (Sutton, Haworth, Pyne-Geithman and Holland, 2013).

6.5. Enhanced Permeability and Retention Effect

UCAs are typically used to study the vasculature in animals and humans. Thus employing them to study the aberrant tumor vasculature due to angiogenesis is a natural transition. For example, perfluoropentane filled silica nanoshells and microshells have been used to selectively image a tumor in a mouse ovarian tumor model (Ta, Liberman, Paul Martinez *et al.*, 2012). Tumor angiogenesis is characterized by branching vessels with irregular diameters ranging from 10 to 200μm (Li, 2000) and a lack of defining structures such as arterioles, capillaries, or venules (Wheatley and Lewandowski, 2010). Tumors induce angiogenesis to increase their nutrient and oxygen supply. The particular property of angiogenic vessels is that their rapid growth from established vessels renders them "leaky" and defective. According to Pasqualini *et al.,* (Pasqualini, Arap and McDonald, 2002) and Li *et al.,* (Li, 2000), the tumor microvasculature has a vascular pore cutoff size from as low as 380nm up to 780nm, and the endothelial cells are misaligned or have large fenestrations. This phenomenon which is generally referred to as the Enhanced Permeability and Retention (EPR) effect, can achieve high local concentrations of nano-encapsulated drugs at a tumor site (10- to 50-fold higher than in normal tissue) (Cavalieri, Zhou, Tortora, Lucilla and Ashokkumar, 2012). US exposure can enhance the size of these leaky vascular pores allowing for micron sized bubbles to collect at the tumor site. Then at the breast cancer (SK-BR-3) tumor site Zhao *et al.,* (Zhao, Luo, Lu *et al.*, 2008) with phospholipid MBs showed membrane pore diameter of 1-2μm with US exposure of 30 sec, diameter of 2-3μm with US exposure of 60 seconds and diameter of 3-5μm with US exposure greater than 60 seconds. Thus the EPR effect seen in tumors can be extremely beneficial in treating cancer.

Submicron bubbles could show higher intracellular uptake than microsized bubbles, allowing drug-release in different cellular compartments such as cytoplasm and nucleus (Cavalieri, Zhou, Tortora, Lucilla and Ashokkumar, 2012). The ability to synthesize nanobubbles has opened up further opportunities to deliver therapeutic agents which require targeted extravasation into the tissues as micrometer sized MBs are typically too large to exit the vasculature. A prerequisite for this process is that the nanocarrier stays in the blood long enough to slowly accumulate in the tissue of interest with affected and leaky vasculature (Cavalieri, Zhou, Tortora, Lucilla and Ashokkumar, 2012). Nanometer sized bubbles can potentially exhibit an improved circulating lifetime (Wheatley and Lewandowski, 2010). The radiation force generated by insonofication (Dayton, Klibanov, Brandenburger and Ferrara, 1999) with the medical ultrasonography equipment can force the nanobubbles or MBs towards pores in these vessels and induce penetration of nanobubbles or MBs through the pores. This results in a higher concentration of contrast in the tumor, a better visualization of the acoustic imaging and a targeted delivery of drug payload. In addition, the drug containing nanobubbles can be made slowly biodegradable, thus delivering their payload at a controlled rate (Cavalieri, Zhou, Tortora, Lucilla and Ashokkumar, 2012). These properties of the micro- or nano- bubbles make them an efficient drug delivery system for treating cancer. The most successful nano-bubble system consist of liquid paclitaxel loaded into perfluorocarbon emulsions that become echogenic when accumulated at the site of interest such as ovarian, breast and pancreatic cancer (Rapoport, Kennedy, Shea, Scaife and Nam, 2009, Wickline and Lanza, 2002).

7. USES OF MICROBUBBLES

Cavitation of MBs and its subsequent bio-effects on the vasculature and tissue cells shows the potential of using MBs as delivery vehicles. The chemical, physical and structural properties of the MBs also enhance the notion of using them to deliver therapeutic agents. Drugs can be incorporated into the MBs in a number of different ways, including binding of the drug to the MB shell and attachment of site-specific ligands (Fig. **16**). Drugs can also be imbedded in the membrane or loaded internally with the therapeutic agents and gas (Fig. **15**).

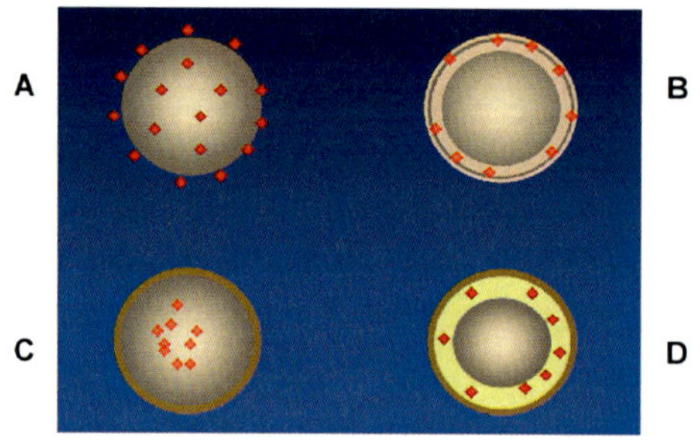

Figure 15: *Manipulation of the microbubble shell for gene and/or drug delivery.* (**A**) Drugs (red diamonds) may be attached to the surrounding microbubble membrane. (**B**) Materials may be imbedded in the membrane. (**C**) Bubbles may be loaded internally with the therapeutic agents and gas. (**D**) Hydrophobic drugs may be incorporated into an oily emulsion that forms a film around the bubble, which is then surrounded by a stabilizing membrane. (Reprinted from European Journal of Radiology, Vol 42, Unger, Matsunaga, McCreery *et al.*, Therapeutic applications of microbubbles, Pages No. 160-168, Copyright (2002), with permission from Elsevier (Unger, Matsunaga, McCreery *et al.*, 2002)).

Subsequently, hydrophobic drugs may be incorporated into an oily emulsion that forms a film around the bubble, which is then surrounded by a stabilizing membrane (Fig. **15**). Perfluorocarbon-filled MBs act as carriers of these agents until the site of interest is reached as they are sufficiently stable for circulating in the vasculature as blood pool agents (Tsutsui, Xie and Porter, 2004). Ultrasound applied over the skin surface can then be used to burst the MBs at this site, causing localized release of the drug (Chen, Shohet, Bekeredjian, Frenkel and Grayburn, 2003, Mukherjee, Wong, Griffin *et al.*, 2000, Shohet, Chen, Zhou *et al.*, 2000, Taniyama, Tachibana, Hiraoka *et al.*, 2002). This lowers the concentrations and reduces the systemic side effects of hazardous drugs like a cytotoxic agents thereby improving the therapeutic index (Tsutsui, Xie and Porter, 2004). Thus, there is an increasing interest in developing noninvasive delivery methods for gene therapy and chemotherapeutics.

7.1. Gene Therapy

Gene therapy shows promise for the treatment of several diseases. However clinical application has been hampered by the process of safe and efficient delivery systems to a site-specific tissue or organ (Koppelhus and Nielsen, 2003). Characterization of genetic diseases and understanding protein transcription has helped relatively little in delivering genetic material to cells for treatment (Liu, Miyoshi and Nakamura, 2006). Recently, UTMD has been proposed as a new technique for local delivery of drugs and genes to specific target tissues, including the heart (Marin, Sun, Husseini *et al.*, 2002). MBs can encapsulate the expressing viral and non-viral vectors until the site of transfection is reached (Fig. **16A**). Once the bubbles reach the specific site an US probe is used to burst the bubbles and distribute the material (Fig. **16C** & **D**). Thus, US can enhance transfection by causing transient non-lethal perforation of the capillary and cell membrane due to the cavitation effects which causes a ballistic effect that drives the MBs across the vessel wall into the target cell (Liu, Miyoshi and Nakamura, 2006). US is known to up-regulate several cell repair genes which also facilitate transfection (Kost, 1993). MB approach has shown to deliver to tissues following microvessel rupture (Fig. **16B**). Thus, US becomes a new effective and safe means for introducing genetic material into the target cells of tissues, thereby enhancing cellular uptake of the therapeutic compound (Stride and Saffari, 2003).

Non-viral gene delivery can be performed by the direct injection of naked DNA, antisense oligonucleotides such as siRNA and miRNA, *etc.* or with fore mentioned macromolecules encapsulated in plasmid vectors. However such an approach is generally associated with a low transfection efficiency and transient expression of the gene product (Calliada, Campani, Bottinelli, Bozzini and Sommaruga, 1998). For example, Azuma *et al.,* (Azuma, Tomita, Sakamoto *et al.*, 2008) used an oligodeoxynucleotide (ODN) decoy to inhibit the activity of a key tumorigenic transcription factor, nuclear factor-kappaB (NFκB), that is known to be associated with cancer progression, apoptotic resistance, cancer cell growth, metastasis and angiogenesis. Azuma *et al.,* (Azuma, Tomita, Sakamoto *et al.*, 2008) used US to induce sonoporation and increased the susceptibility of colon cancer that had metastasized to the liver to paclitaxel. Non-viral gene delivery offers an advantage as they elicit low immunogenic host response. Although there has been successful gene transfer with *in vitro* studies, the *in vivo* studies results have been uninspiring (Howard, 2004). The first *in vivo* study was published by Porter *et al.,* of targeted DNA delivery was performed in 1996, using surface US and intravenously delivered MBs carrying antisense oligonucleotides (Porter, Iversen, Li and Xie, 1996). In 1997, Bao *et al.,* (Bao, Thrall and Miller, 1997) described the use of 0.2MPa US exposure and albumin-coated MBs (Albunex) to enhance the transfection of luciferase reporter plasmid in cultured hamster cells. In subsequent years, Unger and co-workers (Unger, Hersh, Vannan and McCreery, 2001, Unger, Matsunaga, McCreery *et al.*, 2002) performed *in vivo* studies using marker genes that do not exert a therapeutic effect such as p-chloramphenicol acetyl transferase (CAT), beta-galactosidase (β-Gal), and green fluorescent protein (GFP). They prepared 2 μm cationic phospholipid-coated perfluorobutane MBs that bind to the CAT gene by gentle agitation of DNA. The MBs were administered through the peripheral vein and US was applied to the dogs heart using a 1 MHz transducer with a Sonos Model 5500 US system and an insonation energy level of 1.7MPa. CAT gene expression was assayed from the excised heart after 48hrs. The insonated region of the myocardium showed high CAT levels, but the region that was not exposed to US showed no CAT expression (Liu, Miyoshi and Nakamura, 2006). Thus, these reporter plasmids became the proof-of-principle for the use of MBs to enhance the transfection efficiency of gene therapy.

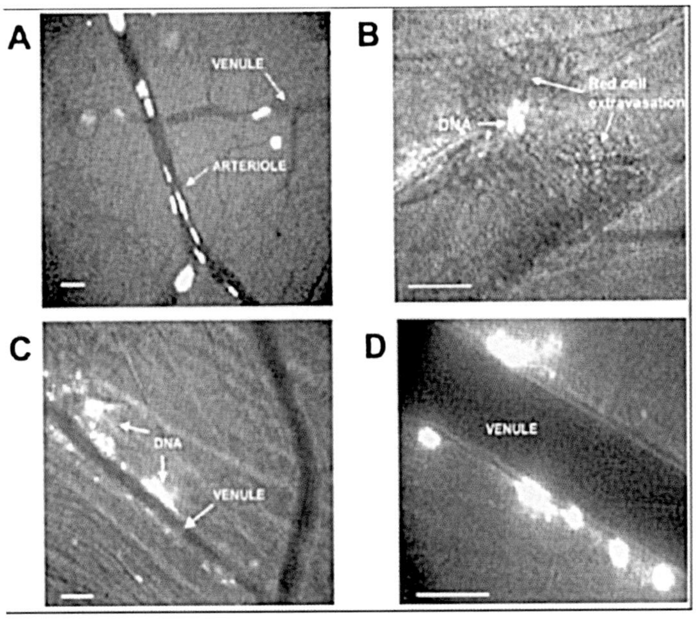

Figure 16: Intravital microscopy of the cremaster muscle in mice following intravascular injection of cationic microbubbles bearing YOYO-1-labeled plasmid. (**A**) Cremaster microcirculation 1 min after IV injection of microbubbles illustrating stable conjugation of plasmid to microbubbles during microvascular transit. All microbubbles in the field transited unimpeded. (**B**) Microvessel rupture and peri-vascular hemorrhage with fluorescent DNA deposition at a site of microbubble destruction. (**C,D**) Deposition of fluorescent plasmid DNA in the perivascular tissue of cremasteric venules following US-mediated destruction of microbubbles without vessel rupture. Scale bar - 20 μm. (Reprinted from Ultrasound in Medicine & Biology, Vol 29, Issue 12, Christiansen, French, Klibanov, Kaul and Lindner, Targeted tissue transfection with ultrasound destruction of plasmid-bearing cationic microbubbles, Pages No. 1759-1767, Copyright (2003), with permission from Elsevier (Christiansen, French, Klibanov, Kaul and Lindner, 2003)).

Liu *et al.,* (Liu, 2005, Liu, Yang and Sakanishi, 2006) and colleagues demonstrated the successful introduction of beta-galactosidase (β-Gal) gene into HeLa-S3, C-127 & NIH/3T3 mammalian cells by US exposure with different percent duty cycles. They subsequently showed 6-fold enhancement of β-Gal transfection by Levovist MBs in vascular smooth muscle cells (VSMCs) than the control. These results were found comparable to transfections of β-Gal by Albunex and Optison MBs in the same mammalian cells. Similar increase in transfection efficiency has been shown in the study where UTMD of albumin coated MBs containing DNA, significantly increased the gene expression in human embryonic kidney (HEK) cells (Frenkel, Chen, Thai, Shohet and Grayburn, 2002). Thus, sonoporation is efficient in facilitating gene transfer. This was further confirmed by Feril *et al.,* (Feril, Ogawa, Tachibana and Kondo, 2006) who showed that sonoporation of HeLa cells led to 19 fold increase in luciferase gene expression in comparison to electroporation. Sonoporation translates well *in vivo* studies where Anwer *et al.,* (Anwer, Kao, Proctor *et al.*, 2000) demonstrated enhancement of cationic lipid-mediated gene transfer into primary lung cancer tumors following systemic administration. His studies on plasmid quantitation and fluorescence microscopy showed that US increased tumor uptake of the plasmid and that uptake was limited to the tumor vasculature. Thus, allowing for a site-specific delivery. Similarly, Taniyama *et al.,* (Taniyama, Tachibana, Hiraoka *et al.*, 2002) have also shown an effective transfection of a luciferase and wt-p53 plasmid DNA to endothelial and vascular smooth muscle cells with albumin-coated MBs (Optison) and US in a balloon injury model for gene therapy of restenosis with significant increase in the p53 protein. The successful transfection of p53 plasmid by this method should be useful for safe clinical gene therapy without a viral vector system. Concern about the functional integrity of the transfected endothelial cell layer after US treatment was negated by Teupe *et al.,* (Teupe, Richter, Fisslthaler *et al.*, 2002) who showed efficient transfer of plasmids encoding either β-Gal or endothelial nitric oxide synthase to the endothelial cells of conductance arteries while preserving its functionality.

Viral vectors such as retroviruses, lentiviruses, adenoviruses (Ads), *etc.* can significantly increase the efficacy of transfection. The viral machinery has evolved significantly over the last decade that has allowed for the introduction of foreign DNA into mammalian cells. However, viral proteins elicit an immune response within the targeted host/tissue (Anderson, 1998) and known to cause an intense inflammatory activation of endothelial cells (Newman, Dunn, Owens *et al.*, 1995). Yet transfection by the viral vectors has relegated its use to only intratumoral injections which has limited its dosage and potential in humans. A recent study showed that transfection of a reporter gene, beta-galactosidase (β-Gal), in a mouse heart model was increased 10-fold using MBs loaded with an adenovirus gene vector (Shohet, Chen, Zhou *et al.*, 2000). They also showed that intravenously injected recombinant Ad vectors encoding a β-Gal reporter gene were successful in delivering to normal rat myocardium using MBs and transthoracic 1.3 MHz diagnostic US, at a mechanical index of 1.5, delivered at a burst of 3 frames of ultrasound every 4 to 6 cardiac cycles (Tsutsui, Xie and Porter, 2004). This protection allows us to use intravenous injection rather than direct target organ delivery by catheter-based approaches (Beeri, Guerrero, Supple *et al.*, 2002).

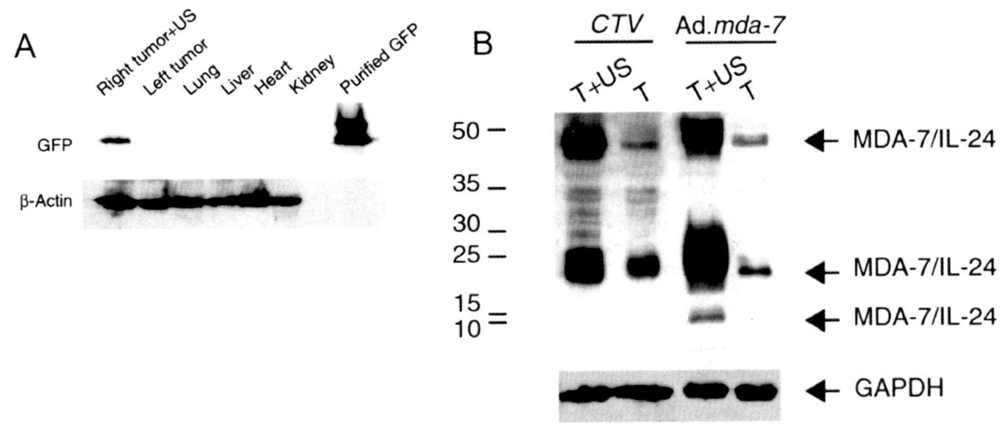

Figure 17: (**A**) *Western blot analysis of Ad-GFP/microbubble–transduced DU-145 tumor xenografts.* Immunoblot showing the expression levels of green fluorescent protein (GFP) in DU-145 cells following ultrasound-targeted microbubble/Ad transduction of GFP at 96 hours. Only the tumor on the right flank was sonoporated for 10 minutes resulting in the delivery and expression of GFP. The left tumor, heart, lung, liver, and kidney were negative for GFP expression. Purified glutathione-S-transferase–GFP was used as a positive control. Protein gel loading was normalized using β-actin as a control. (**B**) Western blot analysis of protein extracts from representative DU-145 tumor samples treated with Ad.mda-7 or CTV. The immunoblot was reacted with anti-MDA-7/IL-24. Arrowheads point at the various glycosylated forms of MDA-7/IL-24. Protein gel loading was normalized using anti-GAPDH as a control. (Reprinted by permission from Macmillan Publishers Ltd: Molecular Therapy, (Greco, Di Benedetto, Howard *et al.*, 2010), copyright (2010)).

Adenoviruses (Ads) can be bound to the surface of various MBs or internalize due to the perfluorocarbon gas that acts as an osmotic agent. Our lab previously (Howard, Forsberg, Minimo *et al.*, 2006) demonstrated that Ad bound to the MB surface can still elicit a immune response or shed intravenously due to shear flow. This would lead to unspecific binding and result in unspecific transfection which is an undesirable trait. To avoid this trait, Howard *et al.,* (Howard, Forsberg, Minimo *et al.*, 2006) used fetal bovine serum (FBS) or complement fraction to inactivate and wash the bound Ad particles from the MB surface resulting in a clean bubble with only active Ads inside the MBs. This process protects the viruses from rapid degradation by the immune system and stops the indiscriminant binding of Ads to other cell surfaces. Our *in vivo* studies demonstrated a site specific enhanced Ad transfection of GFP (Fig. **17A**) and melanoma differentiation–associated gene 7/interleukin-24 (mda-7/IL-24) (Fig. **17B**) in a DU-145 prostate tumor xenograft flank model (Greco, Di Benedetto, Howard *et al.*, 2010).

In our study, we used Targeson CAs reconstituted with either Ad.GFP, Ad.mda7 or CTV (cancer terminator virus) Mda7 that were cleaned, injected in the tail vein of nude mice xenografted with the DU-145 prostate cancer cell line and exposed to a 0.7 MI, 1.8 MPa US for 10 minutes only on the right flank tumor with a Micro-Maxx SonoSite (SonoSite) US machine equipped with the transducer L25. Thus, only the right tumor flank that was sonoporated released the Ads from the Targeson MBs allowing for a site specific delivery. This specificity is clearly observed from the western blot studies in Fig. **17A** & **B**. In our study, you can also observe in the B-mode US imaging of DU-145 tumor xenografts treated with MB/US-guided Ad.mda-7 and therapy resistant DU-Bcl-xL tumor xenografts that were treated with MB/US-guided cancer terminator virus (CTV) (Fig. **18**) a reduction of volume of the tumors after 2 and 4 weeks of treatments with Ad or CTV/MB complexes and US (Greco, Di Benedetto, Howard *et al.*, 2010).

We also studied the transfection efficiency and measured the tumor volume reduction of intravenously (IV) delivered MBs complexed with Ad.p53, Ad.RB and Ad.p130 *versus* intratumorally (IT) delivered Ads to sonoporated tumors in combination with external beam radiation (Nande, Greco, Gossman *et al.*, 2013). We observed the highest uptake of Ads and highest transgene expression in tumors that were sonoporated and irradiated. Additionally, we observed a better reduction of tumor volume in tumors that were sonoporated, irradiated and transduced with MBs complexed with Ad.p53 and Ad.RB delivered intravenously (Nande, Greco, Gossman *et al.*, 2013).

A disadvantage of using intratumoral injections is that the viral particles are collected in the injection tract. Thus, Ads only transfect the cells that surround the

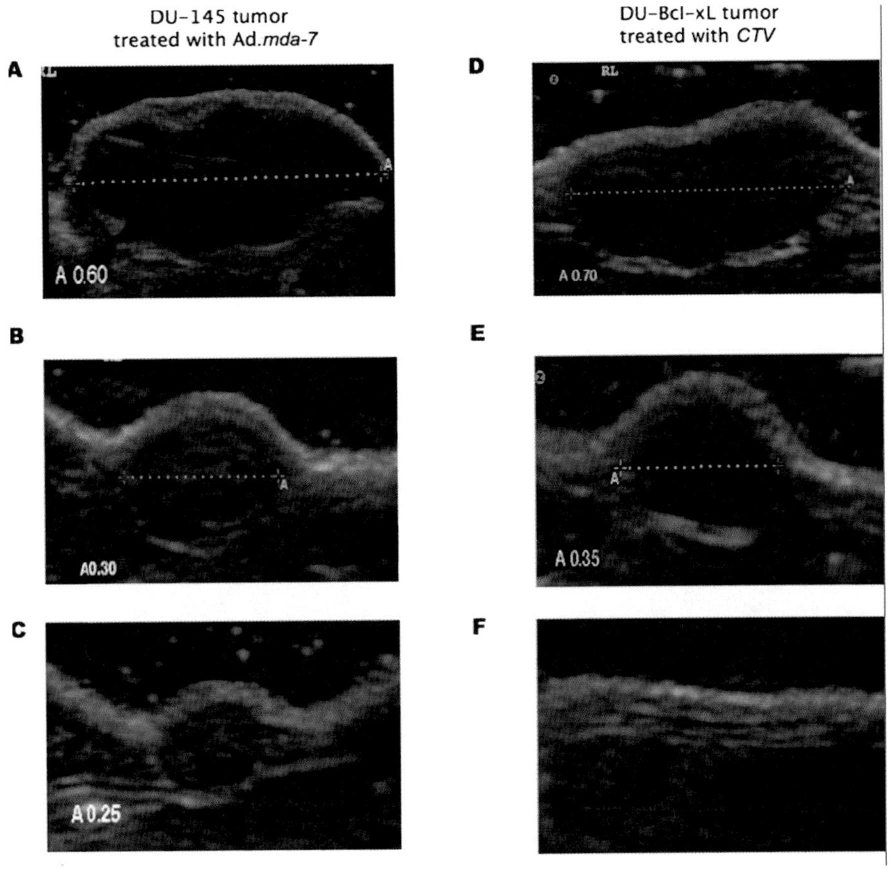

Figure 18: B-mode ultrasound (US) imaging of DU-145 tumor xenografts treated with microbubble/US-guided Ad.mda-7 and therapy resistant DU-Bcl-xL tumor xenografts treated with microbubble/US-guided cancer terminator virus (CTV). Subcutaneous tumor xenografts from DU-145 and DU-Bcl-xL cells were established in athymic nude mice in both right and left flanks and only tumors on the right side were sonoporated following tail-vein injection of the indicated microbubble/Ad complexes during a course of 4 weeks. Tumor volumes were determined by measuring twice a week the tumors with either a caliper or by US measurements of the tumor axes. (**a**) Ultrasound image and measurement of a DU-145 tumor before treatment with Ad.mda-7/microbubble complexes and US. (**b**) US image and measurement of the same DU-145 tumor 2 weeks following treatments with Ad.mda-7/microbubble complexes and US. (**c**) US image and measurement of the same DU-145 tumor 4 weeks following treatments with Ad.mda-7/microbubble complexes and US. (**d**) US image and measurement of a DU-Bcl-xL tumor before treatment with CTV/microbubble complexes and US. (**e**) US image and measurement of the same DU-Bcl-xL tumor 2 weeks following treatments with the CTV/microbubble complexes and US. (**f**) US image and measurement of the same DU-Bcl-xL tumor 4 weeks following treatments with CTV/microbubble complexes and US. Complete eradication of the DU-Bcl-xL tumor occurs 4 weeks after initiating the therapeutic treatment protocol. Ad, adenovirus; GFP, green fluorescent protein. (Reprinted by permission from Macmillan Publishers Ltd: Molecular Therapy, (Greco, Di Benedetto, Howard *et al.*, 2010), copyright (2010)).

injection tract while the remaining ads are exposed to both the cellular and humoral immune responses shortening the life span of transgene expression. Ads are either neutralized by anti-Ad neutralizing antibodies or eliminated by sequestering in macrophages, dendritic and Kupffer cells. Thus, MBs can hide the away the ads until the point of delivery, as well as, make use of the vasculature that surrounds the tumor to deliver drugs to the entire tumor site. MBs may also limit the amount of inflammatory response to the viruses and may allow repeated injections (Howard, 2004).

All forementioned studies show that US in combination with MBs could be feasible for a non-invasive control of drug deposition at specific target sites in the body. A strategy such as viral vector gene therapy has been limited due to the host immune response which is circumvented by UTMD. There exist possibilities to improve the potential of gene therapy by combining it with US mediated destruction.

7.2. Chemotherapy

Current strategies to treat cancer involve surgery, radiation and chemotherapy. Chemotherapeutic strategies to treat cancer have many deleterious side-effects on the human body. MBs-US assisted delivery of chemo-drugs to tumors represents one clever approach for enhancing the limited transport of drugs within solid tumors (Cavalieri, Zhou and Ashokkumar, 2010). There exists different ways in which MBs can be used as chemo-drug carriers. Four concepts have been outlined by Mayer *et al.,* (Mayer, Geis, Katus and Bekeredjian, 2008) in which MBs have primarily been used to combine chemotherapeutics: i) Drugs and MBs are co-administred (Iwanaga, Tominaga, Yamamoto *et al.*, 2007, Price, Skyba, Kaul and Skalak, 1998, Song, Chappell, Qi *et al.*, 2002, Treat, McDannold, Vykhodtseva *et al.*, 2007); ii) Modified Lipid shelled MBs are loaded with a drug (Fang, Hung, Liao and Chien, 2007, Ho, Barbarese, D'Arrigo, Smith-Slatas and Simon, 1997, May, Allen and Ferrara, 2002, Shortencarier, Dayton, Bloch *et al.*, 2004, Tartis, McCallan, Lum *et al.*, 2006, Unger, McCreery, Sweitzer, Caldwell and Wu, 1998); iii) MBs are linked to drug-loaded lipospheres (Kheirolomoom, Dayton, Lum *et al.*, 2007); and iv) drugs are incorporated inside the non-permeable shell of a biodegradable polymer (*e.g.* nano-emulsions) (Gao, Fain and

Rapoport, 2004, Gao, Kennedy, Christensen and Rapoport, 2008, Rapoport, Gao and Kennedy, 2007, Shive and Anderson, 1997). It is thought that pulsed high-intensity focused ultrasound (HIFU) energy disrupts tumor vessel endothelial cell barriers, and this disruption improves vascular permeability. HIFU also reduces hydrostatic pressures in tissues which enhances diffusion of drugs through the interstitium (Yuh, Shulman, Mehta *et al.*, 2005). These effects are summarized in Fig. **19**.

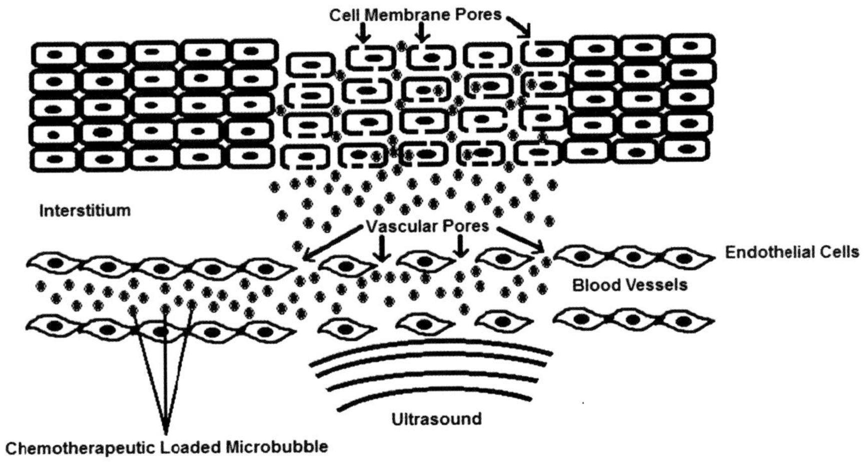

Figure 19: Chemotherapeutic agents can be packaged in microbubbles and delivered through the vaculature. Ultrasound causes pore formation in the endothelial lining of the blood vessel thereby inceasing the permeability. This leads to the extravasation of the therapeutic agent and microbubbles into the interstitium. Ultrasound leads to the cavitation of the microbubbles which results in the release of the chemotherapeutic agent into the targeted region.

The widespread use of chemotherapeutic drugs for brain tumors has been limited because they have limited success in crossing the blood brain barrier (BBB) (Cavalieri, Zhou and Ashokkumar, 2010). Doxorubicin (DOX) has shown to be critical for central nervous system (CNS) cancers but the BBB often prevents cytotoxic levels to be achieved in the brain (Treat, McDannold, Vykhodtseva *et al.*, 2007). Treat *et al.,* (Treat, McDannold, Vykhodtseva *et al.*, 2007) showed that the co-administration of DOX and Optison MBs delivered through the BBB achieved DOX concentrations of 886 +/- 327 ng/g tissue in the brain with minimal tissue effects. These results suggest that despite previous accessibility limitations, targeted delivery by focused ultrasound may render DOX chemotherapy a viable treatment option against CNS tumors (Treat, McDannold, Vykhodtseva *et al.*, 2007). The transient increase in the vascular permeability was investigated with Evans Blue by UTMD for small molecules in hepatoma liver cancer model (Bekeredjian, Kroll, Fein *et al.*, 2007) and for large 8.5-nm diameter fluorescein isothiocyanate-labelled dextran molecules evaluated in the vasculature of a chick CAM model (Stieger, Caskey, Adamson *et al.*, 2007). Thus, an increased intracellular uptake of the drugs can be ascribed to the sonoporation of the cell membranes (Cavalieri, Zhou, Tortora, Lucilla and Ashokkumar, 2012).

The commercially available contrast agent, Sonovue, was used to reduce the LD_{50} of camptothecin on HeLa cells by 70% when co-administered and irradiated with ultrasound of 1 MHz and 270 J/cm^2 (Li, Reid and McHale, 2008). Sonoda *et al.*, co-injected bleomycin (BLM) with Optison MBs in two mouse tumor models. The combination of BLM and US alone could reduce the dose for tumor regression to 0.5 mg/ml and with the addition of MBs to 0.06 mg/ml in a murine eyelid B-16 melanoma tumor model (Mayer, Geis, Katus and Bekeredjian, 2008). These results show that US and MB promote efficient bleomycin uptake by cells (Sonoda, Tachibana, Uchino *et al.*, 2007). Additionally, a complete regression of gingival squamous carcinoma cell (Ca9-22) tumors was achieved by Iwanaga *et al.,* in nude KSN/slc mice treated with low dosage of BLM and sonoporation (Iwanaga, Tominaga, Yamamoto *et al.*, 2007). Thus, MBs have reduced the drug dosage required to elicit tumor reduction. The drop in drug concentration may be beneficial in reducing the side-effects on the human body.

The first studies with drug-loaded MBs were made by Unger *et al.,* with Paclitaxel, a hydrophobic drug with a strong mitosis-inhibiting effect (Mayer, Geis, Katus and Bekeredjian, 2008). Unger and coworkers at the ImaRx Corporation developed an acoustically active liposphere (AALs) agent known as MRX-552 that is a soybean oil-filled phospholipid MBs with a thick fluid shell (~500 nm) loaded with paclitaxel which were tested for cytotoxicity with HeLa cells and for toxicity in mice (Liu, Miyoshi and Nakamura, 2006, Unger, McCreery, Sweitzer, Caldwell and Wu, 1998). This thick shell permits a relatively large payload of drugs to be carried compared to previous thin-shell designs or the nongaseous nanoparticle delivery systems (Liu, Miyoshi and Nakamura, 2006). These results showed a 100-fold lower toxicity in mice with a comparable cytotoxic effect in HeLa cells compared to free paclitaxel (Unger, McCreery, Sweitzer, Caldwell and Wu, 1998). Additionally, US assisted release of drugs can be addressed to the forces associated with the cavitation of MBs (Cavalieri, Zhou, Tortora, Lucilla and Ashokkumar, 2012). Similarly, different non-aqueous soluble cancer drugs such as resveratrol (Fang, Hung, Liao and Chien, 2007) can be suspended in different oils (*e.g.* coconut or soybean) to form AALs that can be used to deliver cancer toxic drugs systemically to a tumor site with US, proving MBs to be very versatile.

In order to improve the intracellular delivery and extravasation of drugs, a synergistic effect can be obtained by the co-injection of drug-loaded liposomes and MBs. However, co-injection of drug loaded liposomes and MBs can induce extravasation and accumulation of drug in undesired tissue, thus resulting in a severe drawback. This effect could be overcome by coupling liposomes to MBs (Cavalieri, Zhou, Tortora, Lucilla and Ashokkumar, 2012). In a recent work, Lentacker *et al.,* (Lentacker, Geers, Demeester, De Smedt and Sanders, 2010) prepared "doxorubicin (DOX)-loaded MBs" through the avidin-biotin binding of DOX containing liposomes attached onto the lipid shell of MBs. They observed that compared to DOX-liposomes, DOX-loaded MBs eradicated at least two times more melanoma cells (Lentacker, Geers, Demeester, De Smedt and Sanders, 2010) while DOX-liposomes-MBs were by far more toxic to the cells after US application than DOX-liposomes or DOX-loaded MBs (Cavalieri, Zhou, Tortora, Lucilla and Ashokkumar, 2012). DOX-liposome-MBs delivered DOX almost exclusively to the nuclei when melanoma cells were treated with US while DOX was found in the cytoplasm and the nucleus of melanoma cells treated with DOX-liposomes (Lentacker, Geers, Demeester, De Smedt and Sanders, 2010). According to the authors, exposure to US freed DOX from the DOX-liposome-MBs which enters the cells and accumulates in the nucleus because of its high affinity for DNA. Ultrasound also increases the amount of free DOX and DOX-liposomes that enters the cells through the pores formed on the membrane (Lentacker, Geers, Demeester, De Smedt and Sanders, 2010). Also, DOX-liposome-MBs may show lower side effects than free DOX. The micron-sized

DOX-liposome-MBs should stay intact without releasing its contents from the DOX liposome so that there is no extravasation of free DOX into normal tissue. MB cavitation and implosion in the tumor microvasculature may perforate endothelial cells and enhance the extravasation of the released DOX (Cavalieri, Zhou, Tortora, Lucilla and Ashokkumar, 2012).

The avidin-biotin link is immunogenic in nature thus limiting the fore mentioned benefits of DOX-liposome-MBs. To circumvent this main issue the link was made from functionalized (SPDP-) PEG-lipid by Lentacker, Geers and colleagues. DPPC and DSPE-PEG-SPDP were dissolved in glycerine-propyleneglycol-water solvent with perfluorobutane gas (Geers, Lentacker, Cool *et al.*, 2010). The Capmix™ (capsule mixing device) disperses the lipophilic perfluorobutane in the lipid solution forming gas bubbles. DOX-liposomes made from DSPE-PEG-MALEIMIDE were added to a mixture of lipids. The two mixture spontaneously formed DOX-liposome-loaded-MBs (Geers, Lentacker, Sanders *et al.*, 2011). The above mentioned authors showed that liposome-loaded-MBs remained bound to the bubbles after injection into the bloodstream till they were exposed to US (Cavalieri, Zhou, Tortora, Lucilla and Ashokkumar, 2012). DOX-liposome-MBs were clearly more cytotoxic and caused significant tumor cell death when US was applied in comparison to the same concentration of free DOX (Geers, Lentacker, Sanders *et al.*, 2011). These results clearly showed that smaller concentration of chemotherapeutic agent is required for observing significant tumor reduction when used in combination with MBs and US.

Lastly, US-induced transformation of perfluorocarbon liquids (nanodroplets/ nanoemulsion) to gases is of interest in the area of drug and gene delivery. Experimental data by Singh *et al.,* (Singh, Husseini and Pitt, 2012) showed that low frequencies were more effective in forming and collapsing a bubble from nanoemulsions. The nanoemulsions are composed of nanodroplets that are surrounded by a viscous extracellular matrix which extravasate into tumor tissue and vaporized in response to US irradiation (Rapoport, Kennedy, Shea, Scaife and Nam, 2009). There is an inverse relationship that exist between the size of the emulsion droplet and the US intensity required for bubble formation (Singh, Husseini and Pitt, 2012). Perfluoropentane (PFP) nanoemulsions are converted into MBs under heating to hyperthermia conditions or US irradiation (Rapoport, Kennedy, Shea, Scaife and

Nam, 2009). Singh *et al.,* further showed that perfluorohexane emulsions require greater intensity to form cavitating bubbles than perfluoropentane emulsions (Singh, Husseini and Pitt, 2012). Nano-emulsions can be loaded with different anti-cancer drugs such as dacarbazine (DAC) (Tagne, Kakumanu and Nicolosi, 2008), camptothecin (Han, He, Fang *et al.*, 2009), paclitaxel (Rapoport, Kennedy, Shea, Scaife and Nam, 2009) and resveratrol (Hung, Chen, Liao, Lo and Fang, 2006). Drugs such as doxorubicin or PTX are tightly retained by the nanodroplets or MBs *in vivo* but is released under the action of US and effectively internalized by tumor cells. The accumulation of the nanoemulsions in tumor cells can be confirmed by US imaging (Rapoport, Kennedy, Shea, Scaife and Nam, 2009). Intramuscular (IM) injections of nanoemulsions of DAC have showed 5-fold greater efficacies in preventing melanoma tumor growth in mice (Tagne, Kakumanu and Nicolosi, 2008). Paclitaxel-loaded nanoemulsions systemically injected into animals and converted into MBs locally in ovarian, breast, and pancreatic tumors under the action US. A dramatic regression of ovarian, breast, and pancreatic tumors was observed in tumor therapy through US-triggered drug release from tumor accumulated nanobubbles. The US intensity (1-MHz CW, nominal output power density 3.4 W/cm2, exposure duration 1 min 30sec) used in this study suppressed tumor metastasis (Cavalieri, Zhou and Ashokkumar, 2010, Rapoport, Kennedy, Shea, Scaife and Nam, 2009). Similarly, low concentration of camptothecin nanoemulsions suspended in oil exhibited cytotoxicity against melanomas and ovarian cancer cells (Fang, Hung, Hua and Hwang, 2009). 10-methoxy-9-nitrocamptothecin (MONCPT) nanoemulsion exhibited an improved solubility, stability and antitumor activity, providing a promising carrier for cancer chemotherapy agent (Han, He, Fang *et al.*, 2009).

In recent years, the use of chemotherapeutic agents have advanced significantly because of ultrasound assisted MBs. In fact it has been shown that chemo-drugs can be delivered at lower doses which lower the potential side-effects seen in humans. However, the delivery of chemo-drugs at lower concentrations doesn't decrease their antineoplastic efficiency that is they still elicit tumor volume reduction.

8. CONCLUSIONS

In the above chapter, our goal was to emphasize the potential of site-specific therapeutics to cancer treatment. US is a real-time imaging modality that enables monitoring the delivery of drugs *in vivo*. US has shown promise in transiently compromising the tight junctions and inter-endothelial clefts of the membrane such as the BBB that lines the vasculature. This increases the permeability of the endothelial cells to allow the extravasation of high molecular weight drugs into the target tissue. *Trans*-cranial delivery of US has limited its use in dealing with diseases of the brain. But, high frequency ultrasound (HIFU) has changed those dynamics allowing scientists to focus US even with the distortion caused by the skull. By transiently altering the microvasculature of any tissue one can target nearly any US accessible organ to deliver drugs, proteins, nucleotides, inhibitory oligonucleotides and viruses. Thus a wide range of interdisciplinary studies can be developed by combining current therapies with US.

MBs use in ultrasonography has evolved from diagnostic to therapeutic purposes. They have been beneficial in studying the vasculature of the human body. The bubbles are filled with different gases (air or perfluorocarbon) and stabilized with different shells or surfactants such as proteins, lipids or polymers that enable MBs to circulate longer in the vasculature. Typically, the sizes of the bubbles range from 1-10μm but with better understanding and emerging controlled manufacturing methods the MBs size can be further reduced to the nanoscale while maintaining a more uniform bubble size distribution. The surfactant also offers several advantages such as specific targeting by means of ligand attachment to several receptors, antibodies and other drugs. Additionally, several types of cavitation of the MBs have been described and observed *in vitro* and *in vivo* along with the acoustic frequencies that drive these reactions. The cavitation effect that is brought about by the interaction of the MBs and US has been shown to elicit different bio-effects on the endothelial layer. Cavitation is known to cause transient, reversible, mechanical pore and channel formations on the endothelial cells and the neighboring cell membranes allowing for the extravasation of drugs that are loaded onto the MBs into the interstitial layer or the cytoplasm of the cells. Also, hydrophobic drugs can be loaded into the oil layer of the MBs thereby making systemic delivery a possibility. These characteristics of MBs make them strong delivery agents that can protect toxic agents (such as viruses and chemo-drugs) from the immune system resulting in reduced systemic toxicity otherwise seen by these drugs. Therefore, MBs and US could potentially enhance therapeutic efficiency for targeted delivery of clinically approved/disapproved chemo-, immuno- and gene therapies (Deelman, Decleves, Rychak and Sharma, 2010).

However, the use of US and MBs is still in its infancy. In fact, the proof of principle has been limited to several rodent models while there are too few large animal studies. Additionally, the flexibility of the endothelial layer in the vasculature differs greatly between species which may be a problem. The role of US in triggering endocytosis of drugs is still under investigation. It is also necessary to figure out MBs optimal drug loading and delivering strategies without losing its acoustic behavior. There is also a need for the production of different transducers and supporting equipment before its application in humans. The uses of other theranostic agents such as sono-sensitizing chemicals that render the target cell or tissue hypersentivity to relative low intensity US haven't been studied. Also, toxicity of polymer shells or nanoparticles and its degradation still have to be studied in detail, and nanoemulsions that can be loaded with different chemotherapeutic drugs like paclitaxel are still newcomers in this field. Thus, there are several questions that need to be answered by clinicians and scientists before MBs and US can be made available as a drug delivery system. However, this non-invasive strategy for US triggered release of drugs could become in the near future applied to various other diseases beyond cancer as a delivery system for inflammation, pain, wound healing, hormones, *etc.* Thus, a bright future research road is paved ahead to determine the potential applications in medicine of this new theranostic technology.

ACKNOWLEDGEMENTS

We gratefully acknowledge the Marshall University Biochemistry and Microbiology, Surgery, and Oncological Sciences Departments for their support. The present studies were supported by the NASA WV Space Grant Consortium, award #NNX10AK62H, and in part by NIH grants CA131395, CA140024, and WV-INBRE 5P20RR016477. The funders had no role in study design, data collection and analysis, decision to publish, or preparation of the manuscript. The content is solely the responsibility of the authors and does not necessarily represent the official views of the National Cancer Institute or the National Institute of Health.

CONFLICT OF INTEREST

The authors confirm that this chapter content has no conflict of interest.

REFERENCES

Aaronson D.S., Horvath C.M. 2002. A road map for those who don't know JAK-STAT. *Science*, 296, 1653-5.

Ahonen T.J., Harkonen P.L., Laine J., *et al.,* 1999. Prolactin is a survival factor for androgen-deprived rat dorsal and lateral prostate epithelium in organ culture. *Endocrinology*, 140, 5412-21.

Ahonen T.J., Harkonen P.L., Rui H., Nevalainen M.T. 2002. PRL signal transduction in the epithelial compartment of rat prostate maintained as long-term organ cultures *in vitro*. *Endocrinology*, 143, 228-38.

Ahonen T.J., Xie J., LeBaron M.J., *et al.,* 2003. Inhibition of transcription factor Stat5 induces cell death of human prostate cancer cells. *J Biol Chem*, 278, 27287-92.

Alexander W.S., Hilton D.J. 2004. The role of suppressors of cytokine signaling (SOCS) proteins in regulation of the immune response. *Annu Rev Immunol*, 22, 503-29.

Alfano C.M., Imayama I., Neuhouser M.L., *et al.,* 2012. Fatigue, inflammation, and omega-3 and omega-6 fatty acid intake among breast cancer survivors. *J Clin Oncol*, 30, 1280-7.

Alfranca A., Iniguez M.A., Fresno M., Redondo J.M. 2006. Prostanoid signal transduction and gene expression in the endothelium: role in cardiovascular diseases. *Cardiovasc Res*, 70, 446-56.

Alkan-Onyuksel H., Demos S.M., Lanza G.M., *et al.,* 1996. Development of inherently echogenic liposomes as an ultrasonic contrast agent. *J Pharm Sci*, 85, 486-90.

Allen J.S., May D.J., Ferrara K.W. 2002. Dynamics of therapeutic ultrasound contrast agents. *Ultrasound Med Biol*, 28, 805-16.

Alzaraa A., Gravante G., Chung W.Y., *et al.,* 2012. Targeted microbubbles in the experimental and clinical setting. *Am J Surg*, 204, 355-66.

Anderson H.A., Chen Y., Norkin L.C. 1996. Bound simian virus 40 translocates to caveolin-enriched membrane domains, and its entry is inhibited by drugs that selectively disrupt caveolae. *Mol Biol Cell*, 7, 1825-34.

Anderson R.G.W. 1998. The caveolae membrane system. *Ann Rev Biochem*, 67, 199-225.

Anderson R.G.W., Kamen B.A., Rothberg K.G., Lacey S.W. 1992. Potocytosis: sequestration and transport of small molecules by caveolae. *Science*, 255, 410-1.

Anderson W.F. 1998. Human gene therapy. *Nature*, 392, 25-30.

Anwer K., Kao G., Proctor B., *et al.,* 2000. Ultrasound enhancement of cationic lipid-mediated gene transfer to primary tumors following systemic administration. *Gene Ther*, 7, 1833-9.

Arnold C., Konkel A., Fischer R., Schunck W.H. 2010. Cytochrome P450-dependent metabolism of omega-6 and omega-3 long-chain polyunsaturated fatty acids. *Pharmacol Rep*, 62, 536-47.

Arterburn L.M., Hall E.B., Oken H. 2006. Distribution, interconversion, and dose response of n-3 fatty acids in humans. *Am J Clin Nutr*, 83, 1467S-76S.

Aubry J.F., Tanter M., Pernot M., Thomas J.L., Fink M. 2003. Experimental demonstration of noninvasive transskull adaptive focusing based on prior computed tomography scans. *J Acoust Soc Am*, 113, 84-93.

Ayala G.E., Dai H., Tahir S.A., *et al.,* 2006. Stromal antiapoptotic paracrine loop in perineural invasion of prostatic carcinoma. *Cancer Res*, 66, 5159-64.

Azmin M., Harfield C., Ahmad Z., Edirisinghe M., Stride E. 2012. How do microbubbles and ultrasound interact? Basic physical, dynamic and engineering principles. *Curr Pharm Des*, 18, 2118-34.

Azuma H., Tomita N., Sakamoto T., *et al.,* 2008. Marked regression of liver metastasis by combined therapy of ultrasound-mediated NF kappaB-decoy transfer and transportal injection of paclitaxel, in mouse. *Int J Cancer*, 122, 1645-56.

Babitt J., Trigatti B., Rigotti A., *et al.,* 1997. Murine SR-BI, a high density lipoprotein receptor that mediates selective lipid uptake, is N-glycosylated and fatty acylated and colocalizes with plasma membrane caveolae. *J Biol Chem*, 272, 13242-9.

Balkwill F., Coussens L.M. 2004. Cancer: an inflammatory link. *Nature*, 431, 405-6.

Bao S., Thrall B.D., Miller D.L. 1997. Transfection of a reporter plasmid into cultured cells by sonoporation *in vitro*. *Ultrasound Med Biol*, 23, 953-9.

Barahmand-pour F., Meinke A., Eilers A., *et al.,* 1995. Colony-stimulating factors and interferon-gamma activate a protein related to MGF-Stat 5 to cause formation of the differentiation-induced factor in myeloid cells. *FEBS Lett*, 360, 29-33.

Barnes N., Haywood P., Flint P., Knox W.F., Bundred N.J. 2006. Survivin expression in *in situ* and invasive breast cancer relates to COX-2 expression and DCIS recurrence. *Br J Cancer*, 94, 253-8.

Barry B. Goldberg J.S.R. Ultrasound Contrast Agents: Basic Principles and Clinical Applications United Kindom: Martin Dunitz Ltd; 2001.

Baselga J. 2000. Clinical trials of single-agent trastuzumab (Herceptin). *Semin Oncol*, 27, 20-6.

Becker S., Groner B., Muller C.W. 1998. Three-dimensional structure of the Stat3beta homodimer bound to DNA. *Nature*, 394, 145-51.

Beeri R., Guerrero J.L., Supple G., *et al.,* 2002. New efficient catheter-based system for myocardial gene delivery. *Circulation*, 106, 1756-9.

Begin M.E., Ells G., Horrobin D.F. 1988. Polyunsaturated fatty acid-induced cytotoxicity against tumor cells and its relationship to lipid peroxidation. *J Natl Cancer Inst*, 80, 188-94.

Bekeredjian R., Kroll R.D., Fein E., *et al.,* 2007. Ultrasound targeted microbubble destruction increases capillary permeability in hepatomas. *Ultrasound Med Biol*, 33, 1592-8.

Bender F.C., Reymond M.A., Bron C., Quest A.F. 2000. Caveolin-1 levels are down-regulated in human colon tumors, and ectopic expression of caveolin-1 in colon carcinoma cell lines reduces cell tumorigenicity. *Cancer Res*, 60, 5870-8.

Bennett N., Hooper J.D., Lee C.S., Gobe G.C. 2009. Androgen receptor and caveolin-1 in prostate cancer. *IUBMB Life*, 61, 961-70.

Beuvink I., Hess D., Flotow H., *et al.,* 2000. Stat5a serine phosphorylation. Serine 779 is constitutively phosphorylated in the mammary gland, and serine 725 phosphorylation influences prolactin-stimulated *in vitro* DNA binding activity. *J Biol Chem*, 275, 10247-55.

Bloch S.H., Wan, M., Dayton P.A., Ferrara, K.W. 2004. Optical observation of lipid- and polymer-shelled ultrasound microbubble contrast agents. *Applied Physics Letters*, 84, 631-3.

Blomley M., Claudon M., Cosgrove D. 2007. WFUMB Safety Symposium on Ultrasound Contrast Agents: clinical applications and safety concerns. *Ultrasound Med Biol*, 33, 180-6.

Bohmer M.R., Klibanov A.L., Tiemann K., *et al.,* 2009. Ultrasound triggered image-guided drug delivery. *Eur J Radiol*, 70, 242-53.

Bonuccelli G., Casimiro M.C., Sotgia F., *et al.,* 2009. Caveolin-1 (P132L), a common breast cancer mutation, confers mammary cell invasiveness and defines a novel stem cell/metastasis-associated gene signature. *Am J Pathol*, 174, 1650-62.

Bonuccelli G., Tsirigos A., Whitaker-Menezes D., *et al.,* 2010. Ketones and lactate "fuel" tumor growth and metastasis: Evidence that epithelial cancer cells use oxidative mitochondrial metabolism. *Cell Cycle*, 9, 3506-14.

Bonuccelli G., Whitaker-Menezes D., Castello-Cros R., *et al.,* 2010. The reverse Warburg effect: Glycolysis inhibitors prevent the tumor promoting effects of caveolin-1 deficient cancer associated fibroblasts. *Cell Cycle*, 9.

Borden M.A., Caskey C.F., Little E., Gillies R.J., Ferrara K.W. 2007. DNA and polylysine adsorption and multilayer construction onto cationic lipid-coated microbubbles. *Langmuir*, 23, 9401-8.

Borden M.A., Kruse D.E., Caskey C.F., *et al.,* 2005. Influence of lipid shell physicochemical properties on ultrasound-induced microbubble destruction. *IEEE Trans Ultrason Ferroelectr Freq Control*, 52, 1992-2002.

Borden M.A., Zhang H., Gillies R.J., Dayton P.A., Ferrara K.W. 2008. A stimulus-responsive contrast agent for ultrasound molecular imaging. *Biomaterials*, 29, 597-606.

Bouakaz A., Versluis M., de Jong N. 2005. High-speed optical observations of contrast agent destruction. *Ultrasound Med Biol*, 31, 391-9.

Bougnoux P., Germain E., Chajes V., *et al.,* 1999. Cytotoxic drugs efficacy correlates with adipose tissue docosahexaenoic acid level in locally advanced breast carcinoma. *Br J Cancer*, 79, 1765-9.

Bougnoux P., Hajjaji N., Ferrasson M.N., *et al.,* 2009. Improving outcome of chemotherapy of metastatic breast cancer by docosahexaenoic acid: a phase II trial. *Br J Cancer*, 101, 1978-85.

Braun T., Carvalho G., Fabre C., *et al.,* 2006. Targeting NF-kappaB in hematologic malignancies. *Cell Death Differ*, 13, 748-58.

Bray F., Ren J.S., Masuyer E., Ferlay J. 2013. Global estimates of cancer prevalence for 27 sites in the adult population in 2008. *Int J Cancer*, 132, 1133-45.

Brennan M., Wilcken N., French J., Ung O., Boyages J. 2005. Management of early breast cancer--the current approach. *Aust Fam Physician*, 34, 755-60.

Brown D.A., London E. 1998. Functions of lipid rafts in biological membranes. *Ann Rev Cell Dev Biol*, 14, 111-36.

Buchanan F.G., Wang D., Bargiacchi F., DuBois R.N. 2003. Prostaglandin E2 regulates cell migration *via* the intracellular activation of the epidermal growth factor receptor. *J Biol Chem*, 278, 35451-7.

Burns C.P., Halabi S., Clamon G.H., *et al.,* 1999. Phase I clinical study of fish oil fatty acid capsules for patients with cancer cachexia: cancer and leukemia group B study 9473. *Clin Cancer Res*, 5, 3942-7.

Calder P.C. 2009. Polyunsaturated fatty acids and inflammatory processes: New twists in an old tale. *Biochimie*, 91, 791-5.

Calder P.C. 2012. Mechanisms of action of (n-3) fatty acids. *J Nutr*, 142, 592S-9S.

Calliada F., Campani R., Bottinelli O., Bozzini A., Sommaruga M.G. 1998. Ultrasound contrast agents: basic principles. *Eur J Radiol*, 27 Suppl 2, S157-60.

Calviello G., Di Nicuolo F., Gragnoli S., *et al.,* 2004. n-3 PUFAs reduce VEGF expression in human colon cancer cells modulating the COX-2/PGE2 induced ERK-1 and -2 and HIF-1alpha induction pathway. *Carcinogenesis*, 25, 2303-10.

Capozza F., Williams T.M., Schubert W., *et al.*, 2003. Absence of caveolin-1 sensitizes mouse skin to carcinogen-induced epidermal hyperplasia and tumor formation. *Am J Pathol*, 162, 2029-39.

Cathcart M.C., Lysaght J., Pidgeon G.P. 2011. Eicosanoid signalling pathways in the development and progression of colorectal cancer: novel approaches for prevention/intervention. *Cancer Metastasis Rev*, 30, 363-85.

Cavalieri F., Ashokkumar M., Grieser F., Caruso F. 2008. Ultrasonic synthesis of stable, functional lysozyme microbubbles. *Langmuir*, 24, 10078-83.

Cavalieri F., El Hamassi A., Chiessi E., Paradossi G. 2005. Stable polymeric microballoons as multifunctional device for biomedical uses: synthesis and characterization. *Langmuir*, 21, 8758-64.

Cavalieri F., Finelli, I., Tortora, M., Mozetic, P., Chiessi, E., Polizio, F., Brismar, T., Paradossi., G. 2008. Microbubbles as (NO) delivery device. *Chem Matter*, 20, 3254-8.

Cavalieri F., Zhou M., Ashokkumar M. 2010. The design of multifunctional microbubbles for ultrasound image-guided cancer therapy. *Curr Top Med Chem*, 10, 1198-210.

Cavalieri F., Zhou M., Caruso F., Ashokkumar M. 2011. One-pot ultrasonic synthesis of multifunctional microbubbles and microcapsules using synthetic thiolated macromolecules. *Chem Commun (Camb)*, 47, 4096-8.

Cavalieri F., Zhou M., Tortora M., Lucilla B., Ashokkumar M. 2012. Methods of preparation of multifunctional microbubbles and their *in vitro* / *in vivo* assessment of stability, functional and structural properties. *Curr Pharm Des*, 18, 2135-51.

Chan A.T., Ogino S., Fuchs C.S. 2007. Aspirin and the risk of colorectal cancer in relation to the expression of COX-2. *N Engl J Med*, 356, 2131-42.

Chang A. 2011. Chemotherapy, chemoresistance and the changing treatment landscape for NSCLC. *Lung Cancer*, 71, 3-10.

Chatterjee-Kishore M., Wright K.L., Ting J.P., Stark G.R. 2000. How Stat1 mediates constitutive gene expression: a complex of unphosphorylated Stat1 and IRF1 supports transcription of the LMP2 gene. *Embo J*, 19, 4111-22.

Chen H., Brayman A.A., Bailey M.R., Matula T.J. 2010. Blood vessel rupture by cavitation. *Urol Res*, 38, 321-6.

Chen H., Brayman A.A., Kreider W., Bailey M.R., Matula T.J. 2011. Observations of translation and jetting of ultrasound-activated microbubbles in mesenteric microvessels. *Ultrasound Med Biol*, 37, 2139-48.

Chen S., Shohet R.V., Bekeredjian R., Frenkel P., Grayburn P.A. 2003. Optimization of ultrasound parameters for cardiac gene delivery of adenoviral or plasmid deoxyribonucleic acid by ultrasound-targeted microbubble destruction. *J Am Coll Cardiol*, 42, 301-8.

Chen W.S., Matula T.J., Brayman A.A., Crum L.A. 2003. A comparison of the fragmentation thresholds and inertial cavitation doses of different ultrasound contrast agents. *J Acoust Soc Am*, 113, 643-51.

Chen W.S., Matula T.J., Crum L.A. 2002. The disappearance of ultrasound contrast bubbles: observations of bubble dissolution and cavitation nucleation. *Ultrasound Med Biol*, 28, 793-803.

Chen X., Vinkemeier U., Zhao Y., *et al.*, 1998. Crystal structure of a tyrosine phosphorylated STAT-1 dimer bound to DNA. *Cell*, 93, 827-39.

Chiavarina B., Whitaker-Menezes D., Migneco G., *et al.*, 2010. HIF1-alpha functions as a tumor promoter in cancer associated fibroblasts, and as a tumor suppressor in breast cancer cells: Autophagy drives compartment-specific oncogenesis. *Cell Cycle*, 9, 3534-51.

Cho Y.K., Yang, W., Harry, B.L., Klibanov, A.L., Hossack, J.A.. 2006. Dual-targeted contrast enhanced ultrasound imaging of atherosclerosis in apolipoprotein gene knockout mice. *Circulation*, 114, 759.

Choi J.J., Pernot M., Small S.A., Konofagou E.E. 2007. Noninvasive, transcranial and localized opening of the blood-brain barrier using focused ultrasound in mice. *Ultrasound Med Biol*, 33, 95-104.

Chomas J.E., Dayton P., Allen J., Morgan K., Ferrara K.W. 2001. Mechanisms of contrast agent destruction. *IEEE Trans Ultrason Ferroelectr Freq Control*, 48, 232-48.

Chomas J.E., Dayton P., May D., Ferrara K. 2001. Threshold of fragmentation for ultrasonic contrast agents. *J Biomed Opt*, 6, 141-50.

Chomas J.E., Dayton P.A., May, D., Allen, J., Klibanov, A., Ferrara, K. 2000. Optical observation of contrast agent destruction. *Applied Physics Letters*, 77, 1056-8.

Chopin L.K., Veveris-Lowe T.L., Philipps A.F., Herington A.C. 2002. Co-expression of GH and GHR isoforms in prostate cancer cell lines. *Growth Horm IGF Res*, 12, 126-36.

Christensen J.P., Klibanov A.L., Lindner, J.R. 2002. Transfection of plasmid DNA in cardiac and skeletal muscle with ultrasound and intravenous cationic microbubble vehicles.. *Journal of the American College of Cardiology*, 39, 361A.

Christiansen C., Kryvi, H., Sontum, P., Skotland, T. 1994. Physical and biochemical-characterization of albunex (TM): A new ultrasound contrast agent consisting of air-filled albumin microspheres suspended in a solution of human albumin. *Biotechnology and Applied Biochemistry*, 19, 307-20.

Christiansen J.P., French B.A., Klibanov A.L., Kaul S., Lindner J.R. 2003. Targeted tissue transfection with ultrasound destruction of plasmid-bearing cationic microbubbles. *Ultrasound Med Biol*, 29, 1759-67.

Chung C.D., Liao J., Liu B., *et al.,* 1997. Specific inhibition of Stat3 signal transduction by PIAS3. *Science*, 278, 1803-5.

Church C.C., Carstensen EL. 2001. "Stable" inertial cavitation. *Ultrasound Med Biol*, 27, 1435-7.

Clement G.T., Hynynen K. 2002. A non-invasive method for focusing ultrasound through the human skull. *Phys Med Biol*, 47, 1219-36.

Clevers H. 2004. At the crossroads of inflammation and cancer. *Cell*, 118, 671-4.

Cohen A.W., Razani B., Wang X.B., *et al.,* 2003. Caveolin-1-deficient mice show insulin resistance and defective insulin receptor protein expression in adipose tissue. *Am J Physiol Cell Physiol*, 285, C222-35.

Collis J., Manasseh R., Liovic P., *et al.,* 2010. Cavitation microstreaming and stress fields created by microbubbles. *Ultrasonics*, 50, 273-9.

Copeland N.G., Gilbert D.J., Schindler C., *et al.,* 1995. Distribution of the mammalian Stat gene family in mouse chromosomes. *Genomics*, 29, 225-8.

Corsetto P.A., Cremona A., Montorfano G., *et al.,* 2012. Chemical-physical changes in cell membrane microdomains of breast cancer cells after omega-3 PUFA incorporation. *Cell Biochem Biophys*, 64, 45-59.

Couet J., Sargiacomo M., Lisanti M.P. 1997. Interaction of a receptor tyrosine kinase, EGF-R, with caveolins. Caveolin binding negatively regulates tyrosine and serine/threonine kinase activities. *J Biol Chem*, 272, 30429-38.

Coussens L.M., Werb Z. 1996. Matrix metalloproteinases and the development of cancer. *Chem Biol*, 3, 895-904.

Csiki I., Morrow J.D., Sandler A., *et al.,* 2005. Targeting cyclooxygenase-2 in recurrent non-small cell lung cancer: a phase II trial of celecoxib and docetaxel. *Clin Cancer Res*, 11, 6634-40.

Dagvadorj A., Collins S., Jomain J.B., *et al.,* 2007. Autocrine prolactin promotes prostate cancer cell growth *via* Janus kinase-2-signal transducer and activator of transcription-5a/b signaling pathway. *Endocrinology*, 148, 3089-101.

Dagvadorj A., Kirken R.A., Leiby B., Karras J., Nevalainen M.T. 2008. Transcription Factor Stat5 Promotes Growth of Human Prostate Cancer Cells *In Vivo*. *Clinical Cancer Research*, In Press.

Dalecki D. 2007. WFUMB Safety Symposium on Echo-Contrast Agents: bioeffects of ultrasound contrast agents *in vivo*. *Ultrasound Med Biol*, 33, 205-13.

Darnell J.E., Jr. 1997. STATs and gene regulation. *Science*, 277, 1630-5.

Darnell J.E., Jr. 2002. Transcription factors as targets for cancer therapy. *Nat Rev Cancer*, 2, 740-9.

Darnell J.E., Jr., Kerr I.M., Stark G.R. 1994. Jak-STAT pathways and transcriptional activation in response to IFNs and other extracellular signaling proteins. *Science*, 264, 1415-21.

Das U.N., Madhavi N. 2011. Effect of polyunsaturated fatty acids on drug-sensitive and resistant tumor cells *in vitro*. *Lipids Health Dis*, 10, 159.

Das U.N., Madhavi N., Sravan Kumar G., Padma M., Sangeetha P. 1998. Can tumour cell drug resistance be reversed by essential fatty acids and their metabolites? *Prostaglandins Leukot Essent Fatty Acids*, 58, 39-54.

Datta S., Coussios C.C., McAdory L.E., *et al.,* 2006. Correlation of cavitation with ultrasound enhancement of thrombolysis. *Ultrasound Med Biol*, 32, 1257-67.

Dayton P., Klibanov A., Brandenburger G., Ferrara K. 1999. Acoustic radiation force *in vivo*: a mechanism to assist targeting of microbubbles. *Ultrasound Med Biol*, 25, 1195-201.

Dayton P.A., Morgan K.E., Klibanov A.L., Brandenburger G.H., Ferrara K.W. 1999. Optical and acoustical observations of the effects of ultrasound on contrast agents. *IEEE Trans Ultrason Ferroelectr Freq Control*, 46, 220-32.

de Jong N., Cornet, R. and Lancee, C.. 1994. Higher harmonics of vibrating gas-filled microspeheres. Part one: Simulations. *Ultrasonics*, 32, 447-53.

de Jong N., Hoff L. 1993. Ultrasound scattering properties of Albunex microspheres. *Ultrasonics*, 31, 175-81.

de Jong N., Hoff L., Skotland T., Bom N. 1992. Absorption and scatter of encapsulated gas filled microspheres: theoretical considerations and some measurements. *Ultrasonics*, 30, 95-103.

Decker T., Lew D.J., Mirkovitch J., Darnell J.E., Jr. 1991. Cytoplasmic activation of GAF, an IFN-gamma-regulated DNA-binding factor. *Embo J*, 10, 927-32.

Deelman L.E., Decleves A.E., Rychak J.J., Sharma K. 2010. Targeted renal therapies through microbubbles and ultrasound. *Adv Drug Deliv Rev*, 62, 1369-77.

DeGraffenried L.A., Friedrichs W.E., Fulcher L., *et al.,* 2003. Eicosapentaenoic acid restores tamoxifen sensitivity in breast cancer cells with high Akt activity. *Ann Oncol*, 14, 1051-6.

Dekoj T., Lee S., Desai S., *et al.,* 2007. G2/M cell-cycle arrest and apoptosis by n-3 fatty acids in a pancreatic cancer model. *J Surg Res*, 139, 106-12.

Deli M.A. 2009. Potential use of tight junction modulators to reversibly open membranous barriers and improve drug delivery. *Biochim Biophys Acta*, 1788, 892-910.

Deng C.X., Sieling F., Pan H., Cui J. 2004. Ultrasound-induced cell membrane porosity. *Ultrasound Med Biol*, 30, 519-26.

Denkert C., Winzer K.J., Muller B.M., *et al.,* 2003. Elevated expression of cyclooxygenase-2 is a negative prognostic factor for disease free survival and overall survival in patients with breast carcinoma. *Cancer*, 97, 2978-87.

Di Vizio D., Adam R.M., Kim J., *et al.,* 2008. Caveolin-1 interacts with a lipid raft-associated population of fatty acid synthase. *Cell Cycle*, 7, 2257-67.

Di Vizio D., Morello M., Sotgia F., *et al.,* 2009. An absence of stromal caveolin-1 is associated with advanced prostate cancer, metastatic disease and epithelial Akt activation. *Cell Cycle*, 8, 2420-4.

Di Vizio D., Sotgia F., Williams T.M., *et al.,* 2007. Caveolin-1 is required for the upregulation of fatty acid synthase (FASN), a tumor promoter, during prostate cancer progression. *Cancer Biol Ther*, 6, 1263-8.

Ditsworth D., Zong W.X. 2004. NF-kappaB: key mediator of inflammation-associated cancer. *Cancer Biol Ther*, 3, 1214-6.

Duncan R., Vicent M.J., Greco F., Nicholson R.I. 2005. Polymer-drug conjugates: towards a novel approach for the treatment of endrocine-related cancer. *Endocr Relat Cancer*, 12 Suppl 1, S189-99.

Edelman M.J., Watson D., Wang X., *et al.,* 2008. Eicosanoid modulation in advanced lung cancer: cyclooxygenase-2 expression is a positive predictive factor for celecoxib + chemotherapy--Cancer and Leukemia Group B Trial 30203. *J Clin Oncol*, 26, 848-55.

Ehret G.B., Reichenbach P., Schindler U., *et al.,* 2001. DNA binding specificity of different STAT proteins. Comparison of *in vitro* specificity with natural target sites. *J Biol Chem*, 276, 6675-88.

El-Sherif D.M., Lathia J.D., Le N.T., Wheatley M.A. 2004. Ultrasound degradation of novel polymer contrast agents. *J Biomed Mater Res A*, 68, 71-8.

Elder S., Nyborg W.L. 1956. Acoustic Streaming Resulting from A Resonance Bubble. *Journal of the Acoustical Society of America*, 28, 155.

Engelman J.A., Chu C., Lin A., *et al.,* 1998. Caveolin-mediated regulation of signaling along the p42/44 MAP kinase cascade *in vivo*. A role for the caveolin-scaffolding domain. *FEBS Lett*, 428, 205-11.

Engelman J.A., Lee R.J., Karnezis A., *et al.,* 1998. Reciprocal regulation of Neu tyrosine kinase activity and caveolin-1 protein expression *in vitro* and *in vivo*. Implications for mammary tumorigenesis. *J Biol Chem*, 273, 20448-55.

Engelman J.A., Zhang X.L., Razani B., Pestell R.G., Lisanti M.P. 1999. p42/44 MAP kinase-dependent and -independent signaling pathways regulate caveolin-1 gene expression. Activation of Ras-MAP kinase and protein kinase a signaling cascades transcriptionally down-regulates caveolin-1 promoter activity. *J Biol Chem*, 274, 32333-41.

Epstein P.S.a.P., M. S. 1950. On the Stability of Gas Bubbles in Liquid-Gas Solutions. *Journal of Chemical Physics*, 18, 1505-9.

Erbas B., Provenzano E., Armes J., Gertig D. 2006. The natural history of ductal carcinoma *in situ* of the breast: a review. *Breast Cancer Res Treat*, 97, 135-44.

Estabrook N.C., Chin-Sinex H., Borgmann A.J., *et al.,* 2011. Inhibition of NF-kappaB and DNA double-strand break repair by DMAPT sensitizes non-small-cell lung cancers to X-rays. *Free Radic Biol Med*, 51, 2249-58.

Faez T., Emmer M., Kooiman K., *et al.,* 2013. 20 years of ultrasound contrast agent modeling. *IEEE Trans Ultrason Ferroelectr Freq Control*, 60, 7-20.

Fahrmann J.F., Ballester O.F., Ballester G., *et al.,* 2013. Inhibition of Nuclear Factor Kappa B activation in Early-Stage Chronic Lymphocytic Leukemia by Omega-3 Fatty Acids. *Cancer Invest*, 31, 29-43.

Fahrmann J.F., Hardman W.E. 2013. Omega 3 fatty acids increase the chemo-sensitivity of B-CLL-derived cell lines EHEB and MEC-2 and of B-PLL-derived cell line JVM-2 to anti-cancer drugs doxorubicin, vincristine and fludarabine. *Lipids Health Dis*, 12, 36.

Fan L., Liu, Y., Ying, H., Xue, Y., Zhang, Z., Wang, P., Liu, L., Zhang, H. 2011. Increasing of blood-tumor barrier permeability through paracellular pathway by low-frequency ultrasound irradiation *in vitro*. *J Mol Neurosci*, 43, 541-8.

Fan Z., Liu H., Mayer M., Deng C.X. 2012. Spatiotemporally controlled single cell sonoporation. *Proc Natl Acad Sci U S A*, 109, 16486-91.

Fang J.Y., Hung C.F., Hua S.C., Hwang T.L. 2009. Acoustically active perfluorocarbon nanoemulsions as drug delivery carriers for camptothecin: drug release and cytotoxicity against cancer cells. *Ultrasonics*, 49, 39-46.

Fang J.Y., Hung C.F., Liao M.H., Chien C.C. 2007. A study of the formulation design of acoustically active lipospheres as carriers for drug delivery. *Eur J Pharm Biopharm*, 67, 67-75.

Farook U., Zhang H.B., Edirisinghe M.J., Stride E., Saffari N. 2007. Preparation of microbubble suspensions by co-axial electrohydrodynamic atomization. *Med Eng Phys*, 29, 749-54.

Feinstein S.B., Ten Cate F.J., Zwehl W., *et al.,* 1984. Two-dimensional contrast echocardiography. I. *In vitro* development and quantitative analysis of echo contrast agents. *J Am Coll Cardiol*, 3, 14-20.

Felicetti F., Parolini I., Bottero L., *et al.,* 2009. Caveolin-1 tumor-promoting role in human melanoma. *Int J Cancer*, 125, 1514-22.

Feril L.B., Jr., Ogawa R., Tachibana K., Kondo T. 2006. Optimized ultrasound-mediated gene transfection in cancer cells. *Cancer Sci*, 97, 1111-4.

Ferrara K., Pollard R., Borden M. 2007. Ultrasound microbubble contrast agents: fundamentals and application to gene and drug delivery. *Annu Rev Biomed Eng*, 9, 415-47.

Ferrara K.W., Borden M.A., Zhang H. 2009. Lipid-shelled vehicles: engineering for ultrasound molecular imaging and drug delivery. *Acc Chem Res*, 42, 881-92.

Fidler M.J., Argiris A., Patel J.D., *et al.,* 2008. The potential predictive value of cyclooxygenase-2 expression and increased risk of gastrointestinal hemorrhage in advanced non-small cell lung cancer patients treated with erlotinib and celecoxib. *Clin Cancer Res*, 14, 2088-94.

Fong A., Garcia E., Gwynn L., *et al.,* 2003. Expression of caveolin-1 and caveolin-2 in urothelial carcinoma of the urinary bladder correlates with tumor grade and squamous differentiation. *Am J Clin Pathol*, 120, 93-100.

Foxwell B.M., Beadling C., Guschin D., Kerr I., Cantrell D. 1995. Interleukin-7 can induce the activation of Jak 1, Jak 3 and STAT 5 proteins in murine T cells. *Eur J Immunol*, 25, 3041-6.

Frank P.G., Marcel Y.L., Connelly M.A., *et al.,* 2002. Stabilization of caveolin-1 by cellular cholesterol and scavenger receptor class B type I. *Biochemistry*, 41, 11931-40.

Frenkel P.A., Chen S., Thai T., Shohet R.V., Grayburn P.A. 2002. DNA-loaded albumin microbubbles enhance ultrasound-mediated transfection *in vitro*. *Ultrasound Med Biol*, 28, 817-22.

Galbiati F., Razani B., Lisanti M.P. 2001. Emerging themes in lipid rafts and caveolae. *Cell*, 106, 403-11.

Gao Z., Fain H.D., Rapoport N. 2004. Ultrasound-enhanced tumor targeting of polymeric micellar drug carriers. *Mol Pharm*, 1, 317-30.

Gao Z., Kennedy A.M., Christensen D.A., Rapoport N.Y. 2008. Drug-loaded nano/microbubbles for combining ultrasonography and targeted chemotherapy. *Ultrasonics*, 48, 260-70.

Garstecki M.A., Gitlin, I., DiLuzio, W., Whitesides,G.M., Kumacheva, E., Stone, H.A. 2004. Formation of monodisperse bubbles in a microfluidic flow-focusing device. *Applied Physics Letters*, 85, 2649-51.

Geers B., Lentacker I., Cool S., *et al.,* 2010. Ultrasound responsive doxorubicin-loaded microbubbles; towards an easy applicable drug delivery platform. *J Control Release*, 148, e59-60.

Geers B., Lentacker I., Sanders N.N., *et al.,* 2011. Self-assembled liposome-loaded microbubbles: The missing link for safe and efficient ultrasound triggered drug-delivery. *J Control Release*, 152, 249-56.

Geiser E.A., Buss D.D., Wible J.H., Jr., *et al.,* 1996. Evidence for a relation between inspired gas mixture and the left ventricular contrast achieved with Albunex in a canine model. *Clin Cardiol*, 19, 289-95.

Germain E., Chajes V., Cognault S., Lhuillery C., Bougnoux P. 1998. Enhancement of doxorubicin cytotoxicity by polyunsaturated fatty acids in the human breast tumor cell line MDA-MB-231: relationship to lipid peroxidation. *Int J Cancer*, 75, 578-83.

Gerster H. 1998. Can adults adequately convert alpha-linolenic acid (18:3n-3) to eicosapentaenoic acid (20:5n-3) and docosahexaenoic acid (22:6n-3)? *Int J Vitam Nutr Res*, 68, 159-73.

Gessner R., Dayton P.A. 2010. Advances in molecular imaging with ultrasound. *Mol Imaging*, 9, 117-27.

Gewinner C., Hart G., Zachara N., *et al.,* 2004. The coactivator of transcription CREB-binding protein interacts preferentially with the glycosylated form of Stat5. *J Biol Chem*, 279, 3563-72.

Ghitescu L., Fixman A., Simionescu M., Simionescu N. 1986. Specific binding sites for albumin restricted to plasmalemmal vesicles of continuous capillary endothelium: receptor-mediated transcytosis. *J Cell Biol*, 102, 1304-11.

Ghoreishi Z., Esfahani A., Djazayeri A., *et al.,* 2012. Omega-3 fatty acids are protective against paclitaxel-induced peripheral neuropathy: a randomized double-blind placebo controlled trial. *BMC Cancer*, 12, 355.

Ghosh-Choudhury T., Mandal C.C., Woodruff K., *et al.,* 2009. Fish oil targets PTEN to regulate NFkappaB for downregulation of anti-apoptotic genes in breast tumor growth. *Breast Cancer Res Treat*, 118, 213-28.

Gingrich J.R., Barrios R.J., Morton R.A., *et al.,* 1996. Metastatic prostate cancer in a transgenic mouse. *Cancer Res*, 56, 4096-102.

Glenney J.R. 1992. The sequence of human caveolin reveals identity with VIP 21, a component of transport vesicles. *FEBS Lett*, 314, 45-8.

Glover J.A., Hughes C.M., Cantwell M.M., Murray L.J. 2011. A systematic review to establish the frequency of cyclooxygenase-2 expression in normal breast epithelium, ductal carcinoma *in situ*, microinvasive carcinoma of the breast and invasive breast cancer. *Br J Cancer*, 105, 13-7.

Gogineni K., DeMichele A. 2012. Current approaches to the management of Her2-negative metastatic breast cancer. *Breast Cancer Res*, 14, 205.

González-Mariscal L., Betanzos, A., Avila-Flores, A. 2000. MAGUK proteins: structure and role in the tight junction. *Semin Cell Dev Biol*, 11, 315-24.

Gouilleux F., Pallard C., Dusanter-Fourt I., *et al.,* 1995. Prolactin, growth hormone, erythropoietin and granulocyte-macrophage colony stimulating factor induce MGF-Stat5 DNA binding activity. *Embo J*, 14, 2005-13.

Gouilleux F., Wakao H., Mundt M., Groner B. 1994. Prolactin induces phosphorylation of Tyr694 of Stat5 (MGF), a prerequisite for DNA binding and induction of transcription. *Embo J*, 13, 4361-9.

Goureau A., Garrigues A., Tosser-Klopp G., *et al.,* 2001. Conserved synteny and gene order difference between human chromosome 12 and pig chromosome 5. *Cytogenet Cell Genet*, 94, 49-54.

Gramiak R., Shah P.M. 1968. Echocardiography of the aortic root. *Invest Radiol*, 3, 356-66.

Greco A., Di Benedetto A., Howard C.M., *et al.,* 2010. Eradication of therapy-resistant human prostate tumors using an ultrasound-guided site-specific cancer terminator virus delivery approach. *Mol Ther*, 18, 295-306.

Greenberg M.E., Li X.M., Gugiu B.G., *et al.,* 2008. The lipid whisker model of the structure of oxidized cell membranes. *J Biol Chem*, 283, 2385-96.

Greenberg N.M., DeMayo F., Finegold M.J., *et al.,* 1995. Prostate cancer in a transgenic mouse. *Proc Natl Acad Sci U S A*, 92, 3439-43.

Greenhough A., Smartt H.J., Moore A.E., *et al.,* 2009. The COX-2/PGE2 pathway: key roles in the hallmarks of cancer and adaptation to the tumour microenvironment. *Carcinogenesis*, 30, 377-86.

Grinstaff M.W., Suslick K.S. 1991. Air-filled proteinaceous microbubbles: synthesis of an echo-contrast agent. *Proc Natl Acad Sci U S A*, 88, 7708-10.

Guh J.Y., Huang J.S., Chen H.C., *et al.,* 2001. Advanced glycation end product-induced proliferation in NRK-49F cells is dependent on the JAK2/STAT5 pathway and cyclin D1. *Am J Kidney Dis*, 38, 1096-104.

Guidi F., Vos H.J., Mori R., de Jong N., Tortoli P. 2010. Microbubble characterization through acoustically induced deflation. *IEEE Trans Ultrason Ferroelectr Freq Control*, 57, 193-202.

Haddad B., Pabon-Pena C.R., Young H., Sun W.H. 1998. Assignmentl of STAT1 to human chromosome 2q32 by FISH and radiation hybrids. *Cytogenet Cell Genet*, 83, 58-9.

Haeggstrom J.Z., Rinaldo-Matthis A., Wheelock C.E., Wetterholm A. 2010. Advances in eicosanoid research, novel therapeutic implications. *Biochem Biophys Res Commun*, 396, 135-9.

Halmos G., Schally A.V., Czompoly T., *et al.,* 2002. Expression of growth hormone-releasing hormone and its receptor splice variants in human prostate cancer. *J Clin Endocrinol Metab*, 87, 4707-14.

Hamill O.P. 2006. Twenty odd years of stretch-sensitive channels. *Pflugers Arch*, 453, 333-51.

Han E.H., Kim H.G., Hwang Y.P., Song G.Y., Jeong H.G. 2010. Prostaglandin E2 induces CYP1B1 expression *via* ligand-independent activation of the ERalpha pathway in human breast cancer cells. *Toxicol Sci*, 114, 204-16.

Han M., He C.X., Fang Q.L., *et al.,* 2009. A novel camptothecin derivative incorporated in nano-carrier induced distinguished improvement in solubility, stability and anti-tumor activity both *in vitro* and *in vivo*. *Pharm Res*, 26, 926-35.

Hardman W.E., Avula C.P., Fernandes G., Cameron I.L. 2001. Three percent dietary fish oil concentrate increased efficacy of doxorubicin against MDA-MB 231 breast cancer xenografts. *Clin Cancer Res*, 7, 2041-9.

Heller A.R., Rossel T., Gottschlich B., *et al.,* 2004. Omega-3 fatty acids improve liver and pancreas function in postoperative cancer patients. *Int J Cancer*, 111, 611-6.

Hernot S., Klibanov A.L. 2008. Microbubbles in ultrasound-triggered drug and gene delivery. *Adv Drug Deliv Rev*, 60, 1153-66.

Hewamana S., Alghazal S., Lin T.T., *et al.,* 2008. The NF-kappaB subunit Rel A is associated with *in vitro* survival and clinical disease progression in chronic lymphocytic leukemia and represents a promising therapeutic target. *Blood*, 111, 4681-9.

Hewamana S., Lin T.T., Jenkins C., *et al.,* 2008. The novel nuclear factor-kappaB inhibitor LC-1 is equipotent in poor prognostic subsets of chronic lymphocytic leukemia and shows strong synergy with fludarabine. *Clin Cancer Res*, 14, 8102-11.

Hewamana S., Lin T.T., Rowntree C., *et al.,* 2009. Rel a is an independent biomarker of clinical outcome in chronic lymphocytic leukemia. *J Clin Oncol*, 27, 763-9.

Hill C.R., editor. Physical Principles of Medical Ultrasonics: Wiley-Blackwell; 2004.

Hirase T., Staddon, J.M., Saitou, M., Ando-Akatsuka, Y., Itoh, M., Furuse, M., Fujimoto, K., Tsukita, S., Rubin, L.L. 1997. Occludin as a possible determinant of tight junction permeability in endothelial cells. *J Cell Sci*, 110, 1603-13.

Ho S.Y., Barbarese E., D'Arrigo J.S., Smith-Slatas C., Simon R.H. 1997. Evaluation of lipid-coated microbubbles as a delivery vehicle for Taxol in brain tumor therapy. *Neurosurgery*, 40, 1260-6; discussion 6-8.

Holland C.K., Roy R.A., Apfel R.E., Crum L.A. 1992. *In vitro* detection of cavitation induced by a diagnostic ultrasound system. *IEEE Trans Ultrason Ferroelectr Freq Control*, 39, 95-101.

Horvath C.M., Wen Z., Darnell J.E., Jr. 1995. A STAT protein domain that determines DNA sequence recognition suggests a novel DNA-binding domain. *Genes Dev*, 9, 984-94.

Hou J., Schindler U., Henzel W.J., Wong S.C., McKnight S.L. 1995. Identification and purification of human Stat proteins activated in response to interleukin-2. *Immunity*, 2, 321-9.

Howard C.M. 2004. The role of ultrasound contrast agents in gene therapy. *Applied Radiology*, 33, 126.

Howard C.M. 2004. The role of ultrasound contrast agents in gene therapy. *Applied Radiology*, 33.

Howard C.M., Forsberg F., Minimo C., *et al.,* 2006. Ultrasound guided site specific gene delivery system using adenoviral vectors and commercial ultrasound contrast agents. *J Cell Physiol*, 209, 413-21.

Hsieh D.Y., Plesset, M.S. 1961. Theory of rectified diffusion of mass into gas bubbles. *J Acoust Soc Am*, 33, 206-11.

Hu Y.C., Lam K.Y., Law S., Wong J., Srivastava G. 2001. Profiling of differentially expressed cancer-related genes in esophageal squamous cell carcinoma (ESCC) using human cancer cDNA arrays: overexpression of oncogene MET correlates with tumor differentiation in ESCC. *Clin Cancer Res*, 7, 3519-25.

Huang S.L., Hamilton A.J., Pozharski E., *et al.,* 2002. Physical correlates of the ultrasonic reflectivity of lipid dispersions suitable as diagnostic contrast agents. *Ultrasound Med Biol*, 28, 339-48.

Hung C.F., Chen J.K., Liao M.H., Lo H.M., Fang J.Y. 2006. Development and evaluation of emulsion-liposome blends for resveratrol delivery. *J Nanosci Nanotechnol*, 6, 2950-8.

Hyde C.A., Missailidis S. 2009. Inhibition of arachidonic acid metabolism and its implication on cell proliferation and tumour-angiogenesis. *Int Immunopharmacol*, 9, 701-15.

Hynynen K. 2008. Ultrasound for drug and gene delivery to the brain. *Adv Drug Deliv Rev*, 60, 1209-17.

Hynynen K., McDannold N., Vykhodtseva N., Jolesz F.A. 2001. Noninvasive MR imaging-guided focal opening of the blood-brain barrier in rabbits. *Radiology*, 220, 640-6.

Hynynen K., McDannold N., Vykhodtseva N., *et al.*, 2006. Focal disruption of the blood-brain barrier due to 260-kHz ultrasound bursts: a method for molecular imaging and targeted drug delivery. *J Neurosurg*, 105, 445-54.

Ibsen S., Benchimol M., Simberg D., *et al.*, 2011. A novel nested liposome drug delivery vehicle capable of ultrasound triggered release of its payload. *J Control Release*, 155, 358-66.

Ihle J.N. 2001. The Stat family in cytokine signaling. *Curr Opin Cell Biol*, 13, 211-7.

Isaacs J.T., Isaacs W.B. 2004. Androgen receptor outwits prostate cancer drugs. *Nat Med*, 10, 26-7.

Itoh T., Tanioka M., Matsuda H., *et al.*, 1999. Experimental metastasis is suppressed in MMP-9-deficient mice. *Clin Exp Metastasis*, 17, 177-81.

Itoh T., Tanioka M., Yoshida H., *et al.*, 1998. Reduced angiogenesis and tumor progression in gelatinase A-deficient mice. *Cancer Res*, 58, 1048-51.

Iwanaga K., Tominaga K., Yamamoto K., *et al.*, 2007. Local delivery system of cytotoxic agents to tumors by focused sonoporation. *Cancer Gene Ther*, 14, 354-63.

Jalali S., Huang, Y., Dumont, D.J., Hynynen, K. 2010. Focused ultrasound-mediated BBB disruption is associated with an increase in activation of AKT: experimental study in rats. *BMC Neurology*, 10, 114.

Jasmin J.F., Mercier I., Sotgia F., Lisanti M.P. 2006. SOCS proteins and caveolin-1 as negative regulators of endocrine signaling. *Trends Endocrinol Metab*, 17, 150-8.

Jemal A., Siegel R., Ward E., *et al.*, 2008. Cancer statistics, 2008. *CA Cancer J Clin*, 58, 71-96.

Jiang H., Wang J., Zhao W. 2013. Cox-2 in non-small cell lung cancer: A meta-analysis. *Clin Chim Acta*, 419C, 26-32.

John S., Vinkemeier U., Soldaini E., Darnell J.E., Jr., Leonard W.J. 1999. The significance of tetramerization in promoter recruitment by Stat5. *Mol Cell Biol*, 19, 1910-8.

Juffermans L.J., van Dijk A., Jongenelen C.A., *et al.*, 2009. Ultrasound and microbubble-induced intra- and intercellular bioeffects in primary endothelial cells. *Ultrasound Med Biol*, 35, 1917-27.

Kamizono S., Hanada T., Yasukawa H., *et al.*, 2001. The SOCS box of SOCS-1 accelerates ubiquitin-dependent proteolysis of TEL-JAK2. *J Biol Chem*, 276, 12530-8.

Kaplan-Lefko P.J., Chen T.M., Ittmann M.M., *et al.*, 2003. Pathobiology of autochthonous prostate cancer in a pre-clinical transgenic mouse model. *Prostate*, 55, 219-37.

Karuppu D., Kalus A., Simpson E.R., Clyne C. 2002. Aromatase and prostaglandin inter-relationships in breast adipose tissue: significance for breast cancer development. *Breast Cancer Res Treat*, 76, 103-9.

Kato J., Matsushime H., Hiebert S.W., Ewen M.E., Sherr C.J. 1993. Direct binding of cyclin D to the retinoblastoma gene product (pRb) and pRb phosphorylation by the cyclin D-dependent kinase CDK4. *Genes Dev*, 7, 331-42.

Kato K., Hida Y., Miyamoto M., *et al.*, 2002. Overexpression of caveolin-1 in esophageal squamous cell carcinoma correlates with lymph node metastasis and pathologic stage. *Cancer*, 94, 929-33.

Kaufmann B.A., Sanders J.M., Davis C., *et al.,* 2007. Molecular imaging of inflammation in atherosclerosis with targeted ultrasound detection of vascular cell adhesion molecule-1. *Circulation*, 116, 276-84.

Kazansky A.V., Spencer D.M., Greenberg N.M. 2003. Activation of signal transducer and activator of transcription 5 is required for progression of autochthonous prostate cancer: evidence from the transgenic adenocarcinoma of the mouse prostate system. *Cancer Res*, 63, 8757-62.

Keller M.W., Feinstein S.B., Watson D.D. 1987. Successful left ventricular opacification following peripheral venous injection of sonicated contrast agent: an experimental evaluation. *Am Heart J*, 114, 570-5.

Kerr J., Leary J.A., Hurst T., *et al.,* 1996. Allelic loss on chromosome 7q in ovarian adenocarcinomas: two critical regions and a rearrangement of the PLANH1 locus. *Oncogene*, 13, 1815-8.

Kheirolomoom A., Dayton P.A., Lum A.F., *et al.,* 2007. Acoustically-active microbubbles conjugated to liposomes: characterization of a proposed drug delivery vehicle. *J Control Release*, 118, 275-84.

Khuri F.R., Wu H., Lee J.J., *et al.,* 2001. Cyclooxygenase-2 overexpression is a marker of poor prognosis in stage I non-small cell lung cancer. *Clin Cancer Res*, 7, 861-7.

Kikawa K.D., Herrick J.S., Tateo R.E., *et al.,* 2010. Induced oxidative stress and cell death in the A549 lung adenocarcinoma cell line by ionizing radiation is enhanced by supplementation with docosahexaenoic acid. *Nutr Cancer*, 62, 1017-24.

Kim J., Lim S.Y., Shin A., *et al.,* 2009. Fatty fish and fish omega-3 fatty acid intakes decrease the breast cancer risk: a case-control study. *BMC Cancer*, 9, 216.

Kindblom J., Dillner K., Ling C., Tornell J., Wennbo H. 2002. Progressive prostate hyperplasia in adult prolactin transgenic mice is not dependent on elevated serum androgen levels. *Prostate*, 53, 24-33.

Kindblom J., Dillner K., Sahlin L., *et al.,* 2003. Prostate hyperplasia in a transgenic mouse with prostate-specific expression of prolactin. *Endocrinology*, 144, 2269-78.

Kinoshita M., McDannold N., Jolesz F.A., Hynynen K. 2006. Noninvasive localized delivery of Herceptin to the mouse brain by MRI-guided focused ultrasound-induced blood-brain barrier disruption. *Proc Natl Acad Sci U S A*, 103, 11719-23.

Klibanov A.L. 1999. Targeted delivery of gas-filled microspheres, contrast agents for ultrasound imaging. *Adv Drug Deliv Rev*, 37, 139-57.

Klibanov A.L. 2005. Ligand-carrying gas-filled microbubbles: ultrasound contrast agents for targeted molecular imaging. *Bioconjug Chem*, 16, 9-17.

Klibanov A.L. 2007. Ultrasound molecular imaging with targeted microbubble contrast agents. *J Nucl Cardiol*, 14, 876-84.

Klibanov A.L., Hughes M.S., Marsh J.N., *et al.,* 1997. Targeting of ultrasound contrast material. An *in vitro* feasibility study. *Acta Radiol Suppl*, 412, 113-20.

Klibanov A.L., Hughes M.S., Villanueva F.S., *et al.,* 1999. Targeting and ultrasound imaging of microbubble-based contrast agents. *MAGMA*, 8, 177-84.

Klibanov A.L., Hughes M.S., Wojdyla J.K., *et al.,* 1998. Targeting of ultrasound contrast material: selective imaging of microbubbles *in vitro*. *Acad Radiol*, 5 Suppl 1, S243-6.

Klibanov A.L., Rasche P.T., Hughes M.S., *et al.,* 2002. Detection of individual microbubbles of an ultrasound contrast agent: fundamental and pulse inversion imaging. *Acad Radiol*, 9 Suppl 2, S279-81.

Klibanov A.L., Rasche P.T., Hughes M.S., *et al.,* 2004. Detection of individual microbubbles of ultrasound contrast agents: imaging of free-floating and targeted bubbles. *Invest Radiol*, 39, 187-95.

Klibanov A.L., Rychak J.J., Yang W.C., *et al.,* 2006. Targeted ultrasound contrast agent for molecular imaging of inflammation in high-shear flow. *Contrast Media Mol Imaging*, 1, 259-66.

Klyubin I., Walsh D.M., Lemere C.A., *et al.,* 2005. Amyloid beta protein immunotherapy neutralizes Abeta oligomers that disrupt synaptic plasticity *in vivo*. *Nat Med*, 11, 556-61.

Koleske A.J., Baltimore D., Lisanti M.P. 1995. Reduction of caveolin and caveolae in oncogenically transformed cells. *Proc Natl Acad Sci U S A*, 92, 1381-5.

Komarova Y., Malik, A.B. 2010. Regulation of endothelial permeability *via* paracellular and transcellular transport pathways. *Annu Rev Physiol*, 72, 463-93.

Kooiman K., Emmer M., Foppen-Harteveld M., van Wamel A., de Jong N. 2010. Increasing the endothelial layer permeability through ultrasound-activated microbubbles. *IEEE Trans Biomed Eng*, 57, 29-32.

Koppelhus U., Nielsen P.E. 2003. Cellular delivery of peptide nucleic acid (PNA). *Adv Drug Deliv Rev*, 55, 267-80.

Korpanty G., Grayburn P.A., Shohet R.V., Brekken R.A. 2005. Targeting vascular endothelium with avidin microbubbles. *Ultrasound Med Biol*, 31, 1279-83.

Kost J. 1993. Ultrasound for controlled delivery of therapeutics. *Clin Mater*, 13, 155-61.

Krysan K., Dohadwala M., Luo J., *et al.,* 2004. Cyclooxygenase-2-dependent expression of survivin in non-small cell lung cancer. *Chest*, 125, 140S.

Labrie F., Dupont A., Belanger A., *et al.,* 1986. Treatment of prostate cancer with gonadotropin-releasing hormone agonists. *Endocr Rev*, 7, 67-74.

Lauterborn W., Kurz, T. 2010. Physics of bubble oscillations. *Reports on Progress in Physics*, 73, 106501.

Lawrie A., Brisken A.F., Francis S.E., *et al.,* 2000. Microbubble-enhanced ultrasound for vascular gene delivery. *Gene Ther*, 7, 2023-7.

Lee L.M., Pan C.C., Cheng C.J., Chi C.W., Liu T.Y. 2001. Expression of cyclooxygenase-2 in prostate adenocarcinoma and benign prostatic hyperplasia. *Anticancer Res*, 21, 1291-4.

Lee S.W., Reimer C.L., Oh P., Campbel l.D.B., Schnitzer J.E. 1998. Tumor cell growth inhibition by caveolin re-expression in human breast cancer cells. *Oncogene*, 16, 1391-7.

Lee S.W., Reimer C.L., Oh P., Campbell D.B., Schnitzer J.E. 1998. Tumor cell growth inhibition by caveolin re-expression in human breast cancer cells. *Oncogene*, 16, 1391-7.

Leek J.P., Hamlin P.J., Bell S.M., Lench N.J. 1997. Assignment of the STAT6 gene (STAT6) to human chromosome band 12q13 by *in situ* hybridization. *Cytogenet Cell Genet*, 79, 208-9.

Leighton T. The Acoustic Bubble. San Diego: Academic Press; 1994.

Lentacker I., De Smedt, S.C., Demeester J., Van Marck, V., Bracke, M., Sanders, N.N. 2009. Lipoplex-loaded microbubbles for gene delivery: A trojan horse controlled by ultrasound. *Adv Funct Matter*, 17, 1910.

Lentacker I., De Smedt, S.C., Sanders, N.N. 2009. Drug loaded microbubble design for ultrasound triggered delivery. *Soft Matter*, 5, 2161-70.

Lentacker I., Geers B., Demeester J., De Smedt S.C., Sanders N.N. 2010. Design and evaluation of doxorubicin-containing microbubbles for ultrasound-triggered doxorubicin delivery: cytotoxicity and mechanisms involved. *Mol Ther*, 18, 101-8.

Lentacker I., Geers B., Demeester J., De Smedt S.C., Sanders N.N. 2010. Tumor cell killing efficiency of doxorubicin loaded microbubbles after ultrasound exposure. *J Control Release*, 148, e113-4.

Lentacker I., Vandenbroucke R.E., Lucas B., *et al.,* 2008. New strategies for nucleic acid delivery to conquer cellular and nuclear membranes. *J Control Release*, 132, 279-88.

Leonard W.J., O'Shea J.J. 1998. Jaks and STATs: biological implications. *Annu Rev Immunol*, 16, 293-322.

Letsch M., Schally A.V., Busto R., Bajo A.M., Varga J.L. 2003. Growth hormone-releasing hormone (GHRH) antagonists inhibit the proliferation of androgen-dependent and -independent prostate cancers. *Proc Natl Acad Sci U S A*, 100, 1250-5.

Levy D.E., Darnell J.E., Jr. 2002. Stats: transcriptional control and biological impact. *Nat Rev Mol Cell Biol*, 3, 651-62.

Li F., Sethi G. 2010. Targeting transcription factor NF-kappaB to overcome chemoresistance and radioresistance in cancer therapy. *Biochim Biophys Acta*, 1805, 167-80.

Li H., Ahonen T.J., Alanen K., *et al.,* 2004. Activation of signal transducer and activator of transcription 5 in human prostate cancer is associated with high histological grade. *Cancer Res*, 64, 4774-82.

Li H., Zhang Y., Glass A., *et al.,* 2005. Activation of signal transducer and activator of transcription-5 in prostate cancer predicts early recurrence. *Clin Cancer Res*, 11, 5863-8.

Li L., Ittmann M.M., Ayala G., *et al.,* 2005. The emerging role of the PI3-K-Akt pathway in prostate cancer progression. *Prostate Cancer Prostatic Dis*, 8, 108-18.

Li L., Ren C.H., Tahir S.A., Ren C., Thompson T.C. 2003. Caveolin-1 maintains activated Akt in prostate cancer cells through scaffolding domain binding site interactions with and inhibition of serine/threonine protein phosphatases PP1 and PP2A. *Mol Cell Biol*, 23, 9389-404.

Li L., Yang G., Ebara S., *et al.,* 2001. Caveolin-1 mediates testosterone-stimulated survival/clonal growth and promotes metastatic activities in prostate cancer cells. *Cancer Res*, 61, 4386-92.

Li T., Liu G., Li J., *et al.,* 2012. Mechanisms of prostate permeability triggered by microbubble-mediated acoustic cavitation. *Cell Biochem Biophys*, 64, 147-53.

Li T., Sotgia F., Vuolo M.A., *et al.,* 2006. Caveolin-1 mutations in human breast cancer: functional association with estrogen receptor alpha-positive status. *Am J Pathol*, 168, 1998-2013.

Li W.W. 2000. Tumor angiogenesis: molecular pathology, therapeutic targeting, and imaging. *Acad Radiol*, 7, 800-11.

Li Y.S., Reid C.N., McHale A.P. 2008. Enhancing ultrasound-mediated cell membrane permeabilisation (sonoporation) using a high frequency pulse regime and implications for ultrasound-aided cancer chemotherapy. *Cancer Lett*, 266, 156-62.

Lim K., Han C., Dai Y., Shen M., Wu T. 2009. Omega-3 polyunsaturated fatty acids inhibit hepatocellular carcinoma cell growth through blocking beta-catenin and cyclooxygenase-2. *Mol Cancer Ther*, 8, 3046-55.

Lin J.X., Mietz J., Modi W.S., John S., Leonard W.J. 1996. Cloning of human Stat5B. Reconstitution of interleukin-2-induced Stat5A and Stat5B DNA binding activity in COS-7 cells. *J Biol Chem*, 271, 10738-44.

Lindner J.R. 2002. Evolving applications for contrast ultrasound. *Am J Cardiol*, 90, 72J-80J.

Lindner J.R. 2009. Molecular imaging of cardiovascular disease with contrast-enhanced ultrasonography. *Nat Rev Cardiol*, 6, 475-81.

Lindner J.R., Wei, K.. 2002. Contrast echocardiography. *Curr Probl Cardiol* 27, 454–519.

Linton K.D., Hamdy F.C. 2003. Early diagnosis and surgical management of prostate cancer. *Cancer Treat Rev*, 29, 151-60.

Liou Y.A., King D.J., Zibrik D., Innis S.M. 2007. Decreasing linoleic acid with constant alpha-linolenic acid in dietary fats increases (n-3) eicosapentaenoic acid in plasma phospholipids in healthy men. *J Nutr*, 137, 945-52.

Lisanti M.P., Scherer P.E., Tang Z., Sargiacomo M. 1994. Caveolae, caveolin and caveolin-rich membrane domains: a signalling hypothesis. *Trends Cell Biol*, 4, 231-5.

Lisanti M.P., Scherer P.E., Vidugiriene J., *et al.,* 1994. Characterization of caveolin-rich membrane domains isolated from an endothelial-rich source: implications for human disease. *J Cell Biol*, 126, 111-26.

Litterst C.M., Kliem S., Lodrini M., Pfitzner E. 2005. Coactivators in gene regulation by STAT5. *Vitam Horm*, 70, 359-86.

Litterst C.M., Kliem S., Marilley D., Pfitzner E. 2003. NCoA-1/SRC-1 is an essential coactivator of STAT5 that binds to the FDL motif in the alpha-helical region of the STAT5 transactivation domain. *J Biol Chem*, 278, 45340-51.

Liu H.L., Hua, M.Y., Chen, P.Y., Chu, P.C., Pan, C.H., Yang, H.W., Huang, C.Y., Wang, J.J., Yen, T.C., Wei, K.C. 2010. Blood-brain barrier disruption with focused ultrasound enhances delivery of chemotherapeutic drugs for glioblastoma treatment. *Radiology*, 255, 415-25.

Liu J., Lee P., Galbiati F., Kitsis R.N., Lisanti M.P. 2001. Caveolin-1 expression sensitizes fibroblastic and epithelial cells to apoptotic stimulation. *Am J Physiol Cell Physiol*, 280, C823-35.

Liu J.X., Mietz J., Modi W.S., John S., Leonard W.J. 1996. Cloning of human Stat5B. Reconstitution of interleukin-2-induced Stat5A and Stat5B DNA binding activity in COS-7 cells. *J Biol Chem*, 271, 10738-44.

Liu P., Ying Y., Anderson R.G. 1997. Platelet-derived growth factor activates mitogen-activated protein kinase in isolated caveolae. *Proc Natl Acad Sci U S A*, 94, 13666-70.

Liu P., Ying Y., Ko Y.-G., Anderson R.G.W. 1996. Localization of the PDGF-stimulated phosphorylation cascade to caveolae. *J Biol Chem*, 271, 10299-303.

Liu X., Gallego M.I., Smith G.H., Robinson G.W., Hennighausen L. 1998. Functional release of Stat5a-null mammary tissue through the activation of compensating signals including Stat5b. *Cell Growth Differ*, 9, 795-803.

Liu X., Robinson G.W., Gouilleux F., Groner B., Hennighausen L. 1995. Cloning and expression of Stat5 and an additional homologue (Stat5b) involved in prolactin signal transduction in mouse mammary tissue. *Proc Natl Acad Sci U S A*, 92, 8831-5.

Liu Y., Miyoshi H., Nakamura M. 2006. Encapsulated ultrasound microbubbles: therapeutic application in drug/gene delivery. *J Control Release*, 114, 89-99.

Liu Y., Yang H., Sakanishi A. 2006. Ultrasound: mechanical gene transfer into plant cells by sonoporation. *Biotechnol Adv*, 24, 1-16.

Liu Y., Yang, H., Sakanishi, A.. 2005. Gene transfer into vascular smooth muscle cells (VSMCs) by ultrasound and microbubbles. *Chinese Journal of Biomedical Engineering* 22, 91-2.

Llorente A., de Marco M.C., Alonso M.A. 2004. Caveolin-1 and MAL are located on prostasomes secreted by the prostate cancer PC-3 cell line. *J Cell Sci*, 117, 5343-51.

Lum A.F., Borden M.A., Dayton P.A., *et al.,* 2006. Ultrasound radiation force enables targeted deposition of model drug carriers loaded on microbubbles. *J Control Release*, 111, 128-34.

Lundberg A.S., Weinberg R.A. 1998. Functional inactivation of the retinoblastoma protein requires sequential modification by at least two distinct cyclin-cdk complexes. *Mol Cell Biol*, 18, 753-61.

Luo P., Wang M.H. 2011. Eicosanoids, beta-cell function, and diabetes. *Prostaglandins Other Lipid Mediat*, 95, 1-10.

Lv W., Yang T. 2012. Identification of possible biomarkers for breast cancer from free fatty acid profiles determined by GC-MS and multivariate statistical analysis. *Clin Biochem*, 45, 127-33.

Maehle L., Lystad E., Eilertsen E., *et al.,* 1999. Growth of human lung adenocarcinoma in nude mice is influenced by various types of dietary fat and vitamin E. *Anticancer Res*, 19, 1649-55.

Magne S., Caron S., Charon M., Rouyez M.C., Dusanter-Fourt I. 2003. STAT5 and Oct-1 form a stable complex that modulates cyclin D1 expression. *Mol Cell Biol*, 23, 8934-45.

Maillard V., Bougnoux P., Ferrari P., *et al.,* 2002. N-3 and N-6 fatty acids in breast adipose tissue and relative risk of breast cancer in a case-control study in Tours, France. *Int J Cancer*, 98, 78-83.

Marg A., Shan Y., Meyer T., *et al.,* 2004. Nucleocytoplasmic shuttling by nucleoporins Nup153 and Nup214 and CRM1-dependent nuclear export control the subcellular distribution of latent Stat1. *J Cell Biol*, 165, 823-33.

Marin A., Sun H., Husseini G.A., *et al.,* 2002. Drug delivery in pluronic micelles: effect of high-frequency ultrasound on drug release from micelles and intracellular uptake. *J Control Release*, 84, 39-47.

Marmottant P., Biben, T., Hilgenfeldt, S. 2008. Deformation and rupture of lipid vesicles in the strong shear flow generated by ultrasound-driven microbubbles. *Proceedings of the Royal Society A*, 464, 1781-800.

Marmottant P., Biben, T., Hilgenfeldt, S. 2008. Deformation and rupture of lipid vesicles in the strong shear flow generated by ultrsound-driven microbubbles. *Proc R Soc A - Mathl Phys Engng Sci*, 464, 1781-800.

Marmottant P., Hilgenfeldt S. 2003. Controlled vesicle deformation and lysis by single oscillating bubbles. *Nature*, 423, 153-6.

Martinez-Outschoorn U.E., Pavlides S., Whitaker-Menezes D., *et al.,* 2010. Tumor cells induce the cancer associated fibroblast phenotype *via* caveolin-1 degradation: Implications for breast cancer and DCIS therapy with autophagy inhibitors. *Cell Cycle*, 9.

Martinez-Outschoorn U.E., Trimmer C., Lin Z., *et al.,* 2010. Autophagy in cancer associated fibroblasts promotes tumor cell survival: Role of hypoxia, HIF1 induction and NFkappaB activation in the tumor stromal microenvironment. *Cell Cycle*, 9, 3515-33.

Martinez-Outschoorn U.E., Whitaker-Menezes D., Pavlides S., *et al.,* 2010. The autophagic tumor stroma model of cancer or "battery-operated tumor growth": A simple solution to the autophagy paradox. *Cell Cycle*, 9, 4297-306.

Maurer A.B., Wichmann C., Gross A., *et al.,* 2002. The Stat5-RARalpha fusion protein represses transcription and differentiation through interaction with a corepressor complex. *Blood*, 99, 2647-52.

May D.J., Allen J.S., Ferrara K.W. 2002. Dynamics and fragmentation of thick-shelled microbubbles. *IEEE Trans Ultrason Ferroelectr Freq Control*, 49, 1400-10.

Mayer C.R., Geis N.A., Katus H.A., Bekeredjian R. 2008. Ultrasound targeted microbubble destruction for drug and gene delivery. *Expert Opin Drug Deliv*, 5, 1121-38.

McBride K.M., Banninger G., McDonald C., Reich N.C. 2002. Regulated nuclear import of the STAT1 transcription factor by direct binding of importin-alpha. *Embo J*, 21, 1754-63.

McBride K.M., McDonald C., Reich N.C. 2000. Nuclear export signal located within theDNA-binding domain of the STAT1transcription factor. *Embo J*, 19, 6196-206.

McDannold N., Vykhodtseva N., Hynynen K. 2006. Targeted disruption of the blood-brain barrier with focused ultrasound: association with cavitation activity. *Phys Med Biol*, 51, 793-807.

McIntosh D.P., Tan X.Y., Oh P., Schnitzer J.E. 2002. Targeting endothelium and its dynamic caveolae for tissue-specific transcytosis *in vivo*: a pathway to overcome cell barriers to drug and gene delivery. *Proc Natl Acad Sci U S A*, 99, 1996-2001.

McNamara W.B. D.Y.T., Suslick K.S. 1999. Sonoluminescence temperatures during multi-bubble cavitation. *Nature*, 401, 772-5.

Mehier-Humbert S., Bettinger T., Yan F., Guy R.H. 2005. Plasma membrane poration induced by ultrasound exposure: implication for drug delivery. *J Control Release*, 104, 213-22.

Meijering B.D., Juffermans L.J., van Wamel A., *et al.,* 2009. Ultrasound and microbubble-targeted delivery of macromolecules is regulated by induction of endocytosis and pore formation. *Circ Res*, 104, 679-87.

Melen K., Kinnunen L., Julkunen I. 2001. Arginine/lysine-rich structural element is involved in interferon-induced nuclear import of STATs. *J Biol Chem*, 276, 16447-55.

Melino S., Zhou M., Tortora M., *et al.,* 2012. Molecular properties of lysozyme-microbubbles: towards the protein and nucleic acid delivery. *Amino Acids*, 43, 885-96.

Mercier I., Casimiro M.C., Wang C., *et al.,* 2008. Human breast cancer-associated fibroblasts (CAFs) show caveolin-1 downregulation and RB tumor suppressor functional inactivation: Implications for the response to hormonal therapy. *Cancer Biol Ther*, 7, 1212-25.

Mercier I., Jasmin J.F., Pavlides S., *et al.,* 2009. Clinical and translational implications of the caveolin gene family: lessons from mouse models and human genetic disorders. *Lab Invest*, 89, 614-23.

Meyer T., Gavenis K., Vinkemeier U. 2002. Cell type-specific and tyrosine phosphorylation-independent nuclear presence of STAT1 and STAT3. *Exp Cell Res*, 272, 45-55.

Meyer W.K., Reichenbach P., Schindler U., Soldaini E., Nabholz M. 1997. Interaction of STAT5 dimers on two low affinity binding sites mediates interleukin 2 (IL-2) stimulation of IL-2 receptor alpha gene transcription. *J Biol Chem*, 272, 31821-8.

Miglietta A., Toselli M., Ravarino N., *et al.,* 2010. COX-2 expression in human breast carcinomas: correlation with clinicopathological features and prognostic molecular markers. *Expert Opin Ther Targets*, 14, 655-64.

Mihran R.T., Barnes F.S., Wachtel H. 1990. Temporally-specific modification of myelinated axon excitability *in vitro* following a single ultrasound pulse. *Ultrasound Med Biol*, 16, 297-309.

Mihran R.T., Barnes F.S., Wachtel H. 1990. Transient modification of nerve excitability *in vitro* by single ultrasound pulses. *Biomed Sci Instrum*, 26, 235-46.

Moghimi S.M., Hamad, I.. 2009. Factors controlling pharmacokinetics of intravenously injected nanoparticulate systems. *Biotechnology: Pharmaceutical Aspects*, 10, 267-82.

Montesano R., Roth J., Robert A., Orci L. 1982. Non-coated membrane invaginations are involved in binding and internalization of cholera and tetanus toxins. *Nature (Lond)*, 296, 651-3.

Morgan K.E., Allen J.S., Dayton P.A., *et al.,* 2000. Experimental and theoretical evaluation of microbubble behavior: effect of transmitted phase and bubble size. *IEEE Trans Ultrason Ferroelectr Freq Control*, 47, 1494-509.

Morris P.G., Zhou X.K., Milne G.L., *et al.,* 2013. Increased Levels of Urinary PGE-M, a Biomarker of Inflammation, Occur in Association with Obesity, Aging, and Lung Metastases in Patients with Breast Cancer. *Cancer Prev Res (Phila).*

Morse P.M., Ingard K. U. Theoretical Acoustics. Princeton, NJ: Princeton University Press; 1968.

Mui A.L., Wakao H., Harada N., O'Farrell A.M., Miyajima A. 1995. Interleukin-3, granulocyte-macrophage colony-stimulating factor, and interleukin-5 transduce signals through two forms of STAT5. *J Leukoc Biol*, 57, 799-803.

Mui A.L., Wakao H., O'Farrell A.M., Harada N., Miyajima A. 1995. Interleukin-3, granulocyte-macrophage colony stimulating factor and interleukin-5 transduce signals through two STAT5 homologs. *Embo J*, 14, 1166-75.

Mukherjee D., Wong J., Griffin B., *et al.,* 2000. Ten-fold augmentation of endothelial uptake of vascular endothelial growth factor with ultrasound after systemic administration. *J Am Coll Cardiol*, 35, 1678-86.

Murata M., Peranen J., Schreiner R., *et al.,* 1995. VIP21/caveolin is a cholesterol-binding protein. *Proc Natl Acad Sci, USA*, 92, 10339-43.

Murff H.J., Shu X.O., Li H., *et al.,* 2011. Dietary polyunsaturated fatty acids and breast cancer risk in Chinese women: a prospective cohort study. *Int J Cancer*, 128, 1434-41.

Murphy R.A., Mourtzakis M., Chu Q.S., *et al.,* 2011. Nutritional intervention with fish oil provides a benefit over standard of care for weight and skeletal muscle mass in patients with nonsmall cell lung cancer receiving chemotherapy. *Cancer*, 117, 1775-82.

Murphy R.A., Mourtzakis M., Chu Q.S., *et al.,* 2011. Supplementation with fish oil increases first-line chemotherapy efficacy in patients with advanced nonsmall cell lung cancer. *Cancer*, 117, 3774-80.

Nagel-Wolfrum K., Buerger C., Wittig I., *et al.,* 2004. The interaction of specific peptide aptamers with the DNA binding domain and the dimerization domain of the transcription factor Stat3 inhibits transactivation and induces apoptosis in tumor cells. *Mol Cancer Res*, 2, 170-82.

Nakajima H., Brindle P.K., Handa M., Ihle J.N. 2001. Functional interaction of STAT5 and nuclear receptor co-repressor SMRT: implications in negative regulation of STAT5-dependent transcription. *Embo J*, 20, 6836-44.

Nande R., Greco A., Gossman M.S., *et al.,* 2013. Microbubble-Assisted p53, RB, and p130 Gene Transfer in Combination with Radiation Therapy in Prostate Cancer. *Curr Gene Ther*, 13, 163-74.

Narayan P., Wheatley, M.A.. 1999. Preparation and characterization of hollow microcapsules for use as ultrasound contrast agents. *Polymer Engineering and Science*, 39, 2242-55.

Nasu Y., Timme T.L., Yang G., *et al.,* 1998. Suppression of caveolin expression induces androgen sensitivity in metastatic androgen-insensitive mouse prostate cancer cells. *Nat Med*, 4, 1062-4.

Nevalainen M.T., Ahonen T.J., Yamashita H., *et al.,* 2000. Epithelial defect in prostates of Stat5a-null mice. *Lab Invest*, 80, 993-1006.

Nevalainen M.T., Valve E.M., Ahonen T., *et al.,* 1997. Androgen-dependent expression of prolactin in rat prostate epithelium *in vivo* and in organ culture. *Faseb J*, 11, 1297-307.

Nevalainen M.T., Valve E.M., Ingleton P.M., Harkonen P.L. 1996. Expression and hormone regulation of prolactin receptors in rat dorsal and lateral prostate. *Endocrinology*, 137, 3078-88.

Nevalainen M.T., Valve E.M., Ingleton P.M., *et al.,* 1997. Prolactin and prolactin receptors are expressed and functioning in human prostate. *J Clin Invest*, 99, 618-27.

Nevalainen M.T., Valve E.M., Makela S.I., *et al.,* 1991. Estrogen and prolactin regulation of rat dorsal and lateral prostate in organ culture. *Endocrinology*, 129, 612-22.

Nevalainen M.T., Xie J., Bubendorf L., Wagner K.U., Rui H. 2002. Basal activation of transcription factor signal transducer and activator of transcription (Stat5) in nonpregnant mouse and human breast epithelium. *Mol Endocrinol*, 16, 1108-24.

Newman K.D., Dunn P.F., Owens J.W., *et al.,* 1995. Adenovirus-mediated gene transfer into normal rabbit arteries results in prolonged vascular cell activation, inflammation, and neointimal hyperplasia. *J Clin Invest*, 96, 2955-65.

Niki E. 2009. Lipid peroxidation: physiological levels and dual biological effects. *Free Radic Biol Med*, 47, 469-84.

Niles W.D., Malik A.B. 1999. Endocytosis and exocytosis events regulate vesicle traffic in endothelial cells. *J Membr Biol*, 167, 85-101.

Nomikou N., McHale A.P. 2010. Exploiting ultrasound-mediated effects in delivering targeted, site-specific cancer therapy. *Cancer Lett*, 296, 133-43.

Ochiai M., Oguri T., Isobe T., Ishioka S., Yamakido M. 1999. Cyclooxygenase-2 (COX-2) mRNA expression levels in normal lung tissues and non-small cell lung cancers. *Jpn J Cancer Res*, 90, 1338-43.

Ohtsuki S., Sato, S., Yamaguchi, H., Kamoi, M., Asashima, T., Terasaki, T. 2007. Exogenous expression of claudin-5 induces barrier properties in cultured rat brain capillary endothelial cells. *J Cell Physiol*, 201, 81-6.

Okamoto T., Schlegel A., Scherer P.E., Lisanti M.P. 1998. Caveolins, A family of scaffolding proteins for organizing "pre-assembled signaling complexes" at the plasma membrane. *J Biol Chem, (Mini-review)*, 273, 5419-22.

Pai R., Soreghan B., Szabo I.L., *et al.,* 2002. Prostaglandin E2 transactivates EGF receptor: a novel mechanism for promoting colon cancer growth and gastrointestinal hypertrophy. *Nat Med*, 8, 289-93.

Palade G.E. 1953. An electron microscope study of the mitochondrial structure. *J Histochem Cytochem*, 1, 188-211.

Pallard C., Gouilleux F., Benit L., *et al.,* 1995. Thrombopoietin activates a STAT5-like factor in hematopoietic cells. *Embo J*, 14, 2847-56.

Pallard C., Gouilleux F., Charon M., *et al.,* 1995. Interleukin-3, erythropoietin, and prolactin activate a STAT5-like factor in lymphoid cells. *J Biol Chem*, 270, 15942-5.

Paquette B., Bisson M., Baptiste C., *et al.,* 2005. Invasiveness of breast cancer cells MDA-MB-231 through extracellular matrix is increased by the estradiol metabolite 4-hydroxyestradiol. *Int J Cancer*, 113, 706-11.

Parthasarathy S., Santanam N., Ramachandran S., Meilhac O. 2000. Potential role of oxidized lipids and lipoproteins in antioxidant defense. *Free Radic Res*, 33, 197-215.

Parton R.G., Joggerst B., Simons K. 1994. Regulated internalization of caveolae. *J Cell Biol*, 127, 1199-215.

Pasqualini R., Arap W., McDonald D.M. 2002. Probing the structural and molecular diversity of tumor vasculature. *Trends Mol Med*, 8, 563-71.

Patterson E., Wall R., Fitzgerald G.F., Ross R.P., Stanton C. 2012. Health implications of high dietary omega-6 polyunsaturated Fatty acids. *J Nutr Metab*, 2012, 539426.

Patterson R.E., Flatt S.W., Newman V.A., *et al.,* 2011. Marine fatty acid intake is associated with breast cancer prognosis. *J Nutr*, 141, 201-6.

Paukku K., Yang J., Silvennoinen O. 2003. Tudor and nuclease-like domains containing protein p100 function as coactivators for signal transducer and activator of transcription 5. *Mol Endocrinol*, 17, 1805-14.

Pavlides S., Tsirigos A., Migneco G., *et al.*, 2010. The autophagic tumor stroma model of cancer: Role of oxidative stress and ketone production in fueling tumor cell metabolism. *Cell Cycle*, 9, 3485-505.

Pavlides S., Tsirigos A., Vera I., *et al.*, 2010. Loss of stromal caveolin-1 leads to oxidative stress, mimics hypoxia and drives inflammation in the tumor microenvironment, conferring the "reverse Warburg effect": A transcriptional informatics analysis with validation. *Cell Cycle*, 9.

Pavlides S., Whitaker-Menezes D., Castello-Cros R., *et al.*, 2009. The reverse Warburg effect: aerobic glycolysis in cancer associated fibroblasts and the tumor stroma. *Cell Cycle*, 8, 3984-4001.

Pender-Cudlip M.C., Krag K.J., Martini D., *et al.*, 2013. Delta-6-desaturase activity and arachidonic acid synthesis are increased in human breast cancer tissue. *Cancer Sci.*

Peng B., Sutherland K.D., Sum E.Y., *et al.*, 2002. CPAP is a novel stat5-interacting cofactor that augments stat5-mediated transcriptional activity. *Mol Endocrinol*, 16, 2019-33.

Pepper C., Mahdi J.G., Buggins A.G., *et al.*, 2011. Two novel aspirin analogues show selective cytotoxicity in primary chronic lymphocytic leukaemia cells that is associated with dual inhibition of Rel A and COX-2. *Cell Prolif*, 44, 380-90.

Perrone G., Santini D., Vincenzi B., *et al.*, 2005. COX-2 expression in DCIS: correlation with VEGF, HER-2/neu, prognostic molecular markers and clinicopathological features. *Histopathology*, 46, 561-8.

Pianetti S., Arsura M., Romieu-Mourez R., Coffey R.J., Sonenshein G.E. 2001. Her-2/neu overexpression induces NF-kappaB *via* a PI3-kinase/Akt pathway involving calpain-mediated degradation of IkappaB-alpha that can be inhibited by the tumor suppressor PTEN. *Oncogene*, 20, 1287-99.

Porter T.R., Iversen P.L., Li S., Xie F. 1996. Interaction of diagnostic ultrasound with synthetic oligonucleotide-labeled perfluorocarbon-exposed sonicated dextrose albumin microbubbles. *J Ultrasound Med*, 15, 577-84.

Porter T.R., Xie F. 1995. Visually discernible myocardial echocardiographic contrast after intravenous injection of sonicated dextrose albumin microbubbles containing high molecular weight, less soluble gases. *J Am Coll Cardiol*, 25, 509-15.

Postema M., Bouakaz A., Versluis M., de Jong N. 2005. Ultrasound-induced gas release from contrast agent microbubbles. *IEEE Trans Ultrason Ferroelectr Freq Control*, 52, 1035-41.

Postema M., Schmitz G. 2007. Ultrasonic bubbles in medicine: influence of the shell. *Ultrason Sonochem*, 14, 438-44.

Postema M.A.B. Medical Bubbles. Veenendaal: Universal Press; 2004.

Predescu S.A., Predescu D.N., Palade G.E. 1997. Plasmalemmal vesicles function as transcytotic carriers for small proteins in the continuous endothelium. *Am J Physiol*, 272, H937-49.

Prentice P., Cuschieri, A., Dholakia, K., Prausnitz, M., Campbell, P. 2005. Membrane disruption by optically controlled microbubble cavitation. *Nature Physics*, 1, 107-10.

Price R.J., Skyba D.M., Kaul S., Skalak T.C. 1998. Delivery of colloidal particles and red blood cells to tissue through microvessel ruptures created by targeted microbubble destruction with ultrasound. *Circulation*, 98, 1264-7.

Racine C., Belanger M., Hirabayashi H., *et al.*, 1999. Reduction of caveolin 1 gene expression in lung carcinoma cell lines. *Biochem Biophys Res Commun*, 255, 580-6.

Rajjayabun P.H., Garg S., Durkan G.C., *et al.*, 2001. Caveolin-1 expression is associated with high-grade bladder cancer. *Urology*, 58, 811-4.

Ram P.A., Waxman D.J. 1999. SOCS/CIS protein inhibition of growth hormone-stimulated STAT5 signaling by multiple mechanisms. *J Biol Chem*, 274, 35553-61.

Rapoport N., Gao Z., Kennedy A. 2007. Multifunctional nanoparticles for combining ultrasonic tumor imaging and targeted chemotherapy. *J Natl Cancer Inst*, 99, 1095-106.

Rapoport N.Y., Kennedy A.M., Shea J.E., Scaife C.L., Nam K.H. 2009. Controlled and targeted tumor chemotherapy by ultrasound-activated nanoemulsions/microbubbles. *J Control Release*, 138, 268-76.

Razani B., Altschuler Y., Zhu L., *et al.*, 2000. Caveolin-1 expression is down-regulated in cells transformed by the human papilloma virus in a p53-dependent manner. Replacement of caveolin-1 expression suppresses HPV-mediated cell transformation. *Biochemistry*, 39, 13916-24.

Reader J., Holt D., Fulton A. 2011. Prostaglandin E2 EP receptors as therapeutic targets in breast cancer. *Cancer Metastasis Rev*, 30, 449-63.

Reich N.C., Liu L. 2006. Tracking STAT nuclear traffic. *Nat Rev Immunol*, 6, 602-12.

Ren S.T., Liao Y.R., Kang X.N., *et al.*, 2013. The antitumor effect of a new docetaxel-loaded microbubble combined with low-frequency ultrasound *in vitro*: preparation and parameter analysis. *Pharm Res*, 30, 1574-85.

Ricciotti E., FitzGerald G.A. 2011. Prostaglandins and inflammation. *Arterioscler Thromb Vasc Biol*, 31, 986-1000.

Riches J.C., Ramsay A.G., Gribben J.G. 2011. Chronic lymphocytic leukemia: an update on biology and treatment. *Curr Oncol Rep*, 13, 379-85.

Riesz P., Kondo T. 1992. Free radical formation induced by ultrasound and its biological implications. *Free Radic Biol Med*, 13, 247-70.

Ristimaki A., Sivula A., Lundin J., *et al.*, 2002. Prognostic significance of elevated cyclooxygenase-2 expression in breast cancer. *Cancer Res*, 62, 632-5.

Rooney J.A. 1970. Hemolysis near an ultrasonically pulsating gas bubble. *Science*, 169, 869-71.

Rothberg K.G., Heuser J.E., Donzell W.C., *et al.*, 1992. Caveolin, a protein component of caveolae membrane coats. *Cell*, 68, 673-82.

Ryan E.P., Pollock S.J., Kaur K., *et al.*, 2006. Constitutive and activation-inducible cyclooxygenase-2 expression enhances survival of chronic lymphocytic leukemia B cells. *Clin Immunol*, 120, 76-90.

Rychak J.J., Li B., Acton S.T., *et al.*, 2006. Selectin ligands promote ultrasound contrast agent adhesion under shear flow. *Mol Pharm*, 3, 516-24.

Sargiacomo M., Scherer P.E., Tang Z.-L., *et al.*, 1995. Oligomeric structure of caveolin: Implications for caveolae membrane organization. *Proc Natl Acad Sci, USA*, 92, 9407-11.

Satoh T., Yang G., Egawa S., *et al.*, 2003. Caveolin-1 expression is a predictor of recurrence-free survival in pT2N0 prostate carcinoma diagnosed in Japanese patients. *Cancer*, 97, 1225-33.

Scherer P.E., Lewis R.Y., Volonte D., *et al.*, 1997. Cell-type and tissue-specific expression of caveolin-2. Caveolins 1 and 2 co-localize and form a stable hetero-oligomeric complex *in vivo*. *J Biol Chem*, 272, 29337-46.

Scherer P.E., Lisanti M.P., Baldini G., *et al.*, 1994. Induction of caveolin during adipogenesis and association of GLUT4 with caveolin-rich vesicles. *J Cell Biol*, 127, 1233-43.

Scherer P.E., Okamoto T., Chun M., *et al.,* 1996. Identification, sequence and expression of caveolin-2 defines a caveolin gene family. *Proc Natl Acad Sci, USA*, 93, 131-5.

Schindler C., Darnell J.E., Jr. 1995. Transcriptional responses to polypeptide ligands: the JAK-STAT pathway. *Annu Rev Biochem*, 64, 621-51.

Schindler C.W. 2002. Series introduction. JAK-STAT signaling in human disease. *J Clin Invest*, 109, 1133-7.

Schmidt D., Muller S. 2003. PIAS/SUMO: new partners in transcriptional regulation. *Cell Mol Life Sci*, 60, 2561-74.

Schmitt-Ney M., Doppler W., Ball R.K., Groner B. 1991. Beta-casein gene promoter activity is regulated by the hormone-mediated relief of transcriptional repression and a mammary-gland-specific nuclear factor. *Mol Cell Biol*, 11, 3745-55.

Schmitt-Ney M., Happ B., Ball R.K., Groner B. 1992. Developmental and environmental regulation of a mammary gland-specific nuclear factor essential for transcription of the gene encoding beta-casein. *Proc Natl Acad Sci U S A*, 89, 3130-4.

Schmitt-Ney M., Happ B., Hofer P., Hynes N.E., Groner B. 1992. Mammary gland-specific nuclear factor activity is positively regulated by lactogenic hormones and negatively by milk stasis. *Mol Endocrinol*, 6, 1988-97.

Schmitz G., Ecker J. 2008. The opposing effects of n-3 and n-6 fatty acids. *Prog Lipid Res*, 47, 147-55.

Schnitzer J.E. Vascular Endothelium: Physiology, Pathology and Therapeutic Opportunities.. Born GVR, Schwartz, C.J., editor. Stuttgart: Schattauer; 1997.

Schnitzer J.E., Oh P., Pinney E., Allard J. 1994. Filipin-sensitive caveolae-mediated transport in endothelium: Reduced transcytosis, scavenger endoctytosis, and capillary permeability of select macromolecules. *J Cell Biol*, 127, 1217-32.

Schnitzer J.E., Oh P., Pinney E., Allard J. 1994. Filipin-sensitive caveolae-mediated transport in endothelium: reduced transcytosis, scavenger endocytosis, and capillary permeability of select macromolecules. *J Cell Biol*, 127, 1217-32.

Schutt *E.G.*, Klein D.H., Mattrey R.M., Riess J.G. 2003. Injectable microbubbles as contrast agents for diagnostic ultrasound imaging: the key role of perfluorochemicals. *Angew Chem Int Ed Engl*, 42, 3218-35.

Secchiero P., Barbarotto E., Gonelli A., *et al.,* 2005. Potential pathogenetic implications of cyclooxygenase-2 overexpression in B chronic lymphoid leukemia cells. *Am J Pathol*, 167, 1599-607.

Sekimoto T., Imamoto N., Nakajima K., Hirano T., Yoneda Y. 1997. Extracellular signal-dependent nuclear import of Stat1 is mediated by nuclear pore-targeting complex formation with NPI-1, but not Rch1. *Embo J*, 16, 7067-77.

Sekimoto T., Nakajima K., Tachibana T., Hirano T., Yoneda Y. 1996. Interferon-gamma-dependent nuclear import of Stat1 is mediated by the GTPase activity of Ran/TC4. *J Biol Chem*, 271, 31017-20.

Serhan C.N., Petasis N.A. 2011. Resolvins and protectins in inflammation resolution. *Chem Rev*, 111, 5922-43.

Serini S., Trombino S., Oliva F., *et al.,* 2008. Docosahexaenoic acid induces apoptosis in lung cancer cells by increasing MKP-1 and down-regulating p-ERK1/2 and p-p38 expression. *Apoptosis*, 13, 1172-83.

Seward J.B., Tajik A.J., Hagler D.J., Ritter D.G. 1977. Peripheral venous contrast echocardiography. *Am J Cardiol*, 39, 202-12.

Shanafelt T.D., Call T.G. 2004. Current approach to diagnosis and management of chronic lymphocytic leukemia. *Mayo Clin Proc*, 79, 388-98.

Shang X., Wang, P., Liu, Y., Zhang, Z., Xue, Y. 2011. Mechanism of low-frequency ultrasound in opening blood-tumor barrier by tight junction. *J Mol Neurosci*, 43, 364-9.

Shapira N. 2012. Women's higher risk with N-6 PUFA *vs.* men's relative advantage: an "N-6 gender nutrition paradox" hypothesis. *Isr Med Assoc J*, 14, 435-41.

Sheikov N., McDannold N., Sharma S., Hynynen K. 2008. Effect of focused ultrasound applied with an ultrasound contrast agent on the tight junctional integrity of the brain microvascular endothelium. *Ultrasound Med Biol*, 34, 1093-104.

Shin J.S., Gao Z., Abraham S.N. 2000. Involvement of cellular caveolae in bacterial entry into mast cells. *Science*, 289, 785-8.

Shishodia S., Koul D., Aggarwal B.B. 2004. Cyclooxygenase (COX)-2 inhibitor celecoxib abrogates TNF-induced NF-kappa B activation through inhibition of activation of I kappa B alpha kinase and Akt in human non-small cell lung carcinoma: correlation with suppression of COX-2 synthesis. *J Immunol*, 173, 2011-22.

Shive M.S., Anderson J.M. 1997. Biodegradation and biocompatibility of PLA and PLGA microspheres. *Adv Drug Deliv Rev*, 28, 5-24.

Shohet R.V., Chen S., Zhou Y.T., *et al.*, 2000. Echocardiographic destruction of albumin microbubbles directs gene delivery to the myocardium. *Circulation*, 101, 2554-6.

Shomura Y., Tanigawa N., Shibutani M., *et al.*, 2011. Water-soluble polyvinyl alcohol microspheres for temporary embolization: development and *in vivo* characteristics in a pig kidney model. *J Vasc Interv Radiol*, 22, 212-9.

Shortencarier M.J., Dayton P.A., Bloch S.H., *et al.*, 2004. A method for radiation-force localized drug delivery using gas-filled lipospheres. *IEEE Trans Ultrason Ferroelectr Freq Control*, 51, 822-31.

Shridhar V., Sun Q.C., Miller O.J., *et al.*, 1997. Loss of heterozygosity on the long arm of human chromosome 7 in sporadic renal cell carcinomas. *Oncogene*, 15, 2727-33.

Sicinski P., Donaher J.L., Parker S.B., *et al.*, 1995. Cyclin D1 provides a link between development and oncogenesis in the retina and breast. *Cell*, 82, 621-30.

Silber R., Degar B., Costin D., *et al.*, 1994. Chemosensitivity of lymphocytes from patients with B-cell chronic lymphocytic leukemia to chlorambucil, fludarabine, and camptothecin analogs. *Blood*, 84, 3440-6.

Simopoulos A.P. 1991. Omega-3 fatty acids in health and disease and in growth and development. *Am J Clin Nutr*, 54, 438-63.

Simopoulos A.P. 2000. Human requirement for N-3 polyunsaturated fatty acids. *Poult Sci*, 79, 961-70.

Simopoulos A.P. 2002. The importance of the ratio of omega-6/omega-3 essential fatty acids. *Biomed Pharmacother*, 56, 365-79.

Simopoulos A.P. 2008. The importance of the omega-6/omega-3 fatty acid ratio in cardiovascular disease and other chronic diseases. *Exp Biol Med (Maywood)*, 233, 674-88.

Singh R., Husseini G.A., Pitt W.G. 2012. Phase transitions of nanoemulsions using ultrasound: experimental observations. *Ultrason Sonochem*, 19, 1120-5.

Sirsi S., Borden M. 2009. Microbubble Compositions, Properties and Biomedical Applications. *Bubble Sci Eng Technol*, 1, 3-17.

Skyba D.M., Price R.J., Linka A.Z., Skalak T.C., Kaul S. 1998. Direct *in vivo* visualization of intravascular destruction of microbubbles by ultrasound and its local effects on tissue. *Circulation*, 98, 290-3.

Sloan E.K., Ciocca D.R., Pouliot N., *et al.,* 2009. Stromal cell expression of caveolin-1 predicts outcome in breast cancer. *Am J Pathol*, 174, 2035-43.

Sloan E.K., Stanley K.L., Anderson R.L. 2004. Caveolin-1 inhibits breast cancer growth and metastasis. *Oncogene*, 23, 7893-7.

Smart E.J., Ying Y., Donzell W.C., Anderson R.G. 1996. A role for caveolin in transport of cholesterol from endoplasmic reticulum to plasma membrane. *J Biol Chem*, 271, 29427-35.

Smart E.J., Ying Y.-s., Donzell W.C., Anderson R.G.W. 1996. A role for caveolin in transport of cholesterol from endoplasmic reticulum to plasma membrane. *J Biol Chem*, 271, 29427-35.

Smart E.J., Ying Y.S., Mineo C., Anderson R.G. 1995. A detergent-free method for purifying caveolae membrane from tissue culture cells. *Proc Natl Acad Sci U S A*, 92, 10104-8.

Smith N.B., Lee S., Maione E., *et al.,* 2003. Ultrasound-mediated transdermal transport of insulin *in vitro* through human skin using novel transducer designs. *Ultrasound Med Biol*, 29, 311-7.

Soldaini E., John S., Moro S., *et al.,* 2000. DNA binding site selection of dimeric and tetrameric Stat5 proteins reveals a large repertoire of divergent tetrameric Stat5a binding sites. *Mol Cell Biol*, 20, 389-401.

Soliman O.I., Geleijnse M.L., Meijboom F.J., *et al.,* 2007. The use of contrast echocardiography for the detection of cardiac shunts. *Eur J Echocardiogr*, 8, S2-12.

Song J., Chappell J.C., Qi M., *et al.,* 2002. Influence of injection site, microvascular pressure and ultrasound variables on microbubble-mediated delivery of microspheres to muscle. *J Am Coll Cardiol*, 39, 726-31.

Sonoda S., Tachibana K., Uchino E., *et al.,* 2007. Inhibition of melanoma by ultrasound-microbubble-aided drug delivery suggests membrane permeabilization. *Cancer Biol Ther*, 6, 1276-83.

Sotgia F., Del Galdo F., Casimiro M.C., *et al.,* 2009. Caveolin-1-/- null mammary stromal fibroblasts share characteristics with human breast cancer-associated fibroblasts. *Am J Pathol*, 174, 746-61.

Sotgia F., Rui H., Bonuccelli G., *et al.,* 2006. Caveolin-1, mammary stem cells, and estrogen-dependent breast cancers. *Cancer Res*, 66, 10647-51.

Stangelberger A., Schally A.V., Varga J.L., *et al.,* 2005. Inhibitory effect of antagonists of bombesin and growth hormone-releasing hormone on orthotopic and intraosseous growth and invasiveness of PC-3 human prostate cancer in nude mice. *Clin Cancer Res*, 11, 49-57.

Stieger S.M., Caskey C.F., Adamson R.H., *et al.,* 2007. Enhancement of vascular permeability with low-frequency contrast-enhanced ultrasound in the chorioallantoic membrane model. *Radiology*, 243, 112-21.

Stieger S.M., Caskey, C.F., Adamson, R.H., Qin, S., Curry, F.R., Wisner, E.R., Ferrara, K.W. 2007. Enhancement of vascular permeability with low-frequency contrast-enhanced ultrasound in the chorioallantoic membrane model. *Radiology*, 243, 112-21.

Stocklin E., Wissler M., Gouilleux F., Groner B. 1996. Functional interactions between Stat5 and the glucocorticoid receptor. *Nature*, 383, 726-8.

Stride E., Saffari N. 2003. On the destruction of microbubble ultrasound contrast agents. *Ultrasound Med Biol*, 29, 563-73.

Sun X., Nair J., Linseisen J., Owen R.W., Bartsch H. 2012. Lipid peroxidation and DNA adduct formation in lymphocytes of premenopausal women: Role of estrogen metabolites and fatty acid intake. *Int J Cancer*, 131, 1983-90.

Suslick K.S. 1990. Sonochemistry. *Science*, 247, 1439-45.

Sutton J.T., Haworth K.J., Pyne-Geithman G., Holland C.K. 2013. Ultrasound-mediated drug delivery for cardiovascular disease. *Expert Opin Drug Deliv*, 10, 573-92.

Ta C.N., Liberman A., Paul Martinez H., *et al.*, 2012. Integrated processing of contrast pulse sequencing ultrasound imaging for enhanced active contrast of hollow gas filled silica nanoshells and microshells. *J Vac Sci Technol B Nanotechnol Microelectron*, 30, 2C104.

Tachibana K., Tachibana S. 1995. Albumin microbubble echo-contrast material as an enhancer for ultrasound accelerated thrombolysis. *Circulation*, 92, 1148-50.

Tagne J.B., Kakumanu S., Nicolosi R.J. 2008. Nanoemulsion preparations of the anticancer drug dacarbazine significantly increase its efficacy in a xenograft mouse melanoma model. *Mol Pharm*, 5, 1055-63.

Tahir S.A., Frolov A., Hayes T.G., *et al.*, 2006. Preoperative serum caveolin-1 as a prognostic marker for recurrence in a radical prostatectomy cohort. *Clin Cancer Res*, 12, 4872-5.

Tahir S.A., Ren C., Timme T.L., *et al.*, 2003. Development of an immunoassay for serum caveolin-1: a novel biomarker for prostate cancer. *Clin Cancer Res*, 9, 3653-9.

Tahir S.A., Yang G., Ebara S., *et al.*, 2001. Secreted caveolin-1 stimulates cell survival/clonal growth and contributes to metastasis in androgen-insensitive prostate cancer. *Cancer Res*, 61, 3882-5.

Tahir S.A., Yang G., Goltsov A.A., *et al.*, 2008. Tumor cell-secreted caveolin-1 has proangiogenic activities in prostate cancer. *Cancer Res*, 68, 731-9.

Takalkar A.M., Klibanov A.L., Rychak J.J., Lindner J.R., Ley K. 2004. Binding and detachment dynamics of microbubbles targeted to P-selectin under controlled shear flow. *J Control Release*, 96, 473-82.

Tan S.H., Dagvadorj A., Shen F., *et al.*, 2008. Transcription factor Stat5 synergizes with androgen receptor in prostate cancer cells. *Cancer Res*, 68, 236-48.

Tang D.W., Lin S.C., Chang K.W., *et al.*, 2003. Elevated expression of cyclooxygenase (COX)-2 in oral squamous cell carcinoma--evidence for COX-2 induction by areca quid ingredients in oral keratinocytes. *J Oral Pathol Med*, 32, 522-9.

Tang X., Liu D., Shishodia S., *et al.*, 2006. Nuclear factor-kappaB (NF-kappaB) is frequently expressed in lung cancer and preneoplastic lesions. *Cancer*, 107, 2637-46.

Tang Z.-L., Scherer P.E., Okamoto T., *et al.*, 1996. Molecular cloning of caveolin-3, a novel member of the caveolin gene family expressed predominantly in muscle. *J Biol Chem*, 271, 2255-61.

Taniyama Y., Tachibana K., Hiraoka K., *et al.*, 2002. Local delivery of plasmid DNA into rat carotid artery using ultrasound. *Circulation*, 105, 1233-9.

Tartis M.S., Kruse D.E., Zheng H., *et al.*, 2008. Dynamic microPET imaging of ultrasound contrast agents and lipid delivery. *J Control Release*, 131, 160-6.

Tartis M.S., McCallan J., Lum A.F., *et al.*, 2006. Therapeutic effects of paclitaxel-containing ultrasound contrast agents. *Ultrasound Med Biol*, 32, 1771-80.

ter Haar G. 2009. Safety and bio-effects of ultrasound contrast agents. *Med Biol Eng Comput*, 47, 893-900.

Teupe C., Richter S., Fisslthaler B., *et al.*, 2002. Vascular gene transfer of phosphomimetic endothelial nitric oxide synthase (S1177D) using ultrasound-enhanced destruction of plasmid-loaded microbubbles improves vasoreactivity. *Circulation*, 105, 1104-9.

Thiebaut A.C., Chajes V., Gerber M., *et al.*, 2009. Dietary intakes of omega-6 and omega-3 polyunsaturated fatty acids and the risk of breast cancer. *Int J Cancer*, 124, 924-31.

Thiele C., Hannah M.J., Fahrenholz F., Huttner W.B. 2000. Cholesterol binds to synaptophysin and is required for biogenesis of synaptic vesicles. *Nat Cell Biol*, 2, 42-9.

Thompson T.C., Tahir S.A., Li L., *et al.*, 2010. The role of caveolin-1 in prostate cancer: clinical implications. *Prostate Cancer Prostatic Dis*, 13, 6-11.

Torres V.A., Tapia J.C., Rodriguez D.A., *et al.*, 2007. E-cadherin is required for caveolin-1-mediated down-regulation of the inhibitor of apoptosis protein survivin *via* reduced beta-catenin-Tcf/Lef-dependent transcription. *Mol Cell Biol*, 27, 7703-17.

Tran T.A., Roger, S., Le, J.Y., Guennec, J.Y., Tranquart, F., Bouakaz, A. 2006. Effect of ultrasound activated microbubbles on the cell electrophysiological properties. *Ultrasound Med Biol*, 33, 158-63.

Treat L.H., McDannold N., Vykhodtseva N., *et al.*, 2007. Targeted delivery of doxorubicin to the rat brain at therapeutic levels using MRI-guided focused ultrasound. *Int J Cancer*, 121, 901-7.

Trimmer C., Whitaker-Menezes D., Bonuccelli G., *et al.*, 2010. CAV1 inhibits metastatic potential in melanomas through suppression of the integrin/Src/FAK signaling pathway. *Cancer Res*, 70, 7489-99.

Tsurutani J., Castillo S.S., Brognard J., *et al.*, 2005. Tobacco components stimulate Akt-dependent proliferation and NFkappaB-dependent survival in lung cancer cells. *Carcinogenesis*, 26, 1182-95.

Tsutsui J.M., Xie F., Porter R.T. 2004. The use of microbubbles to target drug delivery. *Cardiovasc Ultrasound*, 2, 23.

Turkson J., Kim J.S., Zhang S., *et al.*, 2004. Novel peptidomimetic inhibitors of signal transducer and activator of transcription 3 dimerization and biological activity. *Mol Cancer Ther*, 3, 261-9.

Turkson J., Ryan D., Kim J.S., *et al.*, 2001. Phosphotyrosyl peptides block Stat3-mediated DNA binding activity, gene regulation, and cell transformation. *J Biol Chem*, 276, 45443-55.

Uittenbogaard A., Ying Y., Smart E.J. 1998. Characterization of a cytosolic heat-shock protein-caveolin chaperone complex. Involvement in cholesterol trafficking. *J Biol Chem*, 273, 6525-32.

Unger E.C., Hersh E., Vannan M., McCreery T. 2001. Gene delivery using ultrasound contrast agents. *Echocardiography*, 18, 355-61.

Unger E.C., Matsunaga T.O., McCreery T., *et al.*, 2002. Therapeutic applications of microbubbles. *Eur J Radiol*, 42, 160-8.

Unger E.C., McCreery T.P., Sweitzer R.H., Caldwell V.E., Wu Y. 1998. Acoustically active lipospheres containing paclitaxel: a new therapeutic ultrasound contrast agent. *Invest Radiol*, 33, 886-92.

Unger E.C., Porter T., Culp W., *et al.*, 2004. Therapeutic applications of lipid-coated microbubbles. *Adv Drug Deliv Rev*, 56, 1291-314.

Ungureanu D., Saharinen P., Junttila I., Hilton D.J., Silvennoinen O. 2002. Regulation of Jak2 through the ubiquitin-proteasome pathway involves phosphorylation of Jak2 on Y1007 and interaction with SOCS-1. *Mol Cell Biol*, 22, 3316-26.

van der Meij B.S., Langius J.A., Spreeuwenberg M.D., *et al.*, 2012. Oral nutritional supplements containing n-3 polyunsaturated fatty acids affect quality of life and functional status in lung cancer patients during multimodality treatment: an RCT. *Eur J Clin Nutr*, 66, 399-404.

Van Liew H.D., Burkard M.E. 1995. Bubbles in circulating blood: stabilization and simulations of cyclic changes of size and content. *J Appl Physiol*, 79, 1379-85.

van Wamel A., Kooiman K., Emmer M., *et al.,* 2006. Ultrasound microbubble induced endothelial cell permeability. *J Control Release*, 116, e100-2.

van Wamel A., Kooiman K., Harteveld M., *et al.,* 2006. Vibrating microbubbles poking individual cells: drug transfer into cells *via* sonoporation. *J Control Release*, 112, 149-55.

Villanueva F.S., Jankowski R.J., Klibanov S., *et al.,* 1998. Microbubbles targeted to intercellular adhesion molecule-1 bind to activated coronary artery endothelial cells. *Circulation*, 98, 1-5.

Villanueva F.S., Lu E., Bowry S., *et al.,* 2007. Myocardial ischemic memory imaging with molecular echocardiography. *Circulation*, 115, 345-52.

Vinkemeier U. 2004. Getting the message across, STAT! Design principles of a molecular signaling circuit. *J Cell Biol*, 167, 197-201.

Vinkemeier U., Moarefi I., Darnell J.E., Jr., Kuriyan J. 1998. Structure of the amino-terminal protein interaction domain of STAT-4. *Science*, 279, 1048-52.

Vinothini G., Nagini S. 2010. Correlation of xenobiotic-metabolizing enzymes, oxidative stress and NFkappaB signaling with histological grade and menopausal status in patients with adenocarcinoma of the breast. *Clin Chim Acta*, 411, 368-74.

Vykhodtseva N., McDannold N., Hynynen K. 2008. Progress and problems in the application of focused ultrasound for blood-brain barrier disruption. *Ultrasonics*, 48, 279-96.

Wakao H., Gouilleux F., Groner B. 1994. Mammary gland factor (MGF) is a novel member of the cytokine regulated transcription factor gene family and confers the prolactin response. *Embo J*, 13, 2182-91.

Wakao H., Schmitt-Ney M., Groner B. 1992. Mammary gland-specific nuclear factor is present in lactating rodent and bovine mammary tissue and composed of a single polypeptide of 89 kDa. *J Biol Chem*, 267, 16365-70.

Walday P., Tolleshaug H., Gjoen T., *et al.,* 1994. Biodistributions of air-filled albumin microspheres in rats and pigs. *Biochem J*, 299 (Pt 2), 437-43.

Wang D., Dubois R.N. 2010. Eicosanoids and cancer. *Nat Rev Cancer*, 10, 181-93.

Wang Z., Prins G.S., Coschigano K.T., *et al.,* 2005. Disruption of Growth Hormone Signaling Retards Early Stages of Prostate Carcinogenesis in the C3(1)/Tag Mouse. *Endocrinology*.

Ward M., Wu J., Chiu J.F. 1999. Ultrasound-induced cell lysis and sonoporation enhanced by contrast agents. *J Acoust Soc Am*, 105, 2951-7.

Wartmann M., Cella N., Hofer P., *et al.,* 1996. Lactogenic hormone activation of Stat5 and transcription of the beta- casein gene in mammary epithelial cells is independent of p42 ERK2 mitogen-activated protein kinase activity. *J Biol Chem*, 271, 31863-8.

Weiss-Messer E., Merom O., Adi A., *et al.,* 2004. Growth hormone (GH) receptors in prostate cancer: gene expression in human tissues and cell lines and characterization, GH signaling and androgen receptor regulation in LNCaP cells. *Mol Cell Endocrinol*, 220, 109-23.

Weller G.E., Villanueva F.S., Klibanov A.L., Wagner W.R. 2002. Modulating targeted adhesion of an ultrasound contrast agent to dysfunctional endothelium. *Ann Biomed Eng*, 30, 1012-9.

Welte T., Garimorth K., Philipp S., Doppler W. 1994. Prolactin-dependent activation of a tyrosine phosphorylated DNA binding factor in mouse mammary epithelial cells. *Mol Endocrinol*, 8, 1091-102.

Wennbo H., Kindblom J., Isaksson O.G., Tornell J. 1997. Transgenic mice overexpressing the prolactin gene develop dramatic enlargement of the prostate gland. *Endocrinology*, 138, 4410-5.

Wheatley M.A., Lewandowski J. 2010. Nano-sized ultrasound contrast agent: salting-out method. *Mol Imaging*, 9, 96-107.

Wheatley M.A., Schrope B., Shen P. 1990. Contrast agents for diagnostic ultrasound: development and evaluation of polymer-coated microbubbles. *Biomaterials*, 11, 713-7.

Wible J.H., Jr., Galen K.P., Wojdyla J.K., *et al.,* 2002. Microbubbles induce renal hemorrhage when exposed to diagnostic ultrasound in anesthetized rats. *Ultrasound Med Biol*, 28, 1535-46.

Wickline S.A., Hughes M., Ngo F.C., *et al.,* 2002. Blood contrast enhancement with a novel, non-gaseous nanoparticle contrast agent. *Acad Radiol*, 9 Suppl 2, S290-3.

Wickline S.A., Lanza G.M. 2002. Molecular imaging, targeted therapeutics, and nanoscience. *J Cell Biochem Suppl*, 39, 90-7.

Wickline S.A., Lanza G.M. 2003. Nanotechnology for molecular imaging and targeted therapy. *Circulation*, 107, 1092-5.

Wiechen K., Diatchenko L., Agoulnik A., *et al.,* 2001. Caveolin-1 is down-regulated in human ovarian carcinoma and acts as a candidate tumor suppressor gene. *Am J Pathol*, 159, 1635-43.

Wiechen K., Sers C., Agoulnik A., *et al.,* 2001. Down-regulation of caveolin-1, a candidate tumor suppressor gene, in sarcomas. *Am J Pathol*, 158, 833-9.

Wiencek J.G., Feinstein S.B., Walker R., Aronson S. 1993. Pitfalls in quantitative contrast echocardiography: the steps to quantitation of perfusion. *J Am Soc Echocardiogr*, 6, 395-416.

Williams T.M., Hassan G.S., Li J., *et al.,* 2005. Caveolin-1 promotes tumor progression in an autochthonous mouse model of prostate cancer: genetic ablation of Cav-1 delays advanced prostate tumor development in tramp mice. *J Biol Chem*, 280, 25134-45.

Williams T.M., Lee H., Cheung M.W., *et al.,* 2004. Combined loss of INK4a and caveolin-1 synergistically enhances cell proliferation and oncogene-induced tumorigenesis: role of INK4a/CAV-1 in mammary epithelial cell hyperplasia. *J Biol Chem*, 279, 24745-56.

Williams T.M., Lisanti M.P. 2005. Caveolin-1 in oncogenic transformation, cancer, and metastasis. *Am J Physiol Cell Physiol*, 288, C494-506.

Williams T.M., Medina F., Badano I., *et al.,* 2004. Caveolin-1 gene disruption promotes mammary tumorigenesis and dramatically enhances lung metastasis *in vivo*. Role of Cav-1 in cell invasiveness and matrix metalloproteinase (MMP-2/9) secretion. *J Biol Chem*, 279, 51630-46.

Wischke C., Schwendeman S.P. 2008. Principles of encapsulating hydrophobic drugs in PLA/PLGA microparticles. *Int J Pharm*, 364, 298-327.

Witkiewicz A.K., Casimiro M.C., Dasgupta A., *et al.,* 2009. Towards a new "stromal-based" classification system for human breast cancer prognosis and therapy. *Cell Cycle*, 8, 1654-8.

Witkiewicz A.K., Dasgupta A., Nguyen K.H., *et al.,* 2009. Stromal caveolin-1 levels predict early DCIS progression to invasive breast cancer. *Cancer Biol Ther*, 8, 1071-9.

Witkiewicz A.K., Dasgupta A., Sotgia F., *et al.,* 2009. An absence of stromal caveolin-1 expression predicts early tumor recurrence and poor clinical outcome in human breast cancers. *Am J Pathol*, 174, 2023-34.

Wood S.C., Antony, S., Brown, R.P., Chen, J., Gordon, E.A., Hitchins, V.M., Zhang, Q., Liu, Y., Maruvada, S., Harris, G.R. 2012. Effects of ultrasound and ultrasound contrast agent on vascular tissue. *Cardiovasc Ultrasound*, 10, 29.

Xu H.X. 2009. Contrast-enhanced ultrasound: The evolving applications. *World J Radiol*, 1, 15-24.

Xu W., Yu F., Yan M., *et al.,* 2004. Geldanamycin, a heat shock protein 90-binding agent, disrupts Stat5 activation in IL-2-stimulated cells. *J Cell Physiol*, 198, 188-96.

Yagi N., Ohta N., Matsuo T. 2009. Structure of amyloid fibrils of hen egg white lysozyme studied by microbeam X-ray diffraction. *Int J Biol Macromol*, 45, 86-90.

Yamamoto K., Kobayashi H., Arai A., *et al.,* 1997. cDNA cloning, expression and chromosome mapping of the human STAT4 gene: both STAT4 and STAT1 genes are mapped to 2q32.2->q32.3. *Cytogenet Cell Genet*, 77, 207-10.

Yamamoto M., Toya Y., Jensen R.A., Ishikawa Y. 1999. Caveolin is an inhibitor of platelet-derived growth factor receptor signaling. *Exp Cell Res*, 247, 380-8.

Yang E., Henriksen M.A., Schaefer O., Zakharova N., Darnell J.E., Jr. 2002. Dissociation time from DNA determines transcriptional function in a STAT1 linker mutant. *J Biol Chem*, 277, 13455-62.

Yang F.Y., Lin Y.S., Kang K.H., Chao T.K. 2011. Reversible blood-brain barrier disruption by repeated transcranial focused ultrasound allows enhanced extravasation. *J Control Release*, 150, 111-6.

Yang G., Addai J., Wheeler T.M., *et al.,* 2007. Correlative evidence that prostate cancer cell-derived caveolin-1 mediates angiogenesis. *Hum Pathol*, 38, 1688-95.

Yang G., Truong L.D., Timme T.L., *et al.,* 1998. Elevated expression of caveolin is associated with prostate and breast cancer. *Clin Cancer Res*, 4, 1873-80.

Yang G., Truong L.D., Wheeler T.M., Thompson T.C. 1999. Caveolin-1 expression in clinically confined human prostate cancer: a novel prognostic marker. *Cancer Res*, 59, 5719-23.

Yang J., Chatterjee-Kishore M., Staugaitis S.M., *et al.,* 2005. Novel roles of unphosphorylated STAT3 in oncogenesis and transcriptional regulation. *Cancer Res*, 65, 939-47.

Yang J., Liao X., Agarwal M.K., *et al.,* 2007. Unphosphorylated STAT3 accumulates in response to IL-6 and activates transcription by binding to NFkappaB. *Genes Dev*, 21, 1396-408.

Yang P., Cartwright C., Chan D., *et al.,* 2013. Anticancer activity of fish oils against human lung cancer is associated with changes in formation of PGE(2) and PGE(3) and Alteration of Akt Phosphorylation. *Mol Carcinog*.

Yee L.D., Lester J.L., Cole R.M., *et al.,* 2010. Omega-3 fatty acid supplements in women at high risk of breast cancer have dose-dependent effects on breast adipose tissue fatty acid composition. *Am J Clin Nutr*, 91, 1185-94.

Yuh E.L., Shulman S.G., Mehta S.A., *et al.,* 2005. Delivery of systemic chemotherapeutic agent to tumors by using focused ultrasound: study in a murine model. *Radiology*, 234, 431-7.

Zagzebski J. Essentials of Ultrasound Physics. Mosby, St. Louis1996.

Zeng Z.Z., Yellaturu C.R., Neeli I., Rao G.N. 2002. 5(S)-hydroxyeicosatetraenoic acid stimulates DNA synthesis in human microvascular endothelial cells *via* activation of Jak/STAT and phosphatidylinositol 3-kinase/Akt signaling, leading to induction of expression of basic fibroblast growth factor 2. *J Biol Chem*, 277, 41213-9.

Zenklusen J.C., Bieche I., Lidereau R., Conti C.J. 1994. (C-A)n microsatellite repeat D7S522 is the most commonly deleted region in human primary breast cancer. *Proc Natl Acad Sci U S A*, 91, 12155-8.

Zhang D., Jin X., Wang F., *et al.,* 2007. Combined prognostic value of both RelA and IkappaB-alpha expression in human non-small cell lung cancer. *Ann Surg Oncol*, 14, 3581-92.

Zhang J.G., Farley A., Nicholson S.E., *et al.,* 1999. The conserved SOCS box motif in suppressors of cytokine signaling binds to elongins B and C and may couple bound proteins to proteasomal degradation. *Proc Natl Acad Sci U S A*, 96, 2071-6.

Zhang W., Razani B., Altschuler Y., *et al.,* 2000. Caveolin-1 inhibits epidermal growth factor-stimulated lamellipod extension and cell migration in metastatic mammary adenocarcinoma cells (MTLn3). Transformation suppressor effects of adenovirus-mediated gene delivery of caveolin-1. *J Biol Chem*, 275, 20717-25.

Zhang Z., Ma J., Li N., Sun N., Wang C. 2006. Expression of nuclear factor-kappaB and its clinical significance in nonsmall-cell lung cancer. *Ann Thorac Surg*, 82, 243-8.

Zhao Y.Z., Luo Y.K., Lu C.T., *et al.,* 2008. Phospholipids-based microbubbles sonoporation pore size and reseal of cell membrane cultured *in vitro*. *J Drug Target*, 16, 18-25.

Zhong Z., Wen Z., Darnell J.E.J. 1994. Stat3: a STAT family member activated by tyrosine phosphorylation in response to epidermal growth factor and interleukin-6. *Science*, 264, 95-8.

Zhou M., Cavalieri, F. and Ashokkumar, M. 2011. Tailoring the properties of ultrasonically synthesised microbubbles. *Soft Matter*, 7, 623-30.

Zhou Y., Cui J., Deng C.X. 2008. Dynamics of sonoporation correlated with acoustic cavitation activities. *Biophys J*, 94, L51-3.

Zhu M., John S., Berg M., Leonard W.J. 1999. Functional association of Nmi with Stat5 and Stat1 in IL-2- and IFNgamma-mediated signaling. *Cell*, 96, 121-30.

Zmijewski J.W., Landar A., Watanabe N., *et al.,* 2005. Cell signalling by oxidized lipids and the role of reactive oxygen species in the endothelium. *Biochem Soc Trans*, 33, 1385-9.

Zundel W., Swiersz L.M., Giaccia A. 2000. Caveolin 1-mediated regulation of receptor tyrosine kinase-associated phosphatidylinositol 3-kinase activity by ceramide. *Mol Cell Biol*, 20, 1507-14.

Subject Index

Pier Paolo Claudio and Paraskevi Vogiatzi (Eds)

D

E

N

O

P

R